INTRODUCTION TO VASCULAR ULTRASONOGRAPHY

INTRODUCTION TO VASCULAR ULTRASONOGRAPHY

Fourth Edition

William J. Zwiebel, MD
Professor of Radiology
University of Utah
School of Medicine
Salt Lake City, Utah

W.B. SAUNDERS COMPANY
A Harcourt Health Sciences Company
Philadelphia London New York St. Louis Sydney Toronto

W.B. SAUNDERS COMPANY
A Harcourt Health Sciences Company

The Curtis Center
Independence Square West
Philadelphia, Pennsylvania 19106

Library of Congress Cataloging-in-Publication Data

Zwiebel, William J.

Introduction to vascular ultrasonography / William J. Zwiebel. — 4th ed.

p. cm.

Rev. ed. of: Introduction to vascular ultrasonography / edited by William J. Zwiebel. 3rd ed. c1992.

Includes bibliographical references and index.

ISBN 0–7216–6949–2

1. Blood-vessels—Ultrasonic imaging. I. Title.
[DNLM: 1. Vascular Diseases—ultrasonography. 2. Blood Vessels—ultrasonography. WG 500 Z98i 2000]

RC691.6.U47I57 2000 616.1′307543—dc21

DNLM/DLC 98-31218

INTRODUCTION TO VASCULAR ULTRASONOGRAPHY ISBN 0–7216–6949–2

Printed in the United States of America

Last digit is the print number: 9 8 7 6 5 4 3

This text is dedicated to my wife,

Margaret K. Batson, CNM,

who has patiently endured this and other writing projects,

and to our children, Colin and Aaron,

who enrich our lives without measure.

WJZ

Contributors

Carol B. Benson, MD
Associate Professor of Radiology, Harvard Medical School; Co-Director of Ultrasound, Brigham and Women's Hospital, Boston, Massachusetts
Ultrasound and Doppler Evaluation of the Penis

John J. Bergan, MD, FACS, FRCS(Hon)
Professor of Surgery, University of California, San Diego School of Medicine; Attending Surgeon, Scripps Memorial Hospital, La Jolla, California
Definitive Diagnosis and Documentation of Chronic Venous Dysfunction

Warner P. Bundens, MD, MS
Associate Professor of Surgery, University of California, San Diego School of Medicine, La Jolla, California; Attending Physician, UCSD Medical Center, San Diego, California
Definitive Diagnosis and Documentation of Chronic Venous Dysfunction

Gregory K. Call, MD
Assistant Professor of Neurology, Department of Neurology, University of Utah School of Medicine, University of Utah Medical Center, Salt Lake City, Utah
Rationale for Duplex Cerebrovascular Examination

Stefan A. Carter, MD, MSc, FRCP(C)
Professor of Medicine and Physiology, Faculty of Medicine, University of Manitoba; Director, Vascular Laboratory, St. Boniface General Hospital, Winnipeg, Manitoba, Canada
Hemodynamic Considerations in Peripheral Vascular and Cerebrovascular Disease

Edward B. Diethrich, MD
Medical Director, Arizona Heart Institute and Arizona Heart Hospital, Phoenix, Arizona
Normal Cerebrovascular Anatomy and Collateral Pathways

Peter M. Doubilet, MD, PhD
Associate Professor of Radiology, Harvard Medical School; Co-Director of Ultrasound, Brigham and Women's Hospital, Boston, Massachusetts
Ultrasound and Doppler Evaluation of the Penis

James M. Edwards, MD
Associate Professor of Surgery, Department of Surgery, Division of Vascular Surgery, Oregon Health Sciences University; Staff Physician, Portland VA Medical Center, Portland, Oregon
Assessment of Upper Extremity Arteries

Spencer W. Galt, MD
Assistant Professor of Surgery, University of Utah; Staff Surgeon, Salt Lake VA Medical Center, Salt Lake City, Utah
Rationale for Duplex Ultrasonography Assessment of Extremity Veins

Edward G. Grant, MD
Professor of Radiology, UCLA Center for the Health Sciences; Chief of Radiology, Greater Los Angeles VA Healthcare System, Los Angeles, California
Sonographic Contrast Agents

Gregory M. Keck, MD
Chief, Interventional/Vascular Radiology, Lovelace Medical Center, Albuquerque, New Mexico
Arterial Anatomy of the Extremities

Peter F. Lawrence, MD
Professor and Vice Chairman of Surgery, Associate Dean for Program Development, and Vice President for Specialty Services, University of California, Irvine, College of Medicine, Irvine, California
Rationale for Duplex Ultrasonography Assessment of Extremity Veins

Michelle L. Melany, MD
Assistant Professor of Radiology, Chief of Ultrasound, UCLA Department of Radiological Sciences, Los Angeles, California
Sonographic Contrast Agents

Shirley M. Otis, MD
Senior Consultant, Division of Neurology, and Chair, Department of Medicine, Scripps Clinic and Research Foundation; Clinical Member, Scripps Research Institute; Chairman, Department of Medicine, Green Hospital of Scripps Clinic, La Jolla, California
Transcranial Doppler Sonography

E. Bernd Ringelstein, MD
Professor and Direktor, Klinik und Poliklinik für Neurologie, Westfälische Wilhelms-Universität, Münster, Germany
Transcranial Doppler Sonography

D. Eugene Strandness, Jr., MD
Professor of Surgery, Division of Vascular Surgery, University of Washington School of Medicine, Seattle, Washington
The Role of Noninvasive Procedures in the Management of Extremity Arterial Disease; Nonimaging Physiologic Tests for Assessment of Lower Extremity Arterial Disease

James A. Zagzebski, PhD
Professor of Medical Physics, University of Wisconsin, Madison, Wisconsin
Physics and Instrumentation in Doppler and B-Mode Ultrasonography

Brenda K. Zierler, PhD, RN, RVT
Research Assistant Professor, Department of Biobehavioral Nursing and Health Systems, University of Washington School of Nursing; Adjunct Research Assistant Professor, Division of Vascular Surgery, University of Washington School of Medicine, Seattle, Washington
Duplex Sonography of Lower Extremity Arteries

R. Eugene Zierler, MD
Professor of Surgery, Division of Vascular Surgery, University of Washington School of Medicine; Attending Surgeon, University of Washington Medical Center, Seattle, Washington
Nonimaging Physiologic Tests for Assessment of Lower Extremity Arterial Disease; Assessment of Upper Extremity Arteries; Duplex Sonography of Lower Extremity Arteries

William J. Zwiebel, MD
Professor of Radiology, University of Utah School of Medicine; Staff Radiologist, Salt Lake VA Medical Center, Salt Lake City, Utah
Doppler Frequency Spectrum Analysis; Color-Flow Imaging for Vascular Diagnosis; Normal Carotid Arteries and Carotid Examination Technique; Ultrasound Assessment of Carotid Plaque; Doppler Evaluation of Carotid Stenosis; Miscellaneous Carotid Subjects: Occlusion, Dissection, Endarterectomy, Carotid Body Tumor; Ultrasound Vertebral Examination; Arterial Anatomy of the Extremities; Extremity Venous Anatomy; Terminology, Instrumentation, and Characteristics of Normal Veins; Extremity Venous Examination: Technical Considerations; Venous Thrombosis; Arteriovenous Fistula and Nonvenous Extremity Pathology; Anatomy and Normal Doppler Signatures of Abdominal Vessels; Aorta, Iliac Arteries, and Inferior Vena Cava; Ultrasound Assessment of the Splanchnic Arteries; Vascular Disorders of the Liver; Duplex Evaluation of Native Renal Vessels and Renal Allografts

Preface

This edition of *Introduction to Vascular Ultrasonography* is long overdue, and I apologize for the delay in its publication. Many people have asked me when this edition would be ready, which is gratifying evidence that the preceding editions have been appreciated, but these inquiries have also been embarrassing. I greatly regret the lengthy interval that has passed since the publication of the third edition. The delay is a sign, in part, of the difficulties faced by academic radiologists in this time of decreased clinical revenue. When staffing is lean, academic pursuits are sidetracked.

Much has changed in the world of vascular diagnosis since the third edition was published. Color-flow imaging has matured, power Doppler–flow imaging has found a place in the vascular diagnosis repertoire, and ultrasound instrumentation has advanced in many ways. Most importantly, ultrasonography has become the mainstay of the vascular laboratory. Plethysmography continues to have an important role in the diagnosis of extremity arterial insufficiency and vasospastic disease, but virtually all other examinations performed in the vascular laboratory are now ultrasound related.

Another striking change since publication of the previous edition is the extent to which color-flow and Doppler imaging has pervaded diagnostic ultrasound. These modalities are no longer the exclusive province of the vascular laboratory. Instead, they are now used routinely in all areas of ultrasound diagnosis, including abdominal, pelvic, and obstetric imaging. All sonographers must now be familiar with Doppler diagnosis, for blood flow assessment is used virtually every time an ultrasound transducer is placed on a patient's skin.

Also noteworthy since the publication of the third edition is the clarification of the clinical role that vascular ultrasonography plays in cerebrovascular, extremity arterial, and abdominal vascular diagnosis. This edition of the text has been revised accordingly. The cerebrovascular section has been entirely rewritten to reflect the findings of multicenter carotid endarterectomy trials published since the third edition was released. These trials not only proved the efficacy of carotid endarterectomy but also standardized methods for measuring carotid stenoses. The abdominal section has been almost completely rewritten because of technical improvements and increased clinical interest in ultrasound assessment of abdominal vessels. The chapters devoted to extremity arterial diagnosis have also been updated to reflect technical changes and greater understanding of the clinical role of ultrasound in extremity arterial insufficiency.

A cursory examination of the previous edition shows that color-flow imaging was quite primitive at the time of its publication, and methods such as power Doppler–flow imaging were not available at all. As a result, nearly all of the ultrasound images had to be replaced in preparing this edition. Although this was a burden, it was also an opportunity to enter the realm of digital photography. Computer-based digital processing afforded me the opportunity to tightly control the content and appearance of the images. In many cases, I removed extraneous annotations, artifacts, and other distracting material from the images. I also compacted many of the images by moving color bars and scales. This eliminated wasted space and permitted tighter cropping. The purpose of these efforts was to enhance the educational value of the images by making them clearer and more compact. Frequently, the photo-editing process also improved the appearance of the images, but I would like the readers to know that this was not done to make me, my vascular laboratory, or an ultrasound instrument manufacturer look good. The readers should also be aware that it is not possible to consistently obtain images of such good quality clinically, nor is it necessary to do so.

In this edition, the publisher and I have again chosen to concentrate color images in groups rather than to distribute the color images throughout the text. This is necessary to keep the cost of the text within the budget of many purchasers. To publish with dispersed color images would probably double the price of the text. Although this would make the text more user friendly and would enrich the editor somewhat, it would not help to disseminate the information contained.

Vascular ultrasonography continues to evolve from both clinical and technical perspectives. Intravenously administered echo-enhancing agents, harmonic ultrasound imaging, and three-dimensional sonography are but a few diagnostic enhancements that are coming into clinical use as of this writing. It is likely that these advances will be widely applied within a few years, and they may have substantial effects on diagnostic methods and practice patterns. Undoubtedly, this text will once again become outdated quite rapidly, but I hope that I will be able to publish the next edition in a more timely fashion.

WILLIAM J. ZWIEBEL

Acknowledgments

Numerous people assisted in the production of this text, either directly or indirectly. First and foremost, I acknowledge the outstanding work of the authors who contributed chapters for this edition. Many of these authors are world famous, and the availability of their tremendous expertise is greatly appreciated.

After the authors, the person who contributed as much to this text as anyone is my secretary, Mrs. Dixie Zumwalt, who transcribed letters, called authors, proofread, paginated, spell checked, labeled artwork, express mailed, and did myriad other tasks throughout the lengthy course of this project. Without Mrs. Zumwalt's services, the text would never have gotten done.

I am greatly indebted, as well, to my technical colleagues at the Salt Lake City VA Medical Center for assistance with locating illustrations. They are Mrs. Janis McChesney, vascular technologist, and Mrs. Nancy Cottrell, sonographer. I am also indebted to Mr. Tod Peterson and Mr. Sidney Crandall from the Medical Media Division of the Salt Lake City VA Medical Center for their photographic assistance, and to Mr. G. Julian Maack, Jr., Director of the Medical Illustrations Facility at the University of Utah School of Medicine, for his excellent medical illustrations.

WILLIAM J. ZWIEBEL

Contents

SECTION 4

EXTREMITY VEINS 285

SECTION 5

ABDOMINAL VESSELS .. 377

SECTION I

BASICS

Chapter 1

Hemodynamic Considerations in Peripheral Vascular and Cerebrovascular Disease

■ *Stefan A. Carter, MD, MSc, FRCP(C)*

The circulatory system is extremely complex in both structure and function, and blood flow is influenced by many factors, including cardiac function, elasticity of the vessel walls (compliance), the tone of vascular smooth muscle, and the various patterns, dimensions, and interconnections of millions of branching vessels. Some of these factors can be measured and described in reasonably simple terms, but many others cannot be described succinctly because they are difficult to quantify and generally are not well understood.

With these limitations in mind, this chapter presents the basic principles of the dynamics of blood circulation, the many factors that influence blood flow, and the hemodynamic consequences of occlusive disease. These considerations are helpful in understanding the normal physiology of blood circulation and the abnormalities that can occur in the presence of vascular obstruction.

Acknowledgments

The author held grants-in-aid of research from the Manitoba Heart and the St. Boniface Hospital Research Foundations, which supported the studies whose results are discussed in this chapter. He is also grateful to Dr. William J. Zwiebel for the valuable exchange of ideas and assistance and the excellent secretarial work of Mrs. Constance Twomey.

PHYSIOLOGIC FACTORS GOVERNING BLOOD FLOW AND ITS CHARACTERISTICS

Energy and Pressure

For blood flow to occur between any two points in the circulatory system there has to be a difference in the energy level between these two points. Usually, the difference in energy level is reflected by a difference in pressure, and the circulatory system generally consists of a high-pressure, high-energy arterial reservoir and a venous pool of low pressure and energy. These reservoirs are connected by a system of distributing vessels (smaller arteries) and by the resistance vessels of the microcirculation, which consists of arterioles, capillaries, and venules.

During flow, energy is continuously lost from the blood because of the friction between its layers and particles. Both pressure and energy levels therefore decrease from the arterial to the venous ends. The energy necessary for flow is continuously restored by the pumping action of the heart, which forces blood to move from the venous system into the arterial system, and thus maintains the arterial pressure and the energy difference needed for flow to occur.

The high arterial energy level is a result of the large volume of blood in the arterial reservoir. The function of the heart and blood vessels is normally regulated to maintain volume and pressure in the arteries within the limits required for smooth function. This is achieved by maintaining a balance between the amounts of blood that enter and leave the arterial reservoir. The amount that enters the arteries is the cardiac output. The amount that leaves depends on the arterial pressure and on the total peripheral resistance, which is controlled in turn by the amount of vasoconstriction in the microcirculation.

Under normal conditions, flow to all the body tissues is adjusted according to the tissues' particular needs at a given time. This adjustment is accomplished by alterations in the level of vasoconstriction of the arterioles within the organs supplied. Maintenance of normal volume and pressure in the arteries thus allows both for adjustment of blood flow to all parts of the body and for regulation of cardiac output (which equals the sum of blood flow to all the vascular beds).

Forms of Energy in the Blood and Its Dissipation During Flow

This section considers the forms in which energy exists in the circulation and the important factors that govern the dissipation of energy during flow, including friction, resistance, and the influence of laminar and turbulent flow. Poiseuille's law and the equation that summarizes the basic relationships among flow, pressure, and resistance are discussed, as well as the effects of connecting vascular resistances in parallel and in series.

Forms of Energy

POTENTIAL AND KINETIC ENERGY. The main form of energy present in flowing blood is the pressure distending the vessels (a form of potential energy), which is created by the pumping action of the heart. However, some of the energy of the blood is kinetic, namely the ability of flowing blood to do work as a result of its velocity. Usually, the kinetic energy component is small compared with the pressure energy, and under normal resting conditions, it is equivalent to only a few millimeters of mercury or less. The kinetic energy of blood is proportional to its density (which is stable in normal circumstances) and to the square of its velocity. Therefore, important increases in kinetic energy occur in the systemic circulation when flow is high (e.g., during exercise) and in stenotic lesions, in which luminal narrowing leads to high velocities. Kinetic energy is converted back into pressure (potential energy) when velocity is decreased (e.g., in a normal segment of the artery distal to a stenosis).

ENERGY DIFFERENCES RELATED TO DIFFERENCES IN THE LEVELS OF BODY PARTS. There is also variation in the energy of the blood associated with differences in the levels of body parts. For example, the pressure in the vessels in the dependent parts of the body, such as the lower portions of the legs, increases by an amount that depends on the weight of the column of blood resting on the blood in the legs. This hydrostatic pressure increases the transmural pressure and the distention of the vessels. Gravitational potential energy (potential for doing work related to the effect of gravity on a free-falling body), however, is reduced in the dependent parts of the body by the same amount as the increase resulting from hydrostatic pressure. Therefore, differences in the level of the body parts usually do not lead to changes in the driving pressure along the vascular tree unless the column of blood is interrupted, as may be the case when the venous valves close. Changes in energy and pressure associated with differences in level are important under certain conditions, such as with changes in posture or when the venous pump is activated because of muscular action during walking.

Dissipation of Energy

DURING LAMINAR FLOW. In most vessels, blood moves in concentric layers, or laminae; hence, the flow is said to be laminar. Each infinitesimal layer flows with a different velocity. In theory, a thin layer of blood is held stationary next to the vessel wall at zero velocity because of an adhesive force between the blood and the inner surface of the vessel. The next layer flows with a certain velocity, but its movement is delayed by the stationary layer because of friction between the layers, generated by the viscous properties of the fluid. The second layer, in turn, delays the next layer, which flows at a greater velocity. The layers in the middle of the vessel flow with the highest velocity, and the *mean velocity across the vessel is half of the maximal velocity.* Because the rate of change of velocity is greatest near the walls and decreases toward the center of the vessel, a velocity profile in the shape of a parabola exists along the vessel diameter (Fig. 1–1*A*).

Loss of energy during blood flow occurs because of friction, and the amount of friction and energy loss is determined in large part by the dimensions of the vessels. In small vessels, especially in the microcirculation, even the layers in the middle of the lumen are relatively close to the wall and are thus delayed considerably, resulting in a significant opposition or resistance to flow. In large vessels, by contrast, a large central core of blood is far from the walls, and the frictional energy losses are minimal. As indicated later, friction and energy losses increase if laminar flow is disturbed.

Poiseuille's Law and Equation. In a cylindric tube model, the mean linear velocity of laminar flow is directly proportional to the energy difference between the ends of the tube and the square of the radius and is inversely proportional to the length of the tube and the viscosity of the fluid. In the circulatory system, however, volume flow is of more interest than velocity. Volume flow is proportional to the fourth power of the vessel radius, because it is equal to the product of the mean linear velocity and the cross-sectional area of the tube. These important considerations are helpful in understanding Poiseuille's law, as expressed in Poiseuille's equation:

$$Q = \frac{\pi(P_1 - P_2)r^4}{8L\eta} \qquad (1\text{–}1)$$

where Q is the volume flow; P_1 and P_2 are the pressures at the proximal and distal ends of the tube, respectively; r and L are the radius and length of the tube, respectively; and η is the viscosity of the fluid.

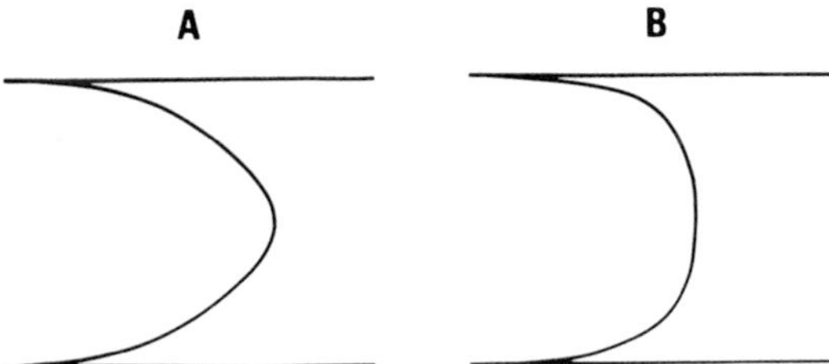

FIGURE 1–1 Flow velocity profiles across a normal arterial lumen. *A*, Parabolic profile of laminar flow. *B*, Flattened profile with a central core of relatively uniform velocity encountered in the proximal portion (inlet length) of arterial branches or with turbulent flow.

Because volume flow is proportional to the fourth power of the radius, even small changes in radius can result in large changes in flow. For example, a decrease in radius of 10% would decrease flow in a tube model by about 35%, and a decrease of 50% would lead to a 95% decrease in flow. *Because the length of the vessels and the viscosity of blood do not change much in the cardiovascular system, alterations in blood flow occur mainly as a result of changes in the radius of the vessels and in the difference in the pressure energy level available for flow.*

Poiseuille's equation can be rewritten, therefore, as follows:

$$\frac{8L\eta}{\pi r^4} = \frac{P_1 - P_2}{Q} \qquad (1\text{–}2)$$

$$R = \frac{8L\eta}{\pi r^4} \qquad (1\text{–}3)$$

$$R = \frac{P_1 - P_2}{Q} \qquad (1\text{–}4)$$

The resistance term (R) depends on the viscous properties of the blood and on the dimensions of the vessels. Although these parameters cannot be measured in a complex system, the pressure difference ($P_1 - P_2$) and the blood flow (Q) can be measured, and the resistance can thus be calculated. Because resistance is equal to the pressure difference divided by the volume flow (the pressure difference per unit flow), it can be thought of as the pressure difference needed to produce one unit of flow and, therefore, can be considered as an index of the difficulty in forcing blood through the vessels.

Vessel Interconnection and Energy Dissipation. Poiseuille's law applies with precision only to constant laminar flow of a simple fluid (such as water) in a rigid tube of a uniform bore. In the blood circulation these conditions are not met. Instead, the resistance is influenced by the presence of numerous interconnected vessels with a combined effect similar to that observed in electrical resistances. In the case of vessels in series, the overall resistance is equal to the sum of the resistances of the individual vessels, whereas in the case of parallel vessels the reciprocal of the total resistance equals the sum of the reciprocals of the individual vessel resistances. Thus, *the contribution of any single vessel to the total resistance of a vascular* *bed, or the effect of a change in the dimension of a vessel, depends on the presence and relative size of the other vessels linked in series or in parallel.*

Deviations from the conditions to which Poiseuille's law applies also occur in relation to changes in blood viscosity, which is affected by hematocrit, temperature, vessel diameter, and rate of flow.

DURING NONLAMINAR FLOW. Various degrees of deviation from orderly laminar flow occur in the circulation under both normal and abnormal conditions. Factors responsible for these deviations include the following: (1) the flow velocity, which changes throughout the cardiac cycle as a result of acceleration during systole and deceleration in diastole; (2) alteration of the lines of flow, which occurs whenever a vessel changes dimensions, including variations in diameter associated with each pulse; and (3) the lines of flow, which are distorted at curves, at bifurcations, and in branches that take off at various angles. For example, the parabolic velocity profile is often not re-established in branches for a considerable distance beyond their origin. Instead, the parabola is flattened so that there is a relatively large central core of blood that flows with a relatively uniform speed (Fig. 1–1*B*).

Because of these and other factors, laminar flow may be disturbed or fully turbulent, even in a uniform tube. The factors that affect the development of turbulence are expressed by the dimensionless Reynolds number (Re):

$$\text{Re} = \frac{vq2r}{\eta} \qquad (1\text{–}5)$$

where v is the velocity, q is the density of the fluid, r is the radius of the tube, and η is the viscosity of the fluid. Because the density (q) and viscosity (η) of the blood are relatively constant, *the development of turbulence depends mainly on the size of the vessels and on the velocity of flow.* In a tube model, laminar flow tends to be disturbed if the Reynolds number exceeds 2000. However, in the circulatory system, disturbances and various degrees of turbulence are likely to occur at lower values because of body movements, the pulsatile nature of blood flow, changes in vessel dimensions, roughness of the endothelial surface, and other factors. Turbulence develops more readily in large vessels under conditions of high flow and can be detected clinically by the finding of bruits or thrills. Bruits may sometimes be heard over the ascending aorta during systolic acceleration in normal individuals at rest and are frequently heard in states of high cardiac output and blood flow, even in more distal arteries, such as the femoral artery.[1] Distortion of laminar flow velocity profiles can be assessed using ultrasound flow detectors, and such assessments can be applied for diagnostic purposes. For example, in arteries with severe stenosis, pronounced turbulence is a diagnostic feature observed in the poststenotic zone. Turbulence occurs because a jet of blood with high velocity and high kinetic energy suddenly encounters a normal diameter lumen or a lumen of increased diameter (because of poststenotic dilatation), where both the velocity and energy level are lower than in the stenotic region.

During turbulent flow, the loss of pressure energy between two points in a vessel is greater than that which would be expected from the factors in Poiseuille's equation, and the parabolic velocity profile is flattened.[2]

Pulsatile Pressure and Flow Changes in the Arterial System

With each heartbeat a stroke volume of blood is ejected into the arterial system, resulting in a pressure wave that travels throughout the arterial tree. The speed of propagation, amplitude (strength), and shape of the pressure wave change as it traverses the arterial system. These alterations are influenced by the varying characteristics of the vessels traversed by the pressure wave. The velocity and, in some parts of the circulation, the direction of flow also vary with each heartbeat. Correct interpretation of noninvasive tests based on recordings of arterial pressure and velocity, as well as pressure and velocity waveforms, requires knowledge of the factors that influence these variables. This section considers these factors as they occur in various portions of the circulatory system.

PRESSURE CHANGES FROM CARDIAC ACTIVITY. As indicated previously, the pumping action of the heart maintains a high volume of blood in the arterial end of the circulation and thus provides the high pressure difference between the arterial and venous ends necessary to maintain flow. Because of the intermittent pumping action of the heart, pressure and flow vary in a pulsatile manner.

During the rapid phase of ventricular ejection, the volume of blood at the arterial end increases, raising the pressure to a systolic peak. During the latter part of systole, when cardiac ejection decreases, the outflow through the peripheral resistance vessels exceeds the volume being ejected by the heart, and the pressure begins to decline. This decline continues throughout diastole as blood continues to flow from the arteries into the microcirculation. Part of the work of the heart leads directly to forward flow, but a large portion of the energy of each cardiac contraction results in distention of the arteries that serve as reservoirs for storing the blood volume and the energy supplied to the system. This storage of energy and blood volume provides for continuous flow to the tissues during diastole.

ARTERIAL PRESSURE WAVE. The pulsatile variations in blood volume and energy occurring with each cardiac cycle are manifested as a pressure wave that can be detected throughout the arterial system. The amplitude and shape of the arterial pressure wave depend on a complex interplay of factors, which include the stroke volume and time course of ventricular ejection, the peripheral resistance, and the stiffness of the arterial walls. In general, an increase in any of these factors results in an increase in the pulse amplitude (i.e., pulse pressure, difference between systolic and diastolic pressures) and frequently in a concomitant increase in systolic pressure. For example, increased stiffness of the arteries with age tends to increase both the systolic and pulse pressures.

The arterial pressure wave is propagated along the arterial tree distally from the heart. The speed of propagation, or pulse wave velocity, increases with stiffness of the arterial walls (the elastic modulus of the material of which the walls are composed) and with the ratio of the wall thickness to diameter. In the mammalian circulation, arteries become progressively stiffer from the aorta toward the periphery. Therefore, the speed of propagation of the wave increases as it moves peripherally. Also, the gradual increase in stiffness tends to decrease wave reflection (discussed later) and has a beneficial effect in that the pulse and systolic pressures in the aorta and proximal arteries are relatively lower than in peripheral vessels. The pressure against which the heart ejects the stroke volume and the associated cardiac work are accordingly reduced.[3]

PRESSURE CHANGES THROUGHOUT THE CIRCULATION. Figure 1–2 illustrates changes in pressure in the systemic circulation from large arteries through the resistance vessels to the veins. Because there is little loss of pressure energy from friction in large and distributing arteries, they offer relatively little resistance to flow, and the mean pressure decreases only slightly between the aorta and the small arteries of the limbs, such as the radial or the dorsalis pedis.[4, 5] The diastolic pressure also shows only minor changes. The amplitude of the pressure wave and the systolic pressure actually increase, however, as the wave travels distally (systolic amplification), because of increasing stiffness of the walls toward the periphery and the presence of reflected waves. These waves arise where the vessels change diameter and stiffness, divide, or branch and are superadded to the oncoming primary pulse wave.[3, 4] The reflected waves, at least in the extremities, are strongly enhanced by increased peripheral resistance.[4] Direct measurements of pressure in small arteries in experimental animals and humans, and indirect measurements of systolic pressure in human digits, have shown that the pulse amplitude and systolic pressure decrease in smaller vessels, such as the digital vessels of the human extremities.[6–9] However, some pulsatile changes in pressure and flow may remain evident even in minute arteries and capillaries, at least under conditions of peripheral vasodilatation, and can be recorded by various methods, including plethysmography. The effect of peripheral vasoconstriction on pulsatility in the microcirculation is opposite to that seen in the proximal small or medium arteries of the ex-

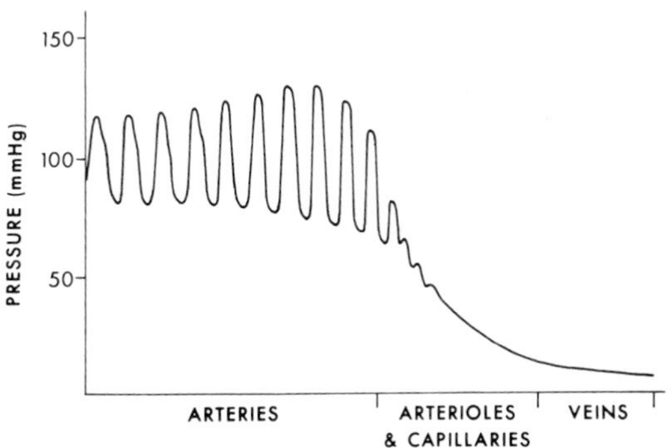

FIGURE 1–2 Schematic representation of normal pressure changes in the systemic circulation. (From Carter SA: Peripheral artery disease: Pressure measurements ease evaluation. Consultant 19[9]:102–115, 1979.)

tremities. *Pulsatile changes in minute arteries, arterioles, and capillaries are reduced by vasoconstriction and enhanced by vasodilatation. In small and medium arteries of the limbs, however, pulsatile changes are increased by vasoconstriction, as a result of enhanced wave reflection, and are decreased by vasodilatation.* Figure 1–3 shows arterial pressure pulses recorded directly from the femoral and dorsalis pedis arteries during peripheral vasoconstriction and vasodilatation induced, respectively, by body cooling and heating.

There is almost a complete disappearance of amplification in the dorsalis pedis artery in response to vasodilatation induced by body heating. Similar changes in the distal pressure waves result from other factors that alter peripheral resistance, for example, reactive hyperemia and exercise. Exercise, by decreasing resistance in the working muscle, would be expected to decrease reflection in the exercising extremity. Because of vasoconstriction in other parts of the body during exercise (the result of cardiovascular reflexes that regulate blood pressure and circulation), however, the reflection may be increased and lead to a high degree of amplification. For example, it has been shown that during walking the pulse pressure in the radial arteries can exceed that in the aorta by perhaps 100%.[10]

These considerations are important for correct interpretation of pressure measurements in peripheral arterial obstruction. For example, brachial systolic pressure corresponds well to aortic or femoral systolic pressure and is used as a standard against which ankle pressure can be compared. The systolic pressure at the ankle usually exceeds brachial pressure in normal subjects; therefore, the finding of ankle systolic pressure that is even slightly lower than brachial systolic pressure indicates a high likelihood of a proximal stenotic lesion. However, systolic pressure in human digits is usually lower than systolic pressure proximal to the wrist or the ankle. This observation has to be taken into account when measurements of digital systolic pressures are used as an index of distal arterial obstruction. In such cases, the appropriate norms for the differences between the proximal and digital systolic pressures have to be applied.[11]

PULSATILE FLOW PATTERNS. Pulsatile changes in pressure are associated with corresponding acceleration of blood flow with systole and deceleration in diastole. Although the energy stored in the arterial walls maintains a positive arteriovenous pressure gradient and overall forward flow in the microcirculation during diastole, temporary cessation of forward flow or even diastolic reversal occurs frequently in portions of the human arterial system. How these phenomena occur may be clarified by considering pulsatile pressure changes at two points along the arterial tree. Figure 1–3 shows arterial pressure pulses in the femoral and dorsalis pedis arteries. The corresponding pressure gradient between the two arteries (Fig. 1–4) varies during the cardiac cycle, not only because of differences in the shape and magnitude of the original pressure waves but

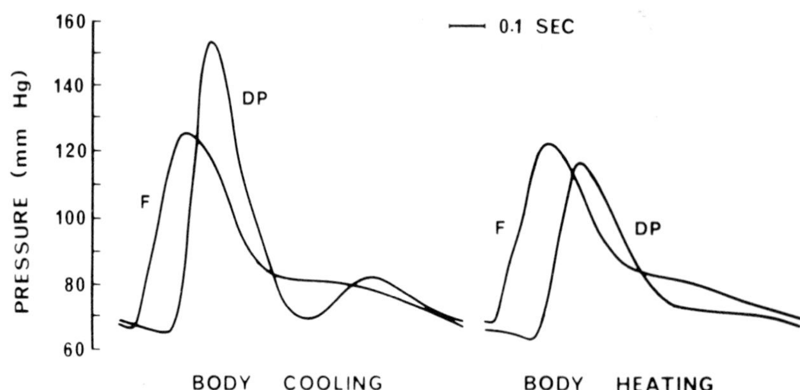

FIGURE 1–3 Pressure waves from the femoral (F) and dorsalis pedis (DP) arteries during heating and cooling. Note that the pulse pressure of the dorsalis pedis artery is greater with vasoconstriction (body cooling) and falls dramatically with vasodilatation (body heating). (From Carter SA: Effect of age, cardiovascular disease, and vasomotor changes on transmission of arterial pressure waves through the lower extremities. Angiology 29:601–616, 1978.)

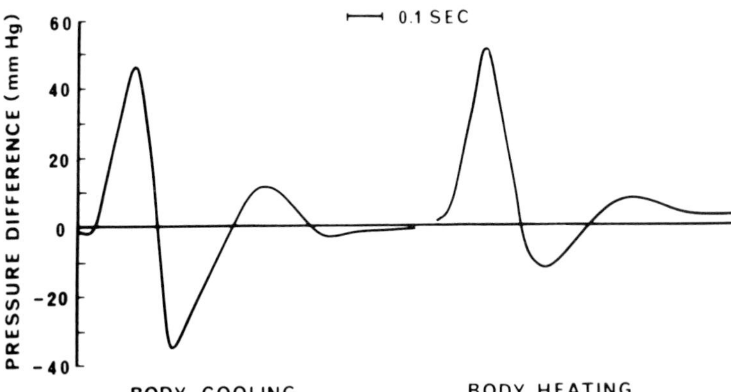

FIGURE 1–4 Pressure differences between the femoral and dorsalis pedis arteries obtained from the waves shown in Figure 1–3. Note the effect of vasodilatation (body heating) on the negative (reverse flow) component.

also, more importantly, because the wave arrives later at the dorsalis pedis. The pressure gradient is greatest during the first half of systole, at which time the peak of the wave arrives at the femoral site. Thereafter, the gradient decreases, and by the time the peak arrives at the dorsalis pedis, the femoral pressure has fallen and a negative pressure gradient appears. Such negative gradients, related to different arrival times of the pressure wave at various sites in the arterial system, are commonly observed along human arteries and are conducive to the reversal of blood flow. Despite the reversal of the pressure gradient, however, the direction of flow may not be reversed if there is a large forward mean flow component.[12]

The presence of reversed flow during diastole can also be understood if one imagines a major arterial segment, with a certain diastolic pressure, that has several branch vessels leading to areas with different levels of resistance. If one of the proximal branches leads to an area with low peripheral resistance, flow during diastole in the main vessel will occur toward this branch, and flow will reverse in the distal portion of the main vessel if distal branches supply areas with higher peripheral resistance. Such situations of transient flow reversal may exist in the limb during cooling (see Fig. 1–4), but during body heating, when peripheral resistance in the distal cutaneous circulation is reduced to a low level, reversed flow is decreased or may be abolished. Diastolic flow reversal is generally present in vessels that supply vascular beds with high peripheral resistance. It tends to be absent in low-resistance vascular beds or when peripheral resistance is reduced by peripheral dilatation, such as that which occurs in the skin with body heating, or in the working muscle during exercise or reactive hyperemia. These principles are important in assessing blood flow in arteries that supply various regions, including the cranial circulation. For example, flow reversal can be observed in the external carotid because extracranial resistance is relatively high, but it is absent in the internal carotid because the cerebrovascular resistance is low.

EFFECTS OF ARTERIAL OBSTRUCTION

Arterial obstruction can result in reduced pressure and flow distal to the site of blockage, but the effects on pressure and flow are greatly influenced by a number of factors proximal and especially distal to the lesion. One must be familiar with these factors when interpreting noninvasive studies, because they affect the pressure and velocity waveforms observed both proximal and distal to the obstructive lesion. In this section of the chapter, the concept of the critical stenosis is considered, as well as the pressure, velocity, and flow manifestations of arterial obstructive disease.

Critical Stenosis

Encroachment on the lumen of an artery by an arteriosclerotic plaque can result in diminished pressure and flow distal to the lesion, but this encroachment on the lumen has to be relatively extensive before hemodynamic changes are manifested, because arteries offer relatively little resistance to flow compared with the resistance vessels with which they are in series. Studies in humans and animals have indicated that about 90% of the cross-sectional area of the aorta has to be encroached upon before there is a change in the distal pressure and flow, whereas in smaller vessels, such as the iliac, carotid, renal, and femoral arteries, the critical stenosis level varies from 70 to 90%.[13, 14] It is important to differentiate between percentage decrease in cross-sectional area and diameter. For example, a decrease in diameter of 50% corresponds to a 75% decrease in cross-sectional area, and a diameter narrowing of 66% is equivalent to about a 90% reduction in area.

Whether a hemodynamic abnormality results from a stenosis, and how severe it may be, depend on several factors, including the following: (1) the length and diameter of the narrowed segment; (2) the roughness of the endothelial surface; (3) the degree of irregularity of the narrowing and its shape (i.e., whether the narrowing is abrupt or gradual); (4) the ratio of the cross-sectional area of the narrowed segment to that of the normal vessel; (5) the rate of flow; (6) the arteriovenous pressure gradient; and (7) the peripheral resistance beyond the stenosis.

The concept of critical stenosis (i.e., a stenosis that causes a reduction in flow and pressure) has been treated extensively in the literature. This concept has been accepted because there is generally little or no change in hemodynamics when an artery is first narrowed by disease, but a relatively rapid decrease in pressure and flow occurs with greater degrees of narrowing. The critical stenosis concept is of practical significance, because lesser degrees of narrowing of human arteries often do not produce significant changes in hemodynamics or clinical manifestations. It must be recognized, however, that the concept of critical stenosis is a gross simplification of a very complex interplay of numerous circulatory factors. In particular, changes in peripheral resistance, such as those occurring with exercise, may profoundly alter the effect of a given stenotic lesion. These considerations dictate that the hemodynamic and clinical significance of stenotic lesions be assessed, whenever possible, by physiologic measurements; otherwise, erroneous conclusions may be reached.[12] In evaluating the hemodynamic effect of stenotic lesions, it is also important to recognize that two or more stenotic lesions that occur in series have a more pronounced effect on distal pressure and flow than does a single lesion of equal total length. This difference is a result of large losses of energy at the entrance, and particularly at the exit, of the lesion resulting from grossly disturbed flow patterns, including jet effects, turbulence, and eddy formation. Thus, the energy losses in tandem lesions far exceed those that result from frictional resistance in a solitary stenosis, as represented in Poiseuille's equation.

Pressure Changes

Experiments with graded stenoses in animals have indicated that, whereas the diastolic pressure does not fall until the stenosis is quite severe, a decrease in systolic pressure is a sensitive index of reduction in both the mean pressure and the amplitude of the pressure wave distal to a relatively minor stenosis (Fig. 1–5).[15, 16] Also, damping of the waveform, increased time to peak, and greater width of the wave at half-amplitude can be detected distal to an arterial stenosis or occlusion.[17, 18]

These abnormal features of the pulse wave correlate well with the results of measurement of systolic pressure and can be demonstrated by noninvasive techniques employing pulse waveforms recorded using various types of plethysmography (Fig. 1–6). In the case of very mild stenotic lesions, however, little or no pressure or pulse abnormality may be evident distal to the lesion when the patient is at rest. The presence of such lesions may be demonstrated if blood flow is in-

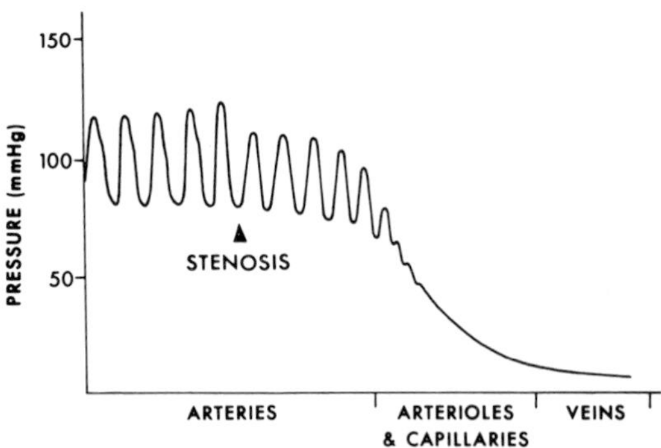

FIGURE 1–5 Decrease in pulse amplitude and systolic and mean pressures distal to a stenosis. In minimal stenosis, alterations in pulse pressure such as this may be evident only during high-volume flow induced by exercise or hyperemia. (From Carter SA: Peripheral artery disease: Pressure measurements ease evaluation. Consultant 19[9]:102–115, 1979.)

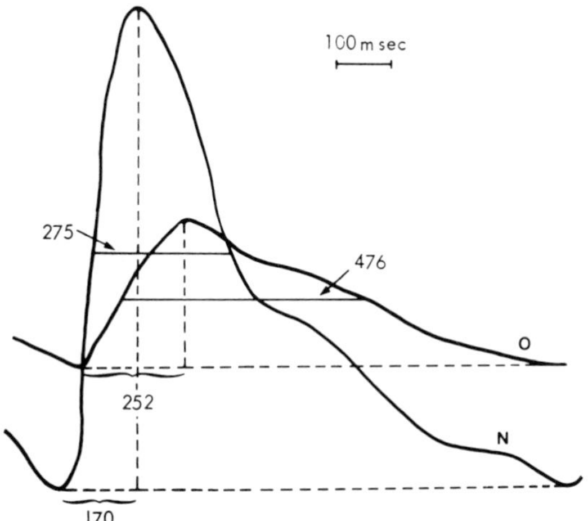

FIGURE 1–6 Dorsalis pedis pulse waves from a normal limb (N) and a limb with a proximal occlusion (O). The wave from the limb with occlusion shows a prolonged time to peak (252 msec) and increased width at half of the amplitude (476 msec). (From Carter SA: Investigation and treatment of arterial occlusive disease of the extremities. Clin Med 79[5]:13–24, 1972 [Part I]; Clin Med 79[6]:15–22, 1972 [Part II].)

creased with exercise or through the induction of hyperemia. Enhanced flow through the stenosis results in increased loss of energy, which can be detected by a decrease in pressure distal to the lesion.[15, 19]

Flow Changes

At rest, the total blood flow to an extremity may be normal in the presence of a severe stenosis or even a complete obstruction of the main artery because of the development of collateral circulation, as well as a compensatory decrease in the peripheral resistance. In such circumstances, measurement of systolic pressure, as discussed earlier, is a better method of assessing the presence and severity of the occlusive or stenotic process than measurement of blood flow.[12, 17] Resting blood flow is reduced only when the occlusion is acute and the collateral circulation has not had a chance to develop or, in the case of a chronic arterial obstruction, when the occlusive process is extensive and consists of two or more lesions in series. Although single lesions might not be associated with symptoms or significant changes in blood flow at rest, such lesions can significantly affect the blood supply when need is increased during exercise. In such cases, the sum of the resistances of the obstructions (stenosis, collateral resistance, or both) and of the peripheral resistance may prevent a normal increase in flow, and symptoms of intermittent claudication may develop.

Arterial obstruction can lead to changes in the distribution of the available blood flow to neighboring regions or vascular beds, depending on the relative resistance and anatomic arrangement of these areas. For example, flow during exercise can increase in the skeletal muscle of the extremity distal to an arterial obstruction, but because the distal pressure is reduced during exercise, the muscle "steals" blood from the skin and the blood supply to the skin of the foot is diminished. Such reduction in flow to the skin may be manifested clinically by numbness of the foot, a common symptom in patients with claudication. In lower extremities with extensive large vessel occlusion and additional obstruction in small distal branches, vasodilator drugs or sympathectomy may divert flow from the critically ischemic distal areas by decreasing resistance in less ischemic regions.[20] Obstruction of the subclavian artery is known to cause cerebral symptoms in some patients because of reversal of flow in the vertebral arteries (the subclavian steal syndrome); similarly, obstructive lesions of the internal carotid artery may lead to reversal of flow in the ophthalmic vessels, which communicate with external carotid branches on the face and scalp.

Velocity Changes

In normal arteries, flow velocity increases rapidly to a peak during early systole and decreases during diastole, when flow reversal can occur. The shape of the resulting pulse velocity wave resembles the pressure gradient shown in Figure 1–4. The character of this velocity profile can be quantified from analogue velocity recordings by calculating various indices of pulsatility and damping.[12, 21] The characteristics of the waveform can also be appreciated by listening to the arterial flow sounds emitted by Doppler flow detectors.[12] Over normal peripheral arteries, double or triple sounds are heard; the second sound represents the diastolic flow reversal and the third sound represents the second forward component. Whether the sounds are double or triple is probably not of practical clinical significance and may be related to a complex interplay of several factors. These factors include the basal heart rate and the shape of the pressure and flow waves. As discussed earlier, the latter factors depend on the degree of peripheral vasoconstriction and elastic properties of the arteries.

Distal to an arterial stenosis the pulse velocity wave is more damped than normal and is similar in pattern to the pressure wave seen in Figure 1–6. Also, flow reversal disappears distal to an arterial stenosis. The calculated wave indices are thus altered, and the audible Doppler signals have a single component rather than the double or triple components usually heard.[12, 21] The disappearance of reversed flow distal to a stenosis probably results from a combination of several factors including the following: (1) the maintenance of a relatively high level of forward flow throughout the cardiac cycle (because of the pressure gradient across the stenosis); (2) resistance to reverse flow created by the stenotic lesion; (3) a decrease in peripheral resistance as a result of relative ischemia; and (4) damping of the pressure wave by the lesion, resulting in attenuated pressure pulses, which are less subject to the reflections and amplification that normally contribute to diastolic flow reversal.

Recordings of flow velocities at and distal to arterial obstructions are useful in the assessment of occlusive processes. The introduction of online frequency spectrum analysis allows better detection and quantification of flow abnormalities resulting from stenotic lesions. This subject is considered in further detail in Chapters 2 and 3, but it is of interest to comment on the physiologic principles illustrated by frequency spectra in normal and abnormal vessels. As noted previously, the velocity pattern across a vessel is flattened by such factors as the effect of branching (see Fig. 1–1*B*). As a result, the particles in the central core of normal arteries flow with relatively uniform and high velocities during systole. This can be demonstrated by spectrum analysis of the arterial velocity Doppler signals, which reveals a narrow band of velocities near the maximum velocity.[22] Stenotic lesions result in marked disturbance of flow with the occurrence of abnormally high velocities, jet effects, irregular travel of particles in various directions and at different velocities, and eddy formation. The change in the direction of particle movement with respect to the axis of the vessel alters the observed Doppler shifts and also contributes to the occurrence of a large range of flow velocities registered with frequency spectral analysis. These effects of arterial stenosis are manifest as widening or dispersal of the band of systolic velocity (spectral broadening) or complete filling in of the spectral tracing, as discussed in Chapter 3.

VENOUS HEMODYNAMICS

As shown in Figure 1–2, the pressure remaining in the veins after the blood has traversed the arterioles and capillaries is low when the subject is in the supine position. Because of their relatively large diameters, medium and large veins offer little resistance to flow, and blood moves readily from the small veins to the right atrium, where the pressure is close to atmospheric pressure. Although the effects of arterial pressure and flow waves are rarely transmitted to the systemic veins, phasic changes in venous pressure and flow do occur in response to cardiac activity and because of alterations of intrathoracic pressure with respiration. Knowledge of these changes is necessary for correct assessment of peripheral veins by noninvasive laboratory studies (see Chapter 21).

The final section of this chapter discusses changes in pressure and flow in various portions of the venous system that are associated with cardiac and respiratory cycles. Also considered are alterations in lower extremity veins that occur with changes in posture, the important consequences of competence or incompetence of venous valves, and the effects of venous obstruction.

Flow and Pressure Changes During the Cardiac Cycle

Figure 1–7 shows changes in pressure and flow in large veins such as the venae cavae that occur during phases of the cardiac cycle. Such oscillations in pressure and flow may, at times, be transmitted to more peripheral vessels. Characteristically, three positive pressure waves (a, c, v) can be distinguished in central venous pressure and reflect corresponding changes in pressure in the atria. The *a wave* is caused by atrial contraction and relaxation. The upstroke of the *c wave* is related to the increase in pressure when the atrioventricular valves are closed and bulge

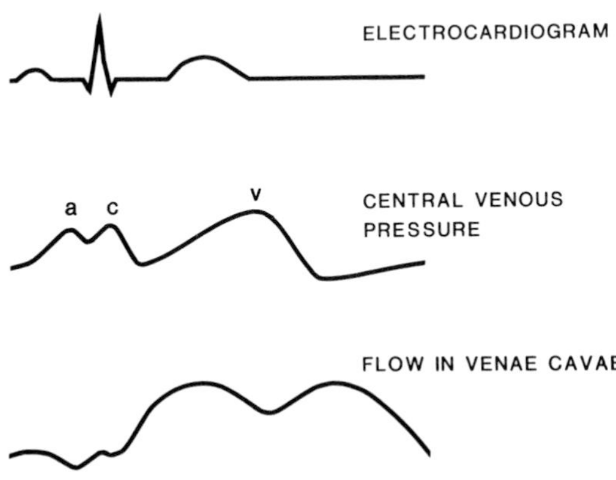

FIGURE 1–7 Schematic representation of normal changes in pressure and flow in the central veins associated with the cardiac cycle. a = a wave; c = c wave; v = v wave.

during isovolumetric ventricular contraction. The subsequent downstroke results from the fall in pressure caused by pulling the atrioventricular valve rings toward the apex of the heart during ventricular contraction, thus tending to increase the atrial volume. The upstroke of the *v wave* results from a passive rise in atrial pressure during ventricular systole when the atrioventricular valves are closed and the atria fill with blood from the peripheral veins. The v wave downstroke is caused by the fall in pressure that occurs when the blood leaves the atria rapidly and fills the ventricles, soon after the opening of the atrioventricular valves, early in ventricular diastole.

The venous pressure waves are associated with changes in flow. There are two periods of increased venous flow during each cardiac cycle. The first occurs during ventricular systole, when shortening of the ventricular muscle pulls the atrioventricular valve rings toward the apex of the heart. This movement of the valve ring tends to increase atrial volume and decrease atrial pressure, thus increasing flow from the extracardiac veins into the atria. The second phase of increased venous flow occurs after the atrioventricular valves open and blood rushes into the ventricles from the atria. Venous flow is reduced in the intervening periods of the cardiac cycle as the atrial pressure rises during and soon after atrial contraction and in the later part of the ventricular systole. Because there are no valves at the junction of the right atrium and venae cavae, some backward flow may actually occur in the large thoracic veins during atrial contraction as blood moves in the reverse direction from the atrium into the venae cavae.

The changes in pressure and flow in the large central veins that are associated with the events of the cardiac cycle are not usually evident in the peripheral veins of the extremities. This is probably the result of damping related to the high distensibility (compliance) of the veins, as well as compression of the veins by intra-abdominal pressure and mechanical compression in the thoracic inlet. Because the effects of right-sided heart contractions are more readily transmitted to the large veins of the arms, the pulsatile changes in venous velocity associated with the events of the cardiac cycle tend to be more obvious in the upper extremities than in the veins of the legs.

In abnormal conditions, such as congestive heart failure or tricuspid insufficiency, venous pressure is increased. This elevation of venous pressure may lead to the transmission of cardiac phasic changes in pressure and flow to the peripheral veins of the upper and lower limbs. Such phasic changes may occasionally be found in healthy, well-hydrated individuals, probably because a large blood volume distends the venous system.

Venous Effects of Respiration

Respiration has profound effects on venous pressure and flow. During inspiration, the volume in the veins of the thorax increases and the pressure decreases in response to reduced intrathoracic pressure. Expiration leads to the opposite effect, with decreased venous volume and increased pressure. The venous response to respiration is reversed in the abdomen, where the pressure increases during inspiration because of the descent of the diaphragm and decreases during expiration as the diaphragm ascends. Increased abdominal pressure during inspiration decreases pressure gradients between peripheral veins in the lower extremities and the abdomen, thus reducing flow in the peripheral vessels. During expiration, when intra-abdominal pressure is reduced, the pressure gradient from the lower limbs to the abdomen is increased and flow in the peripheral veins rises correspondingly.

In the veins of the upper limbs, the changes in flow with respiration are opposite to those in the lower extremities. Because of reduced intrathoracic pressure during inspiration, the pressure gradient from the veins of the upper limbs to the right atrium increases and flow increases. During expiration, flow decreases because of the resulting increase in intrathoracic pressure and the corresponding rise of the right atrial pressure. The respiratory changes in flow in the upper limbs may be influenced by changes in posture. With the upper parts of the body elevated, venous flow tends to stop at the height of inspiration and resumes with expiration, probably because of the compression of the subclavian vein at the level of the first rib during contraction of the accessory muscles of respiration.

The respiratory effects are usually associated with clear phasic changes in venous flow in the extremities; these can be detected by various instruments, including many forms of plethysmographs and Doppler flow detectors. The respiratory changes in venous velocity may be exaggerated by respiratory maneuvers such as the Valsalva maneuver, which increases intrathoracic and abdominal pressures and decreases, abolishes, or even reverses flow in some peripheral veins. Also, the respiratory effects on venous flow may be diminished in the lower limbs in individuals who are chest or shallow breathers and whose diaphragm may not descend sufficiently to elevate intra-abdominal pressure. Venous flow then tends to be more continuous.

Venous Flow and Peripheral Resistance

Blood flow and flow velocity in the peripheral veins, particularly in the extremities, are profoundly influenced by local blood flow, which is in turn largely determined by the peripheral resistance or the state of vasoconstriction or vasodilatation. When limb blood flow is markedly increased as a result of peripheral vasodilatation (e.g., secondary to infection or inflammation), the flow tends to be more continuous, and the respiratory changes in flow are less evident. When there is increased vasoconstriction in the extremities (e.g., when there is a need to conserve body heat, and blood flow through the skin is decreased), venous flow is also markedly decreased and there may be no audible Doppler flow signals over a peripheral vein, such as the posterior tibial vein. Also, severe arterial obstruction may decrease overall blood flow and velocity in the vessels of the extremities and lead to decreased velocity signals over the venous channels.

Effect of Posture

In the upright position, the hydrostatic pressure is greatly increased in the dependent part of the body, particularly in the lower portions of the lower extremities. This increase in hydrostatic pressure, as indicated earlier, is associated with high transmural pressures in the blood vessels and, in turn, leads to greater vascular distention. In the veins, which have low pressure to start with and are distensible, considerable pooling of the blood occurs in the lower parts of the legs. The resulting decrease in venous return to the right atrium is associated with diminished cardiac output. When the normal compensatory reflexes that increase peripheral resistance are impaired, decreased cardiac output can lead to hypotension and fainting.

The movement of the skeletal muscles of the legs, such as that which occurs during walking, leads to decreased venous pressure because of the presence of one-way valves in the peripheral veins. Contraction of the voluntary muscle squeezes the veins and propels the blood toward the heart. Muscular contraction not only increases venous return and cardiac output but also interrupts the hydrostatic column of venous blood from the heart and thus decreases pressure in the peripheral veins (e.g., in the veins at the ankle). Activity of the skeletal muscles of the legs in the presence of competent venous valves therefore results in the lowering of pressure in the veins of the extremity, leading to decreased venous pooling, decreased capillary pressure, reduced filtration of fluid into the extracellular space than would otherwise occur, and increased blood flow because of increased arteriovenous pressure difference.

Effect of External Compression

Sudden pressure on the veins of the extremities, whether caused by an active muscular contraction or external manual compression of the limb, increases venous flow and velocity toward the heart and stops the flow distal to the site of the compression in the presence of competent venous valves.

The responses to sudden pressure changes are affected by venous obstruction and damage to the venous valves. The detection of such changes is important when assessing patients for the presence of venous disease (this is discussed further in Chapter 21).

Venous Obstruction

Venous obstruction can be acute or chronic. In the case of severe chronic obstruction, edema may occur. Also, the nutrition of the skin in the affected region may be impaired, and characteristic trophic changes in the skin and venous stasis ulcers may result. Acute obstruction, usually associated with thrombosis, may lead to potentially fatal pulmonary embolism. Because the clinical diagnosis of acute deep vein thrombosis is unreliable, noninvasive procedures have been developed to enhance the accuracy of this diagnosis.[12] Various forms of plethysmographs, Doppler flow detectors, and duplex ultrasound scanners may be used for this purpose.

An audible Doppler signal should be present over peripheral veins; it can be easily distinguished from an arterial flow signal because of the absence of pulsatility synchronous with the heart. As indicated earlier, a signal may be absent in low-flow states, especially when the limb is cold and auscultation is carried out over small peripheral veins. Squeezing of the limb distal to the site of examination should temporarily increase flow and result in an audible signal if the vein is patent. Spontaneous venous flow signals normally possess clear respiratory phases. However, if there is an obstruction between the heart and the examination site, the respiratory changes in venous velocity are absent or attenuated. Over larger, more proximal veins, such as the popliteal and more proximal vessels, the absence of audible signals after an adequate search is indicative of an obstructed venous segment.

The presence or absence of obstruction is also gauged by increasing flow toward the examination site by squeezing the limb distally or by activating the *distal* muscle groups and thus increasing venous blood flow toward the flow-detecting probe. Absence of increased flow sounds or attenuation of increased flow is associated with obstruction between the probe location and the site from which the enhancement of venous flow is attempted.

Increase in flow is also elicited when manual compression of the limb proximal to the flow-detecting probe is released, because of low filling and pressure in the proximal veins that have been emptied by the compression. If the proximal veins at or near the point of compression are occluded, the augmentation of flow after release of the compression is attenuated.

Venous Valvular Incompetence

When the valves are competent, flow in the peripheral veins is toward the heart. However, flow may be temporarily diminished or stopped soon after assumption of the upright posture, at the height of inspiration, or during the Valsalva maneuver. The peripheral veins normally fill from the capillaries and the rate at which they fill depends on the peripheral resistance and blood flow, as determined by the degree of peripheral vasoconstriction. When there are incompetent veins proximally, there may be retrograde filling of the peripheral veins, such as those in the ankle region, from the more proximal veins, in addition to normal filling from the capillary beds.[12] This retrograde filling may have serious consequences because of a resulting increase in hydrostatic pressure and filtration of fluid into the extravascular spaces in the upright position.

The presence or absence of the retrograde flow may be detected by listening with a Doppler flow detector and squeezing the limb proximally. Also, various plethysmographic methods can detect the rate of filling through measurement of venous volume, which changes with pressure, after the volume and pressure have been reduced by muscular action such as flexion-extension of the ankle in the upright position. After such exercise, the venous volume and pressure increase more rapidly when the valves are incompetent, because the peripheral veins fill as a result of retrograde flow from the more proximal parts of the limbs. The application of a tourniquet or cuff with appropriate pressure compresses the superficial veins and allows localization of incompetent veins, not only to the various segments of the limbs, but also to the superficial veins as opposed to the perforating or deep veins.

REFERENCES

1. Carter SA: Arterial auscultation in peripheral vascular disease. JAMA 246:1682–1686, 1981.
2. Kaufman W: Fluid Mechanics, 2nd ed. New York, McGraw-Hill, 1963, pp 1–432.
3. Taylor MG: Wave travel in arteries and the design of the cardiovascular system. *In* Attinger EO (ed): Pulsatile Blood Flow. New York, McGraw-Hill, 1964, pp 343–372.
4. Carter SA: Effect of age, cardiovascular disease, and vasomotor changes on transmission of arterial pressure waves through the lower extremities. Angiology 29:601–616, 1978.
5. Kroeker EJ, Wood EH: Comparison of simultaneously recorded central and peripheral arterial pressure pulses during rest, exercise and tilted position in man. Circ Res 3:623–632, 1955.
6. Gaskell P, Krisman A: The brachial to digital blood pressure gradient in normal subjects and in patients with high blood pressure. Can J Biochem Physiol 36:889–893, 1958.
7. Lezack JD, Carter SA: Systolic pressures in the extremities of man with special reference to the toes. Can J Physiol Pharmacol 48:469–474, 1970.
8. Nielsen PE, Barras J-P, Holstein P: Systolic pressure amplification in the arteries of normal subjects. Scand J Clin Lab Invest 33:371–377, 1974.
9. Sugiura T, Freis ED: Pressure pulse in small arteries. Circ Res 11:838–842, 1962.
10. Rowell LB, Brengelmann GL, Blackmon JR, et al: Disparities between aortic and peripheral pulse pressure induced by upright exercise and vasomotor changes in man. Circulation 37:954–964, 1968.
11. Carter SA: Role of pressure measurements in vascular disease. *In* Bernstein EF (ed): Noninvasive Diagnostic Techniques in Vascular Disease. St. Louis, CV Mosby, 1985, pp 513–544.
12. Strandness DE Jr, Sumner DS: Hemodynamics for Surgeons. New York, Grune & Stratton, 1975, pp 3–20; 73–120; 209–289; 396–511.
13. May AG, Van de Berg L, DeWeese JA, et al: Critical arterial stenosis. Surgery 54:250–259, 1963.
14. Schultz RD, Hokanson DE, Strandness DE Jr: Pressure-flow and stress-strain measurements of normal and diseased aortoiliac segments. Surg Gynecol Obstet 124:1267–1276, 1967.
15. Carter SA: Peripheral artery disease: Pressure measurements ease evaluation. Consultant 19(9):102–115, 1979.
16. Widmer LK, Staub H: Blutdruck in stenosierten Arterien. Z Kreislaufforsch 51:975–979, 1962.
17. Carter SA: Indirect systolic pressures and pulse waves in arterial occlusive disease of the lower extremities. Circulation 37:624–637, 1968.
18. Carter SA: Investigation and treatment of arterial occlusive disease of the extremities. Clin Med 79(5):13–24, 1972 (Part I); Clin Med 79(6):15–22, 1972 (Part II).
19. Carter SA: Response of ankle systolic pressure to leg exercise in mild or questionable arterial disease. N Engl J Med 287:578–582, 1972.
20. Uhrenholdt A, Dam WH, Larsen OA, et al: Paradoxical effect on peripheral blood flow after sympathetic blockades in patients with gangrene due to arteriosclerosis obliterans. Vasc Surg 5:154–163, 1971.
21. Johnston KW, Taraschuk I: Validation of the role of pulsatility index in quantitation of the severity of peripheral arterial occlusive disease. Am J Surg 131:295–297, 1976.
22. Reneman RS, Hoeks A, Spencer MP: Doppler ultrasound in the evaluation of the peripheral arterial circulation. Angiology 30:526–538, 1979.

Chapter 2

Physics and Instrumentation in Doppler and B-Mode Ultrasonography

James A. Zagzebski, PhD

This chapter presents an overview of the physical and technical aspects of vascular sonography, including the following: (1) a brief review of relevant ultrasound–soft-tissue interactions, (2) pulse-echo principles and display techniques, (3) the Doppler effect as it applies to vascular sonography, (4) continuous-wave (CW) and pulsed Doppler instrumentation, and (5) the common techniques used for displaying Doppler signal spectral information.

SOUND PROPAGATION IN TISSUE

A sound wave can be produced in a medium by placing a vibrating source in contact with it, causing particles in the medium to vibrate. This vibration energy propagates into the medium and is attenuated, scattered, and reflected by interfaces. In medical ultrasonography, a *piezoelectric transducer* (Fig. 2–1) serves as the source and detector of sound waves. The shape of the transducer is chosen so that the sound travels in a beam with a well-defined direction. The reception of reflected and scattered echo signals by the transducer provides information on the acoustic properties of the medium, makes possible the production of ultrasound brightness (B)-mode images, and allows detection of motion using the Doppler effect.

Speed of Sound

The propagation speed for sound waves depends on the medium through which they are traveling. For soft tissues, the average speed of sound has been found to be 1540 m/sec,[1] and most diagnostic ultrasound instruments are calibrated with the assumption that the sound beam propagates at this average speed. As Table 2–1 indicates, the speed of sound in specific soft tissues deviates only slightly from the assumed average. Variations, if any, of speed of sound with frequency and wave amplitude are small and are ignored in ultrasound imaging.

Frequency and Wavelength

The number of oscillations per second of the piezoelectric element in the transducer determines the frequency of the sound wave. Diagnostic ultrasound applications use frequencies in the 1-MHz (1 million cycles/sec) to 30-MHz frequency range. Manufacturers of ultrasound equipment and clinical users strive to use as high a frequency as practical that still allows adequate visualization depth into tissue (see section on Attenuation).

The wavelength λ is the distance over which the acoustic disturbance repeats itself at any instant of time (see Fig. 2–1). It is defined by the equation

$$\lambda = \frac{c}{f} \qquad (2\text{–}1)$$

where c is the speed of sound and f is the frequency. Table 2–2 presents values for the wavelength in soft tissue (sound speed,

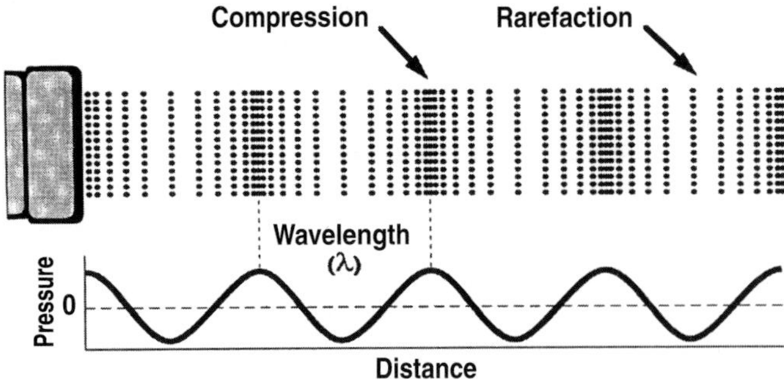

FIGURE 2–1 Sound waves produced by an ultrasound transducer. Vibrations of the transducer send sound waves through the medium, producing fluctuations in tissue pressure. The pressure amplitude is the maximum swing positive or negative. The diagram schematically illustrates compressions and rarefactions at an instant of time.

1540 m/sec) for several frequencies. For example, if the frequency is 5 MHz, the wavelength in soft tissue is about 0.3 mm. Higher frequencies have shorter wavelengths and vice versa.

Wavelength has relevance when describing dimensions of objects, such as reflectors in the body. The size of an object is most meaningfully expressed if given relative to the ultrasonic wavelength for the frequency of the sound beam. Similarly, the width of the ultrasound beam from a transducer depends in part on the wavelength. High frequencies, with their shorter wavelengths, generally permit narrower beams and better resolution.

Amplitude, Intensity, and Power

A sound wave is accompanied by pressure fluctuations as it travels through the medium. The pressure *amplitude* (see Fig. 2–1) is the maximum increase (or decrease) in the pressure due to the presence of the sound wave. The unit for pressure is the pascal (Pa). Pulsed ultrasound scanners can produce peak pressure amplitudes of several megapascals (MPa) in water, when transmit controls are adjusted for maximum levels. As a benchmark for comparison, atmospheric pressure is approximately 0.1 MPa.

The *intensity* I of a sound wave at a point in the medium is estimated by squaring the pressure amplitude P and using $I = P^2/2\rho c$, where ρ is the density and c is the speed of sound. In water, a 2-MPa amplitude during the pulse corresponds to a pulse average intensity of 133 W/cm^2! This is a high intensity, but, fortunately, it is not sustained by a diagnostic ultrasound device because duty factors, that is, the fraction of time the transducer actually emits ultrasound, typically are less than 0.005 sec. Therefore, the time-averaged acoustic intensity from an ultrasound machine, found by averaging over a time that includes transmit pulses as well as the time between pulses, is much lower than the intensity during the pulse. Typical spatial peak time-averaged intensities are on the order of 10 to 20 mW/cm^2 for B-mode imaging. Doppler and color-flow imaging modes have higher duty factors and concentrate the acoustic energy into smaller areas. Time-averaged intensities for these modes may be a few hundred mW/cm^2 for color-flow imaging and as high as 1000 to 2000 mW/cm^2 for pulsed Doppler![2, 2a]

The acoustic *power* produced by a scanner is the rate at which energy is emitted by the transducer. Average acoustic power levels in diagnostic ultrasonography are low because of the small duty factors used in most equip-

TABLE 2–1 SPEED OF SOUND FOR BIOLOGIC TISSUE

Tissue	Speed of Sound (m/sec)	Change from 1540 m/sec (%)
Fat	1450	−5.8
Vitreous humor	1520	−1.3
Liver	1550	+0.6
Blood	1570	+1.9
Muscle	1580	+2.6
Lens of eye	1620	+5.2

From Wells PNT: Propagation of ultrasonic waves through tissues. *In* Fullerton G, Zagzebski J (eds): Medical Physics of CT and Ultrasound. New York, American Institute of Physics, 1980, p 381.

TABLE 2–2 WAVELENGTHS FOR VARIOUS ULTRASOUND FREQUENCIES

Frequency (MHz)	Wavelength* (mm)
1	1.54
2.25	0.68
5	0.31
10	0.15
15	0.103

*Assuming a speed of sound of 1540 m/sec.

ment. Typical power levels are on the order of 10 to 20 mW for most applications.

Decibel Notation

Decibels are frequently used to indicate relative power, intensity, and amplitude levels. They are a way to express the ratio of two signal levels or two intensities. Suppose one wishes to express how much larger (or smaller) an intensity, I_1 is relative to another, I_2. Their relative value in decibels is given by

$$\text{dB} = 10 \log \frac{I_1}{I_2} \quad (2\text{–}2)$$

Thus, the decibel relation between two intensities is just the log of their ratio multiplied by 10. The same equation holds for expressing the ratio of two power levels. If two amplitudes are being compared, A_1 and A_2, their relative value in decibels is

$$\text{dB} = 20 \log \frac{A_1}{A_2}$$

Table 2–3 lists decibel values for various intensity and amplitude ratios. Notice that a 3-dB decrease (or increase) in the power or intensity is the same as halving (or doubling) the quantity.

Attenuation

As a sound beam propagates through tissue, its intensity decreases with increasing distance. This decrease in intensity with path length is called *attenuation.* Sources of attenuation in medical ultrasound imaging include reflection and scatter of the sound wave at boundaries between media having different densities or speeds of sound, and absorption of ultrasonic energy by tissues.

The rate of attenuation in relation to distance is called the *attenuation coefficient,* expressed in decibels per centimeter. The attenuation coefficient depends on both the tissues traversed and the ultrasound frequency. Attenuation is quite high for muscle and skin, an intermediate value for large organs such as the liver, and very low for fluid-filled structures (Fig. 2–2). For the liver, it is approximately 0.5 dB/cm at 1 MHz. An important characteristic of attenuation is its frequency dependence. For most soft tissues, the attenuation coefficient is nearly proportional to the frequency (see Fig. 2–2).[3] Thus, higher frequency sound waves are more severely attenuated than lower frequency waves. Diagnostic studies with higher frequency sound beams (7 MHz and above) are usually limited to superficial regions of the body. Lower frequencies (5 MHz and below) must be used for imaging large organs, such as the liver.

TABLE 2–3 DECIBEL DIFFERENCES CORRESPONDING TO VARIOUS INTENSITY AND AMPLITUDE RATIOS*

Amplitude Ratio (A_1/A_2)	Intensity Ratio (I_1/I_2)	Decibel Difference (dB)
1	1	0
1.41	2	+3
2	4	+6
2.828	8	+9
3.16	10	+10
4.47	20	+13
10	100	+20
100	10,000	+40
1	1	0
0.707	0.5	−3
0.5	0.25	−6

*For example, if I_1 is 10 times I_2, it is 10 dB greater than I_2. A 20-dB difference between 2 signals corresponds to both a ratio of 10 for their amplitude or a ratio of 100 for their intensities, and so forth.

Reflection

Figure 2–3 is an ultrasound image of a Doppler-flow phantom containing a simulated vessel in a tissue-mimicking background material. The wall of the vessel can be seen because of reflection of sound waves from this structure; echoes in the tissue-

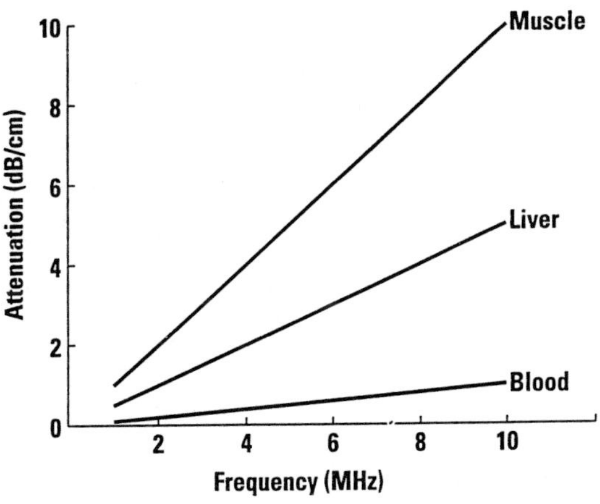

FIGURE 2–2 Variation of attenuation with tissue type and with frequency.

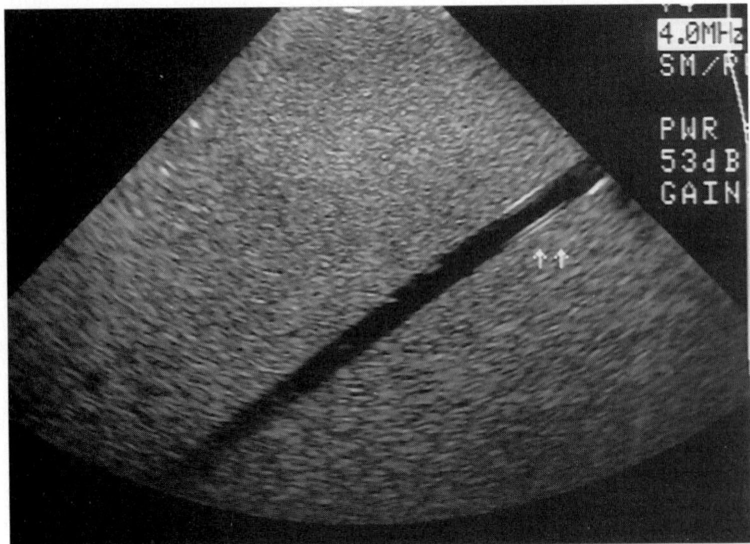

FIGURE 2–3 B-mode image of a Doppler-flow phantom. The interior of the vessel is anechoic because blood-mimicking material has a lower backscatter level than surrounding tissue-like materials. A strong echo is detected from the vessel wall (*arrows*) for ultrasound beams that are perpendicular to the wall, but, being a specular reflector, other beam orientations do not yield a detectable echo.

mimicking background result from ultrasonic scatter. Both reflection and scatter contribute to the detail seen on clinical ultrasound scans.

Whenever an ultrasound beam is incident on an interface formed by two tissues having different acoustic impedances, part of the beam is reflected and part is transmitted. The acoustic impedance Z is the speed of sound c multiplied by the density ρ of a tissue. The amplitude or strength of the reflected wave is proportional to the difference between the acoustic impedances of tissues forming the interface.

For perpendicular incidence of the ultrasound beam on a large, flat interface (Fig. 2–4), the ratio of the reflected to the incident amplitude R is given by

$$R = \frac{Z_2 - Z_1}{Z_2 + Z_1} \qquad (2\text{–}3)$$

where the impedances Z_1 and Z_2 are for the tissues forming the interface. R^2, the ratio of the reflected to the incident power in the beam, is given by

$$R^2 = \frac{(Z_2 - Z_1)^2}{(Z_2 + Z_1)^2} \qquad (2\text{–}4)$$

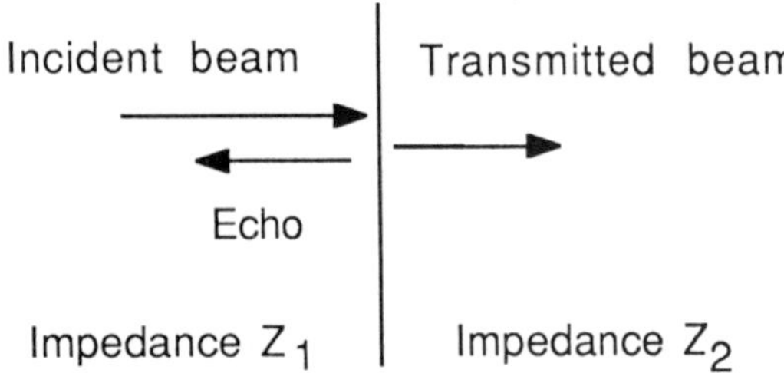

FIGURE 2–4 Reflection at a specular reflector. The echo amplitude depends on the difference between the acoustic impedances Z_1 and Z_2 of the materials forming the interface.

Equations 2–3 and 2–4 show that the echo amplitude at the interface depends on the difference between the acoustic impedances of the tissues forming the interface. The larger the difference between Z_2 and Z_1, the greater the amplitude of the echo and the less power transmitted across the interface. Large impedance mismatches are found at tissue-to-air and tissue-to-bone interfaces. In fact, such interfaces are nearly impenetrable to an ultrasound beam. Significantly weaker echoes originate at interfaces formed by any two soft tissues because, generally, there is not a large difference in impedance between soft tissues.[4]

Large, smooth interfaces, such as depicted in Figure 2–4, are called *specular reflectors*. The direction the reflected wave travels after striking a specular reflector is highly dependent on the orientation of the interface with respect to the sound beam. The wave is reflected back toward the source only when the incident beam is perpendicular or nearly perpendicular to the reflector. The amplitude of an echo detected from a specular reflector thus depends on the orientation of the reflector with respect to the sound beam direction. The ultrasound image in Figure 2–3 was obtained using a sector-scanning probe, which sends individual ultrasound beams into the

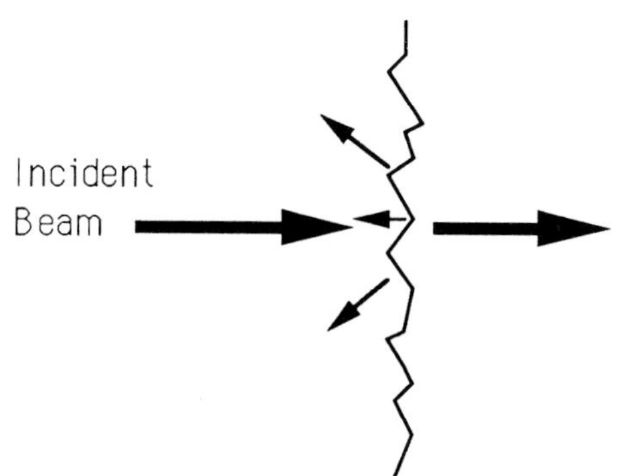

FIGURE 2–5 Diffuse reflection. The reflected waves propagate in various directions.

scanned region at different angles. Only the region for which the ultrasound beams are perpendicular to the vessel wall can be viewed effectively (bright echoes) on the image.

Some soft-tissue interfaces are better classified as *diffuse reflectors* (Fig. 2–5). The reflected waves from a diffuse reflector propagate in various directions with respect to the incident beam. Therefore, the amplitude of an echo from a diffuse interface is less dependent on the orientation of the interface with respect to the sound beam than the amplitude detected from a specular reflector.

Scattering

For acoustic interfaces whose dimensions are small, scattering of the incident sound wave takes place. The scattered energy usually radiates in all directions, as suggested in Figure 2–6. Consequently, there is little angular dependence on the strength of echoes detected from scatterers. The background material in the phantom in Figure 2–3 contains small particles that scatter the ultrasound beam, producing echoes. Unlike the vessel wall, which is best visualized when the ultrasound beam is perpendicular to it, the scatterers are detected with relatively uniform average amplitude from all directions in the phantom. Echoes resulting from scattering within organ parenchyma are clinically important because they provide much of the diagnostic detail seen on ultrasound scans.

In Doppler ultrasonography, blood flow is detected by processing echo signals scattered from red blood cells. The size of a red blood cell is small relative to the ultrasonic wavelength; scatterers of this size range are called *Rayleigh's scatterers.* The scattered intensity from a distribution of Rayleigh's scatterers depends on several factors: (1) the dimensions of the scatterer, with a sharply increasing scattered intensity as the size increases; (2) the number of scatterers present in the beam (e.g., Shung has demonstrated that when the hematocrit is low, scattering from blood is proportional to the hematocrit[5]); (3) the extent, to which the density or elastic properties of the scatterer differ from those of the surrounding material; and (4) the ultrasonic frequency (for Rayleigh's scatterers the scattered intensity is proportional to the frequency to the fourth power).

ULTRASOUND IMAGING

Range Equation

Ultrasound is used to produce images of anatomic structures by using pulse-echo techniques. An ultrasonic transducer is placed in contact with the skin (Fig. 2–7) or is coupled to the skin through a liquid path. The transducer repeatedly emits brief pulses of sound at a fixed repetition rate. After trans-

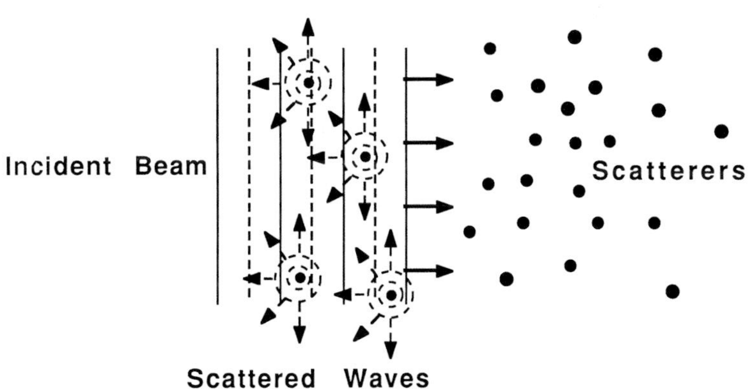

FIGURE 2–6 Scattering of ultrasound by small inhomogeneities.

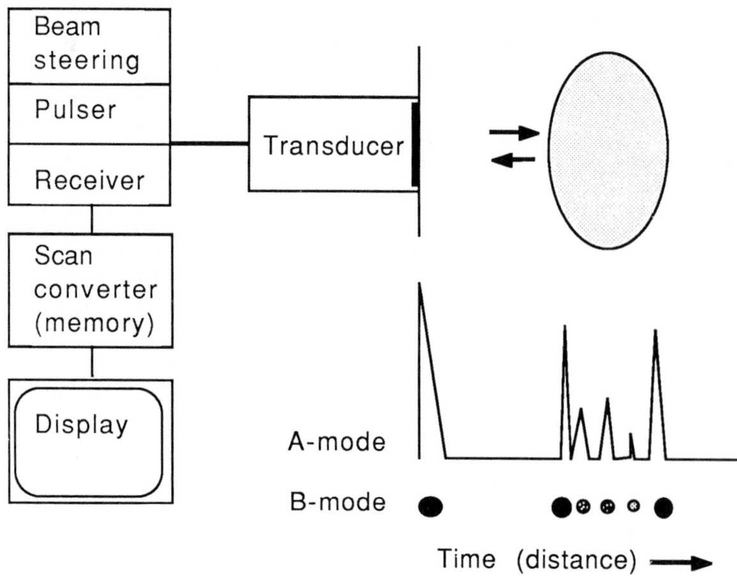

FIGURE 2–7 Simple block diagram of a pulse-echo ultrasound instrument. A-mode and B-mode display methods are also shown for one beam line.

mitting each pulse, the transducer serves as a detector for echoes originating from interfaces and scatterers in the sound beam. Echo signals picked up by the transducer are amplified and processed into a format suitable for display.

With pulse-echo techniques, the distance d to a reflector is determined from the arrival time T of an echo from this structure. Thus,

$$d = \frac{cT}{2} \tag{2–5}$$

where c is the speed of sound and the factor 2 accounts for the roundtrip journey of the sound pulse and echo. Equation 2–5 is called the *range equation* in ultrasound imaging.[6] As mentioned earlier, a speed of sound of 1540 m/sec is assumed in most scanners when converting echo arrival times to reflector distances.

B-Mode Imaging

Two commonly used echo display techniques are also illustrated in Figure 2–7. An amplitude (A)-mode display is a presentation of the echo signal amplitude vs. the time following transmission of the pulse. Because the time is related to the distance from the transducer to the reflector, the A-mode display can also be thought of as a record of the echo amplitude compared with reflector distance. In the B-mode display used for most imaging applications, the reflected signals are converted to a series of dots on the display. With gray-scale processing, the intensity or brightness of each dot is proportional to the echo signal amplitude.

In B-mode scanning, the sound beam is swept across a region, and echoes are placed on the B-mode display in a position that corresponds to their anatomic origin. The displayed position for each B-mode dot is determined from the beam angle at the time of echo detection and the echo return time T. Steps in the generation of a B-mode image are illustrated in Figure 2–8. It is assumed in this illustration that the sound beam is swept by pivoting the ultrasound transducer, as suggested in the two panels on the top of the figure. The two diagrams in the middle show the resultant B-mode line on the display for each beam position. Note that the location of the B-mode line on the display corresponds to the position of the ultrasound beam. Usually, 100 to 200 or more separate ultrasound beam lines are used to construct each image.

Types of Scan Heads

In almost all applications, B-mode imaging is performed with real-time scanners. These scanners automatically sweep ultrasound beams over the imaged region at a rapid rate. The four types of real-time transducer assemblies are illustrated in Figure 2–9.

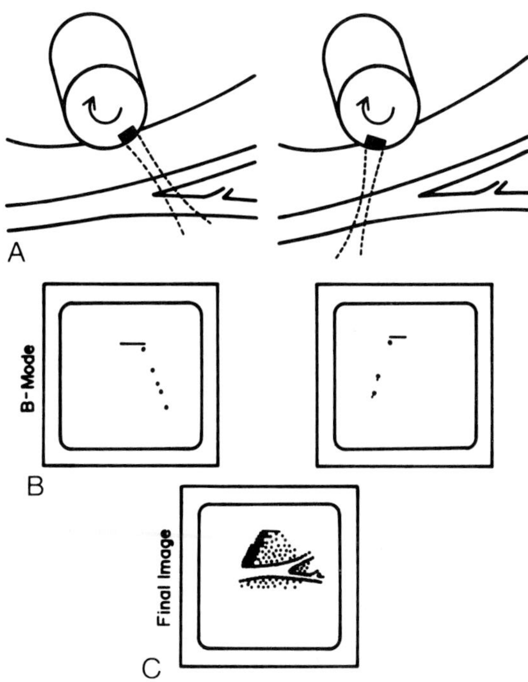

FIGURE 2–8 Ultrasound B-mode scanning. *A,* Pulses of ultrasound are transmitted in various directions. *B,* Echo signals are displayed using the B-mode presentation with the B-mode display line tracking the ultrasound beam axis. *C,* The final image.

MECHANICAL SECTOR SCANNER. A single transducer or several transducers are oscillated within the scan head (transducer assembly), steering the sound beam over the region of interest. Alternatively, the beam from a stationary transducer may be swept by oscillating an acoustic mirror. Each transducer may be a single element, or it may be an annular array,[7] consisting of a central disk surrounded by 5 to 10 annuli.[7]

LINEAR (SEQUENTIAL) ARRAY SCANNER. An array of perhaps 120 separate rectangular transducer elements placed side by side forms the image. Groups of approximately 15 to 20 elements are activated simultaneously to produce each ultrasound beam, with the beam line centered over the central element in the group. Imaging starts with a group of elements on one end of the array, which transmits the first beam line and collects the echo signals. The active element group is shifted (translated) by one element, forming a new element group, and the pulse-echo process is repeated. The active element group progresses from one end of the array to the other by simple element switching. Beam lines are parallel to one another, and the resultant image format is rectangular.

CURVILINEAR ARRAY SCANNER. These arrays are similar to the linear array, only the elements are arranged along a convex scanning surface. The method for image formation is identical to that of the linear array, in which the active element group is switched progressively from one side of the array to the next. Compared with the linear array, the curved array provides a wider image field at depth, from a narrower scanning window on the patient surface.

PHASED ARRAY SCANNER. These consist of an array of 120 or so very narrow elements arranged side by side. All elements are used for each beam line; the ultrasound beam is "steered" by introducing small time delays between the transmit pulses applied to individual elements. Time delays are also applied among echo signals picked up from individual elements during reception, steering the received directionality as well. An image is formed using perhaps 150 beams steered in different directions.

Image Memory

An image memory device called a *scan converter* temporarily retains images for review and photography and converts the image format into one suitable for video monitor viewing and videotape recording. The scan converter is a digital device and may be thought of as a matrix of pixels (image elements); typically 500 or more pixels are arranged vertically and about 500 horizontally. Because the scan converter is digital, capabilities, such as the echo amplitude detail stored at each pixel location, are expressed using digital notation. In particular, each pixel consists of several storage cells called *bits.* A bit can have a value of either 1 or 0, but a multibit storage cell can represent a large range of values because of the different combinations of 1 and 0 that can be accommodated. For example, 6-bit memories divide the echo signal into 64 (2^6) different amplitude levels and store an appropriate level at each pixel location. Eight-bit memories represent the echo amplitude using 256 (2^8) levels, and 10-bit memories will retain 1 out of 1024 (2^{10}) different levels at each pixel location. The more bits (amplitude levels), the more different shades of gray are possible from the stored image, especially during postprocessing (see later). Modern scanners also allow storage of

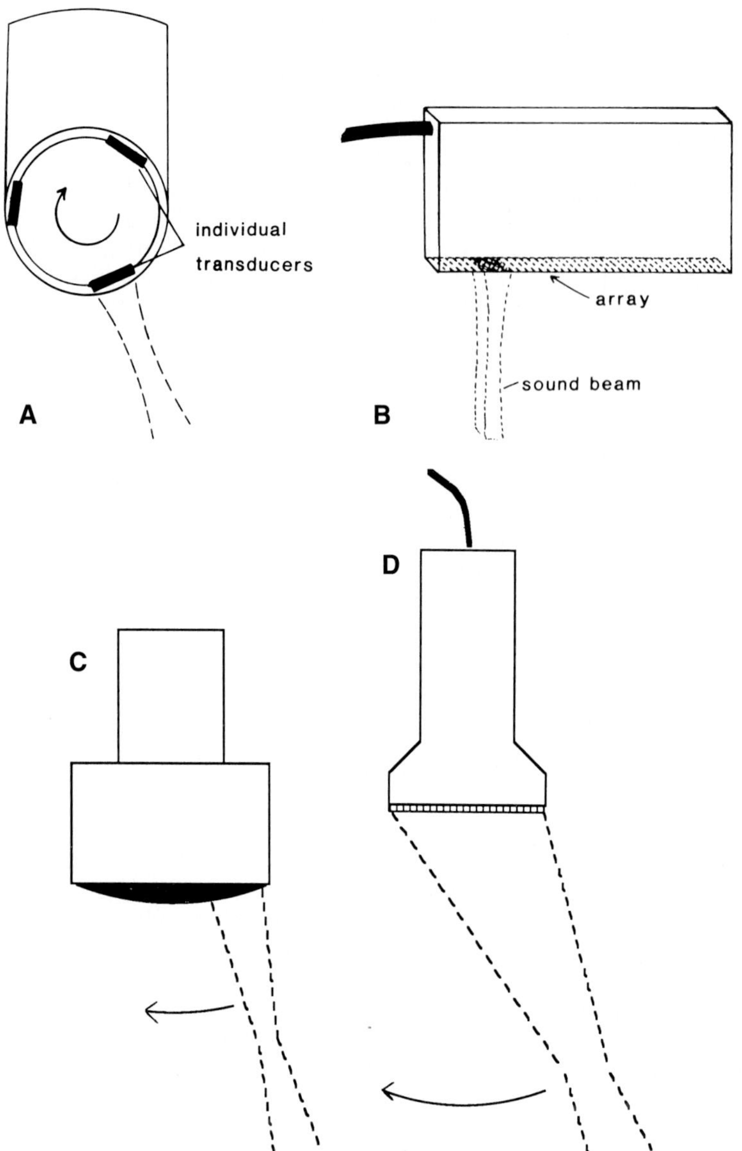

FIGURE 2–9 *A,* Mechanical sector scanner. *B,* Linear array transducer. *C,* Curvilinear array scanner. *D,* Phased array scanner.

cine loops, using a memory that can retain many separate images.

Principal Scanner Controls

Ultrasound scanner operators must be familiar with many instrument controls to produce optimal images with their equipment. Details and examples of different control settings can be found in standard textbooks.[4, 6] The major controls found on scanners include

- Depth setting, to select the size of the imaged field.
- Output power control, to vary the scanner sensitivity. Increasing the transmit power allows the operator to view weaker echo signals from the body. This is accompanied, of course, by higher acoustic exposure to the patient.
- Transducer frequency select, to select the dominant ultrasound frequency coming out of the transducer. Modern transducers can produce ultrasound beams covering a range of frequencies. This control is used to determine which frequencies are used in the image.
- Overall receiver gain, also to vary the scanner sensitivity. Gain describes the amount

of amplification of echoes in the receiver. Higher gains amplify the echo signals picked up by the transducer more than lower gain settings.

- Time gain compensation, to compensate for attenuation of the ultrasound beam in tissue. With time gain compensation the receiver amplification increases automatically with the depth of origin of the echoes, so echo signals from deep structures, which have undergone significant attenuation, are amplified more than signals from shallow structures that have undergone less attenuation. Time gain compensation is controlled in most machines using a set of six to eight gain knobs, each adjusting the receiver gain at a different depth.
- Compression, to vary the amplitude range (dynamic range) of echoes displayed as shades of gray on the image. Most scanners apply logarithmic compression to the echo signals emerging from the receiver; the amount of compression is under user control.
- Other preprocessing, to alter the echo signals before they are sent to the scan converter. Some manufacturers, for example, apply edge-enhancing filters to the signals.
- Postprocessing, to change the appearance of echo signals, already stored in memory, on the image. Various postprocessing curves are available to emphasize different portions of the echo dynamic range.
- Persistence, to include the images from several successive sweeps of the transducer with the current image. High persistence has the effect of smoothing out the image but at the expense of losing some temporal detail.

Frame Rate

The *image frame rate* is the number of complete scans per second carried out by the transducer assembly. It is an important specification of a scanner because it affects the temporal detail that can be resolved. For example, rapidly moving heart valves require high image frame rates to be viewed effectively.

Fundamentally, the image frame rate is limited by the sound propagation speed in tissue. An image is produced by the scanner by sending ultrasound pulses along 100 to 200 different beam directions (beam lines) into the body. For each beam line, the scanner transmits a pulse and waits for the echoes from the maximum depth setting along that line. Then it transmits a pulse along a new beam direction and repeats the process. Beam lines are addressed serially, meaning the scanner cannot transmit a pulse along a new beam line until echoes have been picked up from the maximum depth in the previous line. The speed with which the pulse propagates, the depth setting of the scanner, and the number of beam lines forming the image all conspire to limit the maximum possible image frame rate.

Using the range equation, if the maximum depth setting is D, it takes a time $T = 2D/c$ to receive all echoes from one beam line. The amount of time for a complete image consisting of N beam lines is simply $N \times T$. FR_{max}, the maximum possible frame rate, is the inverse of the time needed for a complete image. This may be written as

$$FR_{max} = \frac{1}{NT} = \frac{c}{2ND} \qquad (2\text{–}6)$$

Because the speed of sound is 1540 m/sec, or 154,000 cm/sec, if the depth setting D is expressed in centimeters, this also works out to

$$FR_{max} = \frac{77{,}000}{ND\,(\text{cm})}\ \text{Hz}$$

For $N = 200$ beam lines and an image depth of 15.4 cm, FR_{max} is 25 Hz. Operators can easily verify that reducing the depth setting (D) on the scanner usually increases the frame rate and vice versa. The scanner is programmed to provide as high a frame rate as practical for the scanning conditions. Some scanners allow the operator to change N, the number of beam lines used to form the image, for example, by increasing the angular separation between beam lines. This also affects the frame rate, as does changing the horizontal size of the image.

DOPPLER EFFECT

The Doppler effect is a change in the frequency of a detected wave when the source or the detector are moving. In medical ultrasonography a Doppler shift occurs when reflectors move relative to the transducer. The frequency of echo signals from moving reflectors is higher or lower than the frequency transmitted by the transducer, depending on whether the motion is toward or away from the transducer. The Doppler shift frequency, or simply the Doppler frequency, is the difference between the received and transmitted frequencies.

Doppler Equation

Ultrasonic Doppler equipment is often used for detecting and evaluating blood flow. A typical arrangement is illustrated in Figure 2–10. An ultrasonic transducer is placed in contact with the skin surface; it transmits a beam whose frequency is f_o. The received frequency f_r will differ from f_o when echoes are picked up from moving scatterers, such as the red blood cells. The Doppler frequency f_D is defined as the difference between the received and transmitted frequencies and is given by

$$f_D = f_r - f_o = \frac{2f_o v\cos\theta}{c} \qquad (2–7)$$

where c is the speed of sound, v is the flow velocity, and θ is the angle between the direction of flow and the axis of the ultrasound beam, looking toward the transducer.

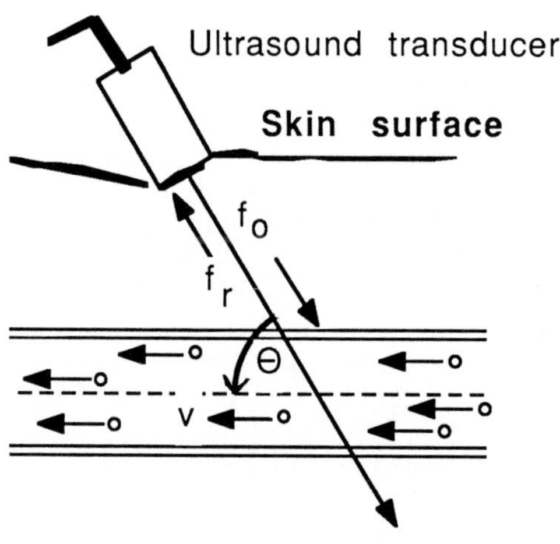

FIGURE 2–10 Arrangement for detecting Doppler signals from blood. The angle θ is the Doppler angle, which is the angle between the direction of motion and the beam axis, looking toward the transducer.

θ is called the *Doppler angle* and strongly influences the detected Doppler frequency for a given reflector velocity. When flow is directly toward the transducer θ is 0 degrees and cos θ is 1. The Doppler frequency detected for this orientation would be the maximum one could obtain for the flow conditions. For the sound beam incident at an angle other than 0 degrees, the detected Doppler frequency is reduced according to the cos θ term. For example, at 30 degrees the Doppler frequency would be 0.87 multiplied by what it is at 0 degrees; at 60 degrees it would be 0.5 multiplied by its 0 degree value. Finally, when the flow is perpendicular to the ultrasound beam direction, $\theta = 90$ degrees and cos $\theta = 0$; there is no detected Doppler shift! In practice, the transducer beam is usually oriented to make a 30- to 60-degree angle with the arterial lumen.

Continuous-Wave Ultrasonic Doppler Equipment

CW Doppler operation is used in a variety of instruments, ranging from simple, inexpensive hand-held Doppler units, to "high-end" duplex scanners, in which CW Doppler may be one of several operating modes. A simplified block diagram of the necessary components of a CW Doppler unit is presented in Figure 2–11. The transmitter continuously excites the ultrasonic transducer with a sinusoidal electrical signal of frequency f_o, producing the incident ultrasound beam. Echoes returning to the transducer have frequency f_r. These signals are amplified in the receiver and then sent to a demodulator to extract the Doppler signal. Here the signals are multiplied by a reference signal from the transmitter, producing a mixture of signals, part having a frequency $(f_r + f_o)$ and part having a frequency $(f_r - f_o)$. The sum frequency, $(f_r + f_o)$, is very high—twice the ultrasound frequency—and is easily removed by electronic filtering. This leaves signals with frequency $(f_r - f_o)$ at the output, which is the Doppler signal!

What are typical Doppler frequencies for blood flow? Suppose $v = 20$ cm/sec; the ultrasound frequency, $f_o = 5$ MHz (5×10^6 cycles/sec); and the speed of sound, $c = 1540$ m/

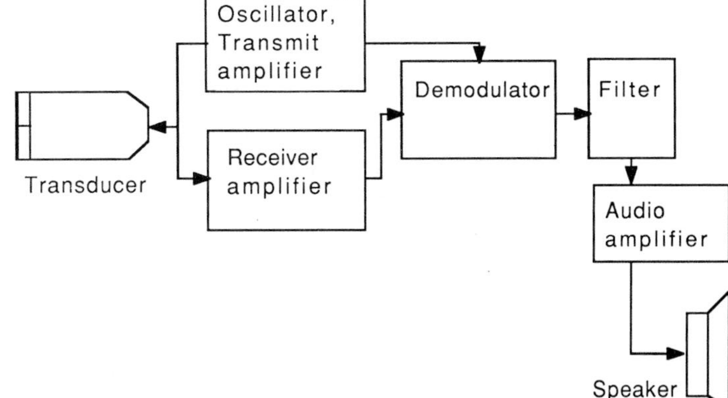

FIGURE 2–11 Schematic representation of a continuous-wave Doppler instrument. The Doppler signal is obtained by demodulating the amplified echo signals and then applying a low-pass filter. Because the signals are generally in the audible range, a loudspeaker may be used to display the Doppler signals.

sec. Furthermore, let $\theta = 0$ degrees so that $\cos\theta = 1$. Using Equation 2–7, we find

$$f_D = \frac{2 \times (5 \times 10^6 \text{ cycles/sec}) \times 0.2 \text{ m/sec}}{1540 \text{ m/sec}}$$
$$= 1299 \text{ cycles/sec}$$

or about 1.3 kHz. This is within the audible frequency range, which is generally the case for most Doppler signals resulting from blood flow. The filtered output Doppler signal can be applied to a loudspeaker or headphones for interpretation by the operator. The signals can also be recorded on audiotape or applied to any of several spectral analysis systems (see later).

It is possible to eliminate signals of certain frequency ranges from the output. This is done in instruments that have additional electrical filters in their circuitry. For example, when studying blood flow, relatively low-frequency Doppler signals originating from movement of vessel walls may be eliminated from the output by applying a high-pass filter. The lower cutoff frequency of such wall filters is usually operator selectable.

Continuous-Wave Doppler Controls

Basic CW Doppler units usually have only a few controls, but operators should be familiar with those on their own equipment. Examples include the following:

- Transmit power, to vary the amplitude of the signal from the transmitter to the transducer, thus changing the sensitivity to weak echoes. Some simple units omit this control, keeping the transmit level constant.
- Gain, to vary the sensitivity of the unit.
- Audio gain, to vary the loudness of Doppler signals applied to loudspeakers.
- Wall filter, to vary the low frequency cutoff frequency of the wall filter.

Directional Doppler

A basic CW Doppler instrument allows detection of the magnitude of the Doppler frequency, but it provides no indication of whether flow is toward or away from the transducer, that is, whether the Doppler shift is positive or negative. A common technique for determining flow direction is to use quadrature detection in the Doppler device. After the received echo signals are amplified, they are split into two identical channels for demodulation. The channels differ only in that the reference signals from the transmitter sent to the two demodulators are 90 degrees out of phase. Two separate Doppler signals are produced. They are identical except for a small phase difference between them, and this phase difference can be used to determine whether the Doppler shift is positive or negative.[8] Clever schemes are used that combine the two quadrature signals to enable presentation of positive and negative flow in stereo speakers.[9]

Pulsed Doppler

With CW Doppler instruments, reflectors and scatterers anywhere within the beam of the transducer can contribute to the instantaneous Doppler signal. A pulsed Doppler instrument provides for discrimination of

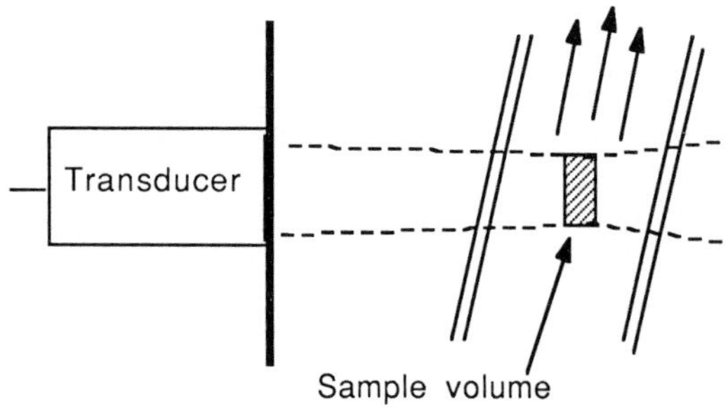

FIGURE 2–12 Sample volume in pulsed Doppler. Echo signals from a fixed depth are selected by a range gate. The size of the sample volume depends on the beam width, the duration of the gate, and the pulse duration from the transducer.

Doppler signals from different depths, allowing for the detection of moving interfaces and scatterers only from within a well-defined sample volume (Fig. 2–12). The sample volume can be positioned anywhere along the axis of the ultrasound beam.

The principal components of a pulsed Doppler instrument[10] are shown in Figure 2–13. The ultrasonic transducer is excited with a short duration burst, rather than continuously as in the CW instrument. Scattered and reflected echo signals are detected by the same transducer, amplified in the receiver, and applied to the demodulator. The output of the demodulator is then applied to a sample-and-hold circuit, which integrates (or averages) a portion of the signal, selected by a range gate. The gate position and duration are controlled by the operator. The gated signal, taken over a series of pulse-echo sequences, forms the Doppler signal heard over the loudspeaker of the device. In Figure 2–13, quadrature detectors are used to form two output channels, enabling the flow direction to be determined.

The Doppler signal produced by a pulsed Doppler instrument is generated from the changes in phase of the echo signals from moving targets from one pulse-echo sequence to the next. Thus the pulse repetition frequency (PRF) of the instrument must be high enough so that important details of the Doppler signal are not lost between transmit pulses (see section on Aliasing in Pulsed Doppler). After each transmit pulse, only a brief portion of the Doppler signal is available within the demodulated echo signals selected by the gated region. Multiple pulse-echo sequences are required to construct the Doppler signal heard over the loudspeakers. By filtering the sample-and-hold output from one pulse-echo sequence to the next, a smooth Doppler signal is formed.

Duplex Instruments

A real-time B-mode imager and a Doppler instrument provide complementary information because the scanner can best outline anatomic structures, whereas a Doppler instrument yields information regarding flow and movement patterns. *Duplex ultrasound in-*

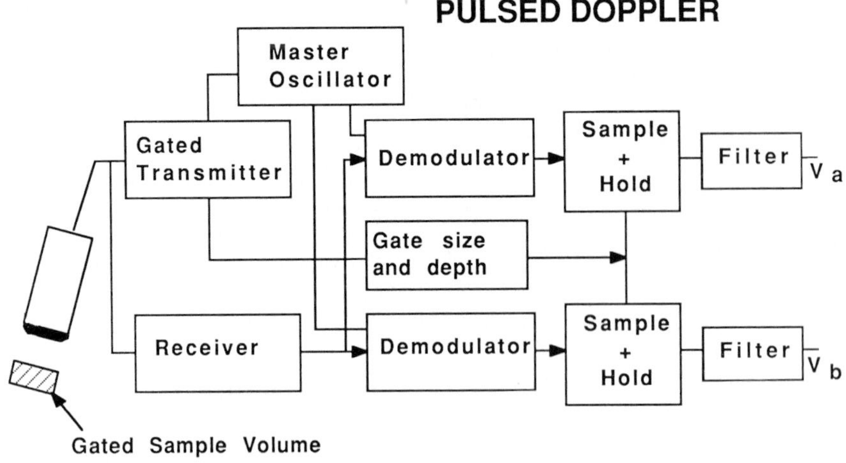

FIGURE 2–13 Principal components of a pulsed Doppler instrument. The transducer is excited by a brief pulse; echo signals are amplified in the receiver and sent to the quadrature demodulators. A portion of the demodulated waveform is held in the sample and hold unit, which forms the Doppler signal by using several pulse-echo sequences. V_a and V_b are signals representing flow toward and away from the transducer.

struments are real-time B-mode scanners with built-in Doppler capabilities. In typical applications, the pulse-echo B-mode image obtained with a duplex scanner is used to localize areas where flow is to be examined using Doppler.

The region of interest for Doppler studies may be selected on the B-mode image by placement of a sample volume indicator, or cursor (Fig. 2–14). Most duplex instruments allow the operator to indicate the Doppler angle or the assumed direction of blood flow with respect to the ultrasound beam. The Doppler angle must be known to estimate flow velocity from the Doppler signal.

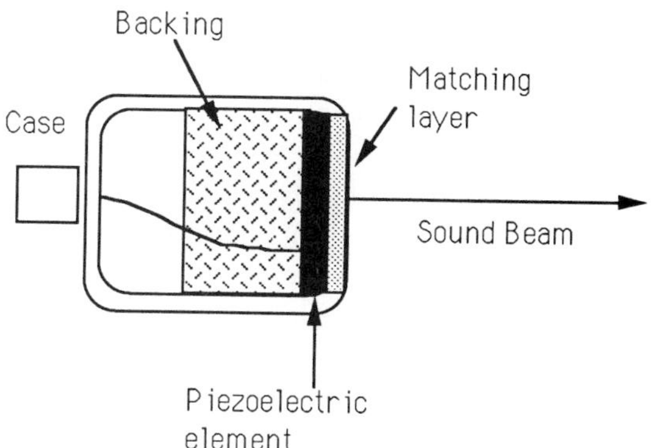

FIGURE 2–15 Drawing of a single-element transducer. The piezoelectric element is a thin circular disk. The view cuts through the axis of symmetry of the transducer.

Transducer Properties

An ultrasound transducer provides the communicating link between the Doppler or pulse-echo imaging instrument and the patient. Medical ultrasound transducers use piezoelectric ceramic materials to generate and detect sound waves. Piezoelectric materials convert electrical signals into mechanical vibrations and pressure waves into electrical signals. Therefore, they are used as both transmitters and detectors of ultrasonic waves.

The internal components of a single-element transducer, used in some mechanical scanners and stand-alone pulsed Doppler systems, are shown in Figure 2–15. The illustration is of a plane circular piezoelectric disk, although other shapes have also been used. In the figure the disk is seen from the side, and the ultrasound beam would be projected to the right. The thickness of the ceramic element governs the resonance frequency of the transducer. Quarter-wave matching layers between the piezoelectric element and a protective outer face plate are used on some transducers. Analogous to special optical coatings on lenses and picture frame glass, the matching layers are employed to improve sound transmission between the transducer and the patient. This improves the sensitivity of the transducer. Backing material is often used in pulse-echo applications to dampen the piezoelectric element vibrations when the transducer is excited. Dampening shortens the duration of the transmitted pulse, improving the axial (or range) resolution.

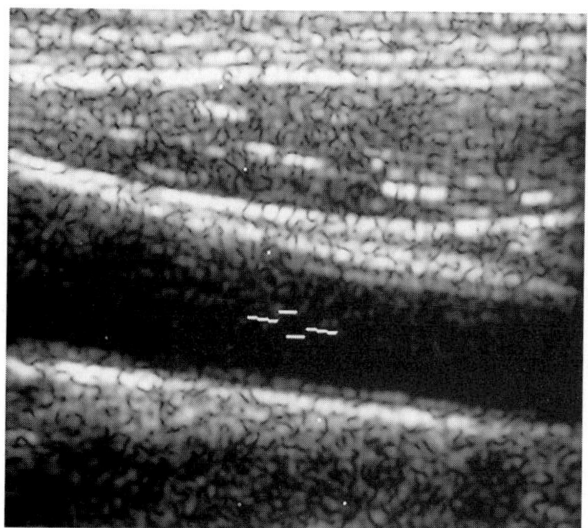

FIGURE 2–14 Image of a carotid artery obtained with a duplex ultrasound machine. A sample volume cursor is positioned to detect Doppler signals from within the artery, and a Doppler angle cursor is oriented to "angle correct" the Doppler signals for displaying the velocity.

Axial Resolution, Lateral Resolution, and Slice Thickness

Spatial resolution describes the minimum spacing between two reflectors for which they can be distinguished on the display. Important factors are the axial resolution, the lateral resolution, and the slice thickness, as illustrated in Figure 2–16.

Axial resolution refers to the ability to resolve reflectors that are closely spaced along the sound beam axis. It is determined by the pulse duration, the length of time the transducer oscillates for each transmit pulse. Short-duration pulses enable the axial resolu-

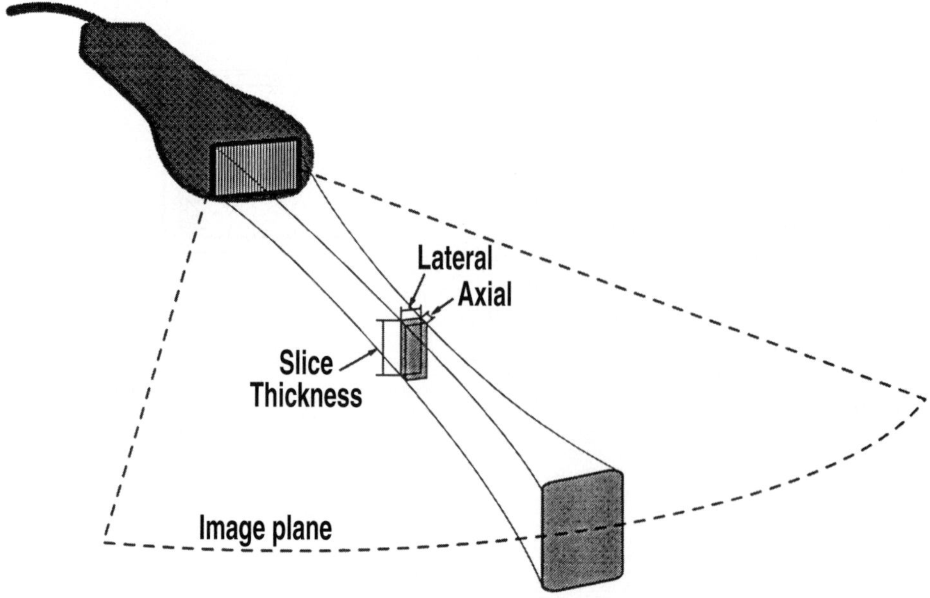

FIGURE 2–16 Typical pulse dimensions emerging from an ultrasound transducer along a single beam line. The pulse duration affects the axial resolution. The width of the beam in the scanning plane determines lateral resolution, whereas the dimensions of the beam perpendicular to the scanning plane determine the slice thickness.

tion to be 1 mm or less in imaging applications. It is better (less) at higher frequencies because pulse durations can be made shorter than at low frequencies.

Lateral resolution refers to the minimum resolvable spacing for reflectors positioned on a line perpendicular to the sound beam axis. It is determined by the width of the ultrasound beam at the location of the reflectors. The sound beam emerging from a diagnostic transducer is directional—that is, its direction of travel conforms to the axis of the transducer (Fig. 2–17). The beam has two components, a near field and a far field. The near field extends outward an axial distance of approximately a^2/λ, where a is the transducer radius and λ is the ultrasonic wavelength. For a transducer whose diameter is 13 mm and whose frequency is 3.5 MHz (3.5×10^6 cycles/sec), the calculated near-field length is 9.6 cm. Within the near field, the amplitude and intensity of the beam fluctuate from one spot to another. Near the point of transition between the near and far fields, the sound beam gradually becomes smooth. It remains smooth throughout the far field, not exhibiting the point-to-point intensity fluctuations found close to the transducer surface. Also, contrary to the near field, where the beam remains collimated, in the

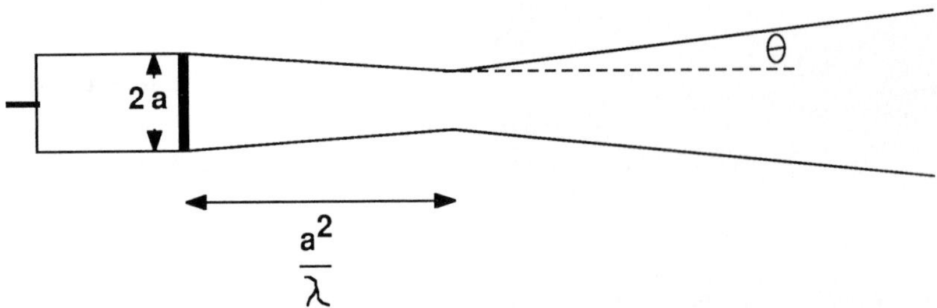

FIGURE 2–17 Representation of the ultrasound beam from a plane disk transducer. The near field extends outward a distance of approximately a^2/λ. Within the near field, the beam remains collimated, but the intensity fluctuates from point to point. In the far field, the beam is smooth but diverges with an angle θ.

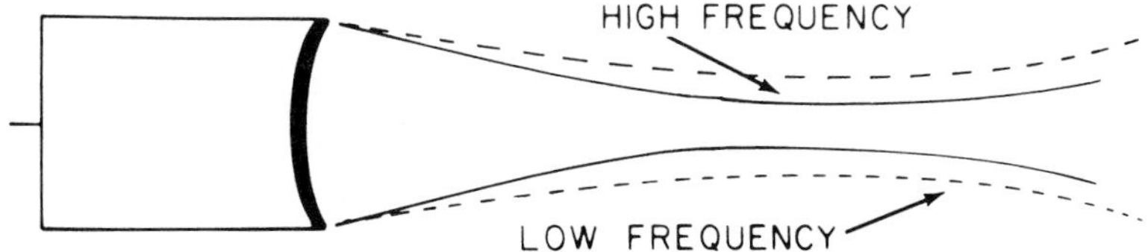

FIGURE 2–18 Sound beam focusing. In this example, focusing is done using a curved piezoelectric element. The beam width at the focal distance depends on the curvature of the lens, the size of the transducer, and the ultrasound frequency.

far field, the beam diverges as the distance from the transducer increases. The divergence angle is greater for lower frequency transducers than for higher frequency transducers of the same diameter. The width of the sound beam at any depth affects the lateral resolution of the ultrasound instrument at that depth.

Focusing of the sound beam is done to improve the lateral resolution. Focusing can be achieved using a lens or a curved piezoelectric element (Fig. 2–18). Focusing reduces the beam width over a volume called the *focal region*. The beam width W in the focal region is approximated by

$$W \approx \frac{1.2\ \lambda\ F}{2a} \qquad (2\text{–}8)$$

where F is the focal distance, $2a$ is the diameter of the radiating surface, and λ is the wavelength. Higher frequency transducers, for which the wavelength is smaller, provide narrower sound beams and better lateral resolution than lower frequency transducers.

Phased, curvilinear, linear, and annular arrays can focus the ultrasound beam electronically. Time delays of the appropriate sequence in the excitation pulses applied to individual elements in the array cause the wavefronts emerging from the array to converge (Fig. 2–19). It is as though a focusing lens or a curved element were producing the beam. An advantage of the array, however, is that the focal region can be varied simply by selecting a different delay sequence for pulses applied to the elements. Most array scanners feature simultaneous multiple

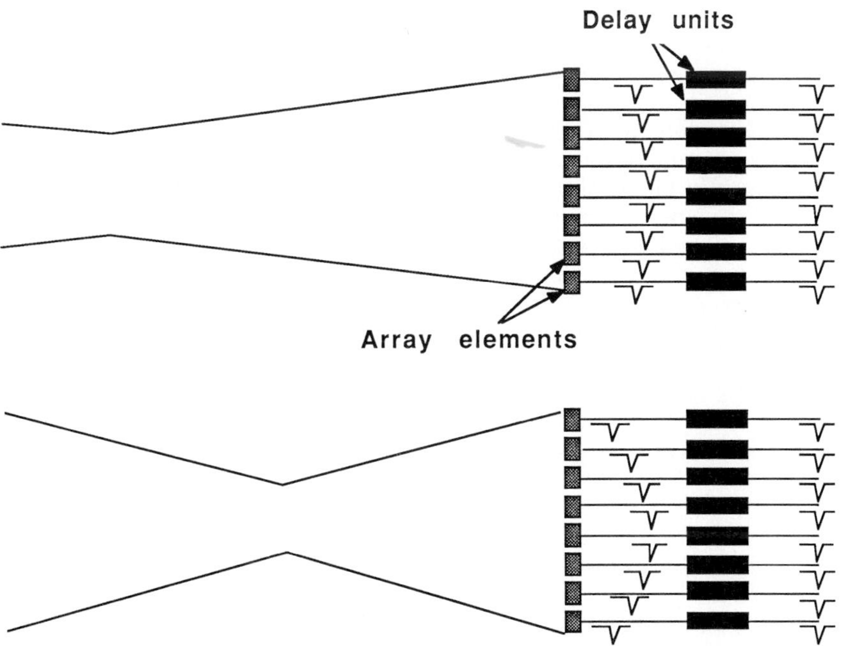

FIGURE 2–19 Electronic focusing of an array during pulse transmission. By exciting the outer elements of an array group slightly before the inner elements in the sequence shown, the waves from individual elements converge, forming a focused beam. The transmit focal distance is user selectable.

transmit focusing, optimizing the lateral resolution over an extended depth. Its use slows the frame rate because a separate transmit pulse must be applied for each focal depth along each beam line.

Array transducers also focus the received echo signals. The reflected wave from a small scatterer along the beam axis arrives at different elements at slightly different times. Delay circuits set appropriately can bring these echo signals into phase, after which the signals from all elements are summed, forming one signal for each reflector. During reception, the focal region changes dynamically, varying automatically with time (and consequently with reflector depth) after the excitation of the transducer. Dynamic focus during reception improves the spatial resolution over the entire range of the image and is done by most instruments that use array transducers. Its use does not slow the frame rate as does multiple transmit focusing.

The *slice thickness* is the thickness of the scanned section that contributes to the image. It depends on the width of the ultrasound beam perpendicular to the image plane (see Fig. 2–16). Phased, linear, and curvilinear array transducers still use a mechanical lens to provide focusing in this direction. Not surprising, this is the worst aspect of the resolution of array transducers. Manufacturers are rapidly developing "1½ dimensional" arrays that will enable electronic focusing in the slice thickness as well as in the lateral direction.

Transducers that are used with stand-alone CW Doppler units are not intended for imaging and therefore are much simpler than imaging transducers. Most employ two elements, one for continuously transmitting and the other for receiving echoes. To detect echo signals from scatterers, the beams from the transmitter and the receiver are caused to overlap. This is done by inclining the transducer elements or by using focusing lenses. The area of beam overlap defines the most sensitive region of the CW transducer.[11]

Choice of Ultrasound Frequency

Competing physical interactions govern the choice of the operating frequency employed in an ultrasound instrument. For Doppler work, the choice is usually dictated by the need to obtain adequate signal strength for reliable interpretation of Doppler signals. For both pulse-echo and Doppler applications, spatial resolution requirements must also be considered.

Signal Strength

It was mentioned previously that the intensity of ultrasonic waves scattered from small scatterers such as red blood cells increases rapidly with increasing frequency, being proportional to the frequency raised to the fourth power. It thus would seem reasonable to use a high ultrasonic frequency to increase the intensity of scattered signals from blood. As the frequency increases, however, the rate of beam attenuation also increases (see Fig. 2–2). In selecting the optimal frequency for detecting blood flow, these competing processes must be balanced, and the choice of operating frequency is often determined by the tissue depth of the vessel of interest. For small, superficial vessels, in which attenuation from overlying tissues is not significant, B-mode and Doppler probes operating at 7 to 10 MHz are commonly used. Doppler applications in the carotid artery usually employ somewhat lower frequencies to avoid significant attenuation losses, and frequencies of 4 to 5 MHz are typical. Frequencies as low as 2 MHz are used for detecting flow in deeper arteries and veins.

Spatial Resolution

For B-mode imaging applications and for some Doppler instruments, the spatial resolution requirements also play a role in dictating the operating frequency. Both the pulse duration, which governs the axial resolution, and the width of beam, which controls lateral resolution, can be made smaller if higher frequency transducers are used. Again, limitations are introduced by the increased tissue attenuation with higher ultrasonic frequencies. Transducer frequencies of 7.5 MHz are commonly used for imaging superficial structures; here, resolution better than 1 mm is obtainable. Attenuation losses dictate the use of lower frequencies when imaging large areas such as the abdomen, but the accompanying spatial resolution is not as good as that obtained for superficial structures.

An additional factor in the choice of the ultrasonic frequency in Doppler applications is the desire to avoid aliasing in the Doppler signal (see later).

Doppler Spectral Analysis

For many structures of interest, the Doppler signal is in the audible frequency range. For some applications, adequate clinical interpretations can be made simply by listening to the signals. The listener then characterizes the flow according to the qualities of the audible signal.

In the case of blood flow, the Doppler signal is fairly complex because of the complicated blood velocity patterns found in most vessels. In a large blood vessel, the blood velocity is not the same at all points but follows some type of flow profile. If the ultrasound beam and the sample volume are large compared with the lumen diameter, scattered ultrasound signals are received simultaneously from blood that is moving at different velocities. The resultant Doppler signal, therefore, is complex.

A complex signal such as that shown in Figure 2–20*A* may be shown to be composed of many single-frequency signals (see Fig. 2–20*B*). Each of these has a particular amplitude and phase so that, when added together, they form the original signal. *Spectral analysis* is a way to separate a complicated signal into its individual frequency components so that the relative contribution of each frequency component to the original signal can be determined (see Fig. 2–20*C*). Often, the relative contribution is denoted by the signal power in a given frequency interval, and the spectrum is referred to as the *power spectrum*.

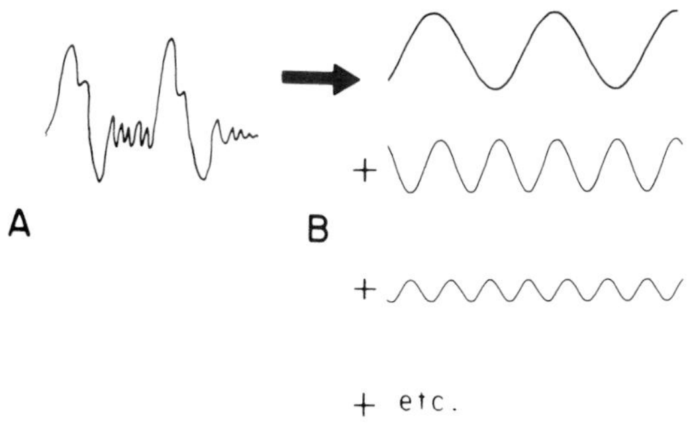

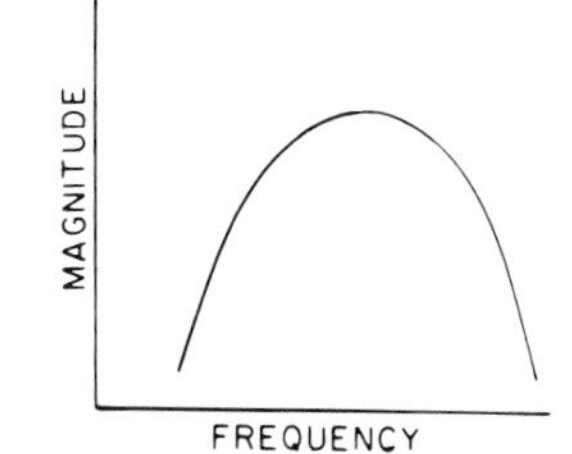

FIGURE 2–20 A complex signal waveform (*A*) can be generated by a combination of single-frequency signals (*B*). *C*, Spectral analysis involves the separation of the complex signal into its frequency components and the display of the magnitude of each frequency component that contributes to the signal.

Most instruments use a digital technique called a fast Fourier transform in spectral analysis of Doppler signals. The Doppler signal is fed into the spectral analyzer in small time segments (e.g., 5 msec). The power spectrum is computed and is displayed along a vertical line, where the height represents a frequency bin and the brightness represents the signal power or intensity for that bin (Fig. 2–21). The relative intensity of Doppler signals depends on the amount of blood generating that signal, so the brightness of each frequency bin indicates the amount of flow at the velocity corresponding to that Doppler frequency. As the spectral signals from one segment are being displayed, a subsequent segment is being analyzed, producing a continuous display.

Duplex instruments display a B-mode image along with a Doppler spectral display. An example is presented in Figure 2–22. The vertical scale on the spectral display can be either Doppler frequency (in Hertz) or velocity (in centimeters per second or meters per second). To display the velocity, the analyzer solves the Doppler equation to derive the velocity from the Doppler signal frequency. The spectral display is considered in detail in Chapter 3.

Zero Crossing Detector

A simple device commonly used to indicate the output Doppler frequency is the zero crossing detector. This device simply counts the number of oscillations per second of the dominant part of the Doppler signal for small time intervals and indicates this value on a display. It is present on many simple, standalone Doppler units, such as ones used in vascular laboratories. The zero crossing detector responds to variations in the Doppler

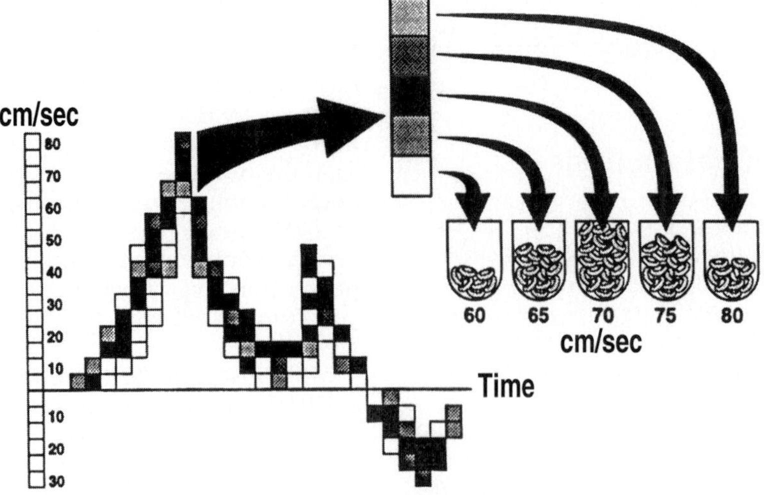

FIGURE 2–21 Information on a spectral Doppler display. Doppler frequency (or reflector velocity) is plotted vertically and time horizontally. For each time segment, the amount of signal within specific frequency bins is indicated by a shade of gray. The amount of signal corresponds to the amount of blood flowing at the corresponding velocity.

frequency during the cardiac cycle and those associated with some abnormal flow conditions. Thus, it may be used as a rough indicator of Doppler signal frequency characteristics. In the presence of a spectrum of Doppler frequencies, however, the output of the zero crossing detector indicates a frequency that is neither the maximum instantaneous frequency (often of clinical interest in the detection of stenosis) nor the mean frequency.[12] Instead, the zero crossing detector output is proportional to the root mean square Doppler frequency.[12] Other disadvantages of zero crossing detectors are (1) they cannot follow fast changes in the flow pattern, and (2) they present false output signals in the presence of electrical noise.

Aliasing in Pulsed Doppler

With a pulsed Doppler instrument, a limitation exists on the maximum Doppler frequency that can be detected from a given depth and on the set of operating conditions. The limitation referred to is *aliasing* and, if present, can lead to anomalies on Doppler signal spectral waveforms.

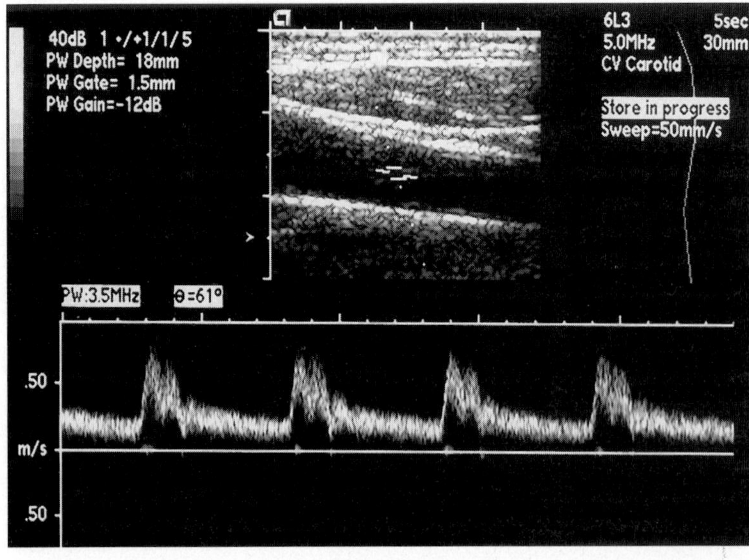

FIGURE 2–22 Spectral display from a carotid artery.

Consider the situation illustrated in Figure 2–23. As mentioned earlier, a pulsed Doppler instrument forms the Doppler signal using multiple pulse-echo sequences. The Doppler signal is said to be sampled, and the sampling frequency is the PRF of the instrument. In Figure 2–23, the Doppler signal is represented by the solid line, and the arrows represent successive samples of this signal. The lower waveform depicts the sampled signal. In this case, the sampled signal is an excellent representation of the original signal because sampling occurred multiple times for each cycle of the original waveform.

Unfortunately, with pulsed Doppler, it is not always possible to have the PRF significantly higher than the frequency of the Doppler signal. As discussed in the next section, we must limit the PRF, so sufficient time is available to collect all signals from one pulsing of the transducer before a subsequent pulsing. This restriction on the PRF depends on the depth of the sample volume. The greater the distance to the sample volume, the longer it takes to pick up echoes from that region and the lower the PRF must be.

At a minimum, the PRF must be at least 2 times the frequency of the Doppler signal to construct the signal successfully. When the PRF equals 2 × F_D, this is known as the *Nyquist sampling rate.* The Nyquist rate is the minimum sampling rate that can be used for a signal of a given frequency. If the sampling rate is lower than the Nyquist rate, aliasing occurs. Aliasing is a production of artifactual, lower frequency signals when the sampling rate (the PRF) is less than twice the Doppler signal frequency.

Aliasing is illustrated schematically in Figure 2–24. The actual Doppler signal (top) is sampled (arrows) at a rate less than 2 times each cycle of the signal. The resulting sampled waveform (see lower part of Fig. 2–24) is one whose frequency is less than that of the actual signal.

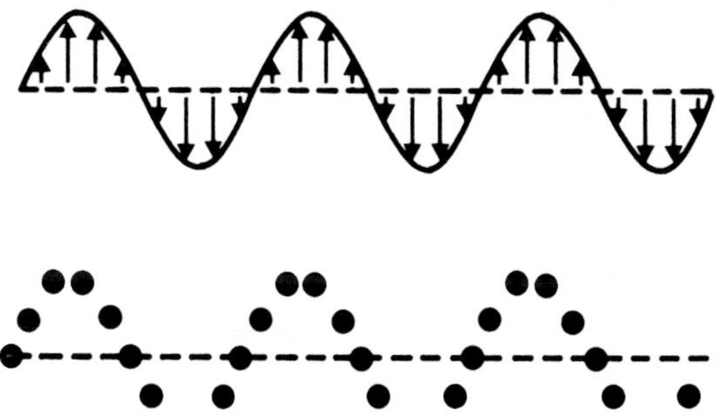

FIGURE 2–23 Sampling a Doppler signal. The *solid line* on top is a sine wave, and *arrows* represent the times when discrete samples of the signal are taken. The *dotted line* on the bottom is the sampled signal.

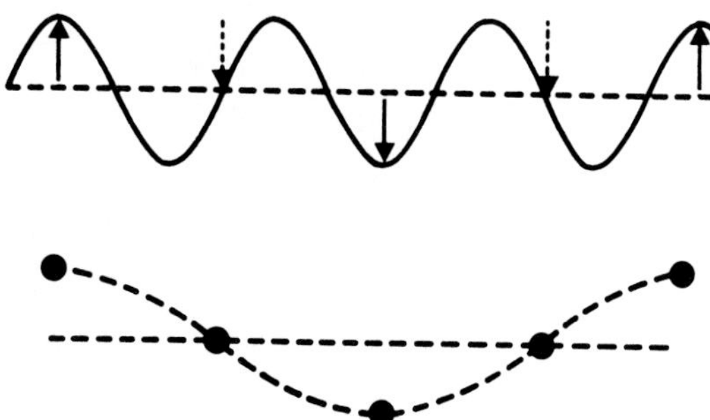

FIGURE 2–24 Production of aliasing when the sampling rate is less than 2 times the frequency of the signal. The upper curve is the signal, which is being sampled at the discrete times indicated by *arrows.* The lower curve is a lower frequency alias of the signal resulting from the inadequate sampling.

A common way that aliasing is manifested on a Doppler spectral display is illustrated in Figure 2–25. The Doppler spectrum wraps around the display, with high velocities being converted to reversed flow immediately at the point of aliasing and still higher velocities in the flow signal appearing as progressively lower velocities.

Several methods are used to eliminate aliasing. It can often be eliminated by increasing the velocity/frequency scale limits of the spectral display (see Fig. 2–25*B*). When the scale is increased, the Doppler instrument increases the PRF, keeping it at the Nyquist limit for the maximum Doppler frequency shown on the spectral scale. The operator can also adjust the spectral baseline, the line representing 0 velocity, assigning the entire spectral display to flow moving in just one direction (see Fig. 2–25*C*). This is successful when flow is in one direction only. Yet another way to eliminate aliasing may be to use a lower frequency transducer. The Doppler frequency is proportional to both the reflector velocity and the ultrasound frequency (f_o), so a lower ultrasound frequency results in a lower frequency Doppler signal for a given velocity.

Maximum Velocity Detectable With Pulsed Doppler

As mentioned earlier, to detect a Doppler signal without aliasing the PRF of the instru-

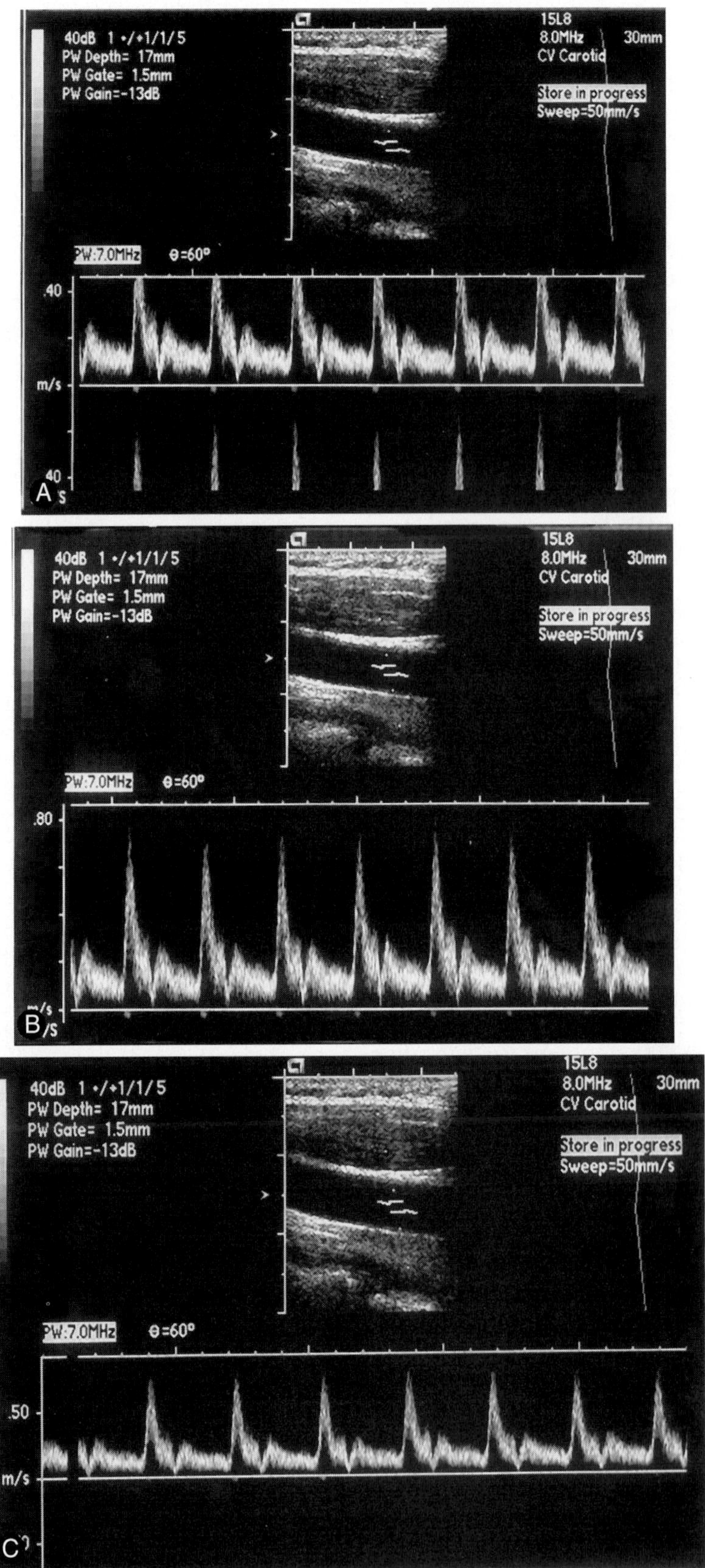

FIGURE 2–25 Manifestation of aliasing on a spectral display. *A,* The spectrum warps around. *B,* Correction of aliasing by increasing the velocity scale on the machine. *C,* Elimination of aliasing by adjusting the baseline.

ment must be at least twice the Doppler frequency. An upper limit on the PRF is established, however, by the time interval required for ultrasound pulses to propagate to the range of interest and return. If the time between pulses is insufficient, "range ambiguities" arise because of overlap of echoes from successive pulses. With the sample volume set at depth *d*, the minimum time needed between pulses T_d is $2d/c$ (from the range equation). The maximum PRF possible, PRF_{max}, is just the inverse of T_d. Thus,

$$PRF_{max} = 1/T_d = c/2d \tag{2-9}$$

What is the highest flow velocity that can be detected, given the limitation expressed in Equation 2–9? The maximum Doppler frequency we can detect without aliasing will now be $PRF_{max}/2 = c/4d$. Using the Doppler equation and substituting for f_D we get

$$\frac{2f_o v_{max}}{c} = \frac{c}{4d}$$

where v_{max} is the maximum velocity detectable without aliasing. Solving for v_{max},

$$v_{max} = \frac{c^2}{8f_o d} \tag{2-10}$$

Assuming a speed of sound of 1540 m/sec, the plots in Figure 2–26 were generated using Equation 2–10, relating the maximum reflector velocity that can be detected to reflector depth for three different ultrasound frequencies. As the sample volume depth increases, the maximum detectable Doppler signal frequency, and hence the maximum reflector velocity that can be detected, decrease. At any depth, lower ultrasound frequencies permit detection of greater velocities than higher frequencies.

In some instruments, higher velocities than those shown in Figure 2–26 can be obtained using a "high PRF" selection. In this mode, the PRF of the instrument is allowed to be increased beyond the limit set by Equation 2–9. Now, range ambiguity is present because the echo data from successive transmit pulses overlap. This is indicated on the display by the presence of multiple sample volumes displayed on the image. In general, however, the range ambiguities are not a problem, because the operator already has the area of flow sampling isolated before activating high PRF, and the exact origin of the Doppler signals is still known.

COLOR-FLOW IMAGING

Color-flow imaging (or color-velocity imaging) is done by estimating and displaying the mean velocity, relative to the ultrasound beam direction, of scatterers and reflectors in a scanned region. Echo signals from moving reflectors are generally displayed so that the color hue, saturation, or brightness indicates the relative velocity. Color-flow image data are superimposed on B-mode data from stationary structures to obtain a composite image.

Several methods for processing echo signals to produce color-flow images have been described. Some of these operate on the signals produced after Doppler signal processing,[13–15] whereas a few process echo signals

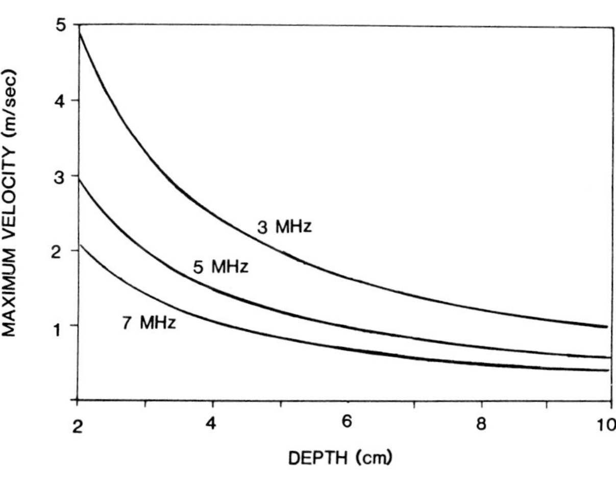

FIGURE 2–26 Maximum velocity detectable with pulsed Doppler vs. sample volume depth for three different ultrasound frequencies.

directly.[16] (Specific mathematical details of the methods are given in the references, especially references 14 and 16.) For each method, a series of pulse-echo sequences are produced along a single-beam axis. With sequential and phased array transducers the beam actually dwells (remains stationary) during this time, but with mechanical transducers the beam continuously sweeps, although often more slowly than for standard imaging. Echo signals from each succeeding transmit pulse are compared with signals from those of the previous pulse, and phase and frequency shifts in the returning signals are estimated. This process is carried out for a series of locations along the beam line. At each location, a mean velocity is computed from the data of all pulse-echo sequences. Then, another beam line is interrogated, and so on. With most instruments, ten or more transmit-receive sequences might be used to produce an estimate of mean reflector velocities along each beam line.

The term *pulse packets* has been adopted to designate the transmit-receive pulse-echo sequences, with *packet size* designating the number of such sequences along each beam line.[17] Some instruments allow the operator to vary the packet size directly; most vary the packet size when the operator changes other control settings, such as color preprocessing.

Because data for each acoustic line that forms a color-velocity image are acquired using multiple pulse-echo sequences, frame rates in color-flow imaging are lower than frame rates in standard B-mode imaging. In color-flow imaging, noticeable tradeoffs are evident among factors affecting color-image quality and scanning speed or frame rate. Most instruments provide signal processing controls that allow the user to optimize imaging parameters for specific applications. Higher frame rates are often accompanied by reduced image quality, because fewer acoustic lines are used to form the image. Very detailed color images, sensitive to low-flow states, are frequently obtained at the expense of lower frame rates.

The direction of blood flow is indicated by the display color; for example, red might encode flow toward the transducer and blue away from the transducer. It should be kept in mind that the color processor displays motion relative to the ultrasound beam direction for each beam line forming the flow image. Different parts of a vessel are often interrogated from different beam directions, either because of the orientation of the vessel or as a result of the transducer scan format. The latter problem is illustrated in Figure 2–27, in which continuous flow through a horizontal vessel appears both blue (away) and red (toward) because of the different beam angles that interrogate the vessel when a sector scanner is used.

Aliasing on Color Displays

The color-velocity image is produced with pulsed Doppler techniques; therefore, the image is subject to aliasing, as discussed previously. A common manifestation of aliasing is a wraparound of the display, resulting in an apparent reversal of the flow direction (Fig. 2–28*A*). For example, aliased flow toward the probe is interpreted as flow moving away. Increasing the color-flow velocity scale essentially increases the PRF of the processor and eliminates the aliasing problem if flow velocities remain within the allowable range of velocities on the instrument (see Fig. 2–28*B*). Also, changing the color baseline (the zero-flow position on the spectral display) can shift the allowable Doppler frequency range; this method is effective when flow signals are only in one direction.

ENERGY-MODE IMAGING

Color-flow imaging displays scatterer velocities relative to the interrogating ultrasound beam direction at positions throughout the scanned field. An alternative processing method ignores the velocity and simply estimates the strength (or power or energy) of the Doppler signal detected from each location. So-called power- or energy-mode imaging[17,18] has both advantages and limitations.

An energy-mode image of the horizontal vessel in the flow phantom depicted in Figure 2–27 is presented in Figure 2–29. The energy-mode image is continuous rather than divided into segments because of the different beam directions. In other words, the energy image is not sensitive to relative flow direction, as is the color-velocity image. Another advantage of the energy-mode image is that it is not affected by aliasing. Figure 2–30 contrasts color-velocity images with energy-mode images of a flow phantom when aliasing is present. The energy-mode image does

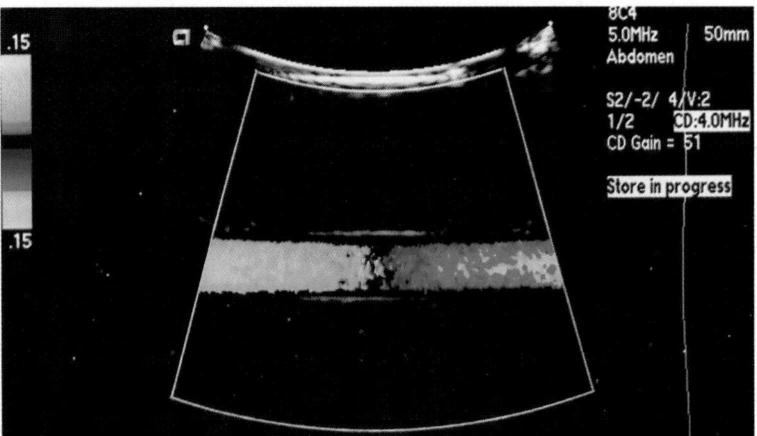

FIGURE 2–27 Color-flow image of a horizontal vessel in a flow phantom. Flow is from left to right on the image, so for the sector transducer it is directed toward the probe on the left-hand side of the image and away from the transducer on the right-hand side.

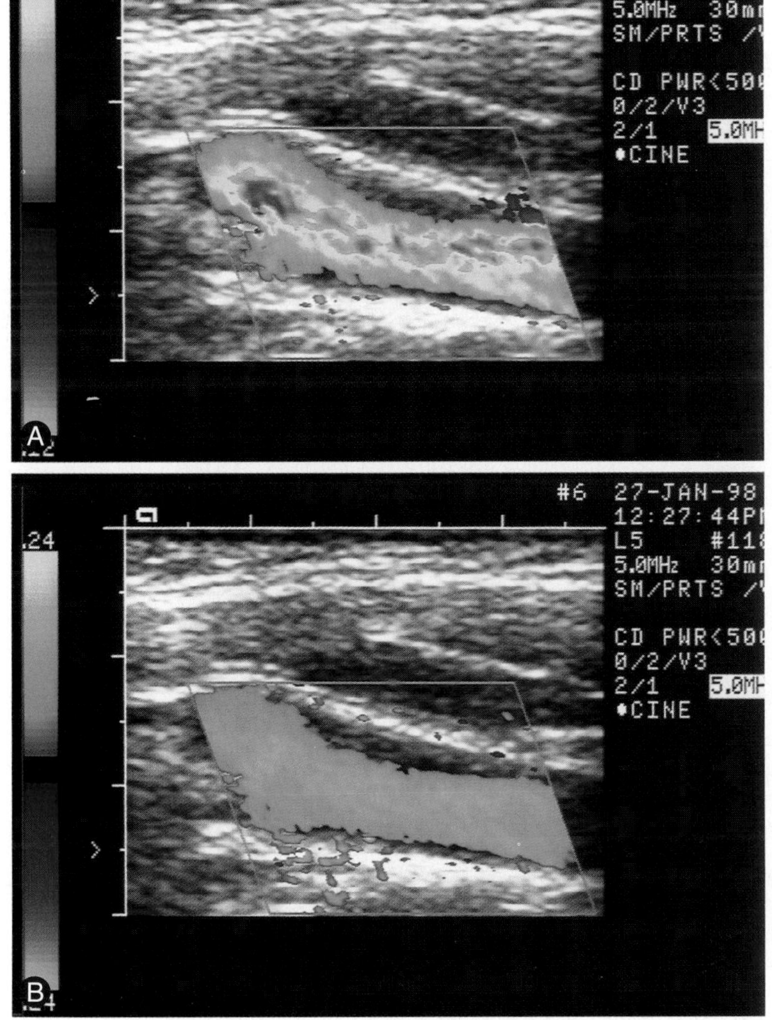

FIGURE 2–28 Elimination of aliasing. *A,* Color-flow image of a carotid artery, with aliasing. *B,* Same as in *A,* only the velocity scale has been adjusted to eliminate aliasing.

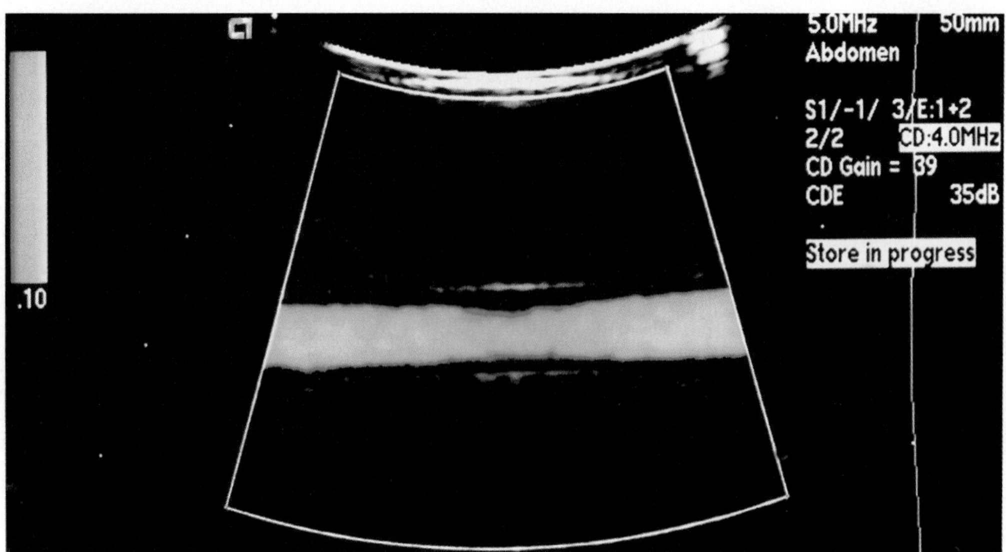

FIGURE 2–29 Power-mode image of the same vessel as in Figure 2–27. The energy-mode image is almost insensitive to the Doppler angle.

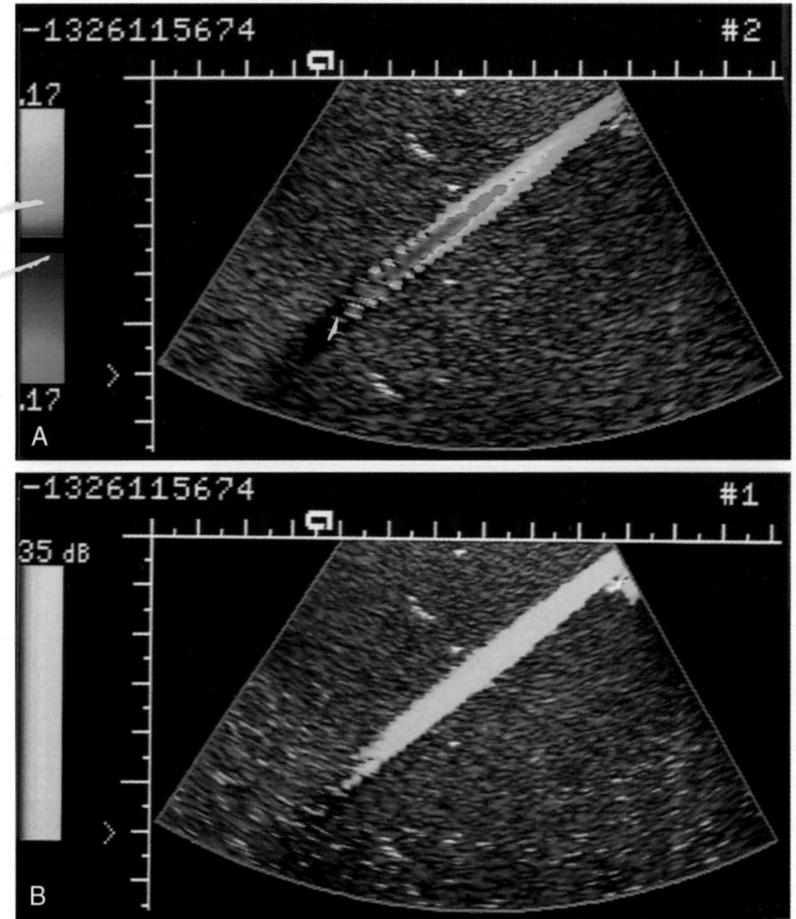

FIGURE 2–30 *A,* Color-velocity image of a vessel in a flow phantom; aliasing is present, resulting in apparent flow reversal. *B,* Energy-mode image of the same vessel.

not depict velocities but only a value related to the strength of the Doppler signal, so the effects of aliasing are not manifested.

The advantages of this modality over color-velocity imaging are, therefore,

1. Energy mode seems to be more sensitive to low- and weak-flow states than color velocity.
2. Angle effects on the Doppler frequency are ignored, unless the angle becomes so close to perpendicular that the Doppler signals are below the flow detectability threshold of the color processor.
3. Aliasing does not affect the energy-mode display.

Thus, a more continuous display of flow, especially in difficult to scan regions, is provided.

Disadvantages of energy-mode imaging are also clear:

1. Information on reflector velocity and flow direction relative to the transducer is not displayed. Sometimes these features are important to a diagnosis.
2. Image build-up tends to be slower and image frame rates lower, because of the use of more signal averaging in energy mode than in velocity mode. Consequently, problems with flash artifact caused by Doppler signals from slowly moving soft tissues are more severe in energy mode than in velocity mode.

ACOUSTIC OUTPUT LABELS ON SCANNERS

In an ultrasound examination, acoustic energy must be transmitted into the tissue. The possibility that the energy could produce a detrimental biologic effect has been considered extensively by bioacoustics researchers; it continues to be studied to this day. At this time, most workers conclude that diagnostic ultrasound equipment is safe and that it is unlikely that bioeffects could result from prudent use of this modality, at least with current scanners. The American Institute of Ultrasound in Medicine's official statement on the clinical safety of diagnostic ultrasound instrumentation reads:

> . . . *There are no confirmed biological effects on patients or instrument operators caused by exposures from present diagnostic ultrasound instruments. Although the possibility exists that such biological effects may be identified in the future, current data indicate that the benefits to patients of the prudent use of diagnostic ultrasound outweigh the risks, if any, that may be present.*[19]

Readers should consult more detailed reports [20, 21] on postulated mechanisms for bioeffects; acoustic exposure parameters of concern; reports of the nature of biologic effects, especially high power and intensity levels; and acoustic output data from current scanners.

Who is responsible for ensuring that diagnostic ultrasonography maintains its good safety record? The responsibility falls on everyone involved in manufacturing, regulating, and using this equipment. Until recently, manufacturers in the United States were required to adhere to "application-specific limits" on the intensity, peak pressure levels, and acoustic power levels of scanners. When a new scanner or a new transducer was planned for marketing, the U.S. Food and Drug Administration considered acoustic output data submitted by the manufacturer of the device. If the intensities were lower than these limits, the product was considered satisfactory as far as acoustic output was concerned. Manufacturers were also required to report in the operator's manual the acoustic intensities for each transducer and each operating mode the transducer could be used in. Users were asked to practice the as low as reasonably achievable (ALARA) rule when scanning.

This method appeared to be effective, but it led to a number of difficulties:

- The application-specific limits were based on records from old scanners that had been used without apparent detrimental effects. However, they were not necessarily based on scientific evidence of safety.
- Demands by clinicians for new applications and capabilities often led to difficulty in the manufacturer getting scanners cleared by regulators. This was especially true for Doppler and color-flow imaging operating modes, for which the intensities are generally the highest!
- For users to practice ALARA generally means scanning with low transmit power and high receiver gain; however, other factors also affect the output levels, and it is

difficult for operators to predict how a specific control changes the output values.
- The reported output levels were not strongly linked to sources of potential biologic effects. For example, the time-averaged intensity is relevant to potential for heating, but the frequency, beam area focal depth, and other parameters must also be included.

To help alleviate these difficulties, a group consisting of ultrasound equipment users, professional organizations, and U.S. and Canadian government regulators developed a real-time output labeling standard.[22] Most equipment manufacturers in the United States and Canada now follow this standard. It requires manufacturers to provide output indicators on their scanners to inform users of levels relevant to potential biologic effects. Two indices have been chosen as labels: a mechanical index (MI) and a thermal index (TI) (Fig. 2–31). MI is computed from the acoustic pressure amplitude and the ultrasound frequency. It is related to the likelihood that a process called *cavitation* could occur in the field of the transducer. Cavitation is one of the postulated mechanisms through which ultrasonography could induce a biologic effect in tissues.[21]

A second potential mechanism for production of bioeffects is heating. The TI is displayed to indicate the possibility of this occurring. The TI value is the acoustic power divided by the power needed to raise the temperature in tissue by 1°C, given some fairly general assumptions regarding the absorption and thermal properties of the medium. Various TIs may be presented, depending on the assumed tissue path. In most cases, TI_S is displayed, where the S stands for soft tissue. This model assumes a uniform soft-tissue path throughout the scanned field. TI_B (B is for bone) is displayed when the operator uses an application that indicates a second- or third-trimester fetus will be imaged; it is assumed that developing fetal bones will be in the field. Bone has a higher absorption coefficient than soft tissue, and calculations suggest that some modes (e.g., Doppler) could heat regions that are very close to the bone. Finally, when scanning the skull for a transcranial Doppler study, TI_C (C is for cranium) is displayed. The high absorption of ultrasound waves by the skull bone would lead to this entity as being the target for the greatest amount of heating during a transcranial Doppler examination.

The advantages provided by this new labeling approach are

- Standardization of output specification information among the different manufacturers. Every scanner labeled according to the standard will have the MI and the TI values clearly displayed, rather than arbitrary designations, such as percent of maximum output or decibels.
- Presentation of acoustic output quantities that are relevant to the possibility of bio-

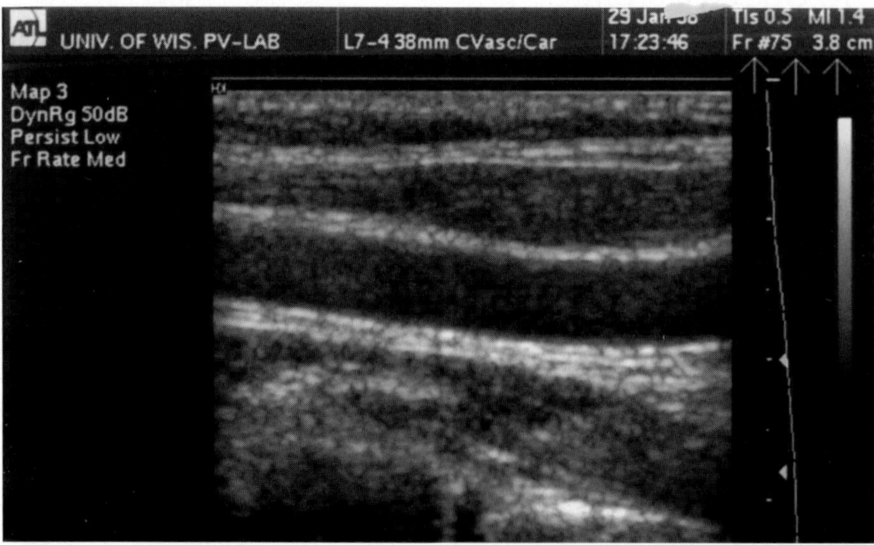

FIGURE 2–31 Ultrasound image with the thermal index (TI_S) and mechanical index (MI) displayed; note arrows at upper right-hand corner.

logic effects from the ultrasound exposures. These quantities enable users to implement the ALARA principle.

- Although the regulators continue to impose a 720 mW/cm^2 limit on the time-average intensity, and a limit of 1.9 on the MI value, regulators may loosen these limits in the future. Presumably, this would open up the potential of still further diagnostic capabilities with medical ultrasonography. It would, of course, also place greater responsibility for clinical safety on the operator and physician responsible for the ultrasound examination.

Some individuals are concerned that the removal of application-specific intensity limits will not be recognized by ultrasound equipment users, and they may operate a scanner at an unnecessarily high output setting. As the new labels become more familiar to ultrasonographers, the likelihood of this occurring will diminish.

REFERENCES

1. Wells PT: Biomedical Ultrasonics. New York, Academic Press, 1977, pp 124–125.
2. 1993 Acoustical Data for Diagnostic Ultrasound Equipment. Laurel, MD, American Institute of Ultrasound in Medicine, 1993.
2a. Duck FA: Output data from European studies. Ultrasound Med Biol 15(suppl 1):61–64, 1989.
3. Wells PT: Biomedical ultrasonics. New York, Academic Press, 1977, pp 120–126.
4. Zagzebski JA: Essentials of Ultrasound Physics. St. Louis, CV Mosby, 1996, pp 7–9.
5. Shung KK: In vitro experimental results on ultrasonic scattering in biological tissues. *In* Shung KK, Thieme GA (eds): Ultrasonic Scattering in Biological Tissues. Boca Raton, FL, CRC Press, 1993.
6. Kremkau F: Diagnostic Ultrasound Principles, Instrumentation and Exercises, 5th ed. Orlando, FL, Grune & Stratton, 1993.
7. Zagzebski JA: Essentials of Ultrasound Physics. St. Louis, CV Mosby, 1996, pp 34–35.
8. Taylor KJW, Wells PNT, Burns PN: Clinical Applications of Doppler Ultrasound. New York, Raven Press, 1995, pp 19–23.
9. Beach K, Philips D: Doppler instrumentation for the evaluation of arterial and venous disease. *In* Jaffe C (ed): Clinics in Diagnostic Ultrasound. New York, Churchill Livingstone, 1984.
10. Zagzebski JA: Essentials of Ultrasound Physics. CV Mosby, St. Louis, 1996, pp 39–41.
11. Zagzebski JA: Essentials of Ultrasound Physics. CV Mosby, St. Louis, pp 93–95.
12. Lunt MJ: Accuracy and limitations of the ultrasonic Doppler blood velocimeter and zero crossing detector. Ultrasound Med Biol 2:1–10, 1975.
13. Omoto R, Kasai, C: Basic principles of Doppler color flow imaging. Echocardiography 3:463, 1986.
14. Evans D: Doppler ultrasound physics instrumentation and clinical applications. New York, John Wiley & Sons, 1989, pp 53–61, 102–106.
15. Zagzebski JA: Essentials of Ultrasound Physics. St. Louis, CV Mosby, 1996, pp 109–120.
16. Embree P, O'Brien W: Volumetric blood flow via time-domain correlation: Experimental verification. IEEE Trans Ultrasonics Ferroelec Frequency Con 37:176–185, 1990.
17. Kisslo J, Adams AB, Belkin RN: Doppler Color Flow Imaging. New York, Churchill Livingstone, 1988.
18. Rubin JM, Bude RO, Carson PL, et al: Power Doppler US: A potentially useful alternative to mean frequency-based color Doppler US. Radiology 190: 853–856, 1994.
19. 1997 Statement on Clinical Safety. Laurel, MD, American Institute of Ultrasound in Medicine, 1997.
20. Bioeffects and Safety of Diagnostic Ultrasound. Laurel, MD, American Institute of Ultrasound in Medicine, 1993.
21. Medical Ultrasound Safety, Part 1: Bioeffects and Bioeffects; Part 2: Prudent Use; Part 3: Implementing ALARA. Laurel, MD, American Institute of Ultrasound in Medicine, 1994.
22. Standard for real time display of thermal and mechanical acoustic output indices on diagnostic ultrasound equipment. Laurel, MD, American Institute of Ultrasound in Medicine, 1991.

Chapter 3

Doppler Frequency Spectrum Analysis

■ *William J. Zwiebel, MD*

If blood flow were continuous rather than pulsatile, if blood vessels followed straight lines and were uniform in caliber, if blood flowed at the same velocity at the periphery and in the center of the lumen, and if vessels were disease free, then each blood vessel would produce a single Doppler ultrasound frequency shift, and frequency spectrum analysis would be unnecessary. However, blood flow is pulsatile, vessels are not always straight or uniform in size, flow is slower at the periphery than in the center of the vessel, and the vessel lumen may be distorted by atherosclerosis and other pathology. For these reasons, blood flow produces a mixture of Doppler frequency shifts that changes from moment to moment and from place to place within the vessel lumen. Spectrum analysis is needed to sort out the jumble of Doppler frequencies generated by blood flow and to provide quantitative information that is critical for diagnosis of vascular pathology.

SPECTRUM ANALYSIS

The word *spectrum,* as derived from Latin, means *image.* The Doppler spectrum is, in fact, an image of the Doppler frequencies generated by moving blood.[1–8] The spectrum shows the mixture of Doppler frequencies present in echoes from the vessel at each moment in time.[1–3] As illustrated in Figure 3–1, the key elements of the Doppler spectrum are *time, frequency, velocity,* and Doppler signal *power.* Please review Figure 3–1 at this time, directing particular attention to these four key elements.

THE POWER SPECTRUM

The Doppler frequency spectrum that you have just reviewed in Figure 3–1 is sometimes called a *power spectrum,*[1–3] because the power, or strength, of each frequency is shown by the *brightness* of the pixels. The power of a given frequency shift, in turn, is proportionate to the *number* of red blood cells producing that frequency shift. If a large number of blood cells are moving at a certain velocity, the corresponding Doppler frequency shift is powerful, and the pixels assigned to that frequency are bright. Conversely, if only a small number of cells are causing a certain frequency shift, the pixels assigned to that frequency are dim. The power spectrum concept is important for understanding power Doppler flow imaging, which is discussed in Chapter 4. As the name implies, power Doppler images are based on the *power* of the Doppler spectrum. These images show the cumulative power of the Doppler signal at all points in a blood vessel.

FREQUENCY VS. VELOCITY

The Doppler spectrum displays both velocity (cm/sec or m/sec) and frequency (kHz) information, as shown in Figure 3–1, yet only frequency shift data are present in the echoes that return to the transducer from the patient. How, then, does the instrument convert the Doppler frequency shift to velocity? The conversion occurs when the sonographer "informs" the duplex instrument of the Doppler

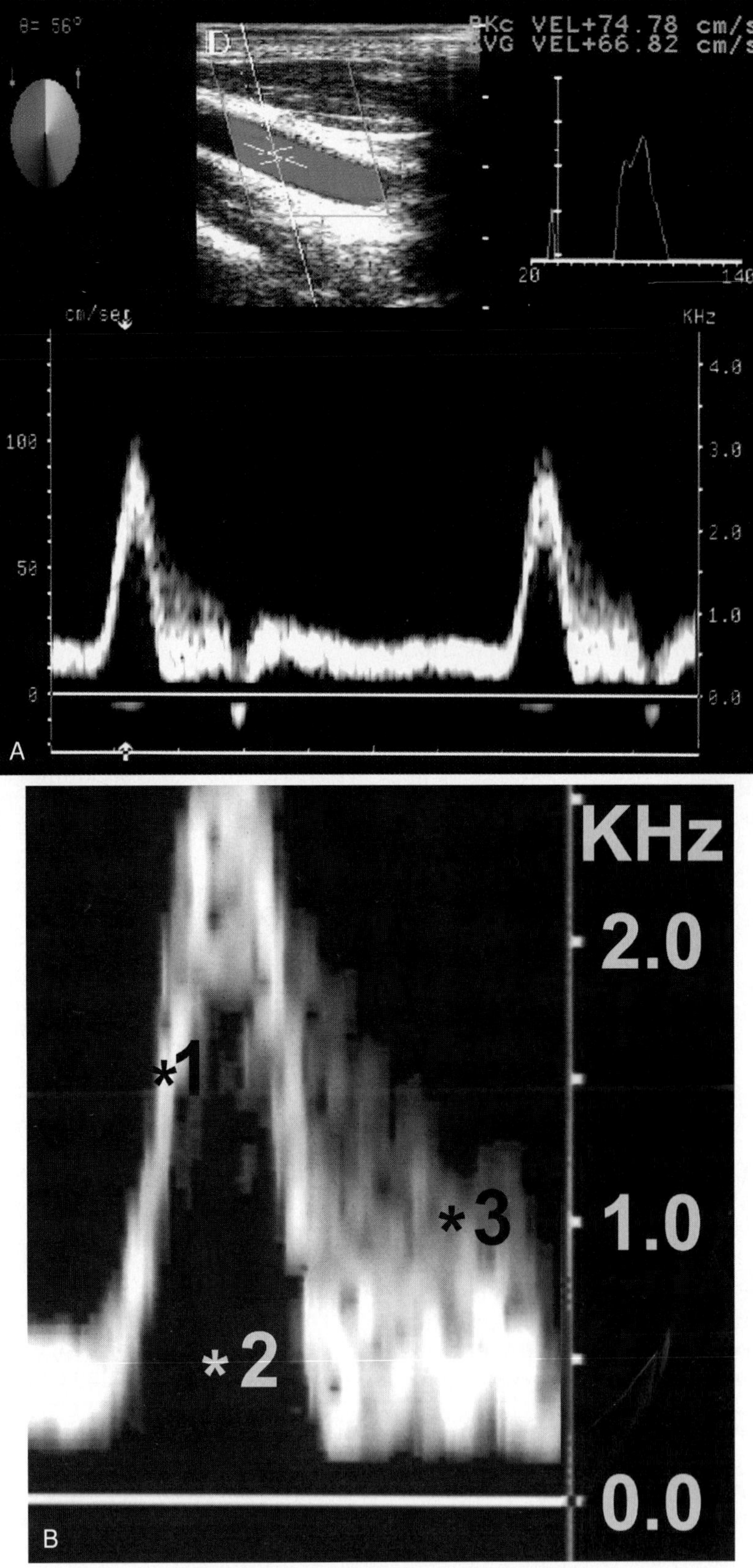

FIGURE 3–1 *See legend on opposite page*

FIGURE 3–1 The Doppler spectrum display. The following information is presented on the display screen (*A,* entire display; *B,* magnified Doppler spectrum).

B-mode image: The image of the vessel, the sample volume, and the Doppler line of sight are shown at the top of the display screen.

Color-flow information: The "color wheel" in the upper left corner indicates the relationship between the colors in the flow image and the flow direction. In this case, colors on the left side of the wheel correspond to flow away from the transducer (*down arrow*), and vice versa for colors on the right side of the wheel. Many manufacturers use a color bar to show flow direction. It is important to recognize that flow is shown relative to the transducer, as discussed in Chapter 4.

Doppler angle: The Doppler angle appears in the left upper corner of the display screen, above the color wheel.

Time: The time is represented on the horizontal (x) axis of the Doppler spectrum in divisions of a second.

Frequency shift and velocity: The Doppler frequency shift (kHz) and the velocity (cm/sec) are shown on the vertical (y-axis) scales of the spectrum.

Flow direction: The direction of flow is shown in relation to the spectrum baseline. For peripheral vascular work, flow away from the transducer is shown above the baseline, and flow toward the transducer is shown below the baseline. This relationship may be reversed by the operator.

The distribution of velocities within the sample volume is illustrated by the brightness of the spectral display (z-axis). To better understand the z-axis concept, examine the magnified spectrum shown in *B* and imagine that the spectral display is made up of tiny squares called *pixels* (for picture elements). You cannot see the pixels in this image, because they are purposely blurred together to smooth the picture. The pixels are there, however, and each corresponds to a specific moment in time and a specific frequency shift and velocity. *The brightness of a pixel (z-axis) is proportionate to the number of blood cells causing that frequency shift at that specific point in time.* In this example, the pixels at asterisk 1 are bright white, meaning that at that moment, a large number of blood cells have a velocity corresponding to a frequency shift of +1.5 kHz (scale at right). The pixels at asterisk 2 are black, meaning that at that moment, no (or very few) blood cells have a velocity corresponding to a frequency shift of +0.5 kHz. The pixels at asterisk 3 are gray, meaning that a moderate number of blood cells have a velocity corresponding to a +1.5 kHz frequency shift at that moment. Got it? If not, read this again and remember that the brightness of each pixel is proportionate to the *relative* number of blood cells with a specific velocity at a specific moment in time.

Graph of velocities: The graph at the upper right in part *A* illustrates the *distribution* of velocities in the sample volume at the time indicated by the small vertical *arrow* at the bottom of the image. In essence, this is a graphic illustration of spectral broadening. Each mark on the scale is 10 cm/sec. In this case, the velocities fall in a moderately narrow range between 40 and 90 cm/sec. The numbers above the graph in *A* are the peak velocity (PKc VEL) and the average velocity (AVG VEL). The operator can move the cursor (*arrow*) to derive numerical information from other portions of the spectrum. (Not all instruments graph the velocity range.)

angle,[1, 2, 9] which is shown in Figure 3–2. If the instrument "knows" the Doppler angle, it can then compute the blood flow velocity via the Doppler formula (see Chapter 2). Voila! The frequency spectrum becomes a velocity spectrum. A Doppler angle of *60 degrees or less* is required to derive accurate velocity (or, for that matter, frequency) measurements. If the angle is greater than 60 degrees, velocity measurement is unreliable, and some instruments do not calculate velocity if the angle is too great.

It is desirable to operate the duplex instrument in the velocity mode, rather than the frequency mode, for two reasons.[1, 2, 9] First, velocity measurements compensate for variations in vessel alignment relative to the skin surface, as shown in Figure 3–3. Second, the Doppler frequency shift is inherently linked to the output frequency of the transducer, but velocity is independent of the transducer frequency. For instance, if the output frequency goes from 5 to 10 MHz, the frequency shift is doubled. Imagine the clinical consequences of such frequency changes; different diagnostic parameters would be needed for different ultrasound transducers (e.g., 3.5, 5, or 7.5 MHz). This problem is eliminated when the instrument converts the "raw" frequency information to velocity data. Flow velocity is a function of the blood vessel, not the ultrasound transducer.

AUDITORY SPECTRUM ANALYSIS

The human ear was the spectrum analysis instrument used initially for Doppler blood flow studies. The ear is a highly capable spectrum analysis instrument, which is evident in its ability to distinguish one person's voice from another. Even though duplex ultrasound instruments are equipped with electronic spectrum analysis devices, an audible Doppler output is provided as well, to take advantage of the capabilities of the ear. Certain features of the Doppler flow signal can be appreciated aurally that are difficult or impossible to display electronically, and as a result, the audible Doppler signal remains important in ultrasound vascular diagnosis. The drawbacks of the human ear, however, are two-fold. First, the ear is a purely qualitative device, and second, it is not equipped with a hard copy output for permanent storage! Electronic spectrum analysis overcomes these obstacles.

THE SAMPLE VOLUME

The frequency spectrum shows blood flow information from a specific location called the *Doppler sample volume,* which is illus-

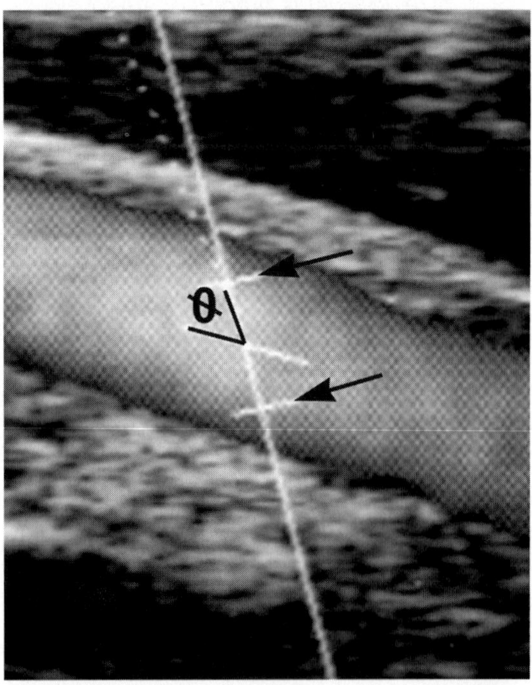

FIGURE 3–2 The Doppler angle and sample volume. The nearly vertical line is the Doppler line of sight. The line in the center of the blood vessel indicates the axis of blood flow. The angle formed by these two lines is the Doppler angle (θ). The parallel lines (*arrows*) indicate the length of the Doppler sample volume.

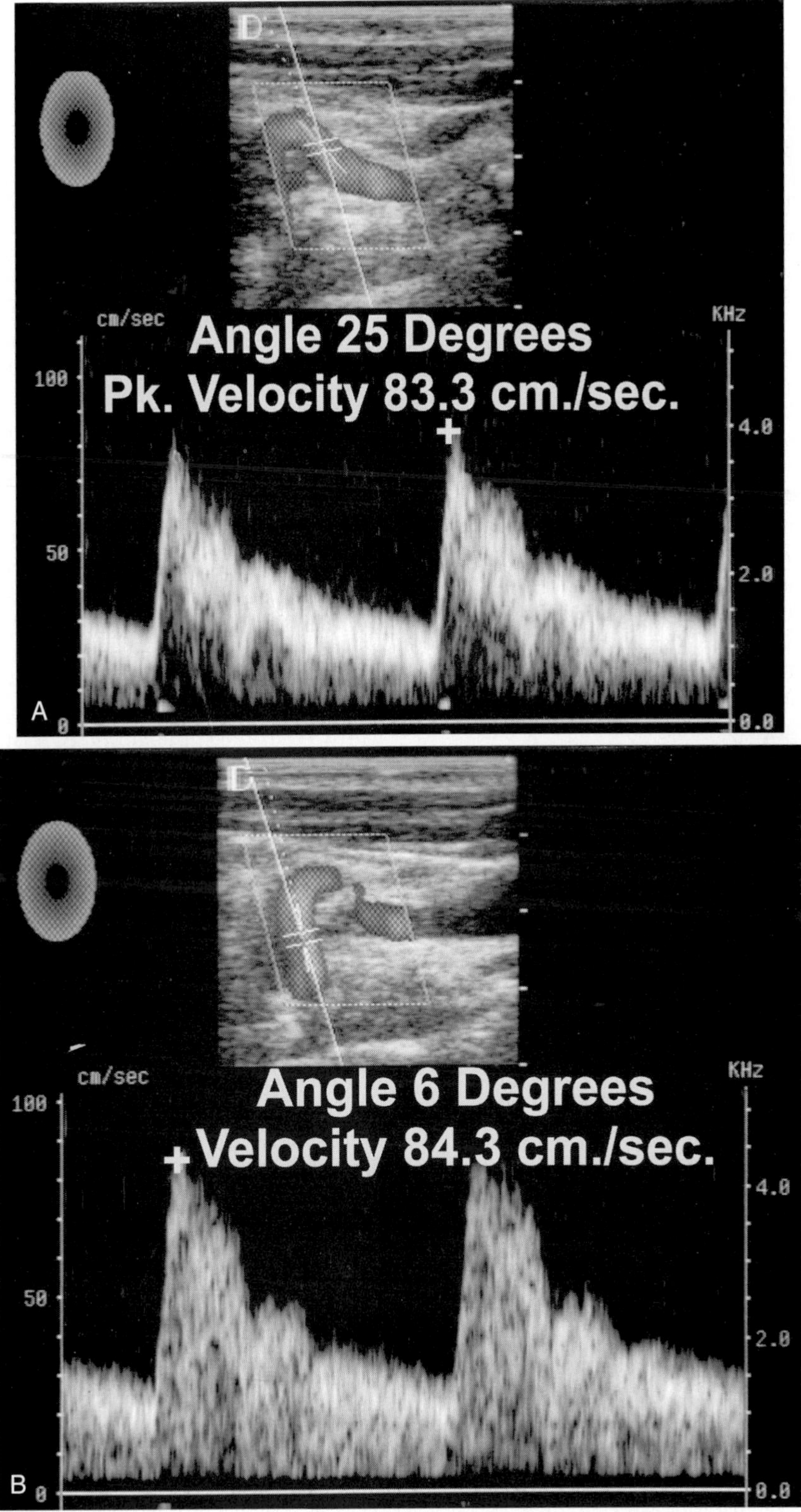

FIGURE 3–3 The importance of velocity measurements. The illustrated peak systolic velocity measurements (*A, B*) are virtually identical, even though the Doppler angles are quite different.

trated in Figure 3–2. You should be aware of the following three characteristics regarding the Doppler sample volume: First, it is, in fact, a volume (three dimensions), even though only two of its dimensions are shown on the duplex image. The "thickness" of the sample volume cannot be shown on the two-dimensional spectrum display, and this can sometimes lead to errors of localization. Doppler signals may be obtained from vessels that are marginally within the sample volume but are not shown on the two-dimensional display. For instance, the ultrasound image may show the internal carotid artery, but you may actually be receiving flow signals from an adjacent external carotid branch. Second, the actual shape and size of the sample volume may be somewhat different from the linear representation shown on the duplex image. Third, and most important, the Doppler spectrum displays flow information only within the sample volume and does not provide information about flow in other portions of the blood vessel that are visible on the ultrasound image. Therefore, if the sample volume is positioned incorrectly, key diagnostic information may be overlooked.

FLOW DIRECTION

The frequency spectrum shows blood flow *relative to the transducer.* Flow in one direction, with respect to the transducer, is displayed above the spectrum baseline, and flow in the opposite direction is shown below the baseline. One must always remember that the flow direction is *relative* to the transducer and is not absolute. The apparent direction of flow can be reversed by turning the transducer around or by pressing a button on the instrument! The arbitrary nature of this arrangement can lead to significant diagnostic error. When accurate determination of flow direction is necessary, a comparison should be made with a reference vessel in which the flow direction is known (e.g., when working in the abdomen, the aorta is a handy reference vessel).

WAVEFORMS AND PULSATILITY

In arteries, each cycle of cardiac activity produces a distinct "wave" on the Doppler frequency spectrum that begins with systole and terminates at the end of diastole. The term *waveform* refers to the shape of each of these waves. The Doppler waveform, in turn, defines a flow property called *pulsatility,*[1, 2, 10–28] which is influenced by a number of hemodynamic factors. In general terms, Doppler waveforms have low, moderate, or high pulsatility features, as illustrated in Figure 3–4.

Low pulsatility Doppler waveforms have broad systolic peaks and forward flow throughout diastole. The carotid, vertebral, renal, and celiac arteries all have low-pulsatility waveforms in normal individuals, principally because these vessels feed circulatory systems with low resistance to flow (low peripheral resistance). Low-pulsatility waveforms are also *monophasic,* meaning that flow is always forward, and the entire waveform is either above or below the Doppler spectrum baseline (depending on the perspective of the ultrasound transducer).

Moderate pulsatility Doppler waveforms have an appearance somewhere between the low- and high-resistance patterns (see Fig. 3–4*B*). With moderate flow resistance, the systolic peak is tall and sharp, but *forward flow is present throughout diastole* (perhaps interrupted by early-diastolic flow reversal). Examples of moderate pulsatility waveforms are found in the external carotid artery and the superior mesenteric artery (during fasting).

High pulsatility Doppler waveforms have tall, narrow, sharp systolic peaks and reversed or absent diastolic flow. The classic example of high pulsatility is the triphasic flow pattern seen in an extremity artery of a resting individual (see Fig. 3–4). A sharp

FIGURE 3–4 Pulsatility. *A,* Low pulsatility is indicated by a broad systolic peak and persistent forward flow throughout diastole (e.g., the internal carotid artery). *B,* Moderate pulsatility is indicated by a tall, sharp, and narrow systolic peak and relatively little diastolic flow (e.g., the external carotid artery). *C,* High pulsatility is characterized by a narrow systolic peak, flow reversal early in diastole, and absence of flow late in diastole. In this classic triphasic example, the first phase (1) is systole, the second phase (2) is brief diastolic flow reversal, and the third phase (3) is diastolic forward flow.

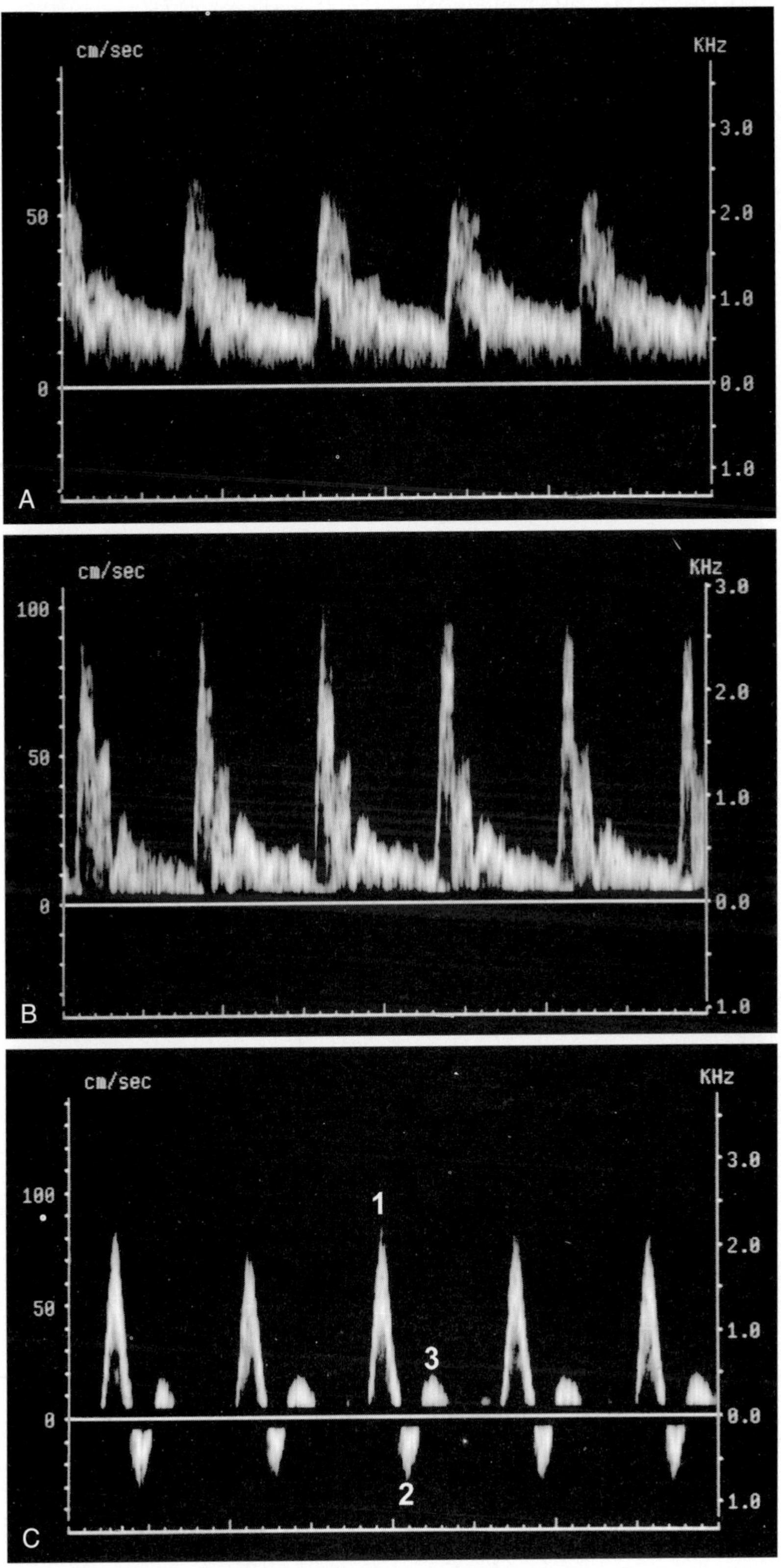

FIGURE 3–4 *See legend on opposite page*

systolic peak (first phase) is followed by brief flow reversal (second phase) and then by brief forward flow (third phase). High pulsatility waveforms are a feature of circulatory systems with high resistance to blood flow (high peripheral resistance).

Pulsatility and flow resistance may be gauged qualitatively, either by visual inspection of the Doppler spectrum waveforms or by listening to the auditory output of a Doppler instrument. Qualitative assessment of pulsatility is often sufficient for clinical vascular diagnosis, but in some situations, quantitative assessment is desirable. A variety of mathematical formulae can be used for this purpose, but the most popular measurements are the pulsatility index (of Gosling), the resistivity index (of Pourcelot), and the systolic/diastolic ratio,[24, 26, 28, 29] all of which are illustrated in Figure 3–5.

Normal values for pulsatility measurements vary from one location in the body to another. Furthermore, both physiology and pathology may alter arterial pulsatility. For example, the normal high-pulsatility pattern seen in extremity arteries during rest converts to a low-resistance, monophasic pattern after vigorous exercise (because the capillary beds open, and flow resistance decreases). Whereas the monophasic pattern is normal after exercise, this pattern is distinctly abnormal in a resting patient and, in that circumstance, indicates arterial insufficiency. The point to be made here is that proper interpretation of pulsatility requires knowledge of the normal waveform characteristics of a given vessel *and* the physiologic status of the circulation at the time of examination. The status of cardiac function is also important; slowed ventricular emptying, valvular reflux, valvular stenosis, and other factors may significantly affect arterial pulsatility.

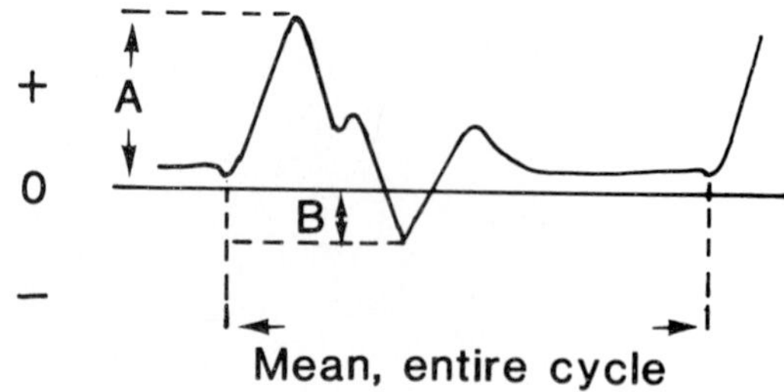

A

$$\text{Pulsatility Index} = \frac{A-B}{\text{mean}}$$

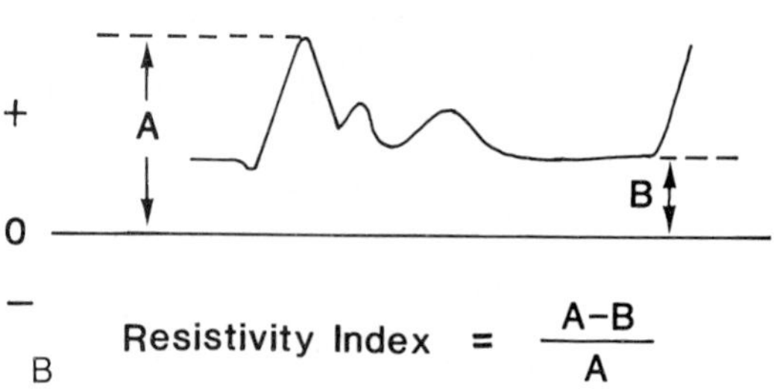

B

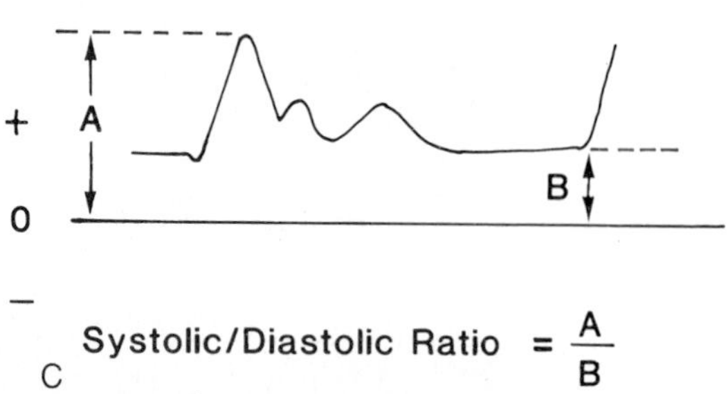

C

FIGURE 3–5 Pulsatility measurements. *A,* The pulsatility index (Gosling). *B,* The resistivity index (Pourcelot). *C,* The systolic/diastolic ratio.

ACCELERATION

Acceleration is another important flow feature evident in Doppler arterial waveforms.[24, 25] In most normal situations, flow velocity in an artery accelerates very rapidly in systole, and the peak velocity is reached within a few microseconds after ventricular contraction begins. Rapid flow acceleration produces an almost vertical deflection of the Doppler waveform at the start of systole (Fig. 3–6*A*). If, however, severe arterial obstruction is present proximal (upstream) to the point of Doppler examination, systolic flow acceleration may be slowed substantially, as shown in Figure 3–6*B*. Quantitative measurement of acceleration is achieved by measuring the acceleration time and the acceleration index, as illustrated in Figure 3–7.

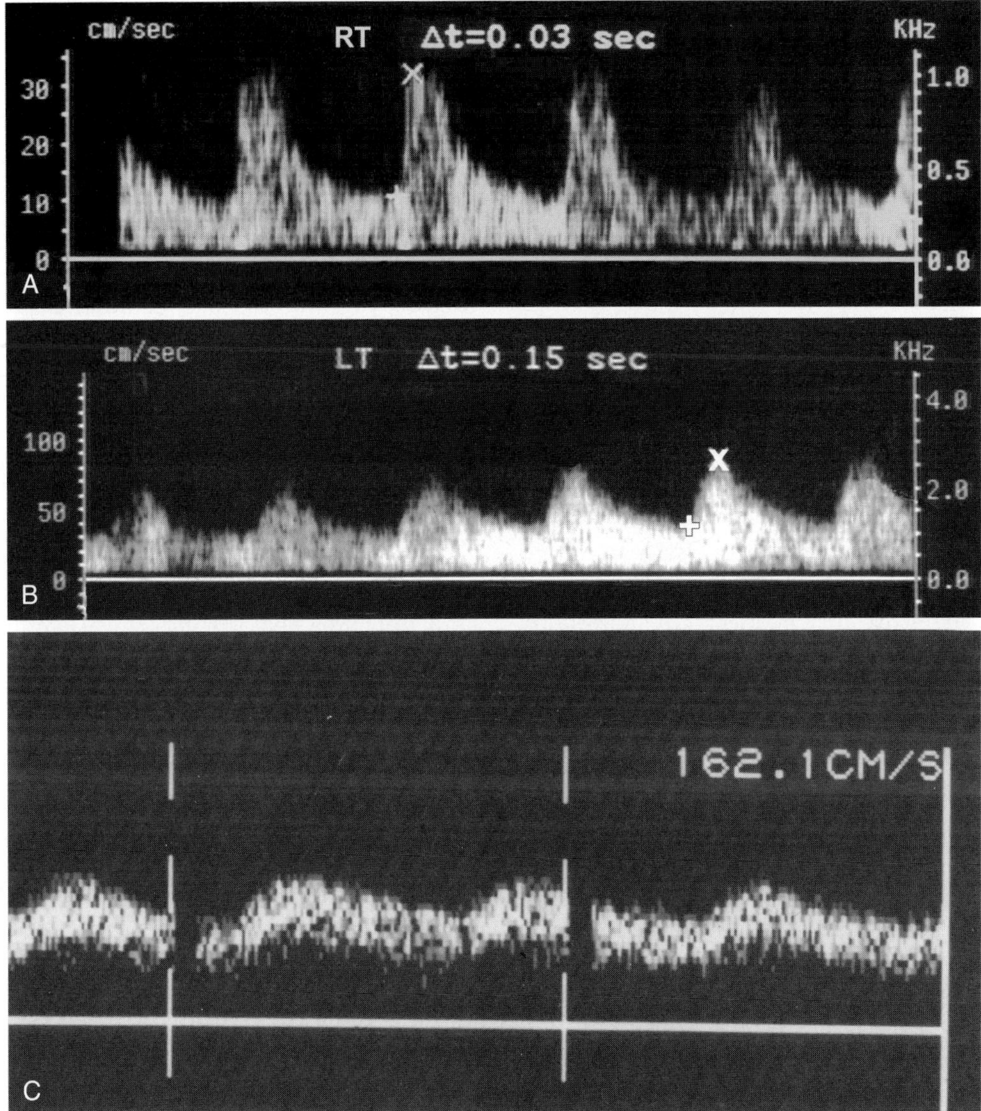

FIGURE 3–6 Acceleration and damping. *A,* The acceleration time (0.03 sec) is normal in the right kidney. *B,* The acceleration time is prolonged (0.15 sec) in the left kidney due to severe proximal renal artery stenosis. (*A* and *B* are from the same patient.) *C,* Severely damped dorsalis pedis artery waveform distal to femoral/popliteal artery occlusion. Normally, this waveform should look like Figure 3–4*C*. Acceleration is severely delayed and a large amount of flow is present throughout diastole, consistent with severe ischemia.

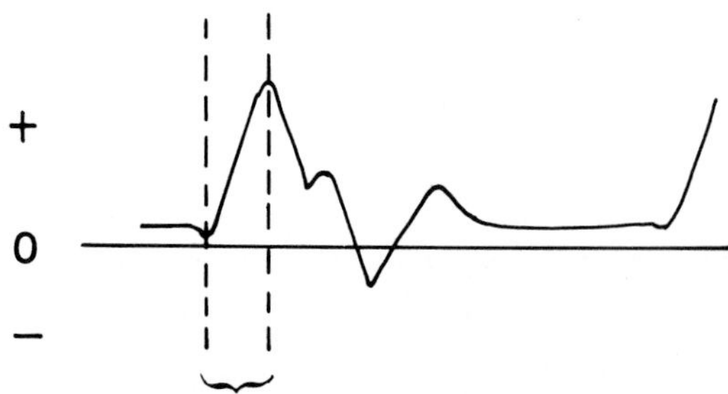

A

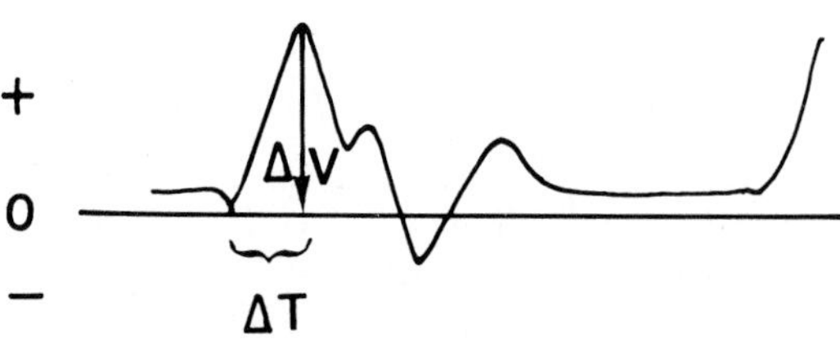

Systolic Acceleration Rate = $\frac{\Delta V}{\Delta T}$
B

FIGURE 3–7 Acceleration measurements: acceleration time (*A*) and acceleration index (*B*).

VESSEL IDENTITY

As you may have already surmised, vessels can be identified by their waveform pulsatility features.[1, 2, 14, 21–23, 26] For example, Doppler waveforms readily differentiate between lower extremity arteries, which are distinctly pulsatile, and veins, which have gently undulant flow features. Doppler waveforms are particularly helpful in identifying the internal and external carotid arteries, which have low and moderate pulsatility, respectively. Pulsatility is also of value for differentiating among the portal veins, hepatic veins, and hepatic arteries within the liver, as discussed in Chapter 26.

LAMINAR AND DISTURBED FLOW

Blood generally flows through arteries in an orderly way—the blood in the center of the vessel moving faster than the blood at the periphery. This flow pattern is described as *laminar,* because the movement of blood is in parallel lines[1, 2, 4, 14, 15] (Fig. 3–8). When flow is laminar, the great majority of blood cells are moving at a uniform speed, and the spectrum display shows a thin line that outlines a clear space called the *spectral window* (see Fig. 3–8*B*).*

In *disturbed flow,* the movement of blood cells is less uniform and orderly than in laminar flow. Disturbed flow is manifested as spectral broadening or widening of the spectral waveform.[1, 2, 4, 15–19] The *degree* of spectral broadening is proportionate to the *severity* of the flow disturbance, as illustrated in Figure 3–9. Although disturbed blood flow often indicates vascular disease, it must be recognized that flow disturbances also occur in normal vessels. Kinks, curves, and arterial branching may produce normal flow disturbances, as illustrated quite vividly in the carotid bulb,[11, 20, 21] where a prominent area of reversed flow is a normal occurrence (Fig. 3–10 [see p 57]). In addition, a spurious disturbed flow appearance may be created in normal arteries through the use of a large sample volume that encompasses both the slow flow area near the vessel wall and more rapid flow at the vessel center (Fig. 3–11 [see p 60]).[16–19]

VOLUME FLOW

Modern duplex instruments are capable of measuring the volume of blood flowing through a vessel (volume flow),[1, 2, 30–32] as illustrated in Figure 3–12 [see p 61]. Although this capability has been available on duplex instruments for more than 15 years and measurement accuracy appears satisfactory, volume flow measurements have not been used widely in a clinical setting.[4–9, 14–16, 30, 31, 33, 34]

DIAGNOSIS OF ARTERIAL OBSTRUCTION

Now that we have covered the basic concepts of Doppler spectral analysis, we can turn to the "heart of the matter," namely, how

* The term *plug flow* is actually more precise for this spectral pattern, as discussed in Chapter 1, but the term *laminar* is used throughout this text, in keeping with common convention.

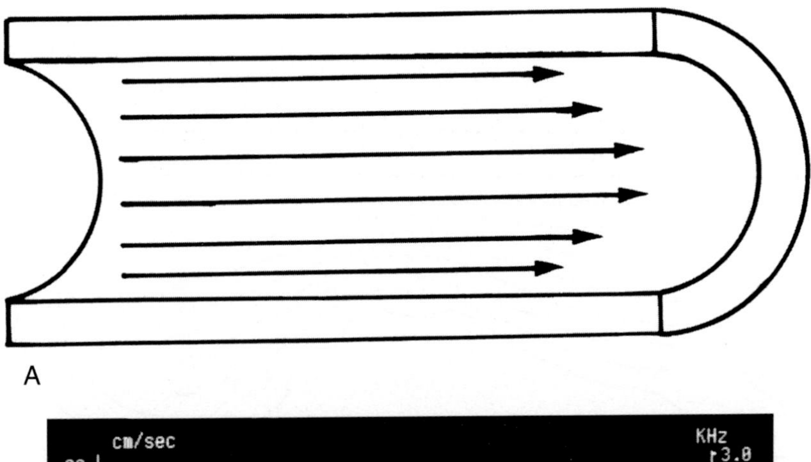

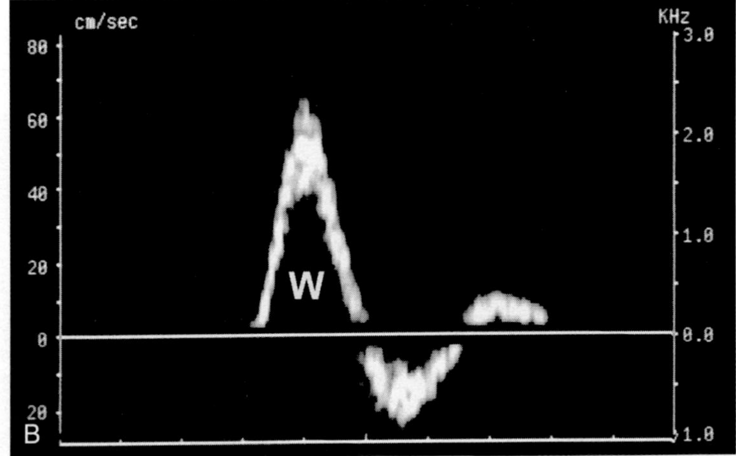

FIGURE 3–8 Laminar flow. *A,* Illustration of parallel lines of blood cell movement. *B,* Doppler spectrum during laminar flow. At all times, the blood cells are moving at similar velocities. As a result, the spectrum is a thin line that encloses a well-defined black "window" (W).

to use Doppler spectral analysis to diagnose arterial obstruction. Five main categories of information are used in this process: increased stenotic zone velocity, disturbed flow in the poststenotic zone, proximal pulsatility changes, distal pulsatility changes, and indirect effects of obstruction, such as collateralization.* These categories are summarized in Table 3–1 (see p 62).

Increased Stenotic Zone Velocity

The term *stenotic zone* refers to the narrowed portion of the arterial lumen. For determining the severity of arterial stenosis, the single most valuable Doppler finding is increased velocity in the stenotic zone (Fig. 3–13*A* and *B* [see p 58]). Flow velocity is increased in the stenotic zone, because blood must move more quickly if the same volume is to flow through the narrowed lumen as through the larger, normal lumen. The increase in stenotic zone velocity is directly proportional to the severity of luminal narrowing.

Three stenotic zone velocity measurements are commonly used to determine the severity of arterial stenoses (see Fig. 3–13): (1) *peak systolic velocity* (peak systole), which is the highest systolic velocity within the stenosis; (2) *end diastolic velocity* (end diastole), which is the highest end diastolic velocity; and (3) *systolic velocity ratio,* which compares peak systole in the stenosis with peak systole proximal to the stenosis (in a normal portion of the vessel). Peak systole in the stenotic zone is the first Doppler parameter to become abnormal as an arterial lumen be-

Text continued on page 62

* References 2, 4–10, 13, 15–19, 22–27, 29, 33, 35.

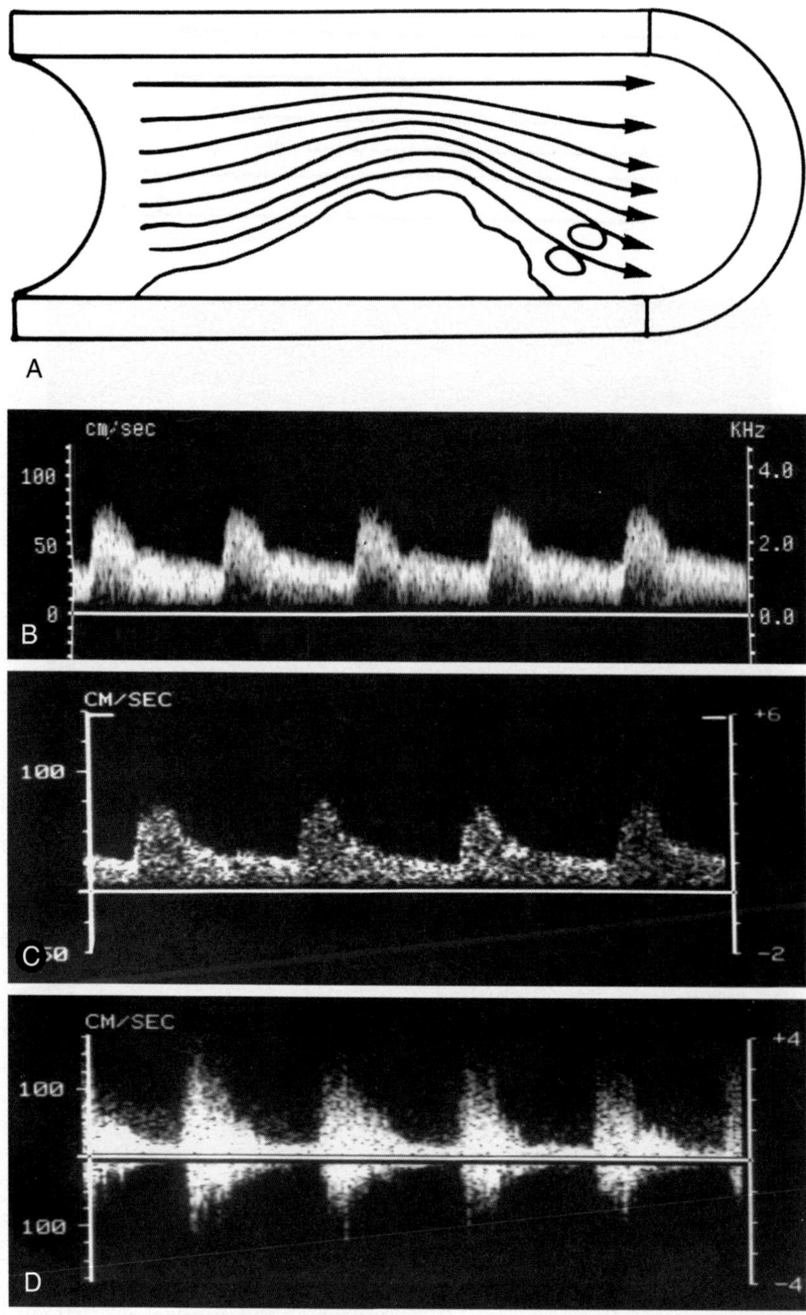

FIGURE 3–9 Disturbed flow. *A,* Disturbed flow illustration. *B,* Minor flow disturbance is indicated by spectral broadening at peak systole and through diastole. *C,* Moderate flow disturbance causes fill-in of the spectral window. *D,* Severe flow disturbance is characterized by spectral fill-in, poor definition of spectral borders, and simultaneous forward and reversed flow. The audible Doppler signal has a loud, gruff character when flow is severely disturbed.

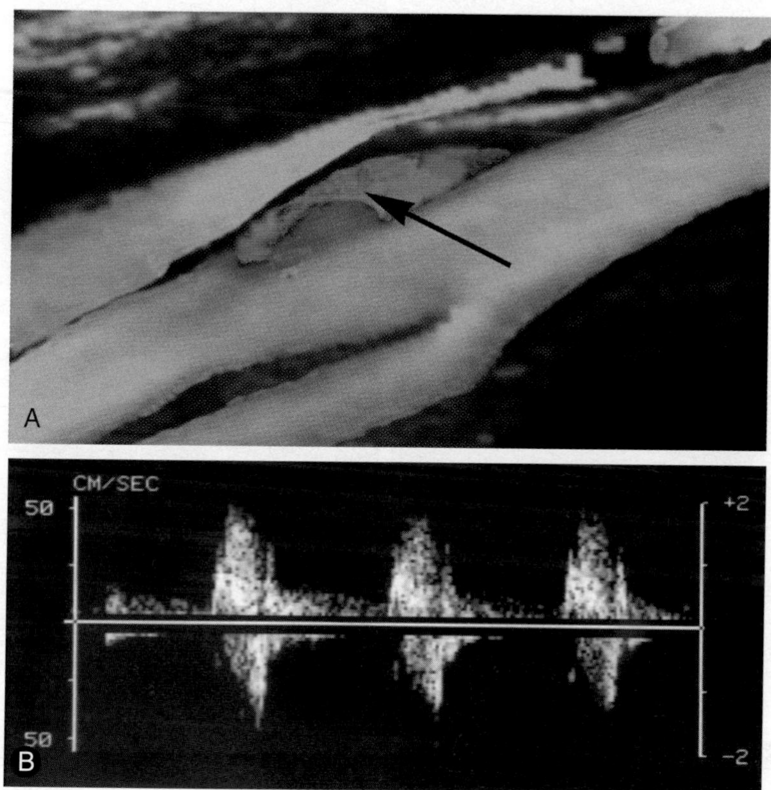

FIGURE 3–10 Normal bifurcation flow disturbance. (See p 54.) *A,* Flow reversal in the bulbous portion of the common and internal carotid arteries causes localized flow reversal (*arrow,* blue color). *B,* Simultaneous forward and reverse flow is evident in the bulbous region on the Doppler spectrum.

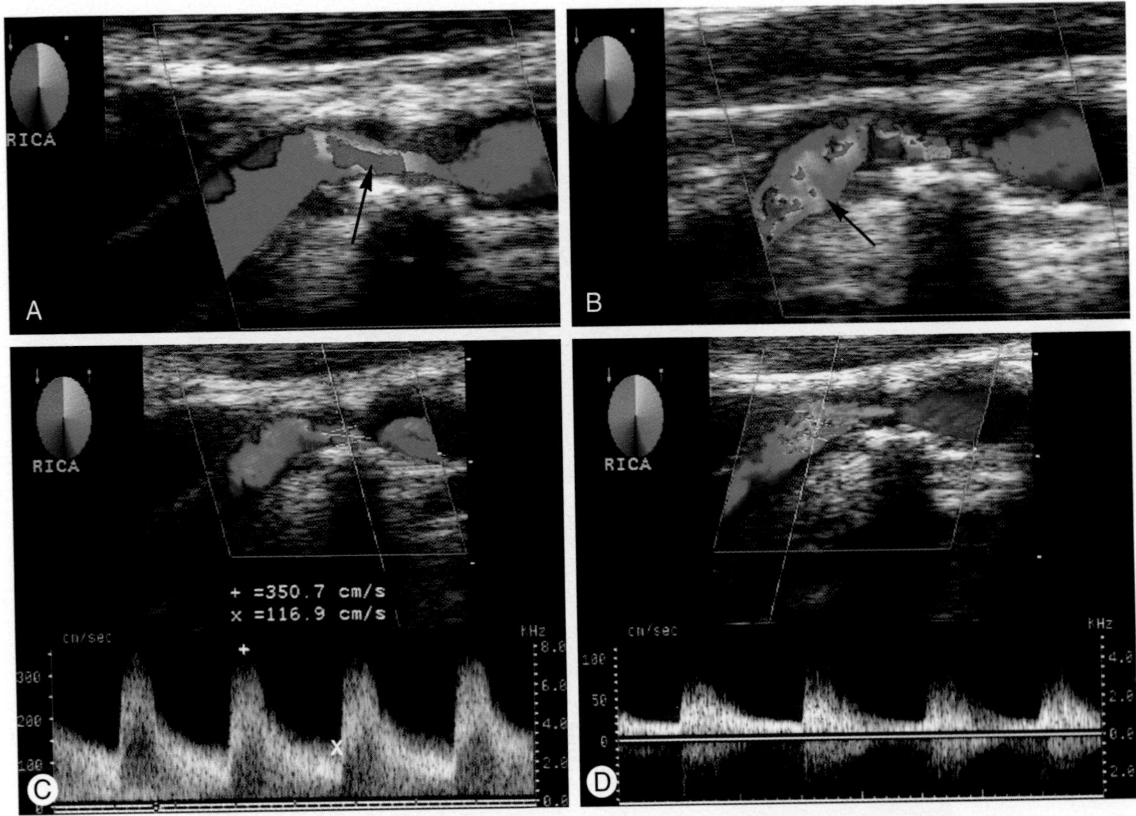

FIGURE 3–13 Local effects of arterial stenosis. *A,* The high velocities present in the narrowed portion of the arterial lumen generate an area of aliasing (*arrow*) within the stenotic lumen. *B,* Disturbed flow in the poststenotic area generates a mixture of colors (*arrow*). *C,* Doppler spectral analysis shows markedly elevated velocity at peak systole (350.7 cm/sec) and end diastole (116.9 cm/sec). *D,* Severe flow disturbance is evident in the poststenotic region, as indicated by simultaneous forward and reverse flow, spectrum fill-in, and poor definition of the spectrum margins.

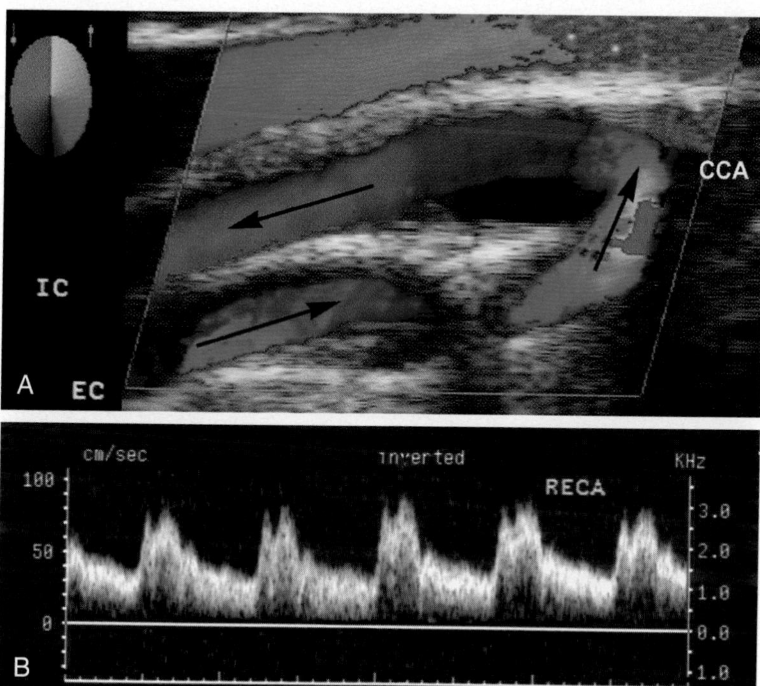

FIGURE 3–16 Effects of arterial collateralization. (See p 64.) *A,* Flow (*arrows*) is reversed in an enlarged external carotid artery (EC) branch that serves as a collateral source for the internal carotid artery (IC). Normally, the flow direction would be the same in both vessels. Flow reversal was caused by occlusion of the common carotid artery (CCA), which is seen at the right of the image. *B,* The external carotid artery waveform also shows the effects of collateralization. The waveform has low resistance features because it is supplying the low resistance circulation of the brain. Compare with the normal external carotid waveform shown in Figure 3–4*B*.

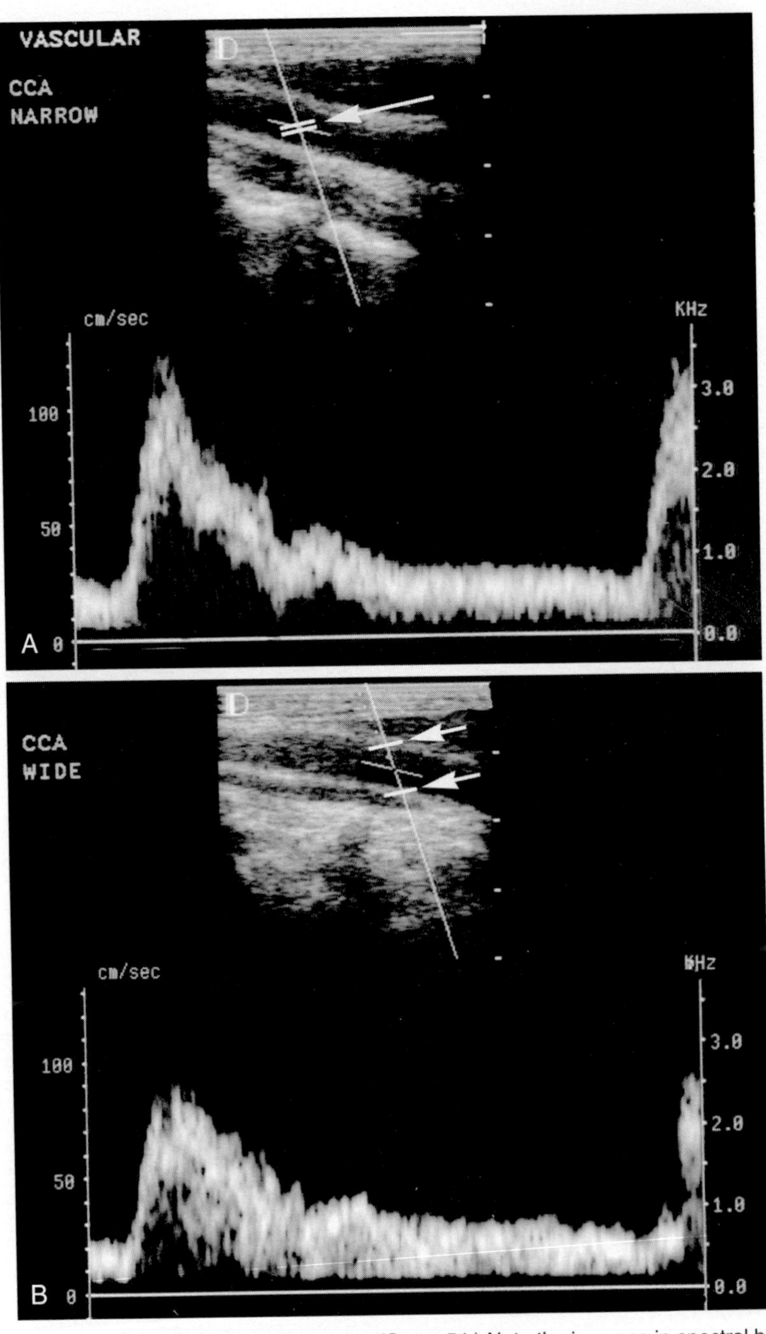

FIGURE 3–11 The effects of sample volume size. (See p 54.) Note the increase in spectral broadening as the sample volume (*arrows*) is enlarged from a small size (*A*) to a large size (*B*). The spectrum is broader in *B* because the sample volume includes slow-moving blood at the periphery of the artery as well as rapidly moving blood nearer the center.

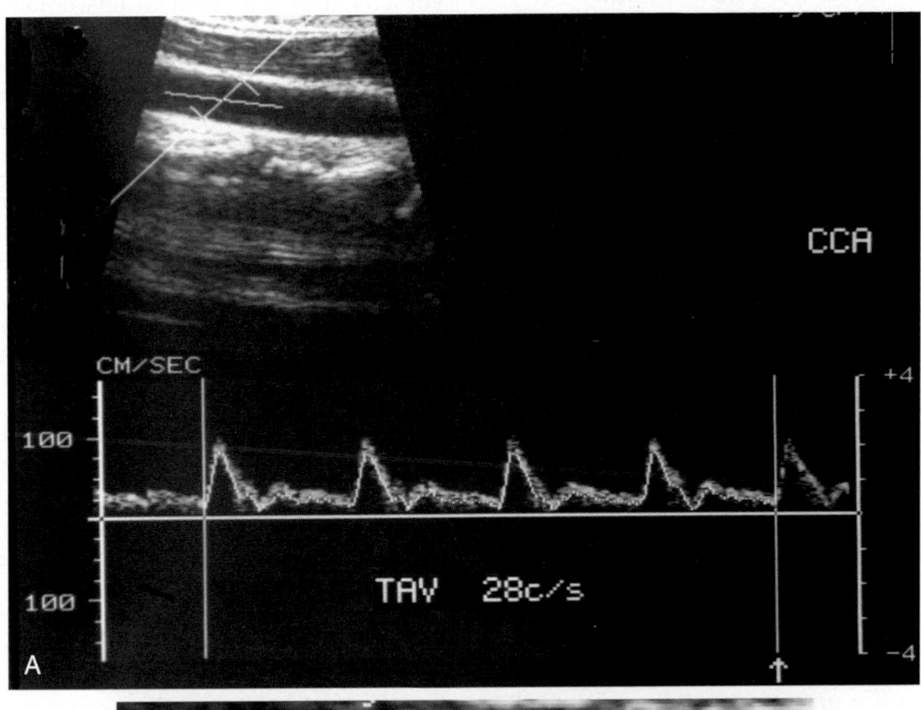

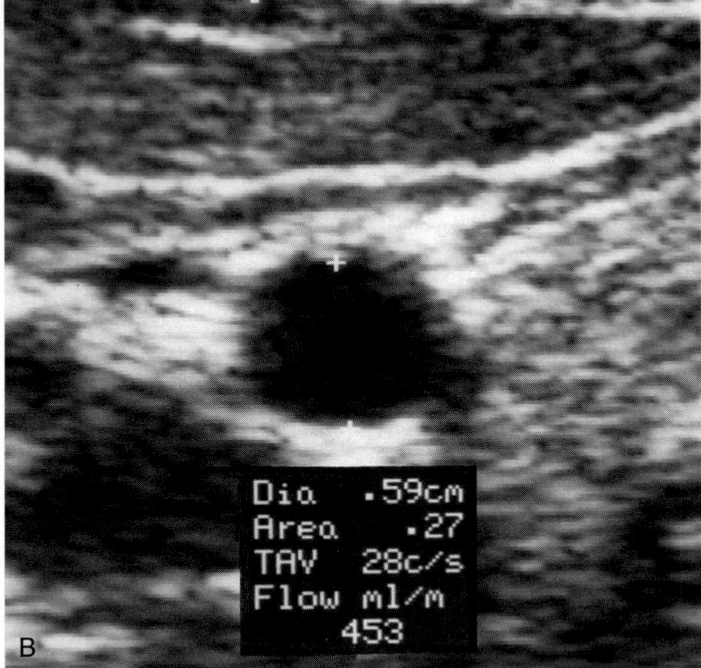

FIGURE 3–12 Duplex volume flow measurement. (See p 54.) *A,* The operator placed the vertical lines to include four complete cardiac cycles. The instrument calculated an average velocity (time average velocity, TAV) of 28 cm/sec (c/s) for the time period within the cursors. *B,* The operator measured the lumen diameter in systole (0.59 cm). The instrument then calculated the cross-sectional area (0.27 cm^2). Using the TAV and the area, the instrument calculated the volume flow at 453 mL/min. Recall that 1 milliliter (mL) = 1 cubic centimeter (cc).

TABLE 3–1 SPECTRAL FEATURES OF ARTERIAL OBSTRUCTION

Local effects
Elevated flow velocity in the stenotic lumen
Poststenotic flow disturbance
Proximal (upstream) pulsatility changes
Increased pulsatility
Decreased velocity overall, due to decreased flow
Distal (downstream) pulsatility changes
Slowed systolic acceleration
Broad systolic peak
Increased diastolic flow (reduced peripheral resistance)
Decreased velocity overall
Secondary (collateral) effects
Increased size, velocity, and volume flow in collateral vessels
Reversed flow in collateral vessels
Decreased pulsatility (flow resistance) in collateral vessels

comes narrowed. As shown in Figure 3–14, peak systole rises steadily with progressive narrowing, but ultimately, the flow resistance becomes so high (at about 80% diameter reduction) that peak systole falls to normal or even subnormal levels. This drop in velocity can cause the unwary to underestimate the severity of a high-grade stenosis. Low flow velocity may also lead to false diagnosis of arterial occlusion, if the flow velocity is so low that Doppler signals cannot be detected with ultrasound. The region of maximum velocity within the stenotic zone may be quite small, and for that reason, the sonographer must "search" the stenotic lumen with the sample volume to locate the highest flow velocity. If the highest flow velocity is overlooked, the degree of stenosis may be underestimated.

The end diastolic velocity (end diastole) in the stenotic zone also increases in proportion to stenosis severity, but end diastole generally remains normal with less than 50% (diameter) narrowing. Below 50%, there is no pressure gradient across the stenosis in diastole. With moderate stenosis (50–70% diameter reduction), however, a pressure gradient exists throughout diastole, and end diastolic velocities are above normal. With severe stenosis (70–90% diameter reduction), a marked pressure gradient exists throughout diastole, and diastolic velocities are high. End diastole is a particularly good marker for

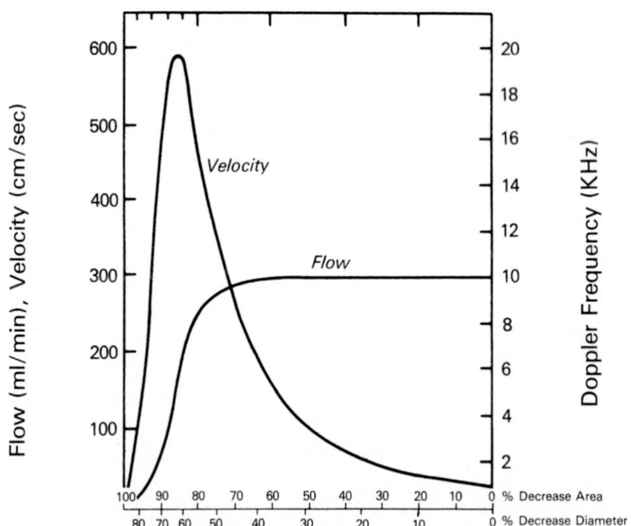

FIGURE 3–14 Relationship among velocity, flow, and lumen size. This graph refers specifically to internal carotid artery stenosis, but the principles illustrated apply to stenoses in other arteries throughout the body. Note that peak systolic velocity in the stenotic internal carotid lumen (labeled *velocity*) increases exponentially as the lumen diameter decreases (from right to left). The highest velocities correspond to approximately 70% diameter reduction. With greater stenosis severity, peak systolic velocity falls off rapidly to zero (because of rapidly increasing flow resistance). In contrast to velocity, volume flow (labeled *flow*) remains stable until the lumen diameter is reduced by about 50%. With further reduction in lumen size, volume flow falls off very rapidly to zero. Finally, note the relationship of percent diameter and area reduction, as shown at the base of the figure. Fifty percent diameter reduction equals about 70% area reduction, and 70% diameter reduction equals about 90% area reduction! (Modified from Spencer MP: Full capability Doppler diagnosis. *In* Spencer MP, Reed JM [eds]: Cerebrovascular Evaluation with Doppler Ultrasound. The Hague, Netherlands, Martinus Nijhoff, 1981, p 213, with kind permission from Kluwer Academic Publishers.)

severe stenosis because this parameter is not elevated in moderate stenosis and increases very rapidly once a "threshold" stenosis level is reached.[9] Beyond this point, end diastole increases, proportionately, at a greater rate than peak systole, and as a result, the difference between peak systole and end diastole decreases.

The systolic velocity ratio, as defined previously, is an additional important parameter for the diagnosis of arterial stenosis. This parameter is used to compensate for patient-to-patient hemodynamic variables, such as cardiac function, heart rate, blood pressure, and arterial compliance. Tachycardia, for instance, tends to increase peak systole in the stenotic zone, whereas poor myocardial function may decrease peak systole. The systolic velocity ratio allows the patient to act as his or her own physiologic "standard," because peak systole in the stenotic zone is compared with peak systole in a normal arterial segment. The systolic velocity ratio is used clinically in a number of circumstances, including the measurement of internal carotid, renal, and extremity artery stenoses.

Poststenotic Flow Disturbance

The poststenotic zone is the region immediately beyond an arterial stenosis, where flow disturbances are commonly present. These flow disturbances are an important diagnostic feature of arterial stenosis. As the flow stream from the stenotic lumen "spreads out" in the poststenotic zone, the laminar flow pattern is lost, and flow becomes disorganized, which generates a disturbed Doppler spectral pattern (see Figs. 3–9 and 3–13). In some cases, frank swirling movements (or vortices) occur in the poststenotic zone, producing simultaneous forward and reverse flow on the Doppler spectrum. The maximal flow disturbance occurs within 1 cm beyond the stenosis,[16] and in very severe stenoses, soft tissues adjacent to this portion of the artery may vibrate, causing a "visible bruit" on color Doppler images, as illustrated in Chapter 4. About 2 cm beyond the stenosis, the flow disturbance becomes less violent and spectral broadening diminishes. An orderly, laminar flow pattern usually is reestablished with 3 cm beyond the stenosis,[4, 16] but this distance is variable.

Poststenotic flow disturbances can be graded,[2, 4, 6, 9, 15–19] as shown in Figure 3–9. In general, minimal and even moderate flow disturbances are of little diagnostic value, because they may occur in both normal and abnormal vessels. Severe flow disturbance, however, with simultaneous forward and reverse flow, generally does not occur in normal vessels and is an important sign of high-grade arterial narrowing. Severe flow disturbance also can be seen occasionally with or without other significant vascular pathology, such as arterial dissection or arteriovenous fistula. Severe flow disturbances are "beacons" for arterial stenosis. Whenever a severe flow disturbance is detected, the sonographer should search carefully for an adjacent stenosis. In some cases, the stenosis may be obscured by plaque calcification (preventing ultrasound visualization), and in such instances, poststenotic disturbed flow may be the only sign of severe arterial stenosis.

Proximal Pulsatility Changes

Arterial obstruction causes increased pulsatility (as defined previously) in portions of the artery proximal to (upstream from) the stenosis, and this finding, therefore, may be important diagnostically. For instance, with severe internal carotid artery obstruction the Doppler spectrum in the common carotid artery has high-pulsatility feature rather than a normal low-pulsatility pattern (Fig. 3–15). To understand why pulsatility is increased proximal to a stenosis, imagine that blood in the common carotid artery is being forced against an internal carotid artery valve that is 90 or 100% closed rather than wide open. How do you think the velocity waveform will look proximal to the valve (upstream)? First, you can imagine that in systole, flow goes forward for only a brief moment when arterial pressure is highest, and then flow slows abruptly; therefore, the systolic peak is sharp and narrow. Second, there is relatively little flow in diastole, because intra-arterial pressure in diastole is insufficient to force blood through the closed valve. Third, back pressure from the blockage may cause a brief flow reversal early in diastole, equivalent to the reflected wave seen in normal extremity arteries. Finally, flow velocity in the common carotid artery is

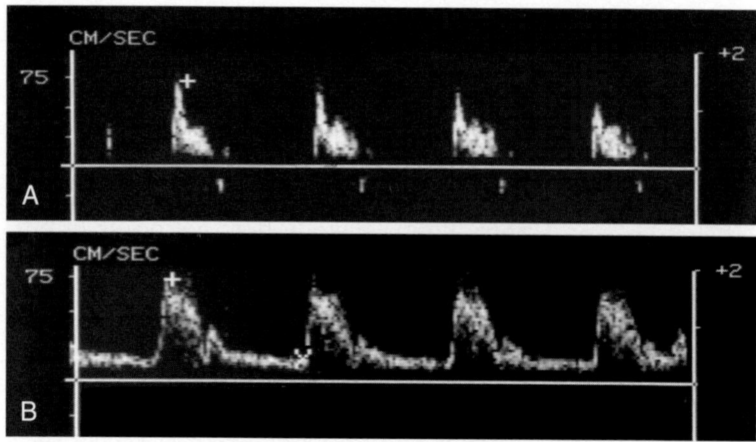

FIGURE 3–15 Increased common carotid artery pulsatility due to internal carotid artery occlusion. *A,* A high-resistance flow pattern is evident in this common carotid artery, consisting of sharp systolic peaks, diastolic flow reversal, and absence of flow throughout most of diastole. The ipsilateral internal carotid artery was occluded. *B,* The contralateral common carotid artery shows normal flow features.

low overall, because blood flow is reduced by the closed internal carotid valve.

Distal Pulsatility Changes

Doppler waveform abnormalities seen distal to a stenosis (downstream) also have considerable value in the diagnosis of arterial stenosis. As noted previously in the section on acceleration, the flow velocity in a normal artery increases abruptly in systole, and the systolic peak is reached quickly (see Fig. 3–6*A*). In contrast, the Doppler waveform distal to a *severe* arterial obstruction has a "damped" appearance (see Fig. 3–6*B,C*), which means that the systolic acceleration is slowed, the systolic peak is rounded, the maximum systolic velocity is lower than normal, and the diastolic flow is increased. There are three explanations for these postobstructive waveform abnormalities. First, it can be imagined that blood is being "squeezed" slowly through the obstructed lumen (or tiny collaterals), rather than "flying" along a broad tube. Therefore, it takes longer to reach peak velocity in systole. Second, overall flow velocity is low, because less blood is moving through the obstructed vessel. Finally, ischemic distal tissues are "begging" for blood, with capillary beds wide open. The resultant decrease in peripheral resistance allows blood to flow throughout diastole, even in vessels that normally would not have diastolic flow (e.g., extremity arteries). The net effect of all three factors is the damped (also called *dampened*) waveform appearance (see Fig. 3–6*B,C*) described previously, which is a significant finding since it clearly indicates arterial insufficiency in the proper setting.

The terms *pulsus tardus* and *pulsus parvus* are also used to describe damped, postobstructive waveforms. Tardus refers to delayed arrival of the systolic peak, and parvus refers to overall low velocity. Waveform damping due to proximal obstruction may be assessed visually, but it also is possible to quantify damping by measuring the acceleration time or acceleration index, as described previously in this chapter.

Secondary (Collateral) Effects of Arterial Obstruction

The final diagnostic features of arterial obstruction of diagnostic importance are flow changes in collateral vessels. Arterial obstruction commonly alters flow in collateral channels that may be near or distant to the site of obstruction. These flow alterations include increased velocity, increased volume flow, reversed flow direction, and pulsatility changes. Figure 3–16 (see p 59) is an example of such changes in the external carotid artery in response to common carotid artery occlusion.

Secondary manifestations of arterial obstruction can be important diagnostically for the following reasons: (1) they may indicate that an obstructive lesion exists that would be inapparent otherwise, for example, when reversed vertebral flow calls attention to subclavian stenosis; (2) the location of collaterals roughly indicates the level of obstruction; and (3) secondary flow changes provide some data, albeit limited, about the adequacy of the collateral system circumventing an obstructive lesion. Such changes are of particular importance in transcranial Doppler applications, as considered in Chapter 13.

REFERENCES

1. Wells PNT, Skedmore R: Doppler developments in the last quinquennium. Ultrasound Med Biol 11:613–623, 1986.
2. Taylor KJW, Holland S: Doppler ultrasound: Part I. Basic principles, instrumentation, and pitfalls. Radiology 174:297–307, 1990.
3. Hutchison KJ, Oberle K, Scott JA, et al: A comparison of Doppler ultrasonic waveforms processed by zero crossing and spectrographic techniques in the diagnosis of peripheral arterial disease. Angiology 32:277–289, 1981.
4. Reneman RS, Spencer MP: Local Doppler audio spectra in normal and stenosed carotid arteries in man. Ultrasound Med Biol 5:1–11, 1979.
5. Johnston KW, deMorais D, Kassam M, et al: Cerebrovascular assessment using a Doppler carotid scanner and real-time frequency analysis. J Clin Ultrasound 9:443–449, 1981.
6. Brown PM, Johnston W, Kassam M, et al: A critical study of ultrasound Doppler spectral analysis for detecting carotid disease. Ultrasound Med Biol 8:515–523, 1982.
7. Zwiebel WJ: Color duplex imaging and Doppler spectrum analysis: Principles, capabilities, and limitations. Semin Ultrasound CT MR 11:84–96, 1990.
8. Zwiebel WJ, Knighton R: Duplex examination of the carotid arteries. Semin Ultrasound CT MR 11:97–135, 1990.
9. Bluth EI, Wetzner SM, Stavros AT, et al: Carotid duplex sonography: A multicenter recommendation for standardized imaging and Doppler criteria. Radiographics 8:487–506, 1988.
10. Feigenbaum H: Doppler color flow imaging. Heart Dis Update 2:25–50, 1988.
11. Zierler RE, Phillips DJ, Beach KW, et al: Noninvasive assessment of normal carotid bifurcation hemodynamics with color-flow ultrasound imaging. Ultrasound Med Biol 13:471–476, 1987.
12. Middleton WD, Foley WD, Lawson TL: Flow reversal in the normal carotid bifurcation: Color Doppler flow imaging analysis. Radiology 167:207–210, 1988.
13. Spencer MP: Frequency spectrum analysis in Doppler diagnosis. *In* Zwiebel WJ (ed): Introduction to Vascular Ultrasonography, 2nd ed. Philadelphia, WB Saunders, 1986, pp 53–80.
14. Smith JJ, Kampine JP: The peripheral circulation and its regulation. *In* Circulatory Physiology: The Essentials. Baltimore, Williams & Wilkins, 1980.
15. Baker D: Application of pulsed Doppler techniques. Radiol Clin North Am 18:79–103, 1980.
16. Douville Y, Johnston KW, Kassam M: Determination of the hemodynamic factors which influence the carotid Doppler spectral broadening. Ultrasound Med Biol 11:417–423, 1985.
17. Campbell JD, Hutchison KJ, Karpinski E: Variation of Doppler ultrasound spectral width in the poststenotic velocity field. Ultrasound Med Biol 15:611–619, 1989.
18. Merode TV, Hick P, Hoeks APG, et al: Limitations of Doppler spectral broadening in the early detection of carotid artery disease due to the size of the sample volume. Ultrasound Med Biol 9:581–586, 1983.
19. Knox RA, Phillips DJ, Breslau PJ, et al: Empirical findings relating sample volume size to diagnostic accuracy in pulsed Doppler cerebrovascular studies. J Clin Ultrasound 10:227–232, 1982.
20. Ku DN, Giddens DP, Phillips DJ, et al: Hemodynamics of the normal human carotid bifurcation: In vitro and in vivo studies. Ultrasound Med Biol 11:13–26, 1985.
21. Phillips DJ, Greene FM, Langlois Y, et al: Flow velocity patterns in the carotid bifurcations of young, presumed normal subjects. Ultrasound Med Biol 9:39–49, 1983.
22. Nimura Y, Matsuo H, Hayashi T, et al: Studies on arterial flow patterns: Instantaneous velocity spectrums and their phasic changes with directional ultrasonic Doppler technique. Br Heart J 36:899–907, 1974.
23. Rutherford RB, Kreutzer EW: Doppler ultrasound techniques in the assessment of extracranial arterial occlusive disease. *In* Nicolaides AN, Yao JST (eds): Investigation of Vascular Disorders. London, Churchill Livingstone, 1981.
24. Rutherford RB, Hiatt WR, Kreutzer EW: The use of velocity wave form analysis in the diagnosis of carotid artery occlusive disease. Surgery 82:695–702, 1977.
25. Nicolaides AN, Angelides NS: Waveform index and resistance factor using directional Doppler ultrasound and a zero crossing detector. *In* Nicolaides AN, Yao JST (eds): Investigation of Vascular Disorders. London, Churchill Livingstone, 1981.
26. Gosling RG: Doppler ultrasound assessment of occlusive arterial disease. Practitioner 220:599–609, 1978.
27. Kotval PS: Doppler waveform parvus and tardus. J Ultrasound Med 8:435–440, 1989.
28. Pourcelot L: Applications cliniques de l'examen Doppler transcutane. *In* Peronneau P (ed): Velocimetrie Ultrasonore Doppler, Vol 34. Paris, INSERM 1974, pp 780–785.
29. Stuart B, Drumm J, Fitzgerald DE, Duignan NM: Foetal blood velocity waveforms in normal pregnancy. Br J Obstet Gynaecol 87:780–785, 1980.
30. Avasthi PS, Greene ER, Voyles WF, et al: A comparison of echo-Doppler and electromagnetic renal blood flow measurements. J Ultrasound Med 3:213–218, 1984.
31. Gill RW: Measurement of blood flow by ultrasound: Accuracy and sources of error. Ultrasound Med Biol 11:625–641, 1985.
32. Burns PN, Jaffe CC: Quantitative flow measurements with Doppler ultrasound: Techniques, accuracy, and limitations. Radiol Clin North Am 23:641–657, 1985.
33. Fei DY, Billian C, Rittgers SE: Flow dynamics in a stenosed carotid bifurcation model. Part I: Basic velocity measurements. Ultrasound Med Biol 14:21–31, 1988.
34. Chang BB, Leather RP, Kaufmann JL, et al: Hemodynamic characteristics of failing infrainguinal in situ vein bypass. J Vasc Surg 12:596–600, 1990.
35. Spencer MP: Full capability Doppler diagnosis. *In* Spencer MP, Reed JM (eds): Cerebrovascular Evaluation with Doppler Ultrasound. The Hague, Netherlands, Martinus Nijhoff Publishers, 1981, p 213.

Chapter 4

Color-Flow Imaging for Vascular Diagnosis

■ *William J. Zwiebel, MD*

One of the more remarkable developments in ultrasound instrumentation is color-flow ultrasound imaging. This imaging method superimposes a blood flow image on a standard gray-scale ultrasound image, permitting instantaneous, visual assessment of blood flow. Color-flow imaging has had significant impact on ultrasound vascular diagnosis; nevertheless, this modality has certain idiosyncrasies and limitations that can cause diagnostic error. It is worthwhile, therefore, to review the capabilities as well as the limitations of color-flow sonography.

PRINCIPLES OF COLOR-FLOW IMAGING

Three ultrasound methods have been developed to display blood flow information visually: "standard" color-Doppler flow imaging, time-domain flow imaging, and Doppler intensity flow imaging (power Doppler). These methods are described briefly later in this chapter. For additional details, please see Chapter 2.

Standard Color-Doppler Imaging

Gray-scale ultrasound instruments use only two pieces of information from each echo that returns from the patient's body: the distance from the echo to the transducer (determined by the time of flight of the ultrasound pulse) and the strength of the echo. The echo signal typically contains other information, such as a Doppler frequency shift, but this information is disregarded. Color-Doppler instruments[1–5] are different from gray-scale instruments because they use the Doppler shift information in addition to time of flight and amplitude information (Fig. 4–1). For each echo shown on the color-Doppler image, the instrument makes five determinations:

1. *How long has it taken for the sound beam to travel to and from the site of the echo?* This "time of flight" of the ultrasound beam indicates the distance of the echo reflector from the transducer.
2. *How strong is the echo?* The strength or amplitude of the ultrasound signal determines how brightly the echo is displayed on the image (for both the gray-scale and the color-Doppler components).
3. *Is a Doppler frequency shift present?* If so, the echo is represented in color; if not, it is represented in shades of gray.
4. *What is the magnitude of the Doppler frequency shift?* The magnitude of the Doppler shift is proportionate to the blood flow velocity and the Doppler angle (shown in Fig. 3–2, Chapter 3). Different frequency levels are shown on the image as different color shades or hues.
5. *What is the direction of the Doppler shift?* The instrument determines whether flow is toward or away from the transducer by noting whether the echo has a higher or lower frequency than the ultrasound beam sent out from the transducer. A higher Doppler frequency means flow is toward the transducer, and a lower Doppler frequency means flow is away from the transducer. It is customary to show flow in one direction in blue and flow in the other direction in red. However, the operator can select other color schemes, if desired.

You should note that both the direction of flow and the velocity of flow (Doppler shift)

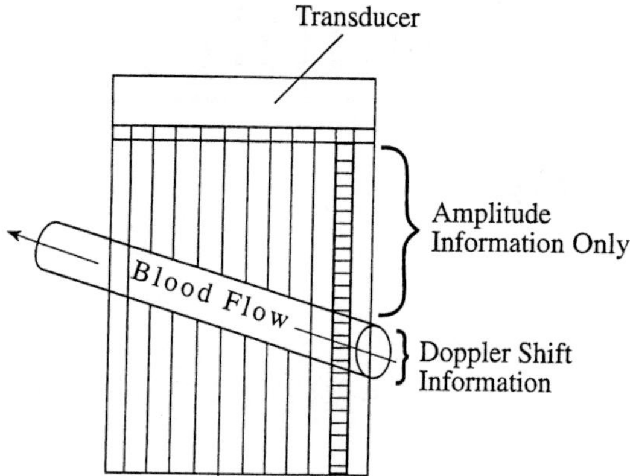

FIGURE 4–1 Color-Doppler instrumentation. Stationary reflectors generate only amplitude information and are represented in shades of gray. Moving reflectors generate a Doppler frequency shift and are shown in color. Different colors can be used to show flow toward the transducer (increased frequency) and away from the transducer (decreased frequency).

are shown on the color-Doppler image (Fig. 4–2). This can be done in two ways. With the shifting hue method, different colors are used to represent different frequency levels (e.g., blue, green, yellow, and white, with increasing frequency). With the changing shade method, the same color is shown, but the color gets lighter as the frequency increases (e.g., dark red, light red, pink, and white). Some sonologists prefer the shifting hue method, believing that it more clearly represents changes in the frequency shift and may demonstrate aliasing more clearly, as considered later.

Time-Domain Color-Flow Imaging

The color-flow images generated with the time-domain method[5a] look like the flow images produced with the Doppler method previously described, but these methods are actually quite different. In the time-domain technique, the ultrasound instrument identifies clusters of echoes (called *speckle*) within the ultrasound image and notes how far these clusters move on successive ultrasound pulses. By repeatedly "testing" echo clusters for movement, the instrument recognizes regions where flow is present. Flow direction and flow velocity are ascertained directly with the time-domain method, by noting which way the clusters move and how fast they move over time.[5a] Time-domain flow imaging is not widely used by ultrasound equipment manufacturers. The most commonly used color-flow methods are color-Doppler and power Doppler.

Power Doppler Flow Imaging

The third method of color-flow imaging that is available commercially is called power Doppler. As its name implies, this is a Doppler method, but it differs from standard Doppler imaging, previously described, in that the *power* or intensity of the Doppler signal is measured and mapped, rather than the Doppler frequency shift per se.[6] Stated differently, the instrument determines how strong the Doppler shift is at all locations within the image field and displays locations where the strength of the Doppler signal exceeds a threshold level (Fig. 4–3). The term *power,* as used here, has the same meaning as in "Doppler power spectrum," as described in Chapter 3. Compared with standard color-Doppler imaging, power Doppler flow imaging is said to be more sensitive in detecting blood flow and less dependent on the Doppler angle.[6] These advantages mean that smaller vessels and vessels with slow flow rates can be imaged; furthermore, even tissue perfusion can be assessed to a limited degree. Increased sensitivity in power Doppler imaging is derived from more extensive use of the dynamic range of the Doppler signal than is possible with standard color-Doppler imaging. More of the dynamic range can be used because noise that would overwhelm the standard color-Doppler image can be assigned a uniform background color (e.g., light blue).[6] Hence anything that represents noise is blue (see Fig. 4–3*C*), and anything that represents flow is another color (usually gold). Furthermore, power Doppler imaging is not affected by aliasing. Even the aliased (wrapped-around) portion of the signal (see Chapter 2) has power and can be displayed as flow.[6]

Power Doppler imaging has one final advantage that has been appreciated since the advent of ultrasound echo-enhancing agents. Power Doppler imaging is less subject to *blooming* than standard color-Doppler imaging. Blooming is the spread of color outside of the blood vessel that occurs when the amplification of the Doppler signal is too great. Blooming is a particular problem when

Text continued on page 73

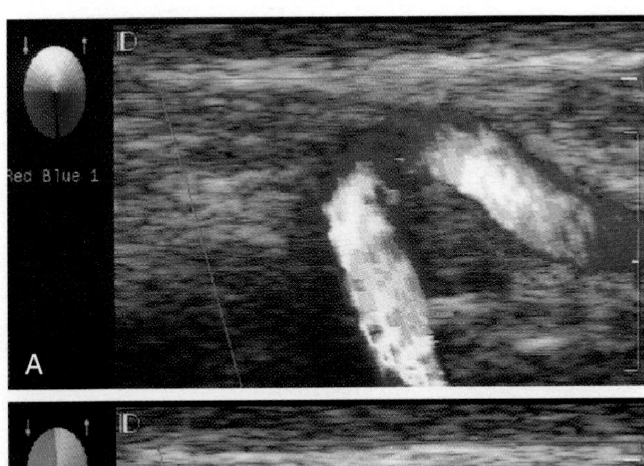

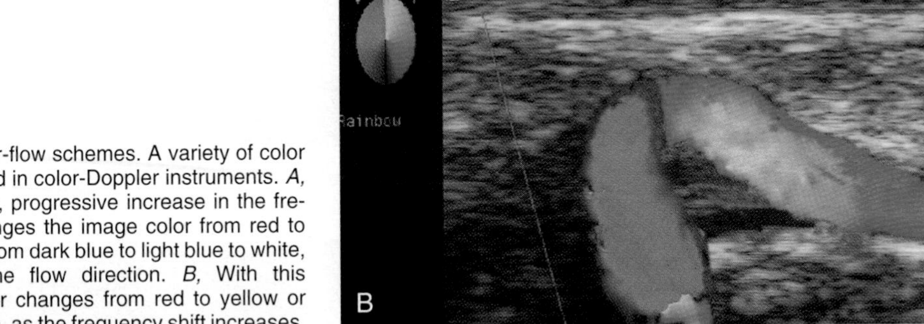

FIGURE 4–2 Color-flow schemes. A variety of color schemes are used in color-Doppler instruments. *A,* With this scheme, progressive increase in the frequency shift changes the image color from red to pink to white, or from dark blue to light blue to white, depending on the flow direction. *B,* With this scheme, the color changes from red to yellow or from blue to green, as the frequency shift increases.

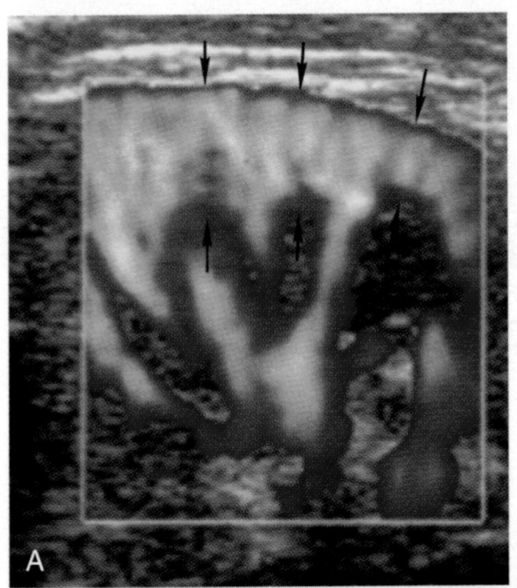

FIGURE 4–3 Power Doppler illustrations. *A,* Renal vessels are seen with striking detail, including small vessels in the renal cortex (*arrows*). Note the absence of flow direction information; all vessels are yellow even though flow in some vessels is toward the cortex (arteries) and in others is toward the renal hilum (veins). *B,* Quantitative spectral information can be obtained in the power Doppler mode. *C,* This power Doppler image of the cranial vasculature uses a blue background, which enhances flow detection because noise is converted to a uniform blue color. With color Doppler, noise would blur the margins of the vessels.

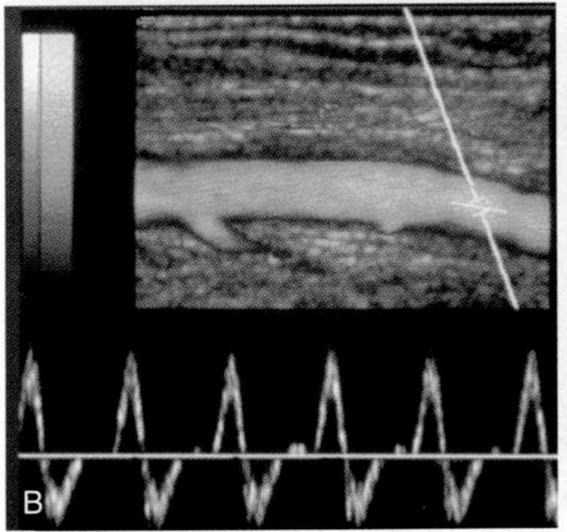

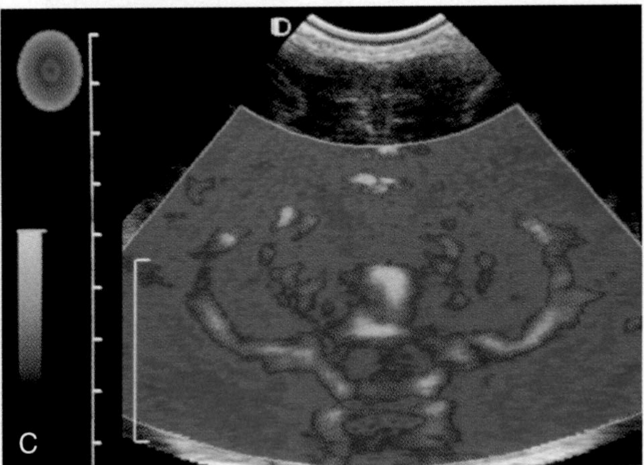

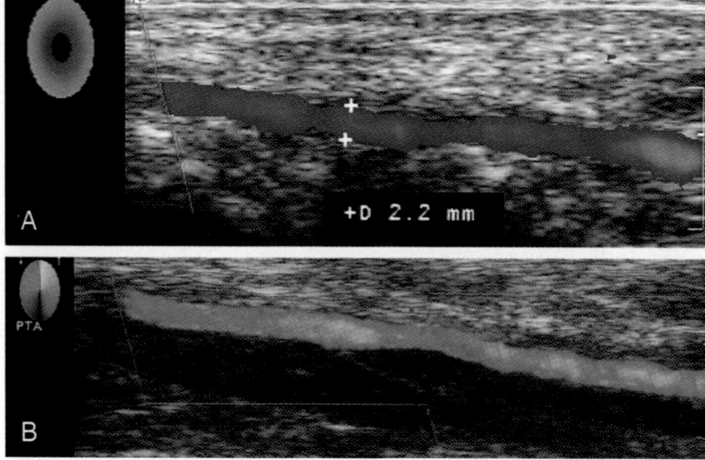

FIGURE 4–4 Technical efficiency. (See p 73.) *A,* Small vessels can be located, such as this 2.2-mm-diameter dorsalis pedis artery (power Doppler image). *B,* Long vascular segments can be traced with color-Doppler imaging. For instance, a 7-cm-long portion of a posterior tibial artery is shown in this composite of two images.

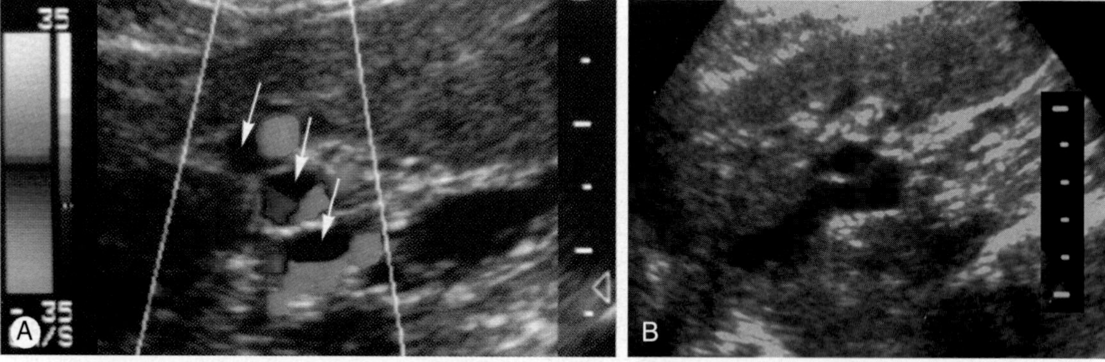

FIGURE 4–5 Color flow clarifies porta hepatis anatomy. (See p 73.) *A,* Dilated bile ducts (*arrows*) can be easily differentiated from the adjacent portal veins because no flow is present in the ducts. *B,* The bile ducts are difficult to identify without color-flow information. Biliary dilatation was not recognized initially in this case but was quite apparent when color-flow imaging was used.

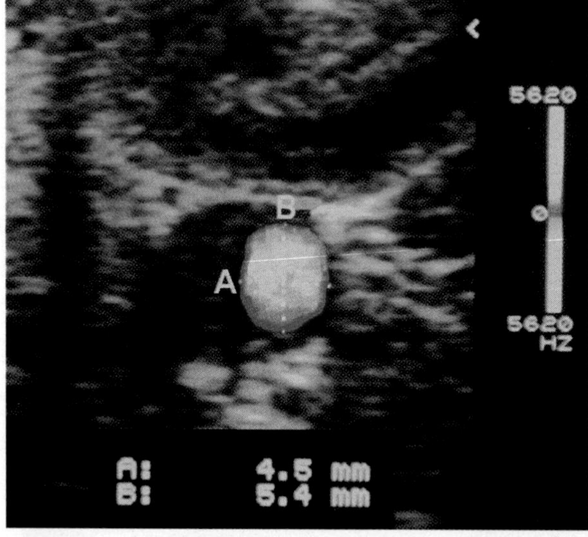

FIGURE 4–6 Enhanced visual stenosis measurement. (See p 74.) The residual lumen (cursors *A* and *B*) is clearly visualized in color, potentially enhancing measurement accuracy.

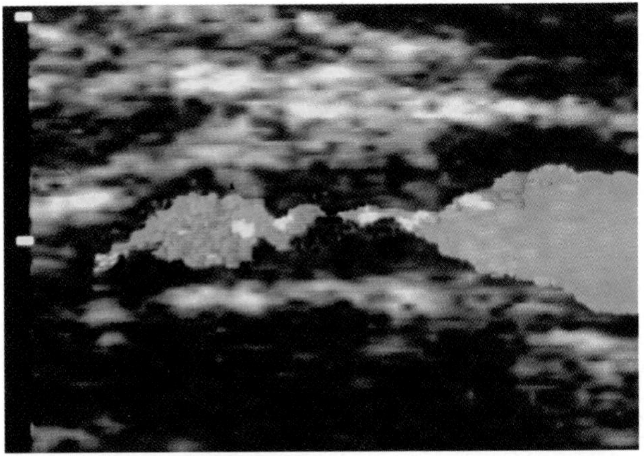

FIGURE 4–7 Stenosis vs. occlusion. (See p 74.) A tiny residual lumen is visualized with color-flow imaging in this internal carotid artery that might be difficult to identify otherwise.

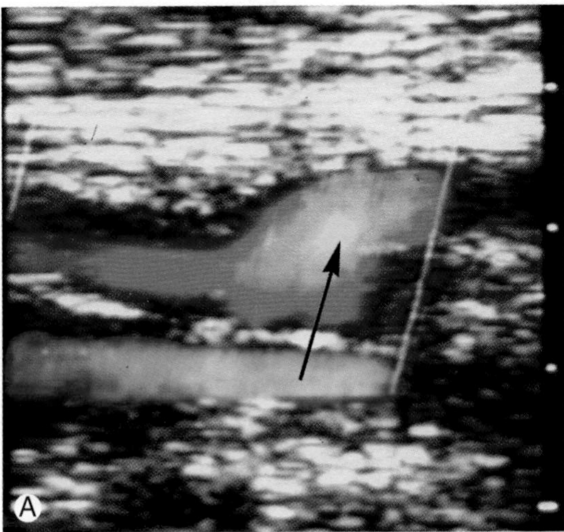

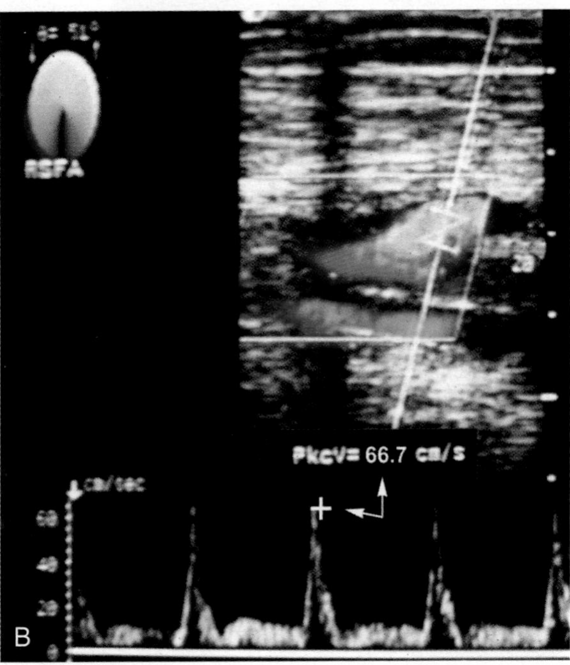

FIGURE 4–8 Color-flow information is qualitative, not quantitative. (See p 74.) *A,* It appears that the flow velocity is elevated at the origin of this arterial bypass graft (*arrow,* yellow color shift) because the color-flow image is not angle corrected. *B,* Angle-corrected spectral Doppler measurement shows a normal peak systolic velocity (66.7 cm/sec).

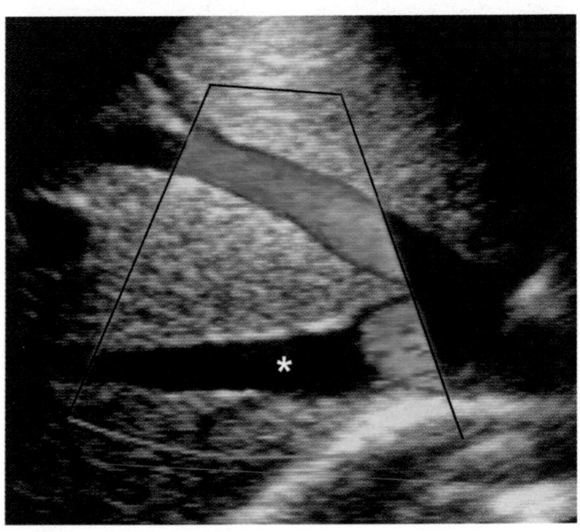

FIGURE 4–10 Spurious absence of flow. (See p 75.) It appears that flow is absent in the right hepatic artery (*asterisk*), because this vessel is perpendicular to the color-Doppler line of sight.

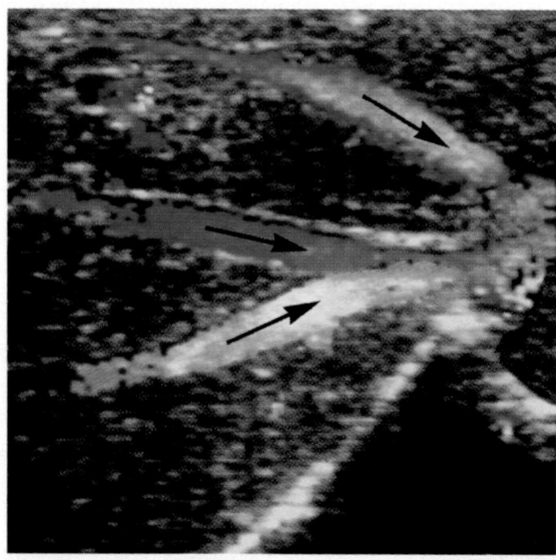

FIGURE 4–11 Color-flow direction is relative to the transducer. (See p 75.) Two of the hepatic veins are blue and one is red, implying that flow in the red vessel is in the opposite direction from the blue vessels. Flow actually is toward the inferior vena cava (*arrows*) in all of the vessels, but flow in the red vessel is relatively toward the transducer (top of image), whereas flow in the other vessels is relatively away from the transducer.

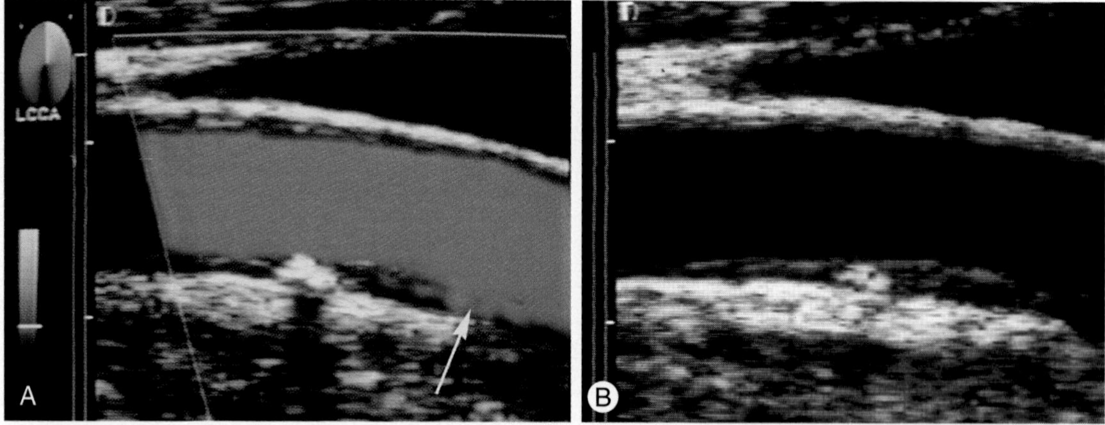

FIGURE 4–12 Color obscures plaque. (See p 75.) *A,* Color blooming obscures part of the plaque (*arrow*). *B,* The plaque is seen optimally with color flow turned off.

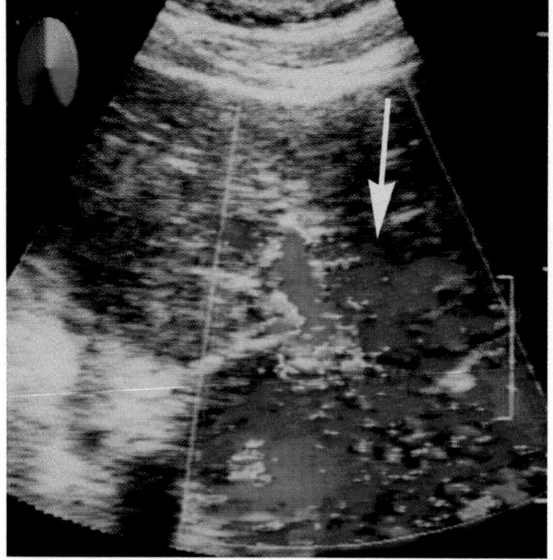

FIGURE 4–13 Color flash (*arrow*), shown in this transverse image of the epigastrium, obscures most of the anatomic detail. (See p 75.) The color flash was generated by aortic pulsations.

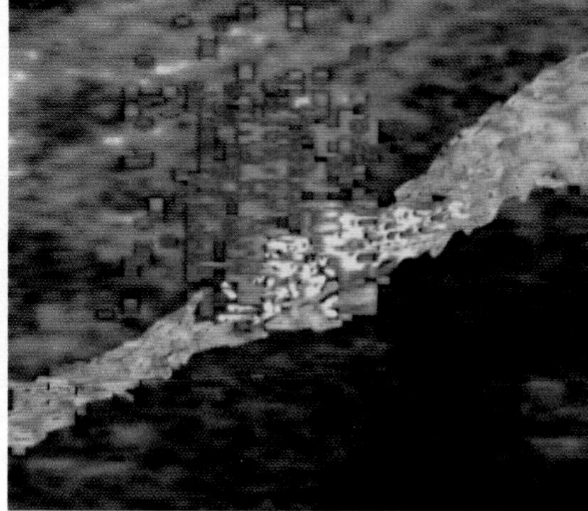

FIGURE 4–14 Visible bruit. (See p 75.) Soft-tissue vibrations cause a montage of color adjacent to this stenotic internal carotid artery.

an echo-enhancing agent (ultrasound contrast agent) is used to improve the detection of blood flow. Intravenous injection of the echo-enhancing agent greatly increases the Doppler signal intensity, causing overamplification and severe blooming. With power Doppler imaging, blooming does *not* occur, however, owing to the way that the flow–no flow determination is made.[6] Power Doppler imaging, therefore, may be the preferred method when echo enhancement is used.

In spite of its potential advantages over color-Doppler, power Doppler imaging has two major limitations. First, the frame rate is agonizingly slow, which renders this imaging method useless for rapidly moving vessels, rapidly moving patients (especially children), and areas subject to respiratory or cardiac motion. Second, power Doppler imaging does not provide flow direction information! (Remember, the Doppler power is imaged, not the Doppler shift, per se.) Without measuring the Doppler shift, the flow direction cannot be determined.

Color Flow vs. Color Doppler

The term *color flow* is broadly applied to all imaging systems that display blood flow in color. *Color Doppler* is correctly applied only to flow imaging methods based on Doppler ultrasound. Time-domain flow imaging (previously described) is not based on Doppler and should be referred to as *color-flow imaging,* not color Doppler. In this chapter, the generic term color flow is generally used.

ADVANTAGES OF COLOR-FLOW IMAGING

Leaving the technical details behind, we now consider color-flow imaging from a clinical perspective: Where does color flow help and where does it have problems? Stated differently, what are the capabilities and limitations of color-flow ultrasound?

Technical Efficiency

Perhaps the greatest advantages of color-flow imaging is technical efficiency. When moving blood is encountered, the vessel "lights up," even if the vessel is too small to be resolved on the gray-scale image (Fig. 4–4*A* [see p 70]). Because vessels stand out in vivid color, they may be located and followed much more easily than with gray-scale instruments. Furthermore, basic judgments about blood flow can be made relatively easily with color-flow imaging. The sonographer can quickly determine the presence of flow, the direction of flow, and the existence of focal flow disturbances. These improvements have expanded the capabilities of duplex sonography. For example, with color-flow imaging, it now is possible to quickly examine long vascular segments (see Fig. 4–4*B*), such as a vascular bypass graft, with relative ease. Furthermore, color-flow imaging facilitates the examination of vessels, such as the calf veins and the renal arteries, which traditionally have been difficult to study.

Assistance in Sorting Out Abdominal Anatomy

Another advantage of color-flow imaging is simplified differentiation between vascular and nonvascular structures, which is particularly useful in the abdomen. One of the most obvious applications (from a radiologist's perspective) is sorting out porta hepatis anatomy (Fig. 4–5 [see p 70]). The bile ducts, which do not exhibit flow, may be differentiated visually from the hepatic artery and portal vein, in which flow is seen.

Flow Assessment in the Entire Lumen

A major advantage of color-flow imaging is the depiction of blood flow throughout a large segment of a vessel, rather than solely at the Doppler sample volume. Because flow features are visible over a large area, localized flow abnormalities are readily apparent and are less likely to be overlooked than with gray-scale duplex methods. The sonographer is immediately made aware of the location of any flow abnormality, which speeds up the examination and permits rapid assessment of long segments of vessels for obstruction and other pathology.

Visual Measurement of Stenoses

As compared with gray-scale ultrasound, color-flow imaging makes it easier to define the residual lumen in stenotic vessels,[7,8] permitting more precise visual (non-Doppler) measurement of arterial stenoses (Fig. 4–6 [see p 70]). Direct, visual stenosis measurement remains problem prone, however, due to vessel tortuosity and acoustic shadows from calcified plaque.

Differentiation of Severe Stenosis and Occlusion

The ability of color-flow imaging to detect low velocity flow in a tiny residual lumen may facilitate the differentiation between occlusion of an artery and near-occlusion with a "trickle" of residual flow (Fig. 4–7 [see p 71]). Personal experience suggests that color-flow imaging is of value in this regard, and studies of the carotid arteries have shown improved results for detecting flow in near-occluded internal carotid arteries.[9,10]

LIMITATION OF COLOR-FLOW IMAGING

Flow Information Is Qualitative

It is most important to recognize that color-flow information is *qualitative* and not quantitative.[1–5] There are three reasons for this: (1) The flow image is based on the *average* Doppler shift within the vessel, rather than the *peak* Doppler shift. Recall that quantitative Doppler spectrum measurements are based on the peak Doppler shift, not the average shift; therefore, the average shift is not helpful for actually putting a *number* on a stenosis. Furthermore, the average Doppler shift is lowered by flow disturbances. (2) Color-flow information is qualitative because it is not corrected for the Doppler angle, which is the case with spectral Doppler measurements. (3) Color-flow information is qualitative because only a few frequency levels are shown. In essence, color-flow imaging is a visual form of Doppler spectrum analysis, but it is a very crude form in which only large frequency "steps" are visible.

Because color-flow images are qualitative, Doppler spectrum analysis must still be used to derive quantitative flow data (Fig. 4–8 [see p 71]). With some time-domain color-flow imaging systems, however, quantitative flow data can be derived from the color-flow display.*

Low Pulse Repetition Frequencies and Frame Rates

A tremendous amount of data must be processed by the color-flow instrument to generate each pixel (picture element) and each television frame. Processing these data take time, and the resultant delay may have serious adverse effects on the gray-scale and color-Doppler images, principally through reduced pulse repetition frequency (PRF, the number of pulses sent out per second) and reduced frame rate (the number of times per second that the television screen is renewed).

Reduced PRF may have the following deleterious effects: (1) The B-mode image may be degraded, because fewer data are available to build up the image (Fig. 4–9). (2) Doppler aliasing may be more common. As explained in Chapter 2, aliasing occurs when a Doppler shift is more than twice the PRF. As the PRF decreases, the Doppler frequency at which aliasing occurs is lowered proportionately. (3) Low PRF and low frame rates may limit the visualization of rapidly moving cardiac or vascular events. For example, cardiac valve motion may be less clearly seen with color-flow scanning than with gray-scale scanning. (4) Low frame rates may produce image flicker. If the frame rate is reduced below 15 frames/sec, the human eye no longer "blurs" the ultrasound images into a moving picture.[11] Instead, each image (or frame) pauses visibly on the screen. These pauses are annoying, but more importantly, they may distort moving objects or cause them to disappear from view.

Flow Detection Is Angle-Dependent

Blood flow is not detected with color-Doppler devices in vessels that are perpendicular to the ultrasound beam. (Color-Doppler devices are similar to spectral Doppler devices in this respect.) A false-positive diagnosis of vascular occlusion may occur if a vessel is approximately perpendicular to the

---

* Philips Medical Systems, Ultrasound Division, Santa Anna, CA.

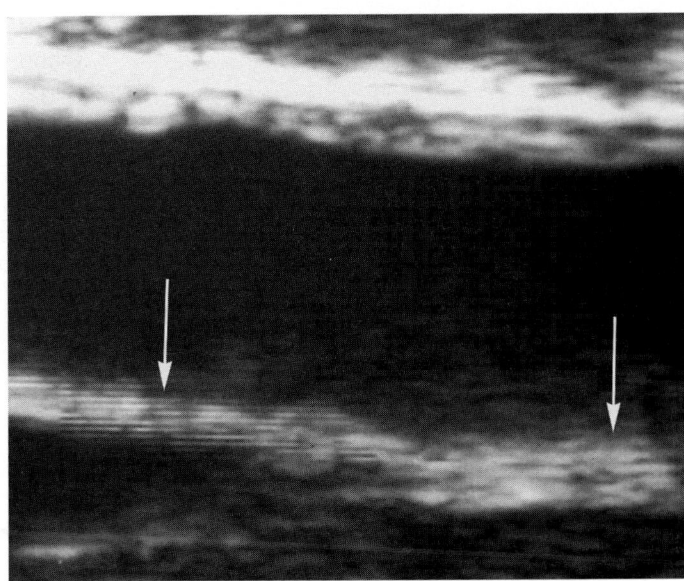

FIGURE 4–9 Low frame rate causes blurring. The margin of this blood vessel is blurred (*arrows*) because the frame rate is only 9 frames/sec.

ultrasound beam (Fig. 4–10 [see p 71]). This is a particularly severe problem when curved array scanners are used for color-Doppler imaging. (Try imaging vessels with a curved array, and you will see what I mean.)

Flow Direction Is Arbitrary

It is crucial to remember that the color of the vessel on the color-flow image is *not* an absolute indication of flow direction. The color is assigned relative to the transducer (Fig. 4–11 [see p 72]). The operator may reverse the color scheme (arteries blue, veins red) simply by reversing the orientation of the transducer or by pushing a button on the instrument. To determine the true direction of flow, the operator must closely observe the orientation of the vessel relative to the transducer or refer to a vessel in which the flow direction is known, such as the aorta.

Color May Obscure Vascular Pathology

If the instrument controls are improperly adjusted, the color-flow information tends to "bloom" into the surrounding gray-scale image (Fig. 4–12 [see p 72]), as mentioned previously. Important vascular pathology, including plaque and venous thrombus, may be obscured by blooming.

Color Flash

With color-flow imaging, anything within the field of view that moves relative to the transducer is shown in color. In the abdomen, peristaltic motion, cardiac motion, or transmitted pulsations from great vessels may generate blotches of color on the ultrasound image called *color flash,* which can obscure structures of interest (Fig. 4–13 [see p 72]). The color flash problem is particularly apparent in the upper abdomen, because of heart motion.

THE STRANGE CASE OF THE VISIBLE BRUIT

The *visible bruit* is a peculiar, but useful, flow phenomenon (Fig. 4–14 [see p 72]) that can be seen with color-flow imaging.[12] A montage of color is seen within the soft tissues adjacent to the blood vessel; this color effect is caused by vibration of the vessel. This vibration, in turn, is caused by a severe flow disturbance within the vessel. A visible bruit suggests severe arterial stenosis, but caution is advised in interpreting this finding, because severe flow disturbances may sometime occur in the absence of significant stenosis. The term *visible bruit* is a misnomer, because a bruit is a sound and is not visible. Nonetheless, I like this term; the tissue vibration seen with color-flow imaging is also the cause of the bruit heard with a stethoscope.

OPTIMIZING COLOR-FLOW IMAGE QUALITY

The color-flow image is derived from relatively weak reflections from red blood cells. Because these reflections are weak, flow detection sensitivity is particularly susceptible to ultrasound instrument settings. The following technical tricks should be tried when it is difficult to obtain an adequate color-flow image. These tricks are summarized in Table 4–1.

1. *Velocity range:* Consider whether the instrument is set for the proper velocity range. If the instrument is set to detect arterial velocities, it is not sensitive to venous velocities, or vice versa. Adjust the PRF or the velocity range to a level appropriate for the vessel of interest.
2. *Doppler angle:* Remember that the Doppler angle (as described in Chapters 2 and 3) profoundly affects the color-flow image. The strength of the color-flow image diminishes as the Doppler angle decreases. So, when flow is absent in a vessel, ask, "Do I have an adequate Doppler angle?" If not, move the color-flow box or the transducer to improve the Doppler angle.
3. *Field of view:* Consider the depth of field shown on the image. Use only as much depth as you need! Greater depth requires a longer roundtrip time for the ultrasound pulses, decreasing the PRF, decreasing the number of pulses per square centimeter of tissue, and increasing the signal-processing time. The net result is diminished ability to display flow (as well as gray-scale image degradation).
4. *Color box size:* Consider the size of the color box. For the same reasons that were stated previously for *Field of view,* pulse-echo information becomes increasingly "diluted" as the color box is enlarged. It is best to use a small color box, especially when examining vessels deep within the body.
5. *Power and gain:* Determine if the output power of the instrument, the time compensated gain, and the color gain are optimal. Insufficient power or gain can result in inadequate color-flow information.
6. *Color priority:* Consider whether the gray-scale or color priority is adjusted correctly. Most (if not all) color-flow instruments permit the operator to determine whether the gray-scale or color image is given more attention. If the gray-scale image is prioritized, then the color image suffers, and vice versa. If you are having trouble detecting flow, shift the image processing priority toward color.
7. *Thump control:* See if the thump control is eliminating too much color-flow information. Thump control refers to electronic filtering that removes color artifacts generated by the heart or vascular pulsations. Thump control is not needed in smaller peripheral vessels and should be set as low as is practical.
8. *Wall filter:* Check the wall filter setting. If the wall filter is set too high, low-frequency signals generated by low velocity flow are eliminated. The wall filter is designed to eliminate low frequency noise, but if it is set too high, it also eliminates flow information. This is not a problem with high velocity flow, but it may be a major problem for detection of venous flow or for evaluating small intrarenal arteries.
9. *Very slow flow:* Finally, remember that flow might be present that simply is too slow for color-flow visualization. Power Doppler or spectral Doppler may be more sensitive to the presence of slow flow than standard color-Doppler imaging, and it may be useful to switch to these modalities when a vessel appears occluded.

TABLE 4–1 WHAT TO CHECK WHEN YOU CANNOT DETECT BLOOD FLOW

Velocity range
Doppler angle
Field of view
Color box size
Power and gain
Color priority
Gray-scale priority
Thump control
Wall filter
Is flow too slow?

REFERENCES

1. Switzer DF, Nanda NC: Doppler color flow mapping. Ultrasound Med Biol 11:403–416, 1985.
2. Merritt CRB: Doppler blood flow imaging: Integrating flow with tissue data. Diagn Imaging 11:146–155, 1986.
3. Powis RL: Color flow imaging: Understanding its science and technology. J Diagn Med Sonograph 4:236–245, 1988.
4. Carroll BA: Carotid sonography: Pitfalls and color flow. Appl Radiol 10:15–21, 1988.

5. Nelson TR, Pretorius DH: The Doppler signal: Where does it come from and what does it mean? AJR Am J Roentgenol 151:439–447, 1988.
5a. Gardiner W, Fox MD: Color-flow ultrasound imaging through the analysis of speckle motion. Radiology 172:866–868, 1989.
6. Murphy KJ, Rubin JM: Power Doppler: It's a good thing. Semin Ultrasound 18:13–21, 1997.
7. Erickson SJ, Mewissen MW, Foley WD, et al: Stenosis of the internal carotid artery: Assessment using color Doppler imaging compared with angiography. AJR Am J Roentgenol 152:1299–1305, 1989.
8. Polak JF, Dobkin GR, O'Leary DH, et al: Internal carotid artery stenosis: Accuracy and reproducibility of color-Doppler assisted duplex imaging. Radiology 173:793–798, 1989.
9. Chang YJ, Lin SK, Ryu SJ, Wai YY: Common carotid artery occlusion: Evaluation with duplex sonography. AJNR Am J Neuroradiol 16:1099–1105, 1995.
10. Lee DH, Gao FQ, Rankin RN, et al: Duplex and color Doppler flow sonography of occlusion and near occlusion of the carotid artery. AJNR Am J Neuroradiol 17:1267–1274, 1996.
11. Powis RL, Powis WD: A Thinker's Guide to Ultrasonic Imaging. Baltimore, Urban & Schwarzenberg, 1984, pp 345–364.
12. Middleton WD, Erickson S, Melson GL: Perivascular color artifact: Pathologic significance and appearance on color Doppler ultrasound images. Radiology 171:647–652, 1989.

Chapter 5

SONOGRAPHIC CONTRAST AGENTS

■ *Michelle L. Melany, MD* ■ *Edward G. Grant, MD*

Contrast agents are used extensively in many forms of modern medical imaging. In general, these compounds are used to change a specific property of an organ with regard to its surrounding tissues. Contrast agents increase the signal-to-noise ratio and allow improved imaging of targeted organ systems. The exact method by which this improved imaging is accomplished depends on the type of examination being performed. With most radiographic examinations, such as that of the upper gastrointestinal (GI) tract, or intravenous pyelography, and computed tomography (CT), it is desirable to increase the density of a specific organ system relative to that of the surrounding tissues. Therefore, high molecular weight elements such as barium or iodine are ingested or injected into the body. With magnetic resonance imaging, iron and other strongly magnetic agents are used to alter the magnetic signal of various structures in the body.

The application of contrast agents to sonographic examinations has received relatively little attention. Clinical use of sonographic contrast agents has been a reality only during the last decade. Although many compounds can theoretically increase echogenicity within the body, most agents use air bubbles to increase reflectivity.

TYPES OF CONTRAST AGENTS

Radiographic contrast agents fall into three broad categories. First, contrast agents may be used to outline a hollow viscus. The most common of these agents, barium and related compounds, are used to evaluate the GI tract. Sonographic GI contrast agents, such as methylcellulose and associated compounds, are under investigation as a means to better outline the upper GI tract sonographically.[1] Several other agents have been used with sonography to define patency of the fallopian tubes[2, 3] and to identify patients with vesicoureteral reflux.[4]

A second broad category of contrast agents includes those compounds that are used to outline the vascular tree. Angiography has long been the prototype for this category of agents. Magnetic resonance angiography and CT angiography have also become popular methods to directly evaluate blood vessels; both rely on the administration of intravenous contrast agents. Most sonographic contrast agents that are injected intravenously have been used for this purpose and enhance visualization of macroscopic blood vessels.

A third broad category of contrast agents provides parenchymal enhancement. Early investigators evaluated several particulate agents including iodipamide ethyl ester[5] and perfluorooctylbromide (PFOB).[6] The exact mechanism by which these compounds increased echogenicity is not entirely understood, but at least in the case of PFOB, it is thought to result from its high density and low acoustic velocity.[7] To some degree, PFOB may also vaporize into microbubbles.[8] These particulate contrast agents function in a similar fashion to those used in nuclear scintigraphy. They are taken up by the Kupffer cells of the liver. Because tumors lack these reticuloendothelial cells, the overall echogenicity of the liver is increased in relation to that of intrahepatic tumors. Although the PFOB compounds do, indeed, increase contrast between normal liver tissue and tumors, they have not come into clinical use due to their high incidence of side effects.[8]

PHYSICAL PROPERTIES

Most contrast agents under investigation rely on echogenicity produced by microbubbles. These agents are distributed throughout the vascular tree and eventually into the microvasculature of parenchymal tissues. Although parenchymal enhancement represents the end organ response to an intravascular injection and is therefore related to the category of vascular agents described previously, the information obtained in the final image (from CT, magnetic resonance imaging, ultrasonography) or radiograph (from intravenous pyelography, angiography) is quite different from simple opacification of large vessels. Investigators are just beginning to evaluate the potential of sonographic contrast agents to facilitate true parenchymal enhancement of visceral organs.[9]

Sonographic contrast agents are not new. The use of rudimentary agents dates back to the late 1960s. The most commonly used agent has been a simple solution of handshaken saline for echocardiography. This material is injected through a superficial vein and is of limited clinical value because the bubbles do not cross into the left side of the heart in normal patients. This application, however, is still used extensively in clinical practice when evaluating the heart for shunts. An interesting adaptation of this simple form of ultrasonic contrast has been used by several Japanese investigators to identify liver tumors. In these studies, carbon dioxide was injected into the hepatic artery, and it successfully outlined hepatomas.[10, 11] Although a novel approach, the necessity for arterial access limits practical applicability. Currently, in the United States, the only Food and Drug Administration (FDA)-approved contrast agents are Albunex* and Optison.* Both agents are approved only for examinations of the heart at this time. However, numerous trials are in progress with Albunex and other agents, several of which will likely receive FDA approval for wider clinical use including radiologic applications.

A clinically useful sonographic contrast agent should possess several specific properties. The most obvious of these is that the agent is nontoxic. Most agents that have been evaluated demonstrate minimal toxicity (with the exception of PFOB as described earlier) with infrequent, minor side effects such as nausea, flushing, or headache. Most sonographic contrast agents are composed of microbubbles that are excreted via the lungs. Pulmonary excretion of sonographic contrast agents avoids the complication of nephrotoxicity, a drawback that plagues iodinated contrast agents.

A successful contrast agent must also be easily injectable through a peripheral vein. Additionally, to be clinically useful, sonographic contrast agents must have the ability to pass through the pulmonary circulation without being destroyed and to remain intact within the body for an extended period. If the compound is filtered by the capillaries of the lungs and unable to pass through the pulmonary vasculature, a venous injection will not provide opacification of the systemic arterial tree, and the agent will be unable to reach the capillary beds of most solid organs, precluding both arterial and parenchymal enhancement. The use of contrast agents that do not pass through the pulmonary vasculature, such as handshaken saline or Albunex, is limited to opacification of veins that have been directly injected or to examination of the right side of the heart for evaluation of intracardiac shunts.[12]

The contrast agent must remain intact for a time period sufficient to allow adequate scanning of the organ of interest. Although a major problem has been filtering by the lungs, the bubbles themselves, regardless of the surrounding shell, tend to be unstable; they burst at various time intervals after injection, limiting their ability to provide arterial contrast enhancement. Albunex, although small enough to pass through the capillary bed of the lungs, is largely destroyed by the rapid pressure changes to which it is subjected as it passes through the heart.[13] Studies also suggest that the interaction of the ultrasound beam with the contrast agent may cause sufficient agitation to burst contrast air bubbles, and therefore the ultrasound examination itself may shorten the half-life of these compounds.[14]

Another desirable property of an ideal contrast agent is uniform particle size. This property extends half-life, allowing consistent passage through the pulmonary capillary bed (assuming the compound is small enough to pass through the pulmonary circulation), and predicts a reasonably consistent duration of enhancement. Particles used in ultrasound contrast agents generally range from 1 to 10 μm.[15] To successfully pass through the pulmonary microcirculation, they must be smaller than the expected diameter of the capillaries, which is approximately 7 μm.

*Mallinckrodt Medical, St. Louis, MO.

ARTIFACTS

A detailed discussion of the physics of contrast agents is beyond the scope of this chapter. However, several important properties are worth reviewing. In general, within the limits of improved imaging, the aim of contrast agents is to increase the ultrasound signal that is returned to the transducer. The ability to increase the signal is proportional to the size of the scatterer, the density of the contrast agent, and the compressibility of the microbubbles.[5, 16–18] All sonographic contrast agents function by increasing backscatter or reflectivity. If one could increase this property infinitely, there would be a practical limit because excessive backscatter leads to shadowing and obscures the organ of interest and the tissues posterior to it.[5, 19]

Organ-selective agents have yet to be developed, and marked enhancement of all vessels and surrounding tissues can degrade ultrasound image quality. This phenomenon is frequently encountered immediately after injection of sonographic contrast agent and is referred to as "blooming"[17] (Fig. 5–1). The amount of backscatter is so overwhelming that the enhancement appears to extend beyond the limits of the vascular structures and parenchymal organs being evaluated. This is a transient phenomenon, and, depending on the severity, it may be diminished by delaying the beginning of the scan until it resolves. Alternatively, one may lower the machine's sensitivity (gain) until adequate vessel appearance is achieved and then gradually increase the gain as the contrast effect diminishes.

Another artifact of contrast agents is termed "bubble noise" (Fig. 5–2). This is a similar phenomenon to the situation described in patients with air in the portal vein, and it refers to an audible "pinging" while scanning. This is translated into a spiked appearance of the spectral signal. According to Forsberg and colleagues,[20] this artifact may be secondary to instability and bursting of bubbles or to the presence of large bubbles in solution. This phenomenon, although worth noting, seems to cause little interference with the ultrasound scan itself.

Finally, several authors have reached divergent conclusions regarding the effect of a contrast agent on perceived spectral velocities. Some investigators have noted an elevation in peak systolic velocity, which they believe may represent an artifact of sonographic contrast agents. Alternatively, a contrast agent may facilitate detection of real, but weak, previously undetected high-velocity Doppler signals. This elevation of velocity may vary depending on the contrast agent under investigation. Forsberg and coworkers[20] have demonstrated elevated velocities of 20 to 45% after the injection of Albunex and Levovist* in rabbits. This phenomenon has not been thoroughly investigated in humans. Our experience in the evaluation of renal artery stenosis has demonstrated little change in peak systolic velocity after injection of the contrast agent EchoGen† in a population of normal humans. In our study, however, patients with stenoses sometimes exhibited marked elevation in peak systolic velocity. This phenomenon did not seem to affect our use of existing diagnostic criteria for renal artery stenosis because it was identified only in patients with stenoses. Patients with stenoses have numerous flow jets and eddies that may be too subtle to be seen with routine sonography but become clinically detectable after injection of a contrast agent. This phenomenon needs further investigation as contrast-induced velocity elevation could affect the application of established velocity criteria for stenosis and other Doppler-related diagnoses. If these agents lead to an elevation in velocity, re-evaluation of Doppler parameters for various disease processes would need to be performed before widespread clinical application of sonographic contrast in the future.

All modes of sonographic imaging have been investigated with regard to the use of a contrast agent. Thus far, the most dramatic effects have been on imaging with spectral and color Doppler. Parenchymal or gray-scale enhancement will likely be realized shortly by newer generations of agents. Although most of the work thus far has been on developing new contrast agents, modification of machine settings for optimum reception of contrast signal will also be necessary and will probably appear routinely as "presets" on machines in the future. Color–power Doppler imaging has been used in conjunction with contrast agents and is believed by some to be more sensitive to contrast agents than conventional color-Doppler imaging.[21]

*Schering AG, Berlin, Germany.
†Sonus Pharmaceuticals, Bothell, WA.

Text continued on page 87

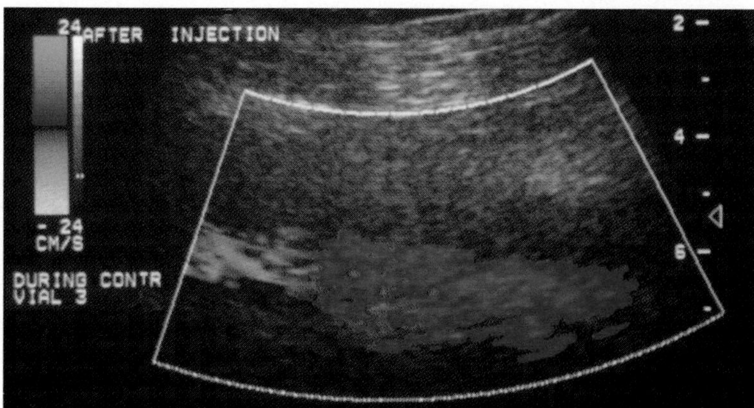

FIGURE 5–1 Sonographic artifact, blooming. Patient with severely swollen right leg suspected of deep venous thrombosis. Veins of the middle and distal thigh could not be visualized with conventional scanning. After injection of Albunex, the distal superficial femoral vein was well visualized. Immediately after injection, however, the contrast response was excessive, producing blooming. Note the extension of color beyond the apparent lumen of the vein. (From Melany ML, Grant EG: Clinical experience with sonographic contrast agents. Semin Ultrasound CT MR 18:3–12, 1997.)

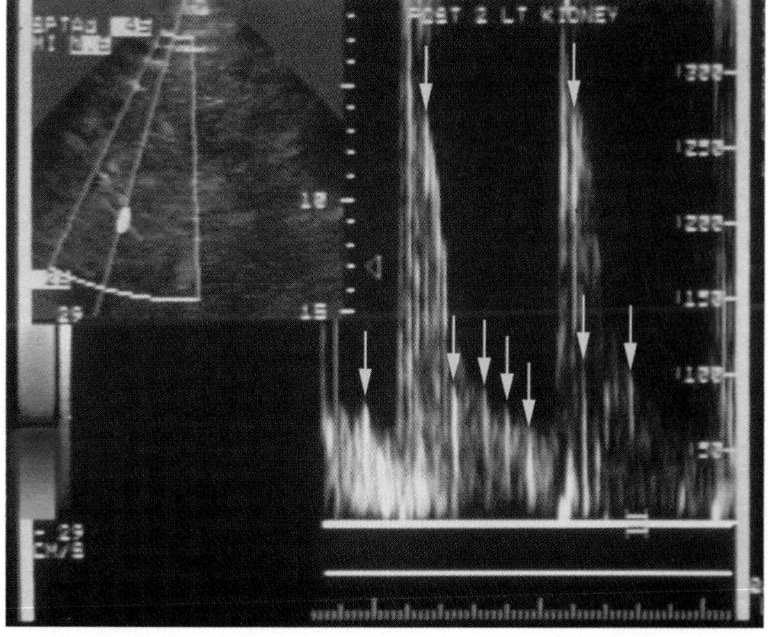

FIGURE 5–2 Sonographic artifact, bubble noise. This sonographic artifact may be secondary to bursting of bubbles within the sonographic field, or multiple large bubbles producing strong echoes. After injection of a contrast agent, a generally "spiky" appearance to the spectral tracing is often found and is probably secondary to numerous strong echoes produced by the contrast. Multiple bright internal lines representing specific, strong bubble noise artifacts are found in this image (*arrows*). (From Melany ML, Grant EG: Clinical experience with sonographic contrast agents. Semin Ultrasound CT MR 18:3–12, 1997.)

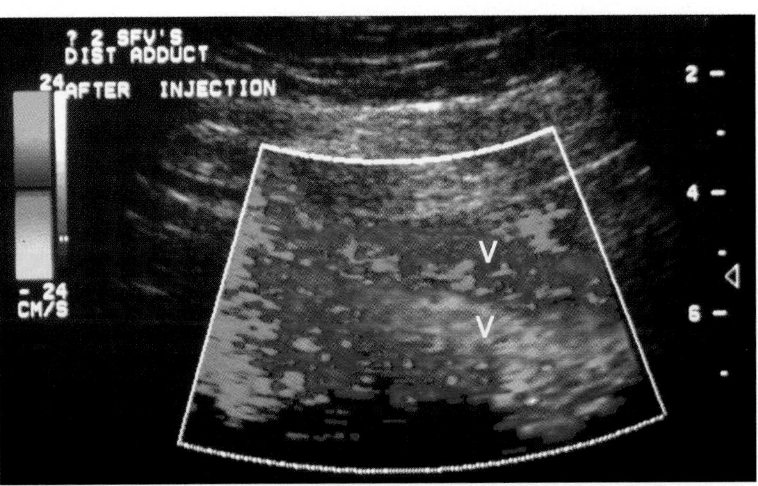

FIGURE 5–4 Improved visualization of venous anatomy with Albunex. Longitudinal image through distal adductor canal was nondiagnostic due to the inability to image the venous structures in this patient with a severely swollen leg. After injection of contrast material through a foot vein, a well-defined double superficial femoral vein (V) was identified. Note considerable degree of blooming in this image. (From Melany ML, Grant EG: Clinical experience with sonographic contrast agents. Semin Ultrasound CT MR 18:3–12, 1997.)

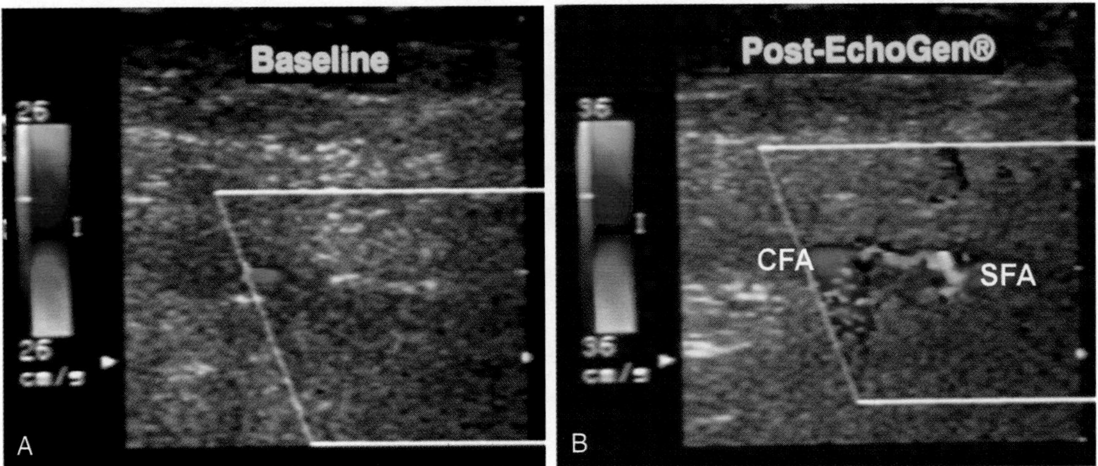

FIGURE 5–5 Improved imaging of a peripheral artery after injection of EchoGen. *A,* Before contrast agent injection, flow could not be identified in the superficial femoral artery. *B,* After injection of EchoGen, flow is well defined in the superficial femoral artery (SFA) and a stenosis is visible. CFA = common femoral artery. (From Melany ML, Grant EG: Clinical experience with sonographic contrast agents. Semin Ultrasound CT MR 18:3–12, 1997.)

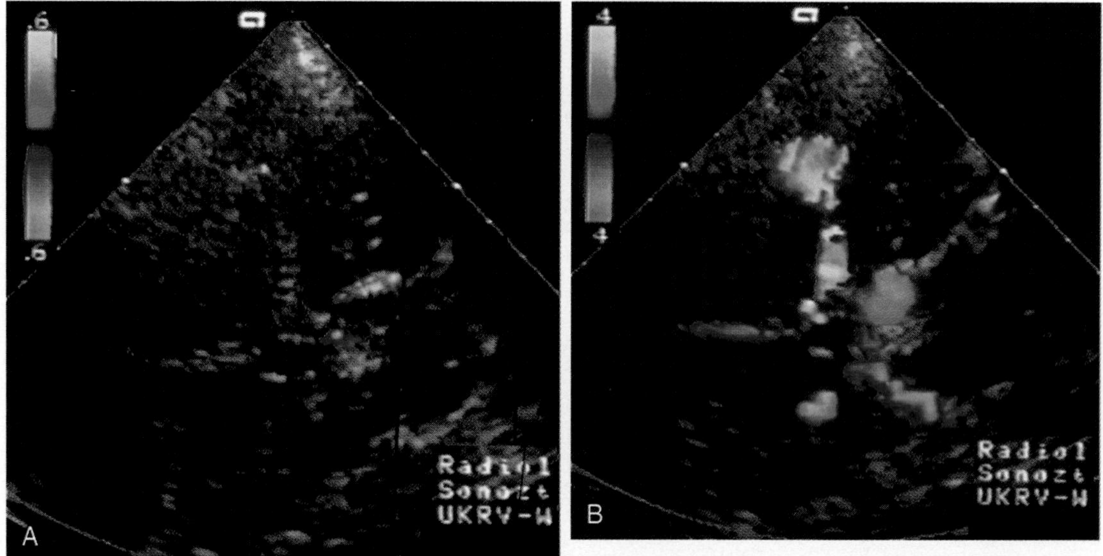

FIGURE 5–6 Transcranial Doppler with contrast. The ability to define the intracranial vasculature may be difficult when scanning through the skull. Suboptimal studies may be obtained in as many as 20% of patients. *A,* Noncontrast scan provides imaging of only a small portion of the posterior cerebral artery and middle cerebral artery. *B,* After injection of Levovist, all major vessels about the circle of Willis are well visualized, including both the ipsilateral and the contralateral middle cerebral arteries, the posterior cerebral arteries, and the anterior cerebral artery. (From Melany ML, Grant EG: Clinical experience with sonographic contrast agents. Semin Ultrasound CT MR 18:3–12, 1997.)

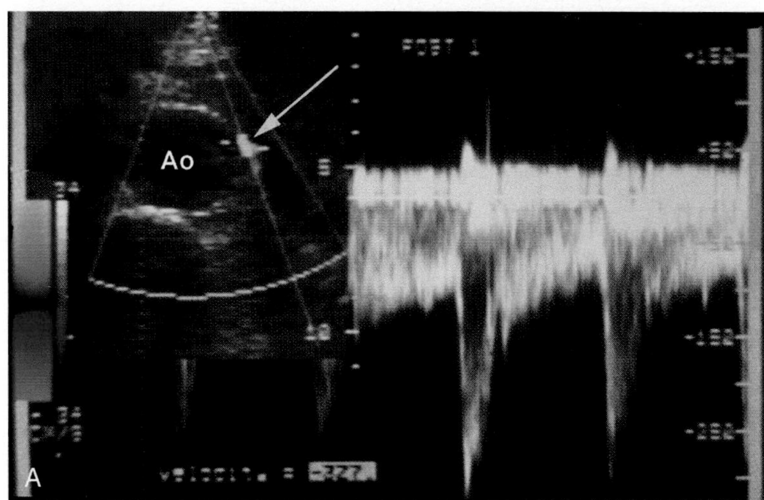

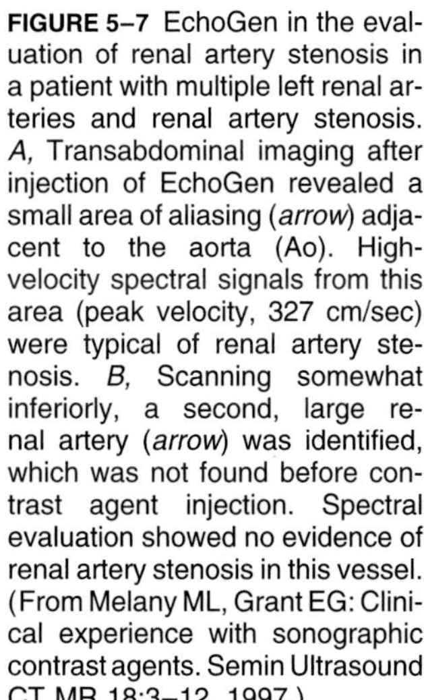
FIGURE 5–7 EchoGen in the evaluation of renal artery stenosis in a patient with multiple left renal arteries and renal artery stenosis. *A,* Transabdominal imaging after injection of EchoGen revealed a small area of aliasing (*arrow*) adjacent to the aorta (Ao). High-velocity spectral signals from this area (peak velocity, 327 cm/sec) were typical of renal artery stenosis. *B,* Scanning somewhat inferiorly, a second, large renal artery (*arrow*) was identified, which was not found before contrast agent injection. Spectral evaluation showed no evidence of renal artery stenosis in this vessel. (From Melany ML, Grant EG: Clinical experience with sonographic contrast agents. Semin Ultrasound CT MR 18:3–12, 1997.)

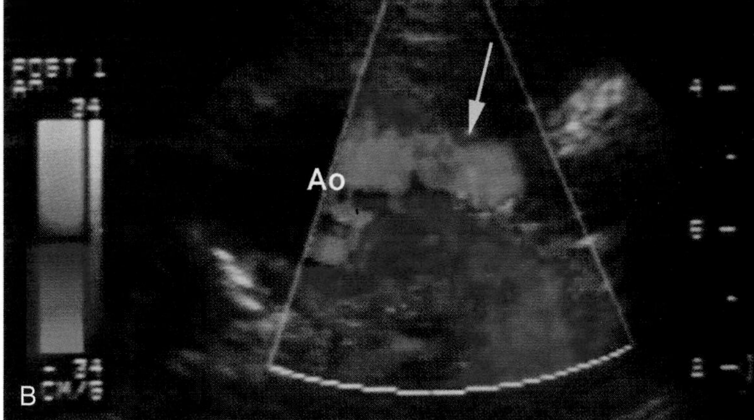

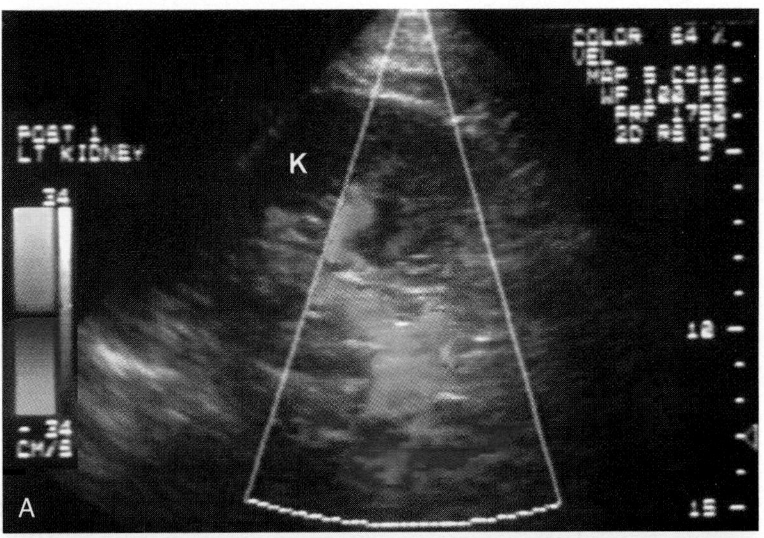

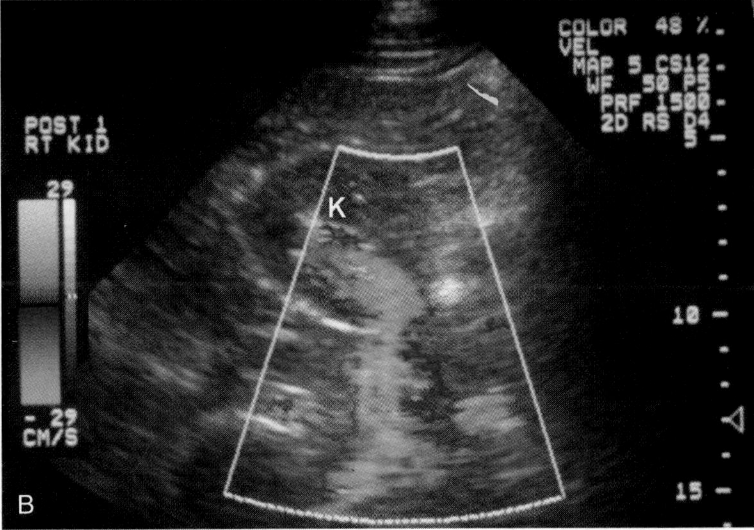

FIGURE 5–8 Normal renal arteries postcontrast. *A, B,* There is excellent visualization of entire right and left renal arteries (red vessels) after injection of EchoGen. These images represented considerable improvement over precontrast scans (not shown). K = kidney. (From Melany ML, Grant EG: Clinical experience with sonographic contrast agents. Semin Ultrasound CT MR 18:3–12, 1997.)

HARMONIC IMAGING

A characteristic of contrast agents that may be used in the future is harmonic imaging (Fig. 5–3), which relies on the inherent property of microbubbles to resonate at specific frequencies once they have encountered the ultrasound beam. Each compound has a specific resonant frequency and various subharmonic frequencies. The resonant frequency is largely dependent on particle size.[21–23] Although harmonic imaging has not been extensively evaluated in humans, animal studies suggest that this may be a method to further enhance the effect of contrast agents. Harmonic imaging requires an ultrasound machine which can transmit the sound beam at a specific frequency and receive it at the resonant frequency. The resonant frequency is twice that of the transmitting frequency. The signal-to-noise ratio is improved because in theory only the echoes arriving back to the transducer from the object (contrast agent) are displayed. This concept is similar to subtraction angiography, in which all is removed from the image except the contrast-filled blood vessels. Research indicates that harmonic imaging may be particularly useful when conventional sonographic imaging is limited by motion artifact. Examples include imaging of the heart and vessels, such as the renal arteries, located deep in the abdomen adjacent to the pulsating aorta.

CLINICAL APPLICATIONS

Most sonographic contrast agents use air bubbles that are injected intravenously into the patient. This is the basis for the original "homemade" contrast agent, agitated saline. The success of more sophisticated contrast agents has been dependent on stabilization of these air bubbles, which are typically short-lived in the peripheral circulation, and to transport them within the body by means of a carrier agent. Albunex relies on albumin and encapsulated microbubbles[24] (Fig. 5–4

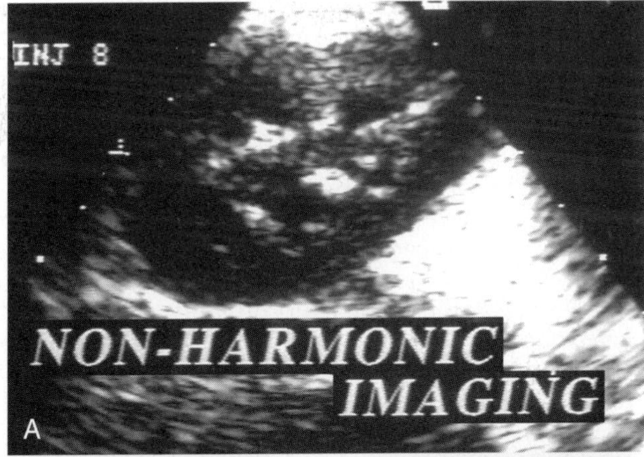

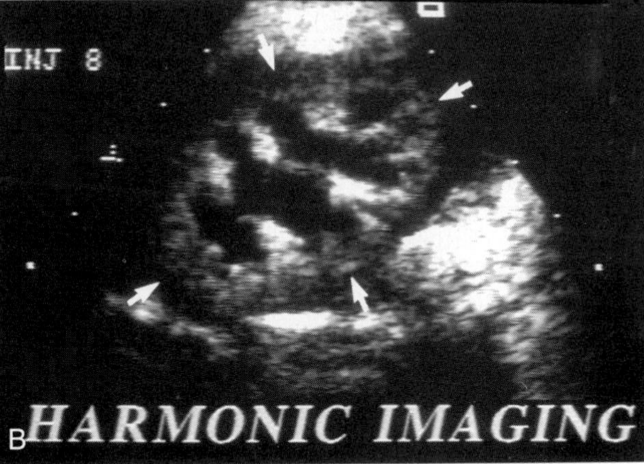

FIGURE 5–3 Harmonic imaging, gray-scale visualization of contrast. *A,* 2.5-MHz scan reveals poor definition of tissue contrast in the kidneys. *B,* Harmonic mode (transmitted frequency, 2.5 MHz; received frequency, 5.0 MHz); contrast within blood vessels can be clearly identified (*arrows*). This effect was far more impressive in real-time as contrast pulsated in vessels. (From Needleman L, Forsberg F: Contrast agents in ultrasound. Ultrasound Q 13:121–138, 1996.)

[see p 83]). Echovist* and Levovist depend on a galactose carrier.[25, 26] Various lipid and surfactant contrast agents are also under investigation.[27, 28] Fluorocarbon shells have been used as carrier agents, and clinical trials are currently under way with EchoGen (perflenapent emulsion), a phase-shift fluorocarbon agent.[29] The latter compound, a liquid at room temperature, has a relatively low boiling point and turns to a gas at body temperature, producing microbubbles. It is likely that additional innovative methods of achieving ultrasound contrast, both with and without bubbles, will be encountered in the future.

Albunex was the first FDA-approved agent in the United States. Thus, there is probably more human experience with this agent than with any other contrast agent to date. Unfortunately, Albunex is largely a single-pass agent. When injected intravenously, it passes through the lungs as evidenced by its appearance in the left atrium and ventricle. However, the stress of pressure changes in the left side of the heart causes Albunex to be largely destroyed while passing through the heart, leaving little to reach the arterial tree.[13] For these reasons, its clinical utility is limited. Echocardiographic uses for this agent include the evaluation of intracardiac shunts and valvular dysfunction and the simple opacification of the cardiac chambers.[12, 30]

Several groups have evaluated Albunex in the peripheral veins of the upper and lower extremities. Indeed, opacification of the lower extremity veins can be achieved with this agent (see Fig. 5–4). Unfortunately, similar to conventional contrast venography, this technique requires injection through a superficial foot or hand vein, which may be difficult to access in patients with severely swollen limbs who are suspected of having deep venous thrombosis. Additionally, because the volume of contrast agent injected is relatively small, the agent may tend to pool in the calf of a patient with either venous reflux or varicose veins. In our experience, increased vessel conspicuity was identified, and anatomically difficult to evaluate regions, such as the calf veins and the adductor canal, were more readily visualized after contrast agent injection. Collaterals were more confidently identified in patients with chronic deep venous thrombosis, and preferential shunting of blood into the superficial veins was identified on postcontrast scans. Variant venous anatomy was also more readily depicted (see Fig. 5–4).[31] Needleman and associates[32] used Albunex in the assessment of upper extremity venous disease, but the number of patients in this series was small. It was postulated in this study that the echogenicity of the thrombus itself might have increased after injection of Albunex, but this effect has not been observed by other groups. Evaluation of the inferior vena cava and vena caval filters has also been undertaken using contrast agents. Vorwerk and colleagues[33] reported improved ability to demonstrate caval blood flow and flow around the filters in 35 patients using Echovist. Although it is technically possible to depict the deep venous structures with a contrast agent, the vast majority of venous examinations are adequate using current ultrasound technology *without* the addition of a contrast agent. This, coupled with cost and the difficulty and discomfort of foot vein injections, probably limits the applicability of contrast agents in venous disease.

The galactose-based contrast agents typified by Levovist and Echovist have been investigated in both the United States and Europe. These agents cause few side effects and are considered to be safe. Approval for clinical use has been granted in many European countries and in Australia. Several large studies, including a multicenter trial in Europe involving more than 1200 patients, have evaluated these agents for both cardiac and vascular uses. This review found improvement in diagnostic confidence after a suboptimal baseline scan in over 80% of cases.[34]

Other studies evaluated the ability of contrast-enhanced sonography to visualize the arterial tree (Fig. 5–5 [see p 83]). Needleman and coworkers[35] revealed improvement in the ability to depict renal, superior mesenteric, and peripheral arteries in 86% of cases. Even better results were demonstrated by Schwartz and associates[36] in a study in which peripheral leg arteries, mitral valve lesions, and intracranial vessels (using transcranial Doppler) were identified. In this population, 100% of patients demonstrated vascular enhancement after injection of a contrast agent. The effect of a contrast agent was further substantiated by the use of time-intensity curves showing appropriate increase then decrease in intensity of blood signals. Diagnostic confidence increased from 35 to 90% and there were no major side effects. Unfortunately, no

*Schering AG, Berlin, Germany.

"gold standard" was used to confirm the accuracy of postcontrast diagnoses in this particular study. Two additional studies have specifically evaluated the effect of Levovist in the peripheral arteries of the legs.[37, 38] Both demonstrated positive results in clinically problematic areas. Vessels that are typically difficult to visualize sonographically, such as the iliac arteries, the superficial femoral artery in the adductor canal, the trifurcation vessels, and the plantar arteries were better seen. Differentiation between patent and nonpatent vessels was also improved in complicated scanning situations such as obesity, edema, or dense vascular calcifications.[37]

In the genitourinary tract, Levovist has been used in the evaluation of renal artery stenosis and tumors of the kidney and prostate. Balen and colleagues[39] reported the results of contrast injection on the *segmental* renal arteries in 26 patients and found that the number of inadequate studies secondary to poor Doppler signal quality decreased from 22 to 0%. As such, accuracy of identifying stenoses greater than 60% improved from 80 to 91%; sensitivity increased to 95%. The time required to perform bilateral examinations dropped from 25 to 14 minutes after administration of a contrast agent. Although these results are impressive, in our experience, the inability to obtain technically satisfactory Doppler waveforms has not been a major limiting factor for using Doppler signals from the intrarenal vasculature to identify renal artery stenosis.

Filippone and coworkers[40] evaluated renal tumor vascularity and the ability to demonstrate renal vein involvement using Levovist in 30 renal tumor patients. Sonographic depiction of internal vascularity improved from 16 of 34 cases precontrast to 28 of 34 cases postcontrast. Unfortunately, benign and malignant lesions were present in both the vascular and the nonvascular groups. Angiomyolipomas were sometimes hypervascular and (as is well known from angiography) four renal carcinomas were avascular. Levovist improved the ability to evaluate the renal veins in difficult patients but did not allow depiction of tumor vascularity in the thrombus itself. Balen and associates[41] also used Levovist to evaluate tumor flow in prostatic nodules. In this study of 20 patients with prostatic disease, the diagnosis was changed from benign to malignant in three patients after the injection of a contrast agent. In general, the detection of abnormal flow seemed considerably enhanced by Levovist.

Levovist has also been used to produce enhancement of the hepatic vessels and increase visibility of tumor vascularity in liver neoplasms. No evidence, however, indicates that this agent causes enhancement of the hepatic parenchyma itself.[42] In a study of 26 patients with suspected portal vein thrombosis, injection of Levovist provided enhancement of portal vein Doppler signals for as long as 420 seconds.[43] The authors reported that the agent allowed exclusion of portal vein thrombosis in 25 cases and a positive diagnosis in one. Earlier work by Tessler and colleagues,[44] however, concluded that color-Doppler examination *without* contrast was also an excellent test for excluding portal vein thrombosis. Several authors have used Levovist in the evaluation of hepatic tumors. Leen and coworkers[45] compared 24 patients with colorectal metastasis to the liver with 28 patients having primary hepatocellular carcinomas (HCC) and 2 patients with carcinoid. Characteristic color patterns were reported for each group: colorectal lesions tended to produce rim enhancement, HCC was associated with marked internal vascularity, and carcinoid tumors showed homogeneous enhancement. In another study of 38 patients with HCC, a similar pattern of internal vascular enhancement was demonstrated[46] after contrast agent administration. The patterns found in these two studies were said to be similar to the "basket" pattern described previously by Tanaka and associates[47] in HCC, but the pattern was more readily seen. Data on the Doppler appearance of benign hepatic lesions after administration of Levovist are limited. As expected, focal nodular hyperplasia and adenomas were hypervascular, whereas hemangiomas showed minimal change.[48]

Galactose-based contrast agents have also been used to assess both the intracranial and extracranial vasculature (Fig. 5–6 [see p 84]). A study by Sitzer and colleagues[49] confirmed that Levovist improved the ability to depict the entire length of carotid stenoses from 52 to 83%. Perhaps more meaningful, however, a "string" sign was identified in a patient previously diagnosed sonographically with a carotid occlusion. The average time of vascular enhancement in this study was approximately 3 minutes. Unfortunately, the gold standard for carotid stenosis in some patients in this study included arteriography; however, only continuous-wave Doppler was performed in other patients. Otis and coworkers[50] evaluated patients with atherosclerotic disease and intracranial arteriovenous malformations using Levovist-enhanced transcranial Doppler. Vascular enhancement was detected in 29 of 30 patients; improved diagnosis was found in 23 patients. The opacification time in this study was also relatively short with an average of 142 seconds.

Transcranial Doppler with Echovist has also been used to identify the presence of a patent foramen ovale.[51, 52] Because Echovist is largely filtered by the lungs, very little of it, if any, will normally be identified on a transcranial Doppler evaluation. After injection, however, if a patent foramen ovale is present, significant amounts of the contrast agent will be identified in the brain. This technique may be useful to evaluate young patients suffering strokes of unknown etiology. Unfortunately, one study did not conclude definitively that Echovist is superior to hand-shaken saline solution for this purpose.

Although Levovist clearly recirculates to a degree that allows arterial enhancement in numerous areas of the body, its half-life is relatively short. The enhancement times given earlier are typical of most published reports and are in the range of several minutes maximum. This amount of time is obviously insufficient for routine scanning, even if vessels are better imaged. A large multicenter study in Europe, however, is ongoing using Levovist in which multiple injections are given to prolong the duration of contrast enhancement.[53] The strict adherence to study protocols has limited most trials to one injection and the potential for multiple doses has been little explored. In the mentioned study, one third of patients experienced side effects, but none were serious or long lasting. In the future, multiple injections or infusion of contrast agent may eliminate the problem of short enhancement times altogether. However, newer agents persist for much longer periods, and a single dose may be sufficient with these compounds.

Phase 2 and 3 clinical trials in the United States using EchoGen for both cardiology and radiology applications are complete and, again, this compound has not been associated with significant side effects.[54] Early studies with this agent by Forsberg and associates[9] were particularly encouraging and actually demonstrated gray-scale enhancement in several animal species. At dosages used in human trials, however, the effect of the compound was limited to enhancement of vessels. A considerable increase in the duration of contrast enhancement has been achieved with this agent. Enhancement times of up to 20 minutes have been reported by many centers, including our own. We identified an average duration of contrast enhancement of 11.4 minutes in our patient population.[55] Among all centers participating in phase 3 trials, contrast enhancement lasted an average of 15.4 minutes.[54]

We used EchoGen to evaluate the renal arteries of 25 patients clinically suspected of having renal artery stenosis. Our study reviewed the ability of the contrast agent to improve visualization of the vessels, to identify multiple renal arteries, and to aid in the diagnosis of renal artery stenosis (Figs. 5–7 and 5–8 [see pp 85 and 86]). Contrast studies were compared with magnetic resonance angiography, catheter angiography, or both. In this study, after the injection of a contrast agent, the number of visualized dual renal arteries increased and detection of renal artery stenosis improved. Most noteworthy, however, was the observation that improved visualization of the main renal artery led to improved confidence in the diagnosis or exclusion of renal artery stenosis. Should this prove true in larger series, ultrasound contrast may decrease the need for more invasive, expensive, and potentially harmful imaging tests by providing a definitive method of ruling out renal artery stenosis. Although not specifically evaluated by this study, we believe that EchoGen shortened the scan time in this often prohibitively lengthy examination and would probably decrease the learning curve for those wishing to undertake scanning for renal artery stenosis. Although clinical utility of EchoGen in renal artery stenosis detection has been demonstrated by our study, the application of this agent to stenosis detection in other areas needs to be more thoroughly investigated. Results of the phase 3 multicenter study, however, were positive and showed that EchoGen facilitated visualization of blood flow and abnormal anatomic structures in 90% of subjects. Increased diagnostic confidence was noted in 56% of cases, and the diagnosis was corrected in 11%. Similar to what we observed in the renal arteries, nondiagnostic studies were reduced by 46%, and additional diagnostic tests were prevented in 13% of cases.[54]

Newer generations of contrast agents may provide routine parenchymal enhancement, opening new frontiers for sonographic imaging. A number of such investigations are now under way and studies in animals by RF Mattrey (Personal communication, 1996) show that in liver tumors, specific enhancement phases can be identified in a fashion similar to that seen with spiral CT scanning. Liver tumors derive most of their blood flow from the hepatic artery. An early arterial phase of peripheral parenchymal enhancement can be identified followed by central enhancement, thought to be secondary to portal venous flow. Finally, an equilibrium phase is reached in which the overall echogenicity of the hepatic parenchyma is increased relative to the echogenicity of the mass. This renders the mass more conspicuous. Should parenchymal enhancement be routinely achieved with future contrast agents, the role of sonography in the detection of liver metastases and other tumors may be dramatically increased.

SUMMARY

Early generations of sonographic contrast agents are beginning to reach the clinician. Research and development of ultrasound contrast agents are progressing at a rapid pace with several new agents approaching FDA approval. Cardiac imaging has been positively affected by the limited availability of contrast agents on the market today, with regard to diagnosis of shunts, chamber opacification, and most recently, actual enhancement of the myocardium. Later generations of contrast agents are capable of providing consistent opacification of both veins and arteries and should prove useful in a variety clinical applications. Thus far, it appears that longer vessel segments may be seen with a contrast agent than without, and flow may be demonstrated in vessels that were not seen or thought to be occluded with conventional color imaging. Improved detection of arterial and venous collaterals and enhanced identification of run-off vessels are demonstrated with sonographic contrast agents. Improved ability to evaluate renal artery stenosis and subtotal occlusion of the carotid artery is a specific advantage of using a contrast agent as well. Several compounds are currently being tested, which may allow routine parenchymal opacification in solid organs.

Ultrasonography is the most commonly performed diagnostic imaging procedure, and therefore sonographic contrast agents have the potential to dramatically alter the practice of clinical medicine.

REFERENCES

1. Bree RL, Platt JF, Bluth EI: Phase III clinical experience with a US contrast agent in the upper abdomen. Radiology 201(suppl):267, 1996.
2. Schlief R, Deichert U: Hysterosalpingo-contrast sonography of the uterus and fallopian tubes: Results of a clinical trial of a new contrast medium in 120 patients. Radiology 178:213–215, 1991.
3. Dietrich M, Suren A, Hinney B, et al: Evaluation of tubal patency by hysterocontrast sonography (HyCoSy, Echovist) and its correlation with laparoscopic findings. Clin Ultrasound 24:523–527, 1996.
4. Wible JH, Adams MD, Sherwin PF, et al: Noncardiac applications of Albunex. Invest Radiol 29(suppl): S145–148, 1994.
5. Parker KJ, Tuthill TA, Lerner RM, Violante MR: A particulate contrast agent with potential for ultrasound imaging of the liver. Ultrasound Med Biol 13:555–566, 1987.
6. Mattrey RF, Scheible FW, Gosink BB, et al: Perfluoroctylbromide: A liver/spleen-specific and tumor imaging ultrasound contrast material. Radiology 145:759–762, 1982.
7. Mattrey RF, Strich G, Shelton RE, et al: Perfluorochemicals as US contrast agents for tumor imaging and hepatosplenography: Preliminary clinical results. Radiology 163:339–343, 1987.
8. Behan M, O'Connell D, Mattrey R, Carney D: Perfluoroctylbromide as a contrast agent for CT and sonography: Preliminary clinical results. AJR Am J Roentgenol 160:399–405, 1993.
9. Forsberg F, Liu JB, Merton DA, et al: Parenchymal enhancement and tumor visualization using a new sonographic contrast agent. J Ultrasound Med 14:949–957, 1995.
10. Matsuda Y, Yabuuchi I: Hepatic tumors: US contrast enhancement with CO_2 microbubbles. Radiology 161:701–705, 1986.
11. Kudo M, Tomita S, Tochio J: Sonography with intraarterial infusion of carbon dioxide microbubbles (sonographic angiography): Value in differential diagnosis of hepatic tumors. AJR Am J Roentgenol 158:65–74, 1992.
12. Schlief R: Ultrasound contrast agents. Curr Opin Radiol 3:198–207, 1991.
13. Schlief R: Developments in echo-enhancing agents. Clin Radiol 51(suppl 1):5–7, 1996.
14. Burns PN, Wilson S, Muradali D, et al: Microbubble destruction is the origin of harmonic signals from FSO69. Radiology 201(suppl):158, 1996.
15. Goldberg BB: Ultrasound contrast agents. *In* Wells PNT (ed): Advances in Ultrasound Techniques and Instrumentation. New York, Churchill Livingstone, 1993, pp 35–46.

16. Newhouse V, Hoover M, Ash S: The detection of blood impurities using ultrasound Doppler. Ultrasonic Imaging 2:370–380, 1980.
17. Goldberg BB, Liu JB, Forsberg F: Ultrasound contrast agents: A review. Ultrasound Med Biol 20:319–333, 1994.
18. Ophir J, Parker KJ: Contrast agents in diagnostic ultrasound. Ultrasound Med Biol 15:353–356, 1989.
19. Fan P, Czuwala P, Nanda N, et al: Comparison of various agents in contrast enhancement of color Doppler flow images: An in-vitro study. Ultrasound Med Biol 19:45–57, 1993.
20. Forsberg F, Liu JB, Burns PN, et al: Artifacts in ultrasound contrast agent studies. J Ultrasound Med 13:357–365, 1994.
21. Burns PN: Harmonic imaging with ultrasound contrast agents. Clin Radiol 51:50–55, 1996.
22. Needleman L, Forsberg F: Contrast agents in ultrasound. Ultrasound Q 13:121–138, 1996.
23. Burns PN, Powers JE, Hope-Simpson D, et al: Power Doppler imaging combined with contrast enhancing harmonic Doppler: New method for small vessel imaging. Radiology 193(suppl):366, 1994.
24. Hilpert PL, Mattrey RF, Mitten RM, Peterson T: IV injection of air-filled human microspheres to enhance arterial Doppler signal: A preliminary study in rabbits. AJR Am J Roentgenol 153:613–616, 1989.
25. Smith MD, Elion JL, McClure RR, et al: Left heart opacification with peripheral venous injection of a new saccharide echo-contrast agent in dogs. J Am Coll Cardiol 13:1622–1626, 1989.
26. Fritzsch TH, Schartl M, Siegert J: Pre-clinical and clinical results with an ultrasonic contrast agent. Invest Radiol 23(suppl):302, 1988.
27. Unger EC, Lund PJ, Shen DK, et al: Nitrogen filled liposomes as a vascular US contrast agent: Preliminary evaluation. Radiology 185:453–456, 1992.
28. Fink IJ, Miller DJ, Shawker TH: Lipid emulsions as contrast agents for hepatic sonography: An experimental study in rabbits. Ultrasound Imaging 7:191–194, 1985.
29. Quay SC: Ultrasound contrast agent development: Phase shift colloids. J Ultrasound Med 13(suppl): 9, 1994.
30. Crouse L, Cheirif J, Hanly D, et al: Opacification and border delineation improvement in patients with suboptimal endocardial border definition in routine echocardiography: Results of a phase III Albunex multicenter trial. J Am Coll Cardiol 22:1494–1500, 1993.
31. Harmon B, Grant EG, Wiegel B, Brown P: An open label study to assess the safety and efficacy of Albunex in lower extremity Doppler in patients with suspected deep venous thrombosis in the lower extremities. Presented at the American Roentgen Ray Society meeting Washington, DC, May, 1995.
32. Needleman L, Nack TL, Feld RI, Goldberg BB: Initial experience with an US contrast agent in upper-extremity venous thrombosis. Radiology 185(suppl):143, 1992.
33. Vorwerk D, Gehl H, Nelles A, Gunther R: Dynamic contrast medium-aided ultrasound venacavography in patients with caval filters. Ultraschall Med 11:146–149, 1990.
34. Schlief R: Galactose based echo-enhancing agents. Proceedings of the Symposium on Ultrasound Contrast Agents. The Leading Edge in Diagnostic Ultrasound. Atlantic City, NJ, 1995, pp 25–26.
35. Needleman L, Goldberg BB, Feld RI, et al: Evaluation of arterial disease in humans using an ultrasound contrast agent. J Ultrasound Med 14(suppl): 48, 1995.
36. Schwartz K, Becher H, Schimpfky C, et al: Doppler enhancement with SHU508A in multiple vascular regions. Radiology 193:195–201, 1994.
37. Langholz J, Schlief R, Schürmann R, et al: Contrast enhancement in leg vessels. Clin Radiol 51(suppl 1):31–34, 1996.
38. Fobbe F, Ohnesorge I, Dahl A, et al: Farbkodierte Duplexsonographie und Ultraschallkontrastmittel zur Untersuchung peripherer Arterien—Erste klinische Erfahrungen. Ultraschall Med 13:193–198, 1992.
39. Balen F, Allen C, Lees W: Ultrasound contrast agents. Clin Radiol 49:77–82, 1994.
40. Filippone A, Muzi M, Basilico R, et al: Color Doppler flow imaging of renal disease. Value of a new intravenous contrast agent: SH U 508 A (Levovist). Radiol Med 87(suppl 1):50–58, 1994.
41. Balen FG, Allen CM, Gardner JE, et al: 3-Dimensional imaging of blood flow in benign and malignant conditions of the prostate. Proceedings of the 51st Annual Congress of the British Institute of Radiology. 1993, p 91.
42. Leen E, McArdle CS: Ultrasound contrast agents in liver imaging. Clin Radiol 51(suppl 1):35–39, 1996.
43. Braunschweig R, Stern W, Dadiban A, et al: Contrast enhanced colour Doppler studies of liver vessels. Abstract of investigators meeting in Berlin 1993. Echocardiography 10:674, 1993.
44. Tessler FT, Gehring BJ, Gomes A, et al: Diagnosis of portal vein thrombosis: Value of color Doppler imaging. AJR Am J Roentgenol 157:293–296, 1991.
45. Leen E, Angerson WG, Warren H, et al: Improved colour Doppler flow imaging of colorectal hepatic metastasis using galactose microparticles: A preliminary report. Br J Surg 81:252–254, 1994.
46. Angeli E, Carpanelli R, Crespi G, et al: Efficacy of SH U 508A in colour doppler ultrasonography of hepatocellular carcinoma vascularization. Radiol Med 87(suppl 1):24–31, 1994.
47. Tanaka S, Kitamura T, Fujita M, et al: Color Doppler flow imaging of liver tumors. AJR Am J Roentgenol 154:509–514, 1990.
48. Maresca G, Barbaro B, Summaria V, et al: Colour Doppler ultrasonography in the differential diagnosis of focal hepatic lesions. The SH U 508A experience. Radiol Med 87(suppl 1):41–49, 1994.
49. Sitzer M, Furst G, Siebler M, Steinmetz H: Usefulness of an intravenous contrast medium in the characterization of high grade internal carotid stenosis with color Doppler assisted duplex imaging. Stroke 25:385–389, 1994.
50. Otis S, Rush M, Boyajian R: Contrast enhanced transcranial imaging. Results of an American phase two study. Stroke 26:203–209, 1995.
51. Jauss M, Kaps M, Keberle M, et al: A comparison of transesophageal echocardiography and transcranial Doppler sonography with contrast medium for detection of patent foramen ovale. Stroke 25:1265–1267, 1994.
52. Kloetzsch C, Janssen G, Berlit P: Transesophageal echocardiography and contrast transcranial Doppler in the detection of patent foramen ovale: Experiences in 111 patients. Neurology 44:1603–1606, 1994.

53. Schlief R, Schurmann R, Niendorf H: Blood pool enhancement with SHU508A: Results of phase II clinical trials. Invest Radiol 26(suppl):188–189, 1991.
54. Robbin ML, Melany ML, Platt JF, et al: Phase III multicenter trial of a US contrast agent for use in diagnostic radiology. Radiology 201(suppl):196, 1996.
55. Melany ML, Grant EG, Duerinckx AJ, et al: Ability of a phase shift ultrasound contrast agent to improve imaging of the main renal arteries. Radiology 205:147–152, 1997.

SECTION 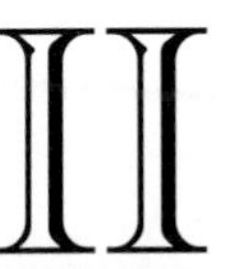

CEREBRAL VESSELS

Chapter 6

Rationale for Duplex Cerebrovascular Examination

■ *Gregory K. Call, MD*

Brain infarction occurs when an artery is occluded or becomes stenotic to the point that an insufficient amount of blood is delivered to a portion of brain. Rupture of an artery or vein allows blood to flow into or around the brain. The resultant hematoma then compresses the brain. Although these etiologies are distinct, both infarction and hemorrhage affect an individual suddenly and so historically have been called *stroke.* This chapter emphasizes the clinical aspects of ischemic brain insults for which ultrasonic examination of the carotid bifurcation was originally developed. Ultrasound applications in cases of hemorrhage are limited, but some examples are mentioned.

In the United States, approximately 500,000 new strokes occur annually, and about 75% of these are ischemic in nature.[1, 2] Among ischemic strokes, no more than 5%, or 25,000 per year, are due to stenosis of the proximal internal carotid artery. The severity of stroke varies over a wide range, extending from fatal to fully recoverable. In many instances, however, stroke alters an individual's emotions, mobility, activities, aspirations, and finances. In the United States, in 1994, the direct and indirect cost of caring for stroke patients was $30 billion.[3] This is 10 times the amount reported in 1976 for about the same incidence of stroke.

BASIC CONSIDERATIONS

Importance of the Carotid Bifurcation

Knowledge of the pathologic status of the internal carotid artery origin is important for a number of anatomic and epidemiologic reasons. About 75% of the brain's substance is nourished by the blood that passes through the two internal carotid arteries.[4, 5] It may also be that the origins of the common carotid arteries are more receptive to emboli. Hence, for anatomic and hemodynamic reasons alone, many strokes are in the carotid territory. Finally, the most common cause of arterial stenosis in occidentals is atherosclerosis, which is most prevalent in the cerebral vasculature at the carotid bifurcation.[6] Because of these factors, it is important to determine the condition of the carotid bifurcation in many patients with stroke. Significant intracranial arterial obstruction from atherosclerosis is less common. The opposite situation seems to be true for some peoples of Asian and African descent.[7] The prevalence of atherosclerosis at the carotid bifurcation does not mean that intracranial disease is unimportant. Intracranial arterial obstruction is the final common pathway in the pathogenesis of most brain infarcts. Furthermore, the impact of carotid and cardiac disease on the nervous system usually occurs in the intracranial arteries in the form of an embolus. Hence, examination of intracranial vessels is important, and improvements in this regard are being made because transcranial Doppler (TCD) examination is being carried out more frequently.

Stroke Syndrome and Transient Ischemic Attack

The stroke syndrome consists of the rapid (generally minutes) development of a focal neurologic deficit that is usually localized to an area of brain supplied by a specific artery.

For example, a prerolandic branch of the middle cerebral artery supplies an area of cerebral cortex and superficial white matter that is necessary for voluntary motor function of the contralateral face and hand. Sudden weakness of the face and hand would therefore be consistent with a stroke in this portion of the contralateral hemisphere. Weakness of a cheek on one side and a hand on the other side would be puzzling and would be less likely to be a result of ischemia.

The word *stroke* implies brain cell death caused by infarction, in which case the deficit endures for days and often longer. The deficit may be fleeting, however, in which case cell death presumably does not occur. Such a brief ischemic episode is called a *transient ischemic attack* (TIA). Most TIAs last from 1 to 30 minutes, but they may be longer.[8] According to common use and for epidemiologic reasons, a neurologic deficit lasting less than 24 hours and otherwise consistent with ischemia is considered a TIA. A longer lasting deficit with full recovery within 3 weeks has been termed a *reversible ischemic neurologic deficit,* or *RIND.* However, the significance of this latter distinction has not been well established, and I do not recall the term being used in a clinical setting. Therefore, it is not used elsewhere in this chapter.

The occurrence of stroke can usually be determined by the physician, because the deficit persists and can be defined by clinical examination. Brain imaging in stroke patients by cranial computed tomography (CT) and magnetic resonance imaging (MRI) allows confirmation of the suspected anatomic location of the injury and usually helps determine its nature (ischemic or hemorrhagic).

The diagnosis of TIA is more difficult. A transient deficit lasting only minutes is often less well appreciated by the person who suffers it. The patient may therefore be unable to give a full account to the physician, who in this case is totally dependent on medical history. By definition, the CT or MRI scan is usually negative, but these studies can help rule out other lesions that may give rise to transient symptoms. In some cases, however, CT or MRI reveals a lesion consistent with infarction, thus suggesting that the current symptoms are also ischemic. More often than not, however, symptoms occur that can be mimicked by other processes, such as multiple sclerosis, disk disease, carpal tunnel syndrome, and sensory or motor seizures. Transient monocular blindness is a prominent example of how difficult it is to explain fleeting symptoms. Transient monocular blindness is known to be associated with carotid stenosis and other less common conditions, but in many cases its cause is not definable.[9–11] Although some of the unexplained cases may yet prove to be ischemic, this example emphasizes that caution is needed when interpreting fleeting symptoms.

Collateral Blood Supply

The cerebral hemispheres are supplied by the anterior and middle cerebral arteries, which arise from the carotid system, and by the posterior cerebral arteries, which arise from the vertebrobasilar system. The areas supplied by these arteries and their branches can extend into adjacent regions if required. For example, the anterior cerebral artery can supply blood to some adjacent middle cerebral regions if the middle cerebral artery is occluded. This form of collateralization may reduce the amount of ischemic tissue distal to an occlusion. Collateralization in this situation is basically an extension of blood flow into an adjacent area through small-caliber vessels that dilate into arterioles.

Another form of collateralization occurs in response to pressure changes in the circle of Willis consequent to a proximal occlusion. Pressure changes may alter the direction of flow. For example, an occlusion proximal to the circle on the left decreases pressure in the left side of the circle, allowing blood to flow from right to left. The final source of cerebral collaterals is extracranial vessels. Connections normally exist among extracranial vessels (e.g., external carotid artery branches) and intracranial vessels. With obstruction of the arteries supplying the intracranial circulation, these vessels increase in flow volume and become a source of supply for the intracranial circulation.

These three principal collateral routes are important in preventing or modifying ischemia. They help explain why a person can sustain carotid occlusion without suffering a persistent neurologic deficit.

ISCHEMIC STROKE

Common Causes

The following are common causes of ischemic stroke:

1. Atherosclerosis (with superimposed thrombosis, with or without distal embolization): carotid bifurcation, distal vertebral artery, proximal and distal basilar arteries, aortic arch
2. Embolus from the heart: atrial fibrillation, mitral stenosis, prosthetic heart valve, cardiomyopathy, acute myocardial infarction, bacterial endocarditis
3. Hypertensive arteriolar sclerosis (lipohyalinosis)
4. Dissection: carotid artery, vertebral artery
5. Prethrombotic states
6. Vasospasm: subarachnoid hemorrhage, idiopathic

There are also many rare causes of ischemic stroke that cannot be covered in this general review. It must be emphasized that a substantial number of strokes, at least 25%, occur without a reasonable working hypothesis as to mechanism or underlying lesion.[12]

Atherosclerosis

Atherosclerosis, with associated intimal disruption or lumen stenosis, is a common cause of stroke, particularly in the elderly. It is the most common finding in persons older than 45 years of age who suffer a stroke. Presumably, the thrombogenic effects of intimal damage and collagen exposure, as well as the hemodynamic effects of severe stenosis, result in thrombus formation with lumen occlusion. Often the thrombus fragments and embolizes distally. Thus, the distinction between thrombo-occlusive and embolic strokes can be misleading, because embolization necessarily implies a proximal thrombus.

Stroke caused by an embolus to carotid territory branches is often a final occurrence in cardiac and arterial diseases. Fibrin emboli always result from proximal thrombosis, which may occur in the heart or in an artery. The origin of the embolus is suspected on the basis of certain aspects of the medical history, most notably the presence or absence of heart disease, a cervical bruit, or preceding TIA.

TIA is an important clue that arterial disease is present in the cerebral vasculature. In population-based studies, only about 10 to 14% of all strokes were found to have been preceded by TIA.[3] In strokes ascribed to carotid disease, however, at least 60% were preceded by TIA.[13] Cardiac conditions such as arterial fibrillation that give rise to stroke are rarely heralded by TIA.[14, 15] Hence, when a stroke occurs in a patient with a history of preceding TIA in the same arterial region, the most likely explanation is arterial disease. If the area is supplied by a carotid branch, the most likely site of disease is the carotid bifurcation.

Finally, recognition of TIA is important because TIAs are followed by stroke within 5 years in 33% of patients, with the greatest risk occurring during the first 2 weeks after the TIA.[16, 17]

Embolus From the Heart

Stroke resulting from cerebral artery occlusion by an embolus from the heart is seen in various situations and at all ages, although certain predisposing conditions are age related. Rhythm disturbances such as atrial fibrillation can result in thrombus formation within the left atrium of the heart, with subsequent embolization to any body part, including the brain. Damaged endocardium of the heart wall or valves can stimulate local thrombosis, which can also give rise to an embolus to the brain.

Hypertension

Hypertension is a condition present in many adults who suffer a stroke. Elevated blood pressure can contribute to heart disease and can also worsen atherosclerosis of the larger arteries. Both these conditions can lead to stroke, as mentioned previously. Hypertension can also injure the small vessels of the kidney and brain, a change known as *arteriolar sclerosis* or *lipohyalinosis.* Arteriolar sclerosis can advance to the point of occlusion of an arteriole, resulting in the formation of a small, localized area of infarction, or lacuna.[18]

Dissection

Dissection refers to hemorrhage and thrombus formation within the arterial wall.[19, 20] This process can occur between the intima and media, within the media, or between the media and adventitia. Dissection of the aorta has long been known to occur consequent to hypertension, cystic medial necrosis, or severe blunt chest trauma (e.g., after an automobile accident). Direct and indirect trauma of the neck can also result in carotid or, less commonly, vertebral artery dissection. The thrombus within the vessel wall, particularly when in a subintimal position, produces some degree of stenosis or even occlusion, possibly with intraluminal thrombus formation. Carotid dissection can also occur in those between the ages of 20 and 50 years without any other obvious medical condition that would predispose to stroke. Carotid dissection often occurs distal to the carotid bifurcation and is frequently limited to the area just below the skull base. Hence, its location is different from that of atherosclerotic disease of the carotid arteries.

Prethrombotic States

Abnormalities in blood coagulation that cause a tendency to thrombosis usually affect the veins but can also involve the arteries, including those that supply the brain. The coagulopathies are still incompletely understood, and, although they may prove to be a significant cause of stroke in the young, they are not considered further here.

Vasospasm

Vasospasm of the intracranial arteries after subarachnoid hemorrhage is a significant cause of stroke and of subsequent morbidity and mortality in those who survive the hemorrhage.[21] Spasm, at least in part, seems to depend both on the amount of blood present around the arteries and on the passage of time. Spasm rarely occurs before the third day after hemorrhage; thus, this form of stroke usually occurs in a sick patient who has already been in the hospital for a few days.

Diagnostic Hypothesis

It can be seen that various common conditions may ultimately lead to stroke. I believe that the treatment of stroke depends on reaching the most accurate diagnosis possible through clinical and laboratory evaluation. Laboratory evaluation, including the noninvasive vascular laboratory results, is used to confirm the clinical impression obtained from the medical history and physical examination. Sometimes the laboratory findings may be used to eliminate a condition that cannot be excluded by clinical characteristics alone. Often, an exact diagnosis is not possible, and the clinician must proceed with the best working hypothesis available.

The natural history of many conditions that cause stroke is unknown. Precise diagnoses help us to obtain a better understanding of the natural histories of these conditions, determine a therapeutic regimen, and reach a suitable prognosis. Diagnosis is therefore important in its own right, even if a specific therapy is not currently available.

Applications of Duplex Sonography and Transcranial Doppler

The ultrasonic evaluation of cerebral arteries is always carried out in a clinical setting with a specific question in mind: what are the anatomic and blood velocity characteristics in the arteries of interest? The gray-scale images provide information about the location and, to some degree, the type of disease present. By combining the gray-scale findings with the Doppler shift frequencies and color Doppler characteristics, information about the severity of stenosis is obtained. In general, the ultrasonic evaluation is not helpful if the nature of the symptoms or signs is uncertain. *The presence of a vascular lesion does not mean that otherwise poorly understood symptoms are ischemic in nature.* This point is stressed because it is known that certain individuals can tolerate carotid stenosis, or even occlusion, without suffering a stroke or TIA.[22, 23] Carotid sonography is therefore most valuable when the symptoms are known to be localized to the carotid territory and are ischemic in nature.

Significant Carotid Lesions

The results of the vascular examination are most meaningful if they are properly interpreted. What is a significant lesion? First, significance generally refers to *hemodynamic significance,* or the degree of stenosis that alters the flow characteristics of blood. This begins to occur when the diameter is reduced by 70%, or the absolute residual lumen diameter is 1.5 mm or less.[24] Such a degree of stenosis would put someone at risk for carotid thrombosis with occlusion and perhaps distal embolization with stroke. It is known, however, that lesser degrees of stenosis can also result in carotid thrombosis with stroke.[25] Plaque characteristics such as ulceration or the presence of plaque contents that could initiate thrombosis are therefore important. Duplex sonography is well suited for determining lumen diameter and velocity characteristics, but it has not been established how well it can define plaque characteristics. Arteriography is also limited with respect to plaque characterization. For example, if ulceration is defined as disruption of the endothelium, then ulceration cannot currently be detected with certainty, with either arteriography or duplex sonography. Irregularity of the vessel wall is a common finding, but it does not necessarily mean that there is currently ulceration with exposure of subintimal tissue.

The term *significant carotid lesion* also relates the lesion to a patient's clinical syndrome. In this sense significance is often incompletely defined because a carotid lesion may be present, but it is not always clear that the lesion is the cause of the stroke or TIA syndrome. The use of the term hemodynamically significant carotid stenosis, as defined previously, which can be anatomically associated with neurologic symptoms, has been widely accepted, because it proposes a way in which thrombosis and subsequent stroke may occur. Several studies have shown that carotid endarterectomy (CEA) can be more effective than medical therapy (usually aspirin) in reducing the incidence of stroke in symptomatic patients with a stenosis of 70% or greater.[26, 27] CEA is not as effective as medical therapy for those patients with a stenosis of less than 30% (trials continue for stenoses between 30 and 69%). Surgery in patients with asymptomatic stenosis can be undertaken fairly safely, but its advantages are debatable.[28] At our institution, we most commonly consider CEA in the asymptomatic person in cases of a high degree of stenosis, such as 80% or more, or when there is contralateral occlusion.

Clinical Examples

With these qualifications in mind, the following case studies are presented to show how the vascular laboratory may be useful in the evaluation of stroke.

EXAMPLE 1

An older (but fit) man suffers two episodes of right-sided face and arm difficulties and has trouble speaking. The episode lasts minutes and is followed by a longer episode, from which recovery takes several days. Physical examination confirms language and motor disturbances, but no other evidence of medical disease is found.

TIA followed by a stroke, as illustrated in this example, is most consistent with a diagnosis of carotid stenosis. A carotid duplex examination should be undertaken in an attempt to confirm the clinical impression. If a significant stenosis is found, angiography is performed next to assess the cerebral vasculature and prepare for surgery. If the patient is not a surgical candidate, duplex sonography still serves the important function of confirming the diagnosis before the institution of medical therapy. Theoretically, if the clinical situation is compelling and the duplex findings are clear, one could bypass arteriography and proceed directly to surgery, because intracranial stenosis of a significant degree is rare. TCD in this instance could help confirm the absence of intracranial arterial disease.

EXAMPLE 2

An older person experiences a shade falling across the right eye with blindness for 5 minutes on three different occasions.

Transient monocular blindness is a common symptom in the atherosclerotic age group. (It also occurs less frequently in the young.) It is sometimes a result of carotid stenosis, but often no cause can be found. Carotid duplex examination is ideal for identifying carotid stenosis in this situation. The use of arteriography, with its inherent discomfort and risk, is not recommended, because many people with transient monocular blindness do not have an identifiable arterial lesion.

EXAMPLE 3

An elderly person develops left-sided face and extremity weakness (arm more than leg), sensory loss, visual field loss, and some confusion. A cranial CT scan reveals a large, right parietal infarct. Atrial fibrillation is detected by physical examination and electrocardiography.

In this case an excellent working diagnosis of stroke caused by cardiac embolus is immediately available. The diagnosis is strengthened further if duplex sonography demonstrates that the carotids are normal or contain only minimal disease. The presence of additional significant carotid bifurcation disease makes the diagnosis of embolization from the heart less certain, and any subsequent therapeutic plans must bear this uncertainty in mind. It might be preferable to treat both the arterial and cardiac problems.

EXAMPLE 4

A hypertensive person awakens with profound weakness and mild sensory changes of the right-sided face, arm, and leg, but with intact language, mentation, and vision. A cranial MRI scan reveals a small lesion in the posterior limb of the internal capsule consistent with infarction. Electrocardiographic evidence of left ventricular hypertrophy is found.

Hypertension can contribute to stroke in a number of ways. The neurologic syndrome and images in this case suggest small-vessel occlusion, which could be a result of hypertensive arteriolar sclerotic changes, but the syndrome could also be caused by an embolus. Carotid duplex evaluation would be most helpful to the diagnosis if completely normal. Even modest carotid disease, however, could serve as a focus for thrombus formation. If severe carotid stenosis is found, the cause of the stroke is even more in doubt. This common situation is one of the more difficult in terms of diagnostic confidence. The presence of hypertensive arteriolar sclerosis can only be suspected and cannot be determined directly on clinical grounds alone.

EXAMPLE 5

A 30-year-old person experiences several days of left-sided neck and hemicranial pain and then develops mild weakness of the right-sided arm and leg. Horner's syndrome is found on examination. No other cardiac or medical disorders are present.

This syndrome strongly suggests carotid dissection. Even in the absence of neck and head pain and Horner's syndrome, the absence of other medical clues in patients of the preatherosclerotic age group should always suggest the possibility of dissection. Arteriography is the diagnostic procedure of choice, though the diagnosis can also often be confirmed by MRI or even CT. Dissection has a characteristic set of arteriographic findings but may not be accessible or definable with a duplex ultrasound probe. In some cases, carotid duplex examination may suggest the diagnosis of dissection, but it does not have a consistently defined role in this condition.

EXAMPLE 6

A hospitalized patient with known subarachnoid hemorrhage resulting from a saccular aneurysm worsens on hospital day 5 with weakness, confusion, and obtundation. A cranial CT scan reveals normal ventricles and no increase in the amount of blood present.

In this setting, clinical suspicion centers on secondary vasospasm, and TCD can confirm this diagnosis. Furthermore, serial TCD evaluation can detect spasm before it is manifested clinically, thus allowing preventive measures to be instituted.

Clinical Indications

The indications for cerebrovascular duplex sonography can be summarized:

1. General indications: whenever anatomic and physiologic information about the carotid bifurcation would be of diagnostic value
2. Specific indications:
   a. Classic TIA (1 to 30 minutes, particularly if stereotyped and repetitious) in the carotid distribution or in border zone territories (border zone—the border of two adjacent vascular territories)
   b. To rule out carotid disease when other explanations are available (e.g., atrial fibrillation), particularly if the presentations are atypical
   c. Transient monocular blindness (amaurosis fugax)

d. Ischemic oculopathy
e. Branch retinal artery occlusion
f. Central retinal artery occlusion
g. Central retinal vein occlusion
h. Hollenhorst's plaque (controversial)
i. Follow-up after endarterectomy (uncertain)
j. Before cardiac, aortic aneurysmal, and perhaps other major surgeries (controversial)
k. Known contralateral carotid occlusion (debatable)

As seen here and mentioned previously, carotid duplex examination is best suited for defining the anatomy and blood velocities at the carotid bifurcation in patients of the atherosclerotic age group, in whom such knowledge is helpful in narrowing the diagnostic possibilities. Duplex sonography is rarely (if ever) helpful in the young patient for whom arteriography is the diagnostic mainstay.

Noninvasive carotid studies are often done in people with asymptomatic neck bruit or in those who are to undergo cardiac, aortic, or peripheral vascular surgery. These are controversial uses of the vascular laboratory, except for carrying out research to determine the natural history of carotid disease. Endarterectomy in the asymptomatic patient is a more individually defined procedure than the more generalizable undertaking in those with symptoms. Even known tight carotid stenosis can run a harmless course in some people. Furthermore, knowledge of the presence of narrowing in the carotid artery can occasion anxiety in the person with such a lesion.

Usually, the vertebral arteries can be imaged over a short segment in the neck, and a Doppler signal may be obtained from the arteries. Duplex vertebral examination has not been shown to have direct clinical use, however, and duplex evaluation in the setting of vertebrobasilar disease is not recommended. TCD may prove to be of some help for vertebrobasilar diagnosis, but this technique is currently beyond the skills of all but a few. Anatomic definition of the vertebrobasilar arteries still requires arteriography.

TCD is gaining widespread use in those with subarachnoid hemorrhage for detecting and monitoring vasospasm. Spasm can be detected before it is clinically evident, its course can be monitored daily (or even more often), and the success or failure of preventive or therapeutic measures may be determined. TCD can also detect intracranial stenoses, collateral blood flow patterns, and arteriovenous malformations. These latter determinations are currently beyond the capability of most laboratories, but this may change.[29]

REFERENCES

1. National Advisory Neurological and Communicative Disorders and Stroke Council: Decade of the Brain. NIH Publ. No. 88-2957, January 1989.
2. Mohr JP, Caplan LR, Melski JW, et al: The Harvard Cooperative Stroke Registry: A prospective registry. Neurology 28:754–762, 1978.
3. Bronner LL, Kanter DS, Manson JE: Primary prevention of stroke. N Engl J Med 333:1392–1400, 1995.
4. Kurtzke JF: Epidemiology and risk factors in thrombotic brain infarction. *In* Harrison MJG, Dyken ML (eds): Cerebral Vascular Disease. London, Butterworth, 1983, pp 27–45.
5. Easton JD: Cerebrovascular disease. *In* Stein JH (ed): Internal Medicine. Boston, Little, Brown, 1983, pp 856–864.
6. Marshall J: The natural history of cerebrovascular disease. *In* Meyer JS (ed): Modern Concepts of Cerebrovascular Disease. New York, Spectrum Publications, 1975, pp 53–62.
7. Caplan LR, Gorelick PB, Hier DB: Race, sex and occlusive cerebrovascular disease: A review. Stroke 17:648–655, 1986.
8. Levy DE: How transient are transient ischemic attacks? Neurology 38:674–677, 1988.
9. Chawluk JB, Kushner MJ, Bank WJ, et al: Atherosclerotic carotid artery disease in patients with retinal ischemic syndromes. Neurology 38:858–863, 1988.
10. Hurwitz BJ, Heyman A, Wilkinson WE, et al: Comparison of amaurosis fugax and transient cerebral ischemia. Ann Neurol 18:698–704, 1985.
11. Guyer DR, Miller NR, Auer CL, Fine SL: The risk of cerebrovascular and cardiovascular disease in patients with anterior ischemic optic neuropathy. Arch Ophthalmol 103:1136–1141, 1985.
12. Mohr JP: Cryptogenic stroke. N Engl J Med 318: 1197–1198, 1988.
13. Pessin MS, Hinton RC, Davis KR, et al: Mechanisms of acute carotid stroke. Ann Neurol 6:245–252, 1979.
14. Sherman DG, Goldman L, Whiting RB, et al: Thromboembolism in patients with AF. Arch Neurol 41:708–710, 1984.
15. Harrison MJG, Marshall J: Atrial fibrillation, TIA and completed stroke. Stroke 15:441–442, 1984.
16. Whisnant JP, Matsumoto N, Elveback LR: The effect of anticoagulant therapy in the prognosis of patients with transient cerebral ischemic attacks in a community: Rochester, Minnesota, 1955 through 1969. Mayo Clin Proc 48:844–848, 1973.
17. Guatier JC, Juillard JBE, Lovon PHL, et al: The interval between transient ischemic attacks and cerebral infarction (Abstract 80). Stroke 18:298, 1987.
18. Fisher CM: Lacunar strokes and infarcts: A review. Neurology 32:871–876, 1982.
19. O'Connell BK, Towfighi J, Brennan RW, et al: Dissecting aneurysms of head and neck. Neurology 35:993–997, 1985.
20. Caplan LR, Baquis GD, Pessin MS, et al: Dissection of the intracranial vertebral artery. Neurology 38: 868–877, 1988.

21. Kistler JP, Crowell RM, Davis KR, et al: The relation of cerebral vasospasm to the extent and location of subarachnoid blood visualized by CT scan: A prospective study. Neurology 33:424–436, 1983.
22. Martin MJ, Whisnant JP, Sayre GPL: Occlusive vascular disease in the extracranial cerebral circulation. Arch Neurol 5:530–538, 1960.
23. Chambers BR, Norris JW: Outcome in patients with asymptomatic neck bruits. N Engl J Med 315:860–865, 1986.
24. Spencer MP, Reid JM: Quantitation of carotid stenosis with continuous-wave (C-W) doppler ultrasound. Stroke 3:326–330, 1979.
25. Brown PB, Zwiebel WJ, Call GK: Degree of cervical carotid artery stenoses and hemispheric stroke. Radiology 170:541–543, 1989.
26. Barnett JM, Taylor DW, Haynes RB, et al: Beneficial effects of carotid endarterectomy in symptomatic patients with high-grade carotid stenosis. N Engl J Med 325:445–453, 1991.
27. European Carotid Surgery Trialist Collaborative Group. MRC European Carotid Surgery Trial: Interim results for symptomatic patients with severe (70–99%) or with mild carotid stenosis. Lancet 337:1235–1243, 1991.
28. Executive Committee for the Asymptomatic Carotid Atherosclerosis study: Endarterectomy for asymptomatic carotid artery stenoses. JAMA 273:1421–1428, 1995.
29. Caplan LR, Brass LM, Dewitt LD, et al: Transcranial doppler ultrasound: Present status. Neurology 40:696–700, 1991.

Chapter 7

Normal Cerebrovascular Anatomy and Collateral Pathways

■ *Edward B. Diethrich, MD*

The vascular system of the human brain differs significantly, both anatomically and physiologically, from other organs in the body. Although it accounts for only 2% of the body weight, the brain receives 15% of the cardiac output and consumes 20% of the body's oxygen supply in the basal state.[1] Cerebral arteries are little influenced by sympathetic nerves, unlike other arteries, but they are markedly affected by chemical changes in the blood.

Obstructive disease afflicting the cerebrovascular system can produce a wide array of sometimes ambiguous symptoms. Clinicians must attempt to identify the exact areas involved in the disease process; however, this is often made difficult by individual variability in the cerebral vasculature. Indeed, the extent of clinical symptoms is entirely dependent on the ability of the collateral circulation to maintain adequate cerebral perfusion. Therefore, understanding the normal and collateral anatomy and the mechanisms of cerebral blood flow is essential to the diagnosis of obstructive disease in the cerebrovascular system.

This chapter addresses the anatomic and physiologic principles that influence the investigation of the vascular supply to the brain. It is important to stress the significance of appreciating the hemodynamics of the brain. Individuals vary considerably in their ability to compensate for alterations in cerebral blood flow, and the physician must be aware of the potential mechanisms for cerebrovascular collateralization to carry out a judicious evaluation protocol.

VASCULAR ANATOMY

The brain is supplied directly by four vessels: the two internal carotid arteries and the vertebral arteries. Any discussion of the cerebrovascular system must begin at the origins of these vessels, because obstructive disease, stenoses, ulcerative plaques, or anomalies anywhere in the cerebrovascular tree may produce a stroke or symptoms of insufficiency.

The blood supply for the central nervous system[1–3] derives from the three great vessels arising from the aortic arch in the superior mediastinum—the innominate, the left common carotid, and the left subclavian arteries (Fig. 7–1). The innominate artery travels upward, slightly posteriorly from the arch to the right of the neck for its 4- to 5-cm length, dividing into the right common carotid artery and the right subclavian artery at the upper border of the right sternoclavicular junction. The left common carotid artery ascends from the arch and passes beneath the left sternoclavicular joint. Neither common carotid has collateral branches, but each divides into the internal and external carotid arteries at the level of the upper border of the thyroid cartilage.

The internal carotids supply most of the anterior circulation to the cerebrum (Fig. 7–2). In their cervical portion, the internal carotid arteries may be relatively straight or may curve tortuously as they travel to the base of the skull. There are no branches of the internal carotid arteries in the neck. As

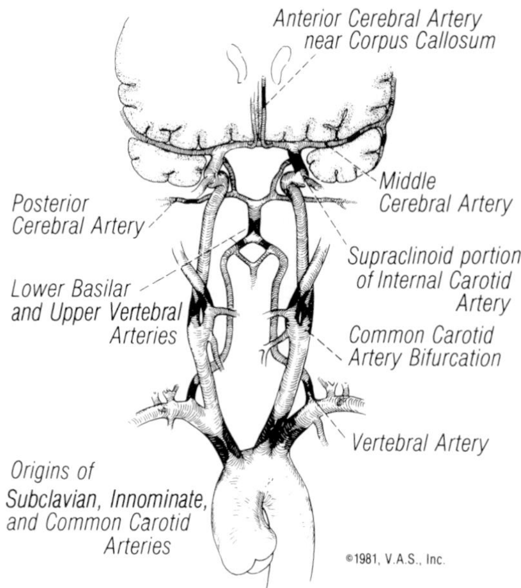

FIGURE 7–1 Extracranial cerebrovascular anatomy showing the areas predisposed to atherosclerotic plaque formation.

they proceed intracranially, the internal carotid arteries give rise to the caroticotympanic branches in the petrous bone, the meningohypophyseal branches in the cavernous sinus region, and the ophthalmic arteries immediately distal to the cavernous sinus. Eight millimeters beyond the clinoid process, within the dura mater, the internal carotid arteries give rise to the posterior communicating arteries, which join with the posterior cerebral arteries. Further cephalad, the internal carotid arteries divide into the middle and anterior cerebral arteries and give rise posteriorly to the anterior choroidal arteries.

The external carotid arteries normally supply no blood to the brain. However, several of their branches can become important collateral pathways if occlusion occurs in the internal carotid or vertebral arteries. The branches of the external carotid artery are the ascending pharyngeal, the superior thyroid, the lingual, the external maxillary, the occipital, the facial, the posterior auricular, the internal maxillary, the transverse facial, and the superficial temporal arteries. The external carotid branches most vital to collateral circulation are those in communication with the ophthalmic artery and those that interconnect between the muscular branches of the occipital and vertebral arteries (Fig. 7–3).

The posterior circulation to the brain is supplied in large part by the vertebral arteries arising from the subclavian arteries. The vertebrals lie within the foramina transversarium of the upper cervical vertebrae and wind anteriorly into the subarachnoid space at the side of the medulla oblongata at the level of

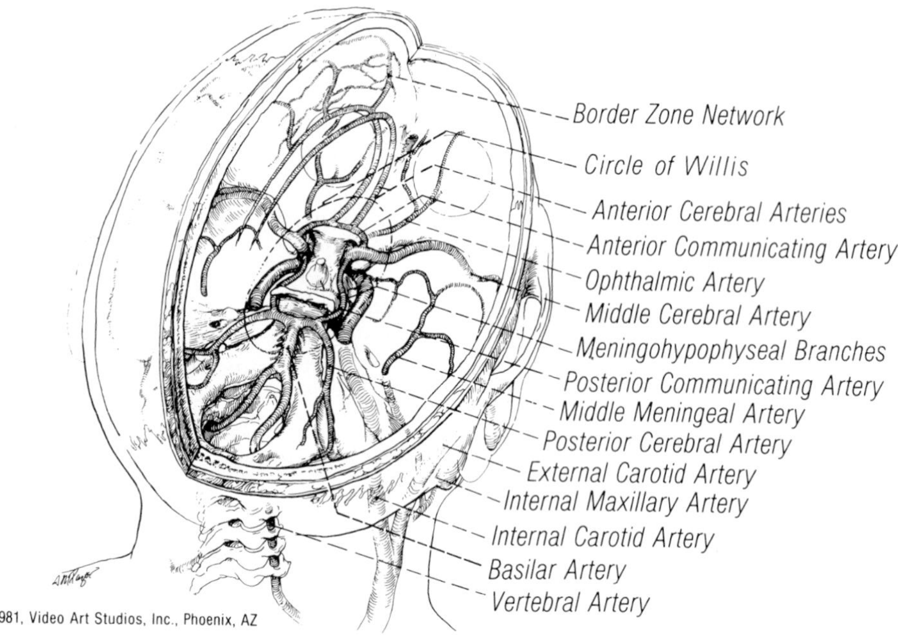

FIGURE 7–2 Intracranial cerebrovascular anatomy showing anastomotic connections of the circle of Willis. Note that the principal blood supply to intracranial structures is through the carotid arteries.

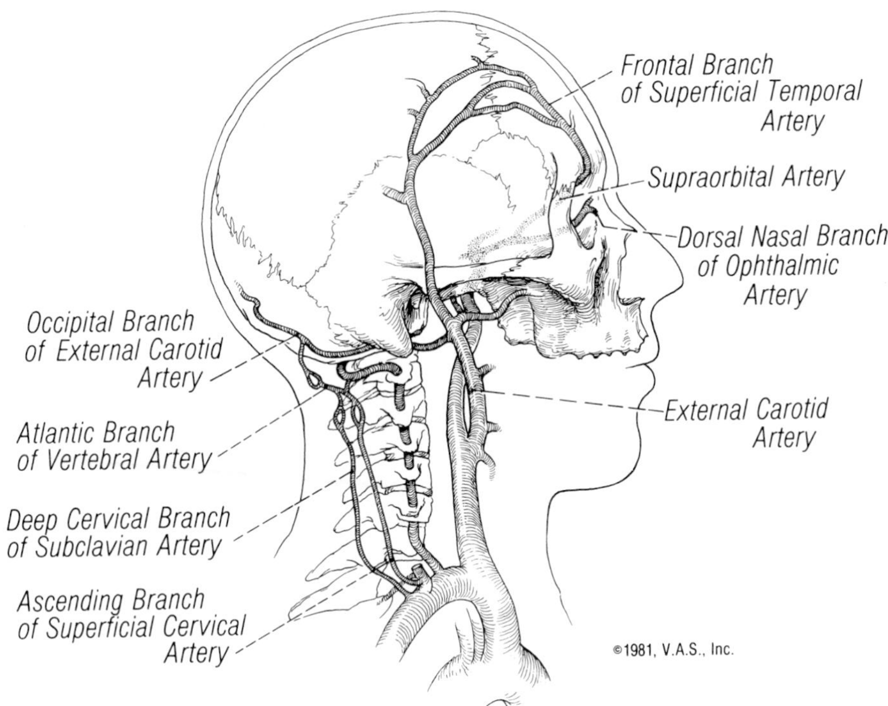

FIGURE 7–3 Extracranial cerebrovascular anatomy. Note the anastomotic connections between the external and internal carotid arteries and among the occipital, cervical, and vertebral arteries.

the atlanto-occipital interspace. They proceed cephalad and anteriorly until they reach the pontomedullary level, where they join to form the basilar artery. Four branches arise from the basilar artery as it courses upward before dividing into the posterior cerebral arteries. Branches of the basilar artery supply the entire pons and the superior and anterior aspects of the cerebellum. Branches of the vertebral arteries supply the medulla and the interior surface of the cerebellum.

The cerebral branches of the internal carotids and vertebral arteries are joined at the base of the brain by an arterial circle known as the circle of Willis. This anastomosis is the most important element in intracranial collateral circulation and is also a common site of aneurysmal formation. It is a hexagonal arrangement of arteries composed of the anterior, middle, and posterior cerebral arteries, which are joined together by the anterior and posterior communicating arteries (see Fig. 7–2). Under normal circumstances, there is usually little mixing of blood through the communicating arteries. However, in instances of arterial occlusion in carotid or vertebrobasilar vessels, this circle opens to function as a vital collateral pathway (see later).

Component arteries of the circle of Willis can vary greatly in size, and there are at least nine congenital variations in the structure of the circle (Fig. 7–4). The most common anomalies involve the absence or hypoplasia of one or both communicating arteries. An anomalous origin of the posterior cerebral artery from one or both internal carotid arteries has also been commonly encountered. Anomalies in the anterior portion of the circle are less commonly found, although among these, absence or hypoplasia of the proximal segment of the anterior cerebral artery between the internal carotid and anterior communicating arteries is more usual. Among the variations, the most significant in terms of decreasing collateral potential are those in which the anterior or posterior communicating arteries are absent or impervious. These conditions may isolate the anterior and posterior circulations or the left and right hemispheric carotid territories.

Anomalous formations can also occur in the extracranial circulation, most commonly involving the origins of the carotid and vertebral arteries. Most frequent is a close association between or a sharing of the origin of the innominate artery with the left common

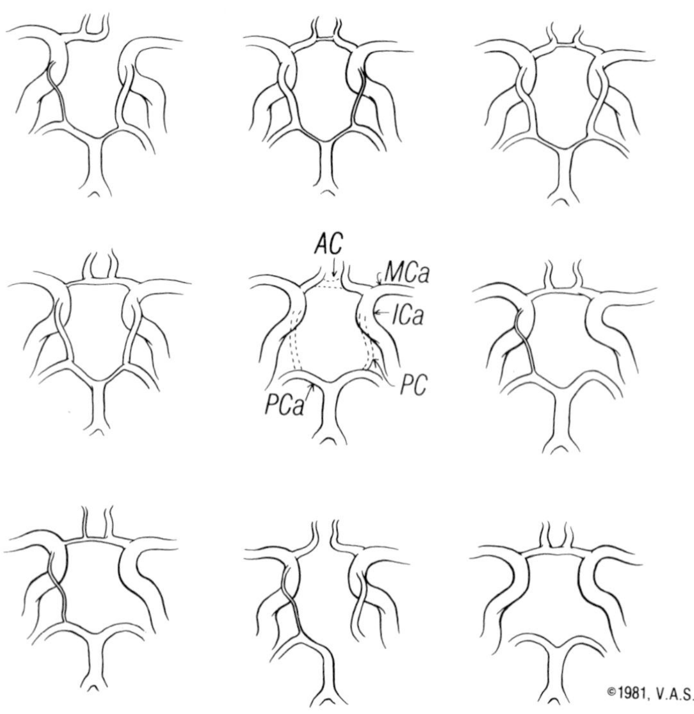

FIGURE 7–4 Nine of the possible configurations of the circle of Willis, the most important cerebrovascular collateral pathway. The center drawing depicts one configuration in which there is no communication between the anterior (AC) and posterior (PC) circulation. MCa = middle cerebral artery; ICa = internal carotid artery; PCa = posterior cerebral artery.

carotid artery. Less often, the left common carotid artery may arise from the innominate artery. Also seen is the anomalous origin of the left vertebral artery on the aortic arch between the left common carotid and subclavian arteries. Rarely, the right subclavian artery may have an aberrant origin on the aortic arch. Other abnormalities may occur in the cervical region, such as agenesis of the internal carotid arteries, but these are rare. Abnormalities in the vertebral arteries are usually limited to variations in size between the left and right, a common occurrence.

CEREBRAL HEMODYNAMICS

Before discussing the potential collateral pathways in the cerebrovascular system, it is best to explain the dynamics of cerebral blood flow[1,4] to help gain an appreciation of the importance of collateralization.

Despite the brain's large apportionment of the body's blood supply (15% of the cardiac output), there is little circulatory reserve because of the brain's high metabolic rate. Furthermore, the brain has no significant oxygen or glucose stores, making it entirely dependent on the vascular system for maintenance.[1,2] This is why even short episodes of interrupted cerebral flow can bring on symptoms of cerebral dysfunction, and cellular death can occur within 3 to 8 minutes of vascular failure.

Extrinsically, cerebral blood flow varies with the effective arterial perfusion pressure. Adequate perfusion relies on systemic blood pressure, cardiac output, and blood volume. Within the range of fluctuation possible for these extrinsic factors, blood flow can be modulated by a group of intrinsic factors that control cerebral vascular resistance. Among these factors are intracranial pressure, arterial oxygen tension, carbon dioxide tension, blood viscosity, and vascular tone. Although the cerebral vessels are supplied with nerves, there has been little evidence that they play other than a minor role in controlling blood flow. Oxygen and carbon dioxide concentrations play the greatest roles in modulating cerebrovascular resistance, with carbon dioxide being the more significant factor.

Variations in cerebral blood gas concentrations serve to provide constant blood flow within a wide range of systemic pressures and also provide local control to areas with varying demands.[1] For instance, if the brain requires more oxygen than is being supplied, it produces more carbon dioxide. This increase in carbon dioxide causes vasodilatation and increases blood flow until enough oxygen has been supplied to reduce the carbon dioxide concentration. This effect can happen either globally or locally.

Compensatory cerebral vasodilatation is also the mechanism that maintains cerebral blood flow when cerebral perfusion pressure drops as a person assumes an upright position. However, if the circulation is compromised by atherosclerotic disease, compensation may be insufficient, leading to symptoms of regional or diffuse hypoxia or anoxia.

COLLATERALIZATION

The vital role of collateral circulation in vascular occlusion has been appreciated for more than a century, but its involvement in cerebrovascular occlusive disease has become an important diagnostic consideration only since the advent of angiography[4–6] and the later development of noninvasive diagnostic techniques. Clinicians evaluating symptoms of cerebrovascular insufficiency and surgeons contemplating ligation of cervical arteries must be aware of the potential for collateral circulation and its influence on diagnostic tests and surgical procedures.

It was once believed that arteries in the brain were end arteries, but it is now known that capillary and precapillary anastomoses are common. To appreciate these collateral pathways better, it should be noted that there are two types of arterial branches supplying the brain. The more important type in terms of neuronal function and nutrient supply for the central nervous system is the penetrating arteries. However, it is the diffuse circumferential or superficial arteries that spread over the entire surface of the cervical hemispheres, brain stem, and spinal cord through which collateral circulation takes place. The circle of Willis and the major arterial trunks are included in this superficial system.

The routes for intracranial collateral circulation can be divided into three categories: large interarterial connections, intracranial-extracranial anastomoses, and small interarterial communications (see Figs. 7–2 through 7–5). The major pathway is the circle of Willis, providing communication between the two carotid arteries or between the basilar artery and the right or left carotid artery. As described earlier, the anatomic variations possible within this arterial circle are normally of little importance unless occlusion in one of the cervical vessels occurs, demanding collateral blood flow.

Second only to the circle of Willis in importance are the complex intracranial-extracranial or prewillisian anastomoses. Perhaps the best known prewillisian anastomosis is that between the external and internal carotid arteries, through the orbital and ophthalmic arteries. Other external-to-internal carotid collaterals include the meningohypophyseal and caroticotympanic branches. Other important prewillisian anastomoses may be encountered clinically, including the following: (1) the occipital branch of the external carotid artery in communication with the atlantic branch of the vertebral artery; (2) the deep cervical and ascending cervical branches of the subclavian artery connecting with branches of the lower vertebral artery, the atlantic branch of the upper vertebral artery, and the occipital branch of the internal carotid artery; and (3) the external carotid arteries communicating across the midline. Also included in the prewillisian group is the rete mirabile or "wonderful net" of transdural anastomoses across the subdural space from the dural arteries to arteries on the surface of the brain.

Of lesser importance are the leptomeningeal collaterals forming the meningeal border zone network. These connect the terminal cortical branches of the main cerebral arteries across the border zones along each vascular territory. Although these are not major collateral pathways, they may be sufficiently developed to interfere with the diagnosis of cerebrovascular insufficiency. Indeed, arterial occlusions may not become symptomatic because of adequate perfusion by the leptomeningeal anastomoses in the portion of the thrombosed artery's distribution. Similarly, excellent collateral flow around a thrombosed cortical vessel may induce rapid clearing of a neurologic deficit, leading the clinician to believe an extracranial occlusive process is involved.

It should be noted that there are no effective anastomotic pathways between neighboring cerebral artery branches, deep penetrating arteries, or the superficial and deep branches of the cerebral arteries.

The opening of collateral pathways is dependent largely on the age of the individual and the time sequence of occlusion. In older individuals, collateral pathways are more likely to be hypoplastic or involved in the

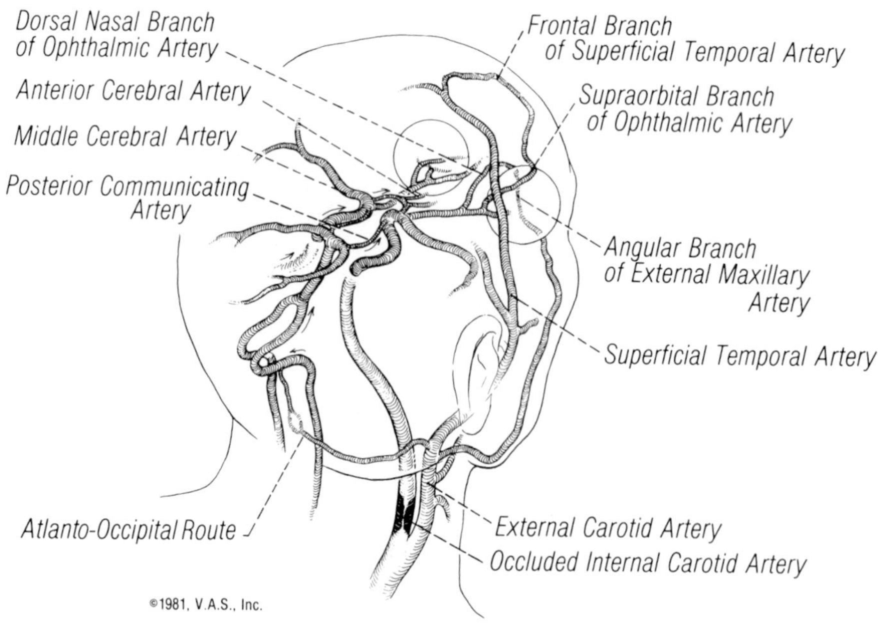

FIGURE 7–5 Major external carotid and vertebral collateral pathways associated with internal carotid occlusion.

atherosclerotic process. Even collateral vessels of sufficient luminal size are often not able to adapt rapidly enough to sudden occlusions, such as from embolism. Hence, collateral flow has a better chance of developing adequately in persons with slowly evolving atherosclerotic occlusions. When multiple atherosclerotic lesions are present, the adequacy of the collateral channels may be greatly lessened. Also affecting the adequacy of a collateral bed are the availability of multiple rather than single collateral sources and the pathologic conditions of the vessels, reducing their capacity for dilation.

Extracranially, there are numerous cervicocranial collaterals. Occlusion of an internal carotid produces collateral circulation to the carotid siphon through the external carotid and ophthalmic arteries (Fig. 7–5). The anterior and middle cerebral arteries in this case are also supplied from the opposite anterior cerebral artery and the posterior cerebral artery through the anterior and posterior communicating arteries. In the case of vertebral occlusion near its origin (Fig. 7–6), flow is shunted to the thyrocervical and costocervical axes, with compensatory enlargement of the opposite vertebral artery. Collateral circulation arising from occlusion of large branches of the aortic arch is through the intercostal and internal mammary arteries to the subclavian, and then through the branches of the thyrocervical and costocervical axes to the vertebral and carotid arteries (Fig. 7–7).

The simplest method of judging intracranial collateral potential is through a 5-minute common carotid compression test. If no

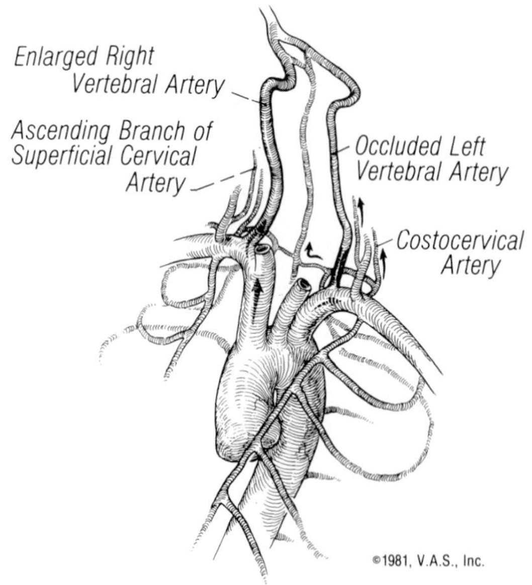

FIGURE 7–6 Major collateral pathways in vertebral occlusion.

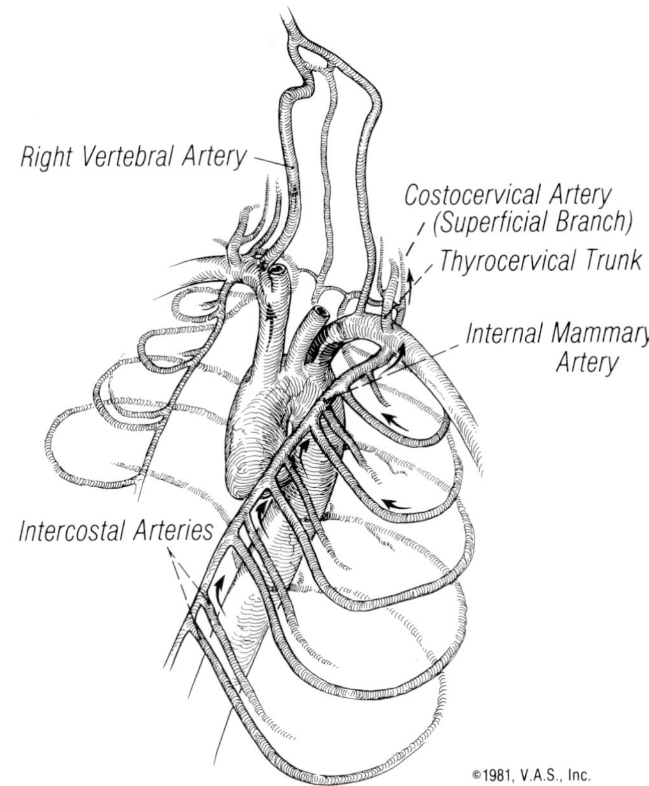

FIGURE 7–7 Major collateral pathways in proximal subclavian occlusion.

changes are noted in consciousness, speech, extremity strength, or fine finger control, then collateral flow can be judged sufficient. More specific information can be obtained by combining carotid compression with serial arteriography, electroencephalography, transcranial Doppler sonography, or duplex scanning with or without Doppler color-flow imaging. Arteriography is a somewhat risky procedure and offers no hemodynamic information, but it does delineate the collateral flow pattern. Carotid compression with electroencephalographic monitoring offers a more discrete result, with the earliest signs of ischemia on the ipsilateral side indicating faulty collateralization. Transcranial Doppler measurement of cerebral blood flow can predict tolerance to carotid ligation fairly well. If the residual blood flow in the middle cerebral artery during carotid compression is >25 cm/sec, the ischemic risk is low. Duplex Doppler ultrasonography with color-flow imaging can be used to determine the direction of blood flow through the ophthalmic artery and also the lumen size of the internal and external carotid arteries. Collateral circulation, however, can interfere with sonographic results. For instance, ophthalmic flow can be in the normal anterior direction, even with an occluded internal carotid artery, either because of stenosis of the ipsilateral external carotid artery or collateral circulation from the contralateral carotid artery through the circle of Willis or the internal maxillary artery.

REFERENCES

1. Stephens RB, Stilwell DL: Arteries and Veins of the Human Brain. Springfield, IL, Charles C Thomas, 1969.
2. McVay CB: Anson and McVay Surgical Anatomy, 6th ed. Philadelphia, WB Saunders, 1984.
3. Clemente CD (ed): Gray's Anatomy of the Human Body, 30th American ed. Philadelphia, Lea & Febiger, 1985.
4. Meyer JS (ed): Modern Concepts of Cerebrovascular Disease. New York, Spectrum Books, 1975.
5. Fields WS, Breutman ME, Weibel J: Collateral Circulation to the Brain. Baltimore, Williams & Wilkins, 1965.
6. Strandness DE Jr: Collateral Circulation in Clinical Surgery. Philadelphia, WB Saunders, 1969.

Chapter 8

NORMAL CAROTID ARTERIES AND CAROTID EXAMINATION TECHNIQUE

■ *William J. Zwiebel, MD*

NORMAL CAROTID WALL STRUCTURE

The walls of all arteries consist of three distinct layers. The innermost layer is the *intima*, or epithelial lining of the artery. The middle layer is the *media*, or muscular layer, which gives the artery its stiffness, elasticity, and strength. The outer layer is the *adventitia*, which is composed of loose connective tissue. As illustrated in Figure 8–1, all three layers are represented on ultrasound images.[1–3] The intima and adventitia produce parallel echogenic lines, with an intervening echo void that represents the media. Please note that the intimal reflection is only a reflection! The thickness of this reflection exceeds the actual thickness of the intima. Histologic studies have shown that the thickness of the media and adventitia are more accurately depicted on ultrasound images.[1]

The intimal reflection should be straight, relatively thin, and parallel to the adventitial layer. Significant undulation and thickening of the intima indicate plaque deposition, or, more rarely, fibromuscular hyperplasia. After endarterectomy, the intimal reflection is missing at the surgical site, because the intima is removed with the plaque.

Seeing the intimal reflection on longitudinal images ensures that the image plane passes through the vessel diameter. Similarly, in transverse sections, visualization of the intima indicates that the image plane is perpendicular to the vessel axis. A false impression of arterial wall thickening may occur with off-diameter longitudinal images, as illustrated in Figure 8–2.

NORMAL FLOW CHARACTERISTICS

In normal arteries that are relatively straight, blood flow is *laminar*, meaning that blood cells move in parallel lines. As shown in Figure 8–3, the laminar flow pattern can sometimes be seen on color-flow images. Slower velocities near the vessel wall and faster velocities near the lumen center are shown in different colors. In some instances, the highest flow velocities may be eccentric within the lumen because of the effects of bifurcations and curves in the vessel. It is important to recognize that flow is not always laminar in normal vessels. As noted in Chapter 3, the laminar pattern may be disturbed by vessel tortuosity, kinks, or branching. These normal flow disturbances are shown by mixtures of colors on color-flow images and by Doppler spectral broadening. The most noteworthy normal flow disturbance occurs at the carotid bifurcation (Fig. 8–4), where a vortex is established in the bulbous portion of the common carotid artery (CCA) and internal carotid artery.[4–7] The size of the vortex appears to be related to anatomic factors, including the diameter of the lumen and the degree of angulation between the internal (ICA) and external (ECA) carotid arteries.

From a spectral Doppler perspective, normal pulsatility features of the CCA, ICA, and ECA are of particular importance and require close attention. Please note these normal features, as presented in Figure 8–5 (see p 117). Normal pulsatility features are used to distin-

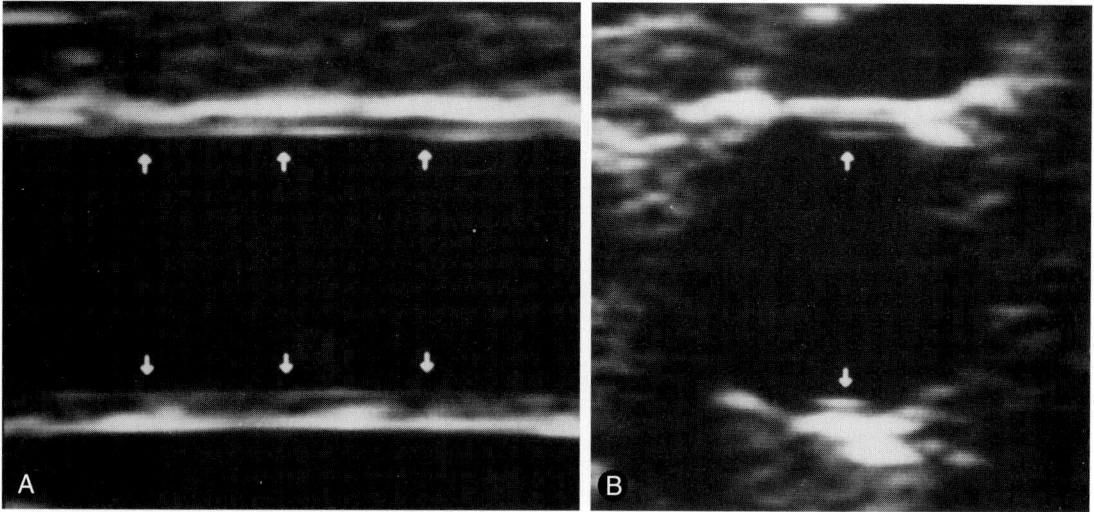

FIGURE 8–1 Normal arterial anatomy. Longitudinal (*A*) and transverse (*B*) images of the common carotid artery demonstrate a sharp line (specular reflection) that emanates from the intimal surface (*arrows*). The black line peripheral to this reflection represents the media of the artery. The outermost white line is the adventitia of the artery.

guish between the ICA and ECA, as discussed in the following section. Furthermore, altered carotid pulsatility is an important clue about the presence of carotid occlusive disease. In some cases, pulsatility changes are the *only* indication of abnormality.

The normal range of velocities in the CCA, ICA, and ECA has not been studied extensively[8–11] and velocities may vary with physiologic differences among individuals. With regard to peak systolic velocity in the ICA, reported mean values for normal adults range from 54 to 88 cm/sec (in the postbulbar region). Peak systolic velocities as high as 120 cm/sec have been reported in some normal individuals, but these values are exceptional and an ICA velocity exceeding 100 cm/sec should be viewed as potentially abnormal. Peak systolic velocity in the ECA is reported as 77 cm/sec (mean) in normal individuals, and the maximum velocity does not normally exceed 115 cm/sec. Considerable patient-to-patient variability occurs in ECA flow velocity, however, particularly if

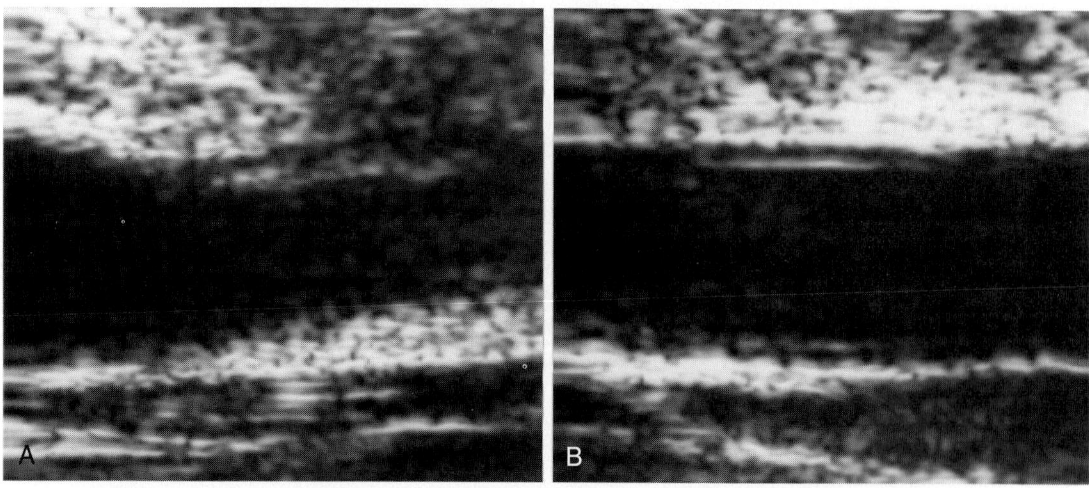

FIGURE 8–2 False-positive plaque diagnosis due to off-diameter image plane. *A*, It appears that plaque is present, resulting in stenosis, in this off-diameter section of the common carotid artery. *B*, The same artery is demonstrated to be normal by moving the transducer very slightly, such that the plane of the section passes through the diameter of the vessel. Note the clearly seen intimal reflections.

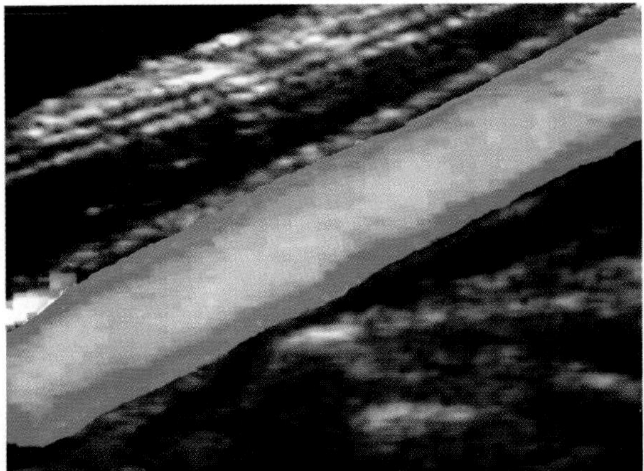

FIGURE 8–3 Laminar flow pattern. Darker red shades are seen at the periphery of this common carotid artery, because flow is slower near the wall. Lighter colors are present throughout the rest of the vessel, in which flow is faster.

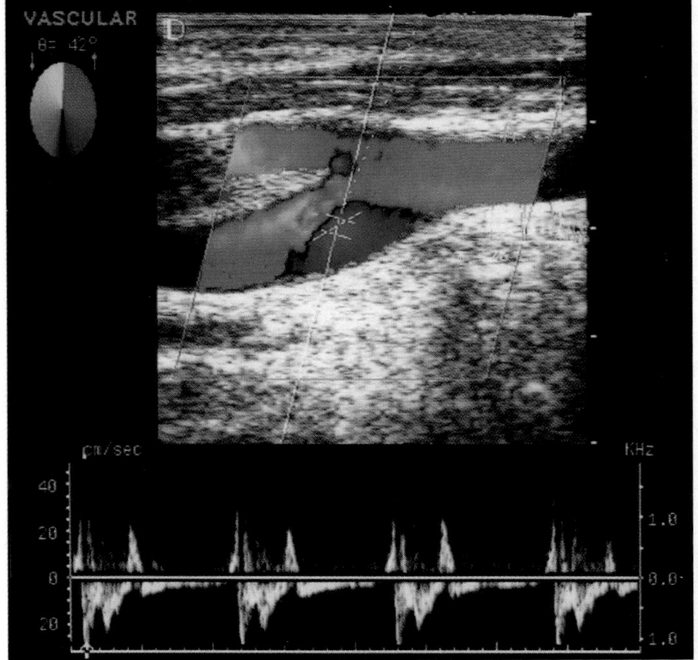

FIGURE 8–4 Long-axis view of the carotid bifurcation. The blue area in the bulbous portion of the internal carotid artery represents the normal flow reversal zone. The Doppler spectrum seen at the base of the image shows a disturbed to-and-fro pattern caused by the combined forward- and reverse-flow components present in the bulbous portion.

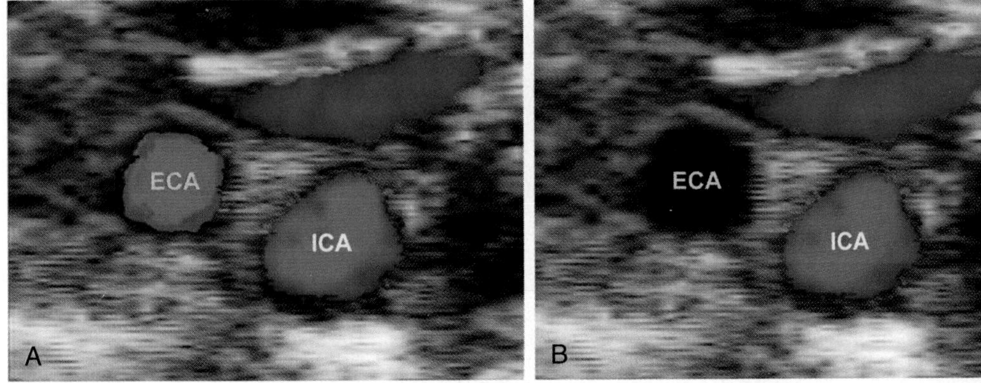

FIGURE 8–8 Color-Doppler visualization of pulsatility patterns. (See p 118.) *A*, In systole, flow (red color) is evident in both the internal (ICA) and external (ECA) carotid arteries. *B*, In diastole, flow is absent in the external carotid artery (ECA) but persists in the internal carotid artery (ICA). When seen in real time, the ECA "blinks" on and off, whereas the ICA undulates in brightness.

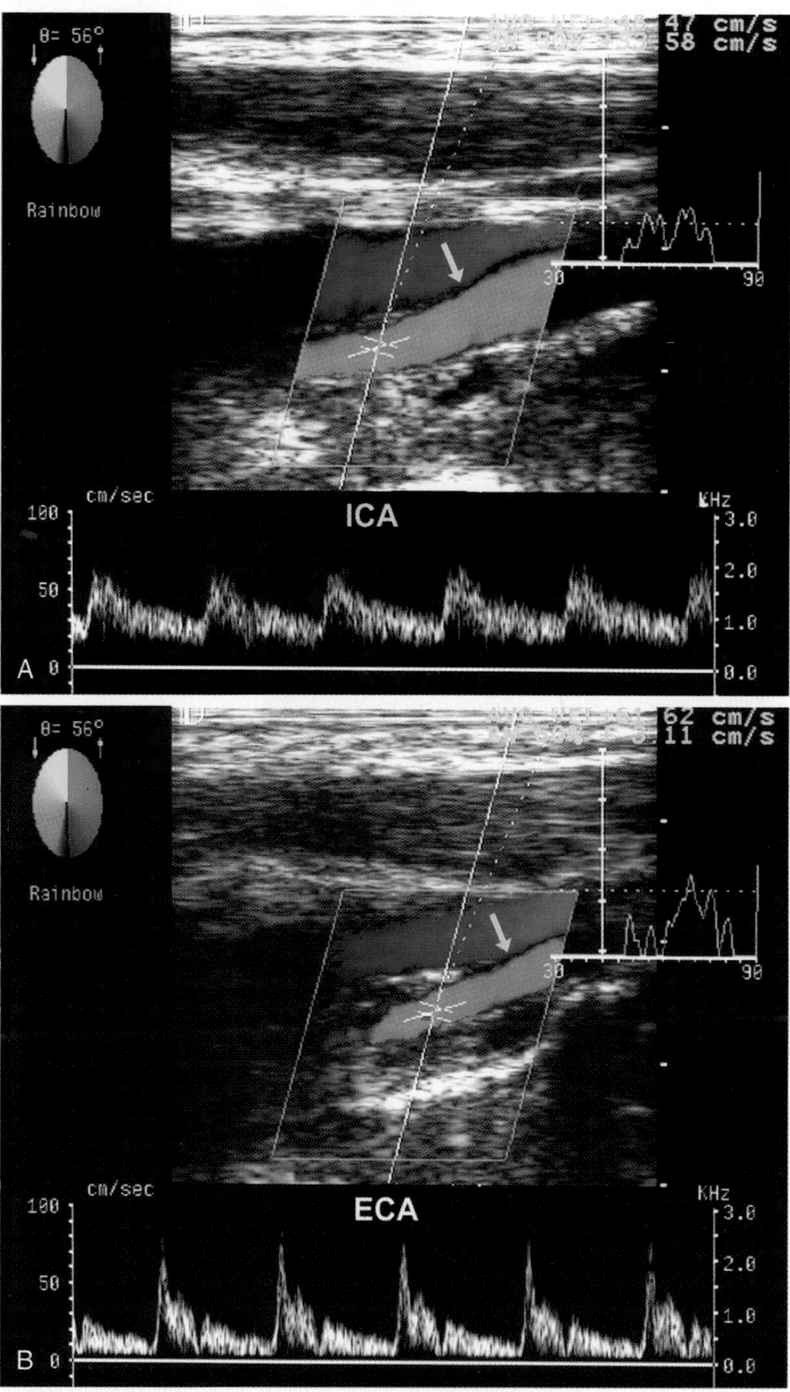

FIGURE 8–13 Identifying the internal and external carotid arteries. (See p 124.) By shifting back and forth between the internal (*A*) and the external (*B*) carotid arteries (ICA and ECA, respectively), the sonographer has determined that the junction of the vessels is at the approximate location of the arrows. The pulsatility of the ICA is clearly different from that of the ECA.

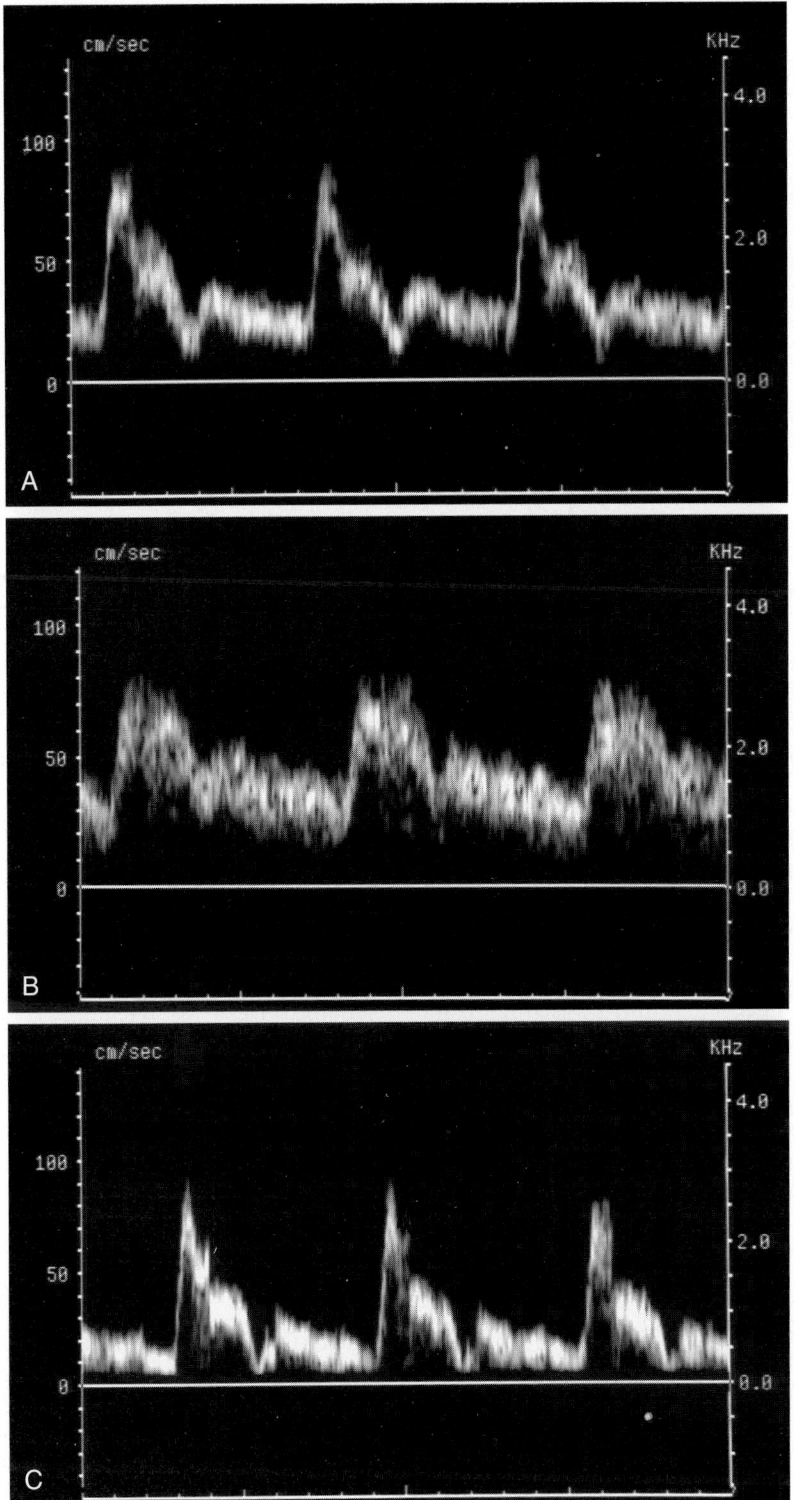

FIGURE 8–5 Normal carotid artery Doppler waveform. (See p 113.) *A*, Waveforms in the common carotid artery have moderately broad systolic peaks and a moderate amount of flow throughout diastole. *B*, The internal carotid artery waveforms have broad systolic peaks and a large amount of flow throughout diastole. Audible Doppler signals in the internal carotid artery have a smoothly undulating sound. *C*, External carotid artery waveforms have sharp systolic peaks and relatively little flow in diastole. The audible signals in the external carotid artery have a whip-like sound that is usually quite different from the sound of the internal carotid artery Doppler signals.

TABLE 8–1 FEATURES THAT IDENTIFY THE EXTERNAL AND INTERNAL CAROTID ARTERIES

Features	Carotid Arteries	
	External	***Internal***
Size	Usually smaller	Usually larger
Branches	Yes	No
Orientation	Proceeds anteriorly, toward the face	Proceeds posteriorly, toward the mastoid process
Doppler characteristics	High-resistance flow pattern	Low-resistance flow pattern
Temporal tap	Waveform deflections	No deflections

the ECA is serving as a collateral that circumvents an ipsilateral or contralateral ICA stenosis. Therefore, higher velocities may be encountered occasionally in the absence of ECA stenosis.

VESSEL IDENTITY

The correct identification of the ECA and ICA is of utmost importance, because significant diagnostic error may occur if these vessels are misidentified. The findings listed in Table 8–1 are all useful for distinguishing between the ICA and ECA, but among these, the Doppler findings are of greatest importance. The ICA has a high-resistance flow pattern, whereas the ECA has a low-resistance pattern. When the identity of the bifurcation branches is uncertain, leave the Doppler device turned on and move back and forth between the branches. The Doppler signals from the two vessels should look and sound *different* if one is the ICA and the other is the ECA. If the Doppler signals look and *sound* the same in both vessels, then you probably have identified two ECA branches, and the ICA is probably occluded (Fig. 8–6). When branch vessel identity is uncertain, do not guess! Indicate to the interpreting sonologist that you are not sure whether you are seeing external carotid branches or the ECA and ICA. It is better to say that you are uncertain than to make a diagnostic error.

Another very helpful means for identifying the ECA is to tap with your finger on the preauricular portion of the temporal artery while obtaining ECA Doppler signals. Because the temporal artery is a branch of the ECA, tapping causes deflections in the spectral waveform of the ECA (Fig. 8–7). Tapping does not affect ICA signals.

Differences in ECA and ICA pulsatility are also manifested in the color-flow image (Fig. 8–8 [see p 115]). Flow continues throughout the entire cardiac cycle in the CCA and ICA. As a result, color is always present in these vessels, although the brightness *undulates* from diastole to systole. In the ECA, flow is markedly diminished or absent in diastole; consequently, color *flickers* off and on in this vessel.

EXAMINATION PROTOCOL

An examination protocol should be established within each vascular laboratory to ensure that carotid sonography is performed consistently, comprehensively, and accurately. The ultrasound protocol used in our department is described here. These techniques may be modified to match the needs of specific patients or vascular laboratories. In all cases, however, the protocol should meet or exceed the standards established by the American Institute of Ultrasound in Medicine or the Intersocietal Commission for the Accreditation of Vascular Laboratories.*,† The standards of these two agencies are substantially the same.

INSTRUMENTATION

The carotid duplex examination should be performed only with appropriate instrumentation. The current standard of practice in the United States includes the following equipment: (1) high-frequency transducers with short focal distances designed for near-field work; (2) color-flow imaging; (3) pulsed, directional Doppler, with velocity measurement capabilities; and (4) frequency spectrum analysis. A large number of instruments are available that provide these features.

---

* American Institute of Ultrasound in Medicine. 14750 Sweitzer Lane, Suite 100, Laurel, MD 20707.

† Intersocietal Commission for Accreditation of Vascular Laboratories. 8840 Stanford Boulevard, Suite 4900, Columbia, MD 21045.

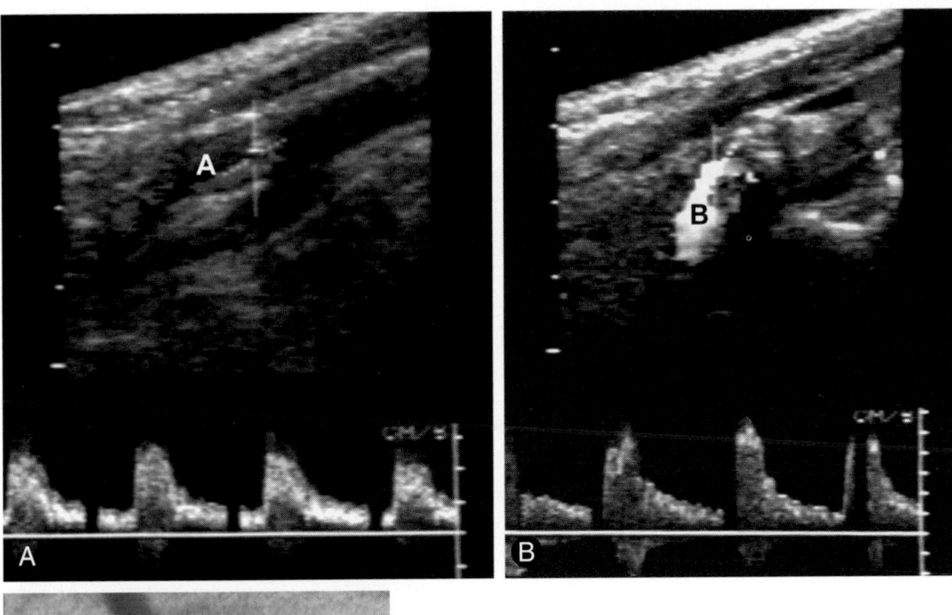

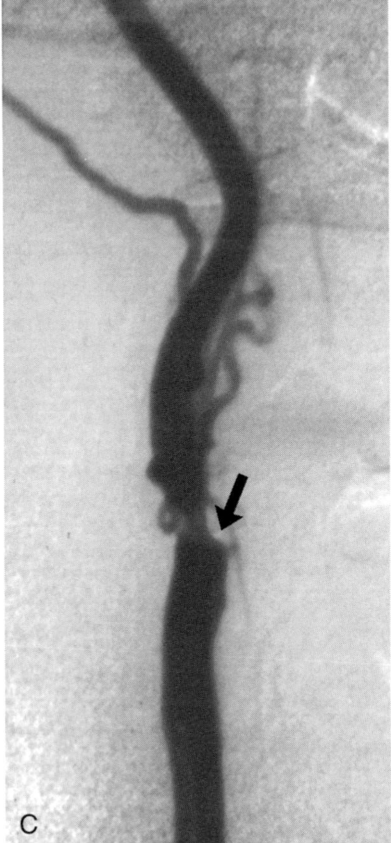

FIGURE 8–6 False-negative diagnosis of internal carotid artery (ICA) occlusion. *A* and *B*, Two branch vessels were identified at the carotid bifurcation, but the Doppler signals look similar. The audible signals were also indistinguishable on review of the tape-recorded study. The waveforms in these vessels do not look like typical external carotid artery (ECA) or ICA signals (see Fig. 8–5). Both vessel *A* and *B* were ECA branches. The atypical waveforms were due to collateral communication of the ECA branches with low-resistance intracranial vessels. *C*, Arteriogram in this patient shows the occluded stump (*arrow*) of the ICA and large ECA branches.

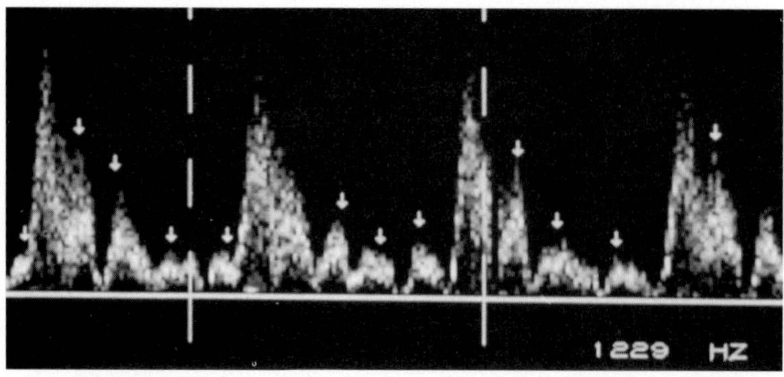

FIGURE 8–7 Temporal artery tapping identifies the external carotid artery (ECA). Each tap of the examiner's finger generates a sharp deflection (*arrows*) on the ECA waveform.

POSITIONING

Patient Position

We examine the carotid arteries with the patient in the supine position and with the examiner seated at the patient's head. In some institutions, the patient is examined in a reclining chair equipped with a headrest, such as a dental chair. In either case, exposure of the neck is maximized by having the patient drop the ipsilateral shoulder as far as possible (tell the patient to "reach down for your hip"). Neck exposure is also enhanced by tilting and rotating the head away from the side being examined (Fig. 8–9). Do not hesitate to vary the position of the head and neck during the examination to facilitate visualization of the vessels. Be creative!

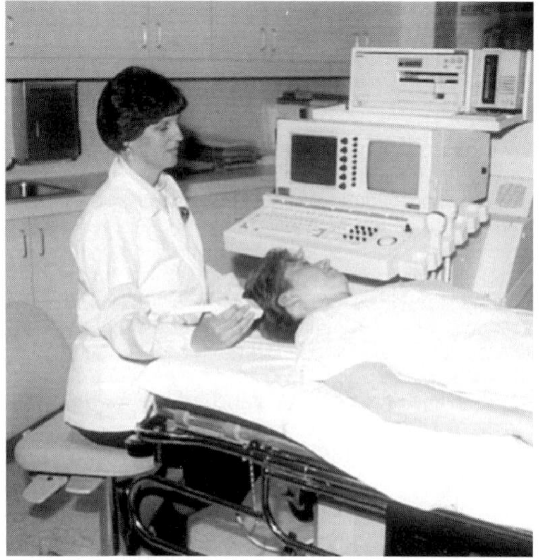

FIGURE 8–9 Patient and technologist positions for carotid ultrasound examination.

Transducer Position

Several transducer positions are used to examine the carotid arteries in long-axis (longitudinal) planes, as illustrated in Figure 8–10. Generally, the posterolateral and far-posterolateral positions are most useful for showing the carotid bifurcation and the ICA, but, in some cases, an anterior or lateral approach works best. Short-axis (transverse) views of the carotid arteries are obtained from an anterior, lateral, or posterolateral approach, depending on which best shows the vessels.

The *far*-posterolateral approach often provides the best images of the distal reaches of the ICA. To use this view effectively, however, it is necessary to turn the patient's head far to the contralateral side and to place the transducer posterior to the sternomastoid muscle (see Fig. 8–10*D*). Neophyte sonographers generally have difficulty imaging the ICA, because they fail to approach the vessel from a sufficiently posterior location.

CAROTID ARTERY VS. JUGULAR VEIN

The CCA lies immediately adjacent to the jugular vein, but the two vessels are easily differentiated. First, flow in the carotid artery is toward the head and pulsatile. In contrast, flow in the jugular vein is toward the feet and has typical venous flow features (low velocity, undulating flow pattern, "windstorm" sound). Also, the caliber of the carotid artery is fairly uniform, whereas the caliber of the jugular vein varies markedly from moment to moment, in response to respiration. Finally, the carotid arteries are thick walled, and a distinct intimal reflection is visible.

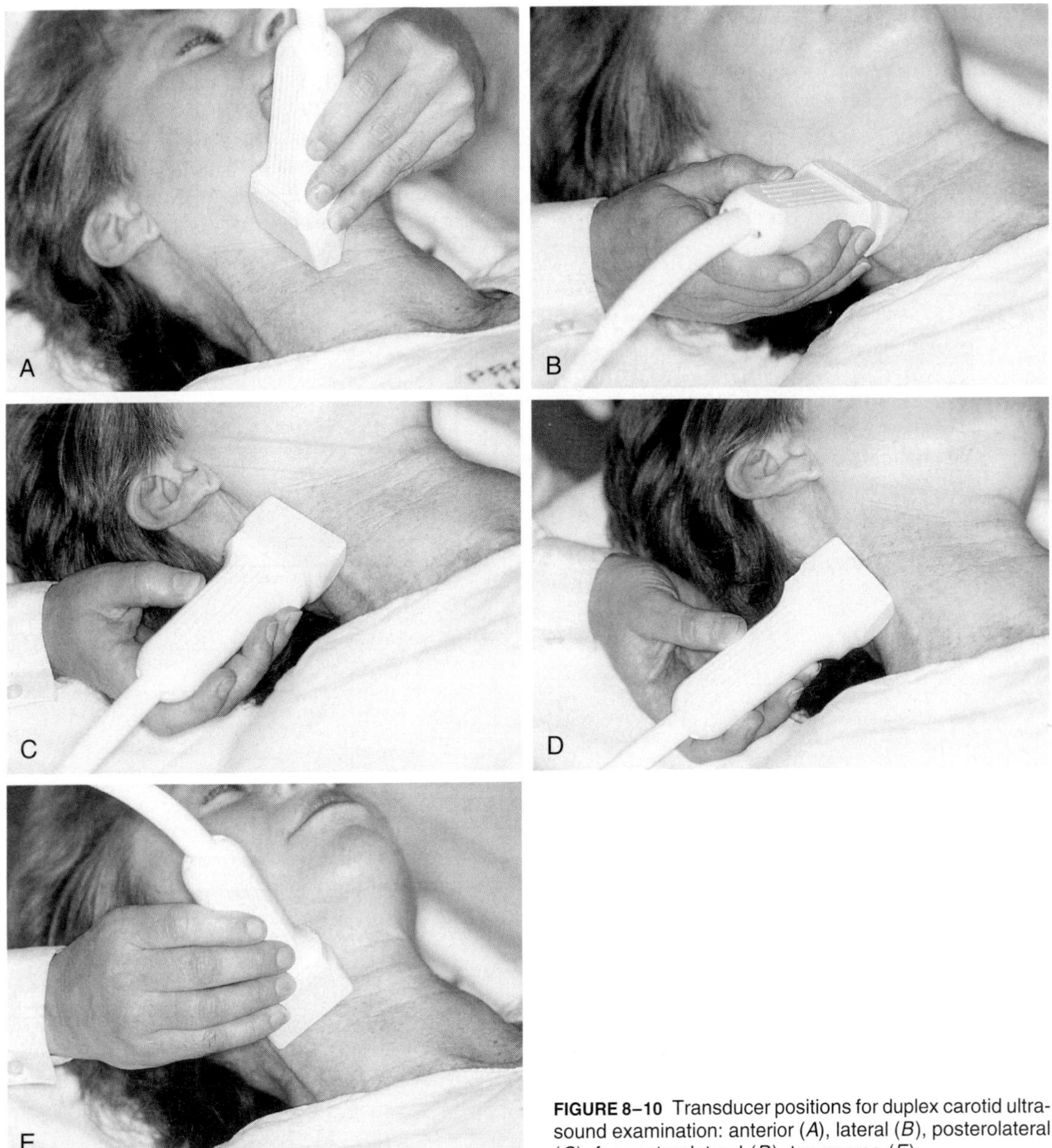

FIGURE 8–10 Transducer positions for duplex carotid ultrasound examination: anterior (*A*), lateral (*B*), posterolateral (*C*), far posterolateral (*D*), transverse (*E*).

The jugular vein wall is thin (invisible), and the vein collapses with slight pressure from the transducer.

IMAGE ORIENTATION

Consistent with internationally accepted conventions, we orient longitudinal images with the patient's head to the left. Likewise, transverse images generally are oriented as if viewed from the patient's feet, with the patient's right side on the left side of the image. Admittedly, we are not terribly particular about transverse image orientation.

RECORDING

In the past, we routinely recorded the entire carotid ultrasound examination on videotape, but we no longer do this, as color hard copy imaging has improved and reviewing taped studies is cumbersome. Our technicians continue to video record difficult or confusing examinations.

We currently use transparent film or color (paper) prints for recording carotid examinations. We conduct the examination in a consistent pattern, starting with the right carotid bifurcation and then going to the left. All segments of the examination are recorded in sequence, beginning with the CCA and proceeding into the ICA and then the ECA. With this patterned approach, hard copy images are recorded in an orderly, predictable way, which greatly simplifies interpretation of the studies. The patterned recording approach, furthermore, reduces the potential for diagnostic error, because the interpreter is less apt

Department of Veterans Affairs

Vascular Laboratory
VA Medical Center
Salt Lake City, Utah

Carotid Artery Duplex Ultrasound

PATIENT IDENTIFICATION

Date:______ Technologist:______ Tape #______ Requested By:______

History:______

Slurred Speech	❑	Amaurosis Fugax	R / L
Vertigo	❑	Blurred Vision	R / L
Drop Attack	❑	Hemiplegia	R / L
Memory Impairment/Confusion	❑	Weakness-Numbness Arm/Leg	R / L
		Previous Carotid Surgery	R / L

Prior Duplex or Angio Resuts______

Right Carotid

______cm/sec
______cm/sec ECA
ICA ______Syst Ratio
CCA ______cm/sec
CCA ______cm/sec

Left Carotid

______cm/sec ECA
______cm/sec
ICA ______Syst Ratio
CCA ______cm/sec
CCA ______cm/sec

Right Vertebral

Diameter ______ mm ______ cm/sec Ante/Retro

Left Vertebral

Diameter ______ mm ______ cm/sec Ante/Retro

Technologist Comments:______

Right	**Preliminary**	**Final**
CCA		
ICA		
ECA		
Progression	Y / N	Y / N

Left	**Preliminary**	**Final**
CCA		
ICA		
ECA		
Progression	Y / N	Y / N

4-Part – White: Radiology - Pink: Preliminary Copy - Yellow: Medical Records - Goldenrod: MD

VA Form 10-44/C (114/660)
August 1994

FIGURE 8–11 Report form for carotid ultrasound examination.

to mistake one Doppler spectrum or vessel for another.

In addition to hard copy images, we routinely use a report form (Fig. 8–11), on which the sonographer writes important information, including the patient history, blood flow velocity data (derived from spectrum analysis), and notations concerning plaque location and severity. The sonographer's preliminary impression and the sonologist's final impression are also recorded on the report form. This form consists of three copies, one for the referring clinician, one for the department records, and one for the hospital medical record. Because all the vital numerical information is included on the report form, the interpreting clinician needs only to dictate a brief report.

THE EXAMINATION SEQUENCE

As a rule, our carotid examinations follow these steps:

Step 1. *Get oriented!* Choose the transducer position that best displays the carotid vessels in a longitudinal view. Generally, the posterolateral approach, as shown in Figure 8–10, is most advantageous.

Step 2. *Record a velocity spectrum* from the CCA (Fig. 8–12). A recording site that is free of disease is preferred, and *care should be taken that the sample volume is squarely within the vessel lumen and that the Doppler angle is sufficient to accurately measure the peak systolic velocity.* This is extremely important, as inadequate sampling of the CCA may artifactually lower the peak systolic velocity and, in turn, may exaggerate velocity ratio calculations used to estimate ICA narrowing (see Chapters 3 and 10). The result could be a false-positive diagnosis of clinically significant carotid narrowing.

Step 3. Survey the carotid bifurcation with color-flow imaging. Begin at the clavicle with longitudinal images, proceed to the carotid bifurcation, and, from there, continue into the ECA and ICA. Then repeat the process with transverse images. The purpose of this survey is to confirm the patency of the arteries, to identify and localize plaque and associated flow abnormalities, and to define the junction of the ECA and ICA (so that plaque location can be determined correctly).

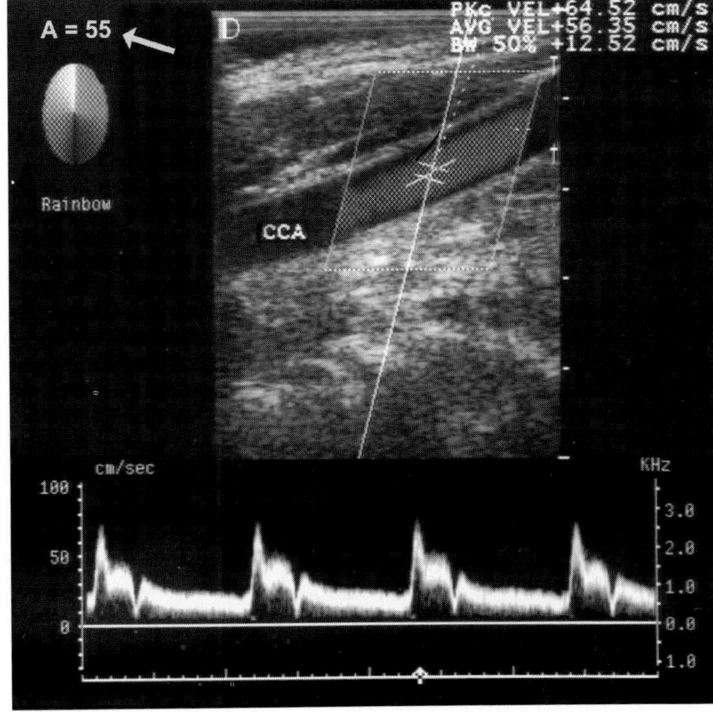

FIGURE 8–12 Accurate common carotid artery (CCA) velocity measurement. The CCA is clearly visualized; the Doppler sample volume is central in the artery and below the bulbous portion. The Doppler angle (*arrow*, left upper corner) is 60 degrees or less, and the Doppler signal (waveform) is strong and clear.

Step 4. Confirm the identity of the ICA and ECA by their Doppler spectral signatures (see Fig. 8–5) and by anatomic features summarized in Table 8–1. Both longitudinal and transverse images are helpful in this regard. The proper identification of the branch vessels is essential, as ECA stenoses usually are *not* treated surgically, whereas significant ICA stenoses usually *are* treated surgically.

Step 5. With the survey completed and the identity of the ICA and ECA confirmed, *scrutinize significant areas of plaque formation,* documenting with hard copy the thickness of plaque, the degree of lumen reduction, and other plaque features, as is discussed in subsequent chapters. Images transverse to the vessel axis are essential for assessment of plaque thickness and luminal narrowing, as shown in Chapter 9. Gray-scale images often show plaque features better than color-flow images.

A view that simultaneously shows both the ECA and the ICA, as seen in Figure 8–4, is very useful for localizing plaque. Unfortunately, this view cannot frequently be achieved (due to an unfavorable orientation of the carotid bifurcation). As an alternative, plaque location may be determined by shifting the image back and forth between the bifurcation branches and noting the point at which they come together (Fig. 8–13 [see p 116]).

Step 6. Most importantly, *record angle-corrected velocity spectra in areas of stenosis* (as discussed in Chapter 10). Also obtain color-flow images that illustrate the location and length of the stenosis, as well as the flow disturbances present in the stenotic and poststenotic regions. If possible, obtain cross-sectional images showing the degree of luminal narrowing, as illustrated in Chapter 9.

Step 7. *Evaluate vertebral artery flow*, as discussed in Chapter 12. During routine examination, we determine only that flow is present in the vertebral arteries and is cephalad in direction.

Step 8. *Assess subclavian artery flow*, to detect stenosis or occlusion of these vessels. Each subclavian artery is imaged from a long-axis perspective, from either a supraclavicular approach or a transpectoral approach. This can be done at the beginning or the end of the ipsilateral carotid examination. A representative Doppler spectral waveform is recorded in each vessel. These waveforms should show a high-resistance flow pattern and should be slightly pulsatile. A low-resistance or damped pattern and lack of pulsatility suggest stenosis or occlusion proximal to the point of Doppler examination. In some cases, a subclavian stenosis may be visualized directly. In such instances, color-Doppler images of the stenosis should be recorded and Doppler spectral measurement should be obtained in and distal to the stenosis, in the same manner as for carotid stenosis.

REFERENCES

1. Wolverson MK, Bashiti HM, Peterson GJ: Ultrasonic tissue characterization of atheromatous plaques using a high resolution real time scanner. Ultrasound Med Biol 6:669–709, 1983.
2. Pignoli P, Tremoli E, Poli A, et al: Intimal plus medial thickness of the arterial wall: A direct measurement with ultrasound imaging. Circulation 6:1399–1406, 1986.
3. Poli A, Tremoli E, Colombo A, et al: Ultrasonographic measurement of the common carotid arterial wall thickness in hypercholesterolemic patients. Atherosclerosis 70:253–261, 1988.
4. Zwiebel WJ: Duplex examination of the carotid arteries. Semin Ultrasound CT MR 11:97–135, 1990.
5. Zierler RE, Phillips DJ, Beach KW, et al: Noninvasive assessment of normal carotid bifurcation hemodynamics with color flow ultrasound imaging. Ultrasound Med Biol 13:471–476, 1987.
6. Merritt CRB: Doppler blood flow imaging: Integrating flow with tissue data. Diagn Imaging 11:146–155, 1986.
7. Middleton WD, Foley WD, Lawson TL: Flow reversal in the normal carotid bifurcation: Color Doppler flow imaging analysis. Radiology 167:207–210, 1988.
8. Blackshear WM, Phillips JD, Chikos PM, et al: Carotid artery velocity patterns in normal and stenotic vessels. 11:67–71, 1980.
9. Zbornikova V, Lassvik C: Duplex scanning in presumably normal persons of different ages. Ultrasound Med Biol 12:371–378, 1986.
10. Ku DN: A review of carotid scanning. Echocardiography 5:53–69, 1988.
11. Paivansalo MJ, Sinituoto TMJ, Tikkakoski TA, et al: Duplex ultrasound of the external carotid artery. Acta Radiol 37:41–43, 1996.

Chapter 9

Ultrasound Assessment of Carotid Plaque

William J. Zwiebel, MD

Diagnostic ultrasound has the unique ability to evaluate the composition of atherosclerotic plaque in vivo.* Considerable controversy exists, however, concerning the accuracy and utility of ultrasound plaque assessment, and this controversy has caused uncertainty about the clinical indications for carotid plaque imaging. It is valuable, therefore, to review this matter in some detail.

DETECTION, EXTENT, SEVERITY, AND FOLLOW-UP

Atherosclerotic plaque is represented sonographically by echogenic material that thickens the intimal reflection and encroaches on the arterial lumen.[1–5] Minimal plaque formation may be detected by measuring the total intimal-medial thickness (Fig. 9–1). A measurement greater than 1.2 mm (lumen to adventitia) appears to accurately indicate the presence of plaque. Reproducibility of plaque detection with ultrasound was found to be only fair to good in a large multicenter study, however.[6] Causes of interobserver variation include level of the technologists' skill, ultrasound image quality, failure to examine the same vascular segment, and lack of a uniform definition of findings that indicate the presence of plaque. Other single-institution studies have shown good intraobserver and interobserver agreement for ultrasound plaque assessment.[7–10]

Having detected carotid plaque, we are faced with the need to describe it in a way that accurately represents its severity. For assessment of plaque progression over time in a clinical or research setting, precise cross-sectional images showing the circumferential extent and thickness of plaque are obtained at specific, repeatable locations. For day-to-day clinical assessment of the carotid arteries for lesions requiring surgery, such detail is unnecessary, and a more general description of plaque severity is adequate. I generally describe two plaque features, extent and severity. By *extent,* I mean the length of the vessel (cephalocaudad) affected by plaque, which is determined with longitudinal images of the carotid arteries. I report plaque extent descriptively (e.g., plaque extends from the distal common carotid artery into the proximal internal carotid artery). By *severity,* I mean the thickness of plaque. This is more difficult to define sonographically, because plaque varies in thickness from one location to another. The best means for assessing carotid plaque thickness is from *transverse* (short-axis) images, which most accurately show the maximum thickness of the plaque and the resultant degree of luminal narrowing. *Plaque severity can be grossly overestimated or underestimated from longitudinal images,* as illustrated in Figure 9–2. The causes for misinterpretation of plaque severity are illustrated in Figure 9–3. When reporting plaque severity, I sometimes use generic terms such as *minimal, moderate,* and *severe.* For situations in which greater precision is desirable, I report the plaque thickness (in millimeters, from transverse images), and whether the plaque is localized or circumferential (i.e., extending around the circumference of the lumen).

In general, I do not follow-up patients on the basis of plaque measurements per se. Instead, I recommend an interval for repeated

* High-resolution magnetic resonance imaging can visualize plaque in detail, but this method is experimental and is not widely used.

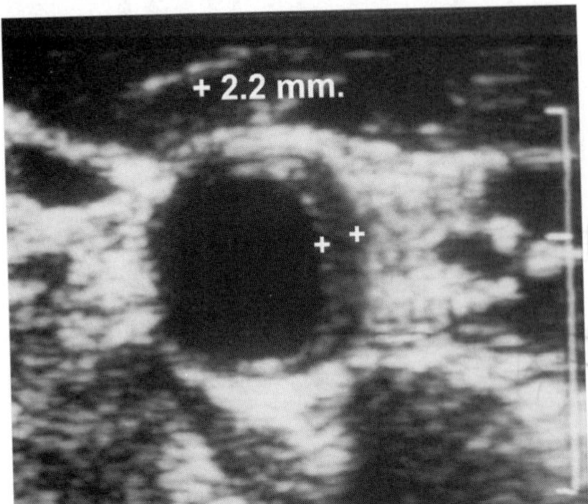

FIGURE 9–1 Intimal-medial thickness. A transverse image shows an area of plaque formation. The intimal-medial thickness is measured.

carotid evaluation as determined by the Doppler-based severity of carotid stenosis. In a sense, this amounts to the same thing, for the degree of stenosis indirectly indicates the severity of plaque formation. The recommended intervals for follow-up are listed in Chapter 10.

PLAQUE PATHOGENESIS

Current theory holds that atherosclerosis is a response to injury and that this response is mediated (or directed) by the endothelial cells that line the arteries.[10–13] Three endothelium-mediated processes occur in the course of plaque formation: the migration of smooth muscle cells into the subendothelial layer; the accumulation of intracellular and extracellular lipid; and the development of a collagenous (fibrous) matrix within the evolving plaque.

There are two main types of atherosclerotic plaque, uncomplicated and complicated (Fig. 9–4). Uncomplicated (or stable) plaque consists of a largely uniform, lipid, and cellular deposit covered by a subendothelial fibrous tissue "cap" (made of smooth muscle cells and connective tissue). The architecture of complicated plaque is disturbed by degenerative processes including

1. Necrosis
2. Hemorrhage
3. Calcification
4. Thinning or disruption of the fibrous cap
5. Disruption of the endothelial layer
6. Ulceration[11–30]

It appears that the most important complications that occur in plaque are fibrous cap disruption, endothelial layer disruption, and intraplaque hemorrhage. Disruption of the fibrous cap and endothelium may lead directly to embolization through the shedding of plaque contents into the blood stream. Alternatively, endothelial disruption may indirectly cause embolization, through the adherence of platelets or thrombus on denuded plaque surface. This material is subsequently shed into the blood stream. Considerable speculation surrounds the role that intraplaque hemorrhage may play in plaque surface disruption. In theory, hemorrhage into plaque (from rupture of vasa vasorum) causes rapid plaque enlargement, which, in turn, causes plaque ischemia and compromises the integrity of both the fibrous cap and the endothelial layer. Subsequent breakdown of the endothelium may lead directly or indirectly to embolization, as discussed previously.

Central to current thinking about plaque evolution is the concept that stable, uncomplicated plaque tends to be transformed into complicated plaque through a largely undefined injury process. It appears, furthermore, that repeated cycles of injury and repair occur in many plaques. Large (hence older) plaques tend to be complicated histologically, whereas small (younger) plaques tend to be uncomplicated.[13] As a correlate, it also is postulated that certain plaque complications (e.g., intraplaque hemorrhage) increase the likelihood of neurologic symptoms because of greater potential for embolization.[14–16, 21]

PLAQUE CHARACTERIZATION

The primary role of carotid sonography is the detection and assessment of carotid stenosis. Nonetheless, much has been made of the ability of ultrasound to characterize plaque, and ultrasound practitioners should be familiar, therefore, with plaque characterization concepts.[14–28] In general terms, plaque can be characterized as *low, medium,* or *high* in echogenicity and as *homogeneous* or *heterogeneous.* The histologic correlates of these characteristics follow.

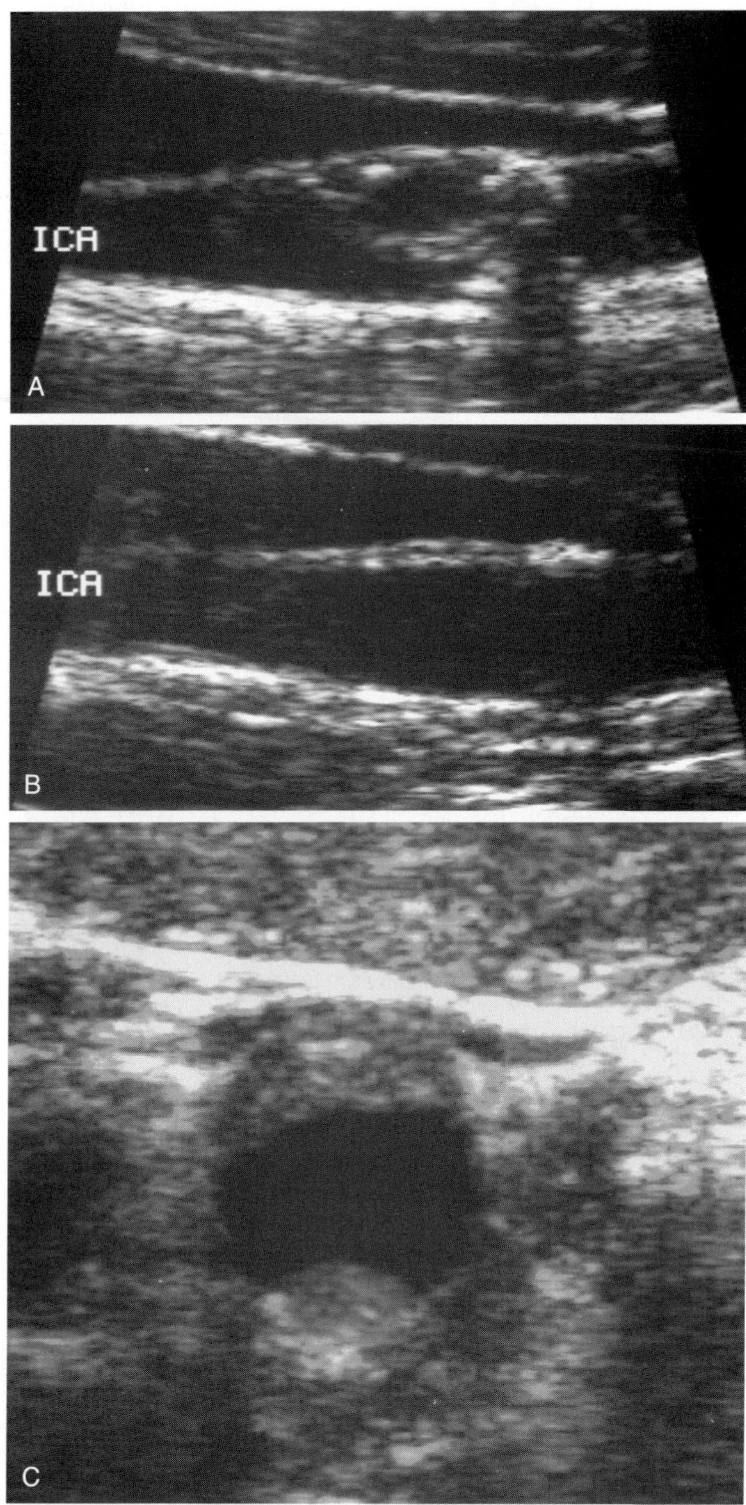

FIGURE 9–2 Incorrect plaque assessment from longitudinal images. *A,* The internal carotid artery (ICA) appears to be largely filled with plaque on this longitudinal image. *B,* Another longitudinal image at the same location shows very little plaque. *C,* Transverse views accurately display the thickness and circumferential extent of plaque.

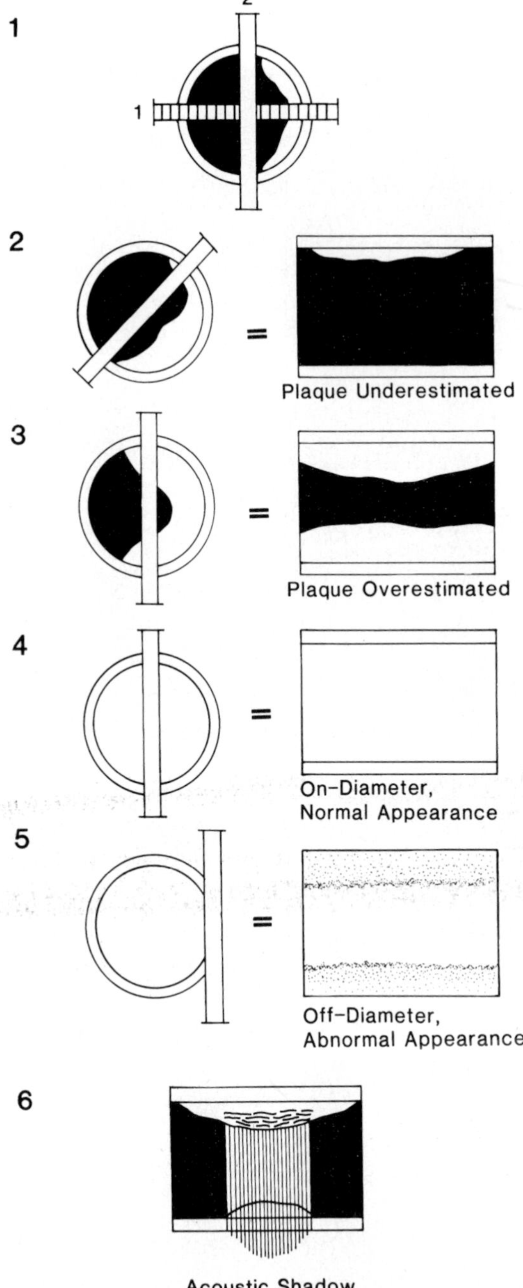

FIGURE 9–3 Causes for misinterpretation of carotid plaque severity. *1,* Plaque is not seen in this example with a horizontal image plane but is accurately represented in the vertical image plane. *2,* This image plane underestimates plaque thickness. *3,* Plaque thickness and luminal narrowing are overestimated in this plane. *4,* A scan through the vessel center generates a normal appearance, but an off-diameter scan (*5*) simulates pathology. *6,* Pathology is obscured by an acoustic shadow.

Low Echogenicity

Fibrofatty plaque (Fig. 9–5*A*), which contains a large amount of lipid material, is low in echogenicity. This type of plaque is less echogenic than the nearby sternomastoid muscle, and in some cases fibrofatty plaque is so echo poor that it is difficult to see with ultrasound. The occasional problem of visualizing fibrofatty plaque is ameliorated with color-flow imaging, because a flow void (and perhaps flow disturbance) is visible, even if the plaque is not well seen.

Moderate Echogenicity

As the collagen content of plaque increases relative to the fat content, ultrasound echogenicity also increases. Hence, fibrous plaque, in which collagen is a prominent component, is moderately echogenic (Fig. 9–5*B*). Fibrous plaque is easy to see with ultrasound. Its echogenicity equals or exceeds that of the sternomastoid muscle, but it is less echogenic than the arterial adventitia.

Strong Echogenicity With Shadowing

Dystrophic calcification occurs in plaque at sites of hemorrhage and necrosis, and such calcification generates strong reflections, accompanied by distal acoustic shadows (Fig. 9–5*C*). These reflections equal or exceed the brightness of any other object in the image. High-resolution sonography is extremely sensitive to the presence of calcification, and areas as small as 1 mm in diameter may be detected. Plaque calcification may be focal or diffuse, and large calcification may generate acoustic shadows that obscure the arterial lumen, interfering with ultrasound diagnosis (Fig. 9–6).

Homogeneous vs. Heterogeneous Plaque

It has long been noted that, from an ultrasound perspective, some plaque is homogeneous, and some plaque is heterogeneous.[15–17, 22–25] Calcification is one cause of heterogeneity, but no correlation has been

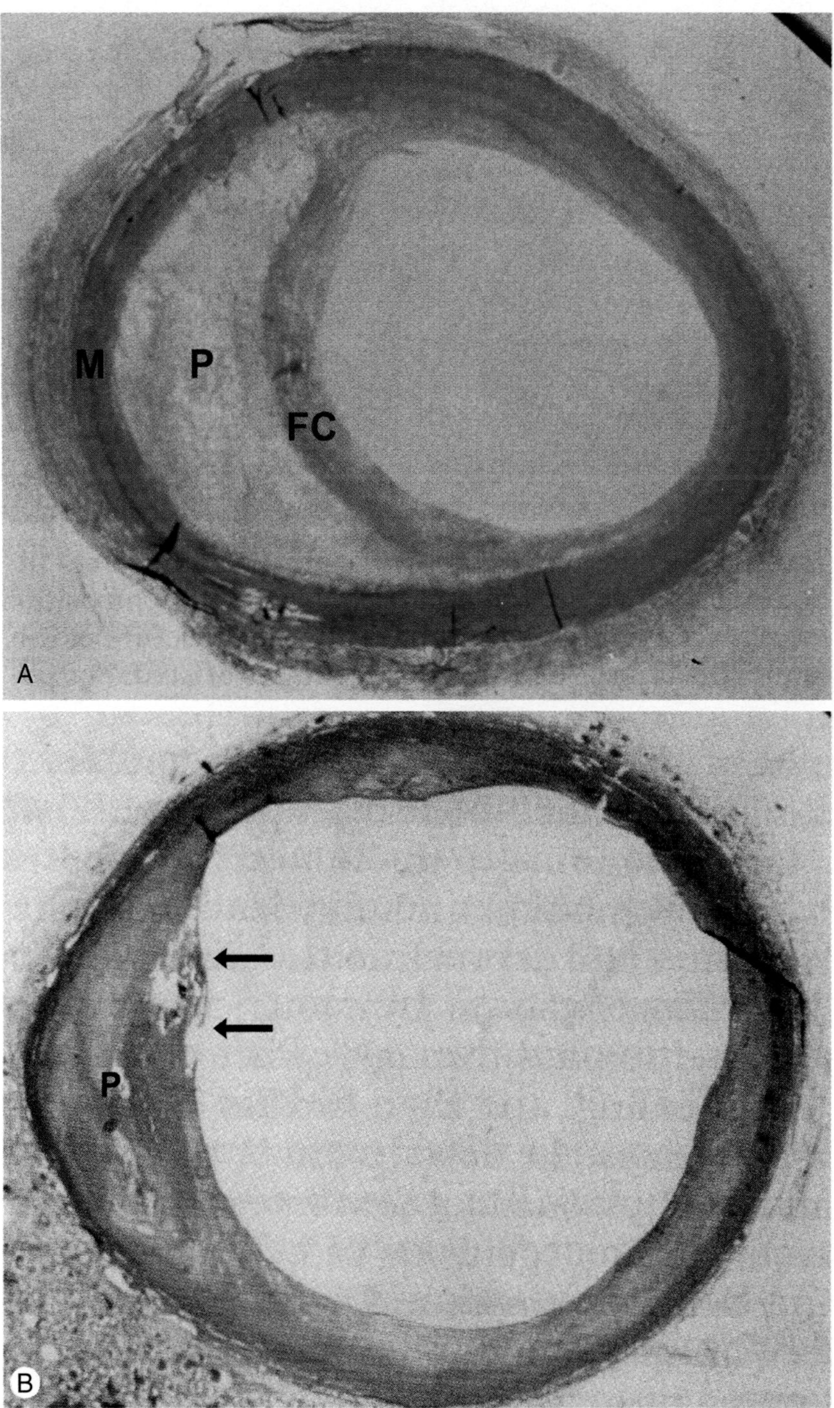

FIGURE 9–4 Plaque histology. *A,* Microscopic section of an uncomplicated plaque (P). The fibrous cap (FC) is intact and the plaque contents (P) are homogeneous. M = muscularis. *B,* Microscopic section of a complicated plaque. The fibrous cap is ruptured and an area of cavitation is present (*arrows*). The plaque contents (P) are heterogeneous. (From O'Leary D, Glagov S, Zarins C, Giddens D: Carotid artery disease. *In* Rifkin MD, Charboneau JW, Laing FC [eds]: Ultrasound 1991: Special Course Syllabus, 77th Scientific Assembly and Annual Meeting. Oak Park, IL, RSNA Publications, 1991, pp 189–200. Reproduced with the kind permission of Daniel O'Leary MD.)

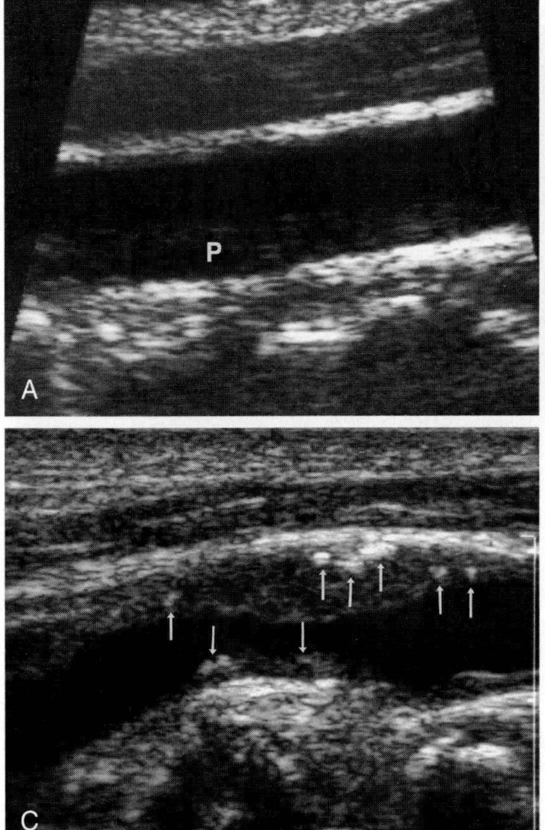

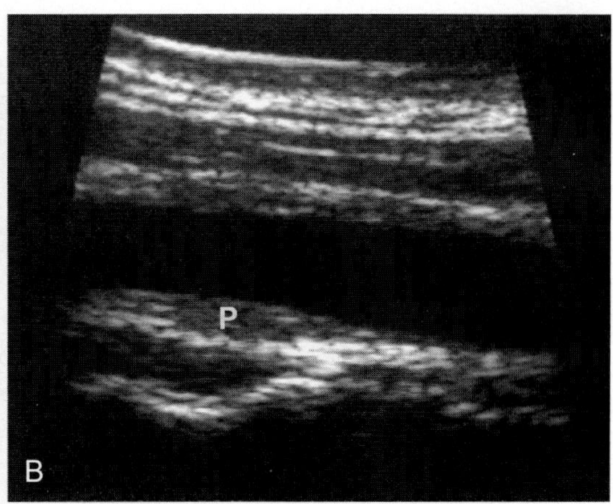

FIGURE 9–5 Ultrasound plaque characterization. *A,* Low echogenicity, fibrofatty, plaque (P). *B,* Moderately echogenic fibrous plaque (P). *C,* Strongly echogenic calcifications (*arrows*) are present throughout the plaque.

reported between the presence of calcification and neurologic symptoms. Two other types of heterogeneity have been discussed widely in the literature, namely, focal and multifocal areas of *low* echogenicity (Fig. 9–7). The focal variety is often called a *focal hypoechoic zone,* and the diffuse variety is called *diffuse nonhomogeneity.* Clinical interest has centered on reports that neurologic

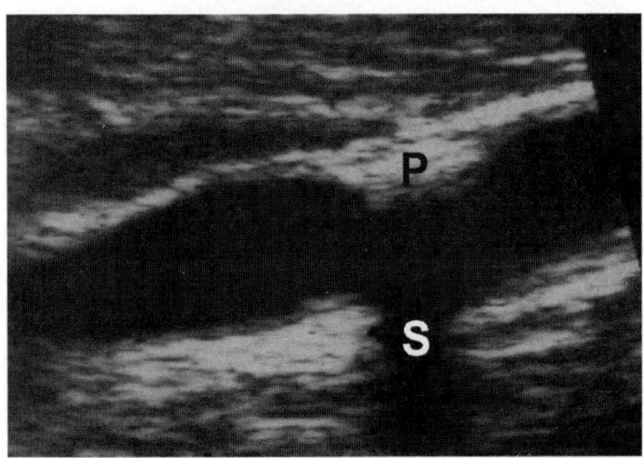

FIGURE 9–6 Acoustic shadow. A large acoustic shadow (S) obscures much of the carotid lumen. P = calcified plaque.

symptoms are more common in patients with these two types of plaque heterogeneity, compared with patients with homogeneous or calcified carotid plaque. In theory, focal or diffuse plaque heterogeneity is caused by intraplaque hemorrhage, which, in turn, may cause embolization, as discussed previously. Plaque heterogeneity, therefore, is postulated as a precursor of hemispheric neurologic symptoms, including transient cerebral ischemia or stroke.[15, 23, 25] These theories are controversial however, for several reasons. First, ultrasound plaque heterogeneity is only about 65% specific for intraplaque hemorrhage, and heterogeneity may also be caused by plaque necrosis or accumulated lipid material.[16, 24] At least two studies have found no correlation between sonographic and histologic findings, casting further doubt on the significance of heterogeneity.[27, 29] Second, the association of heterogeneity with neurologic symptoms has come into question, with several studies showing no association between ultrasound patterns and the incidence of hemispheric symptoms.[13, 16, 30] Third, if

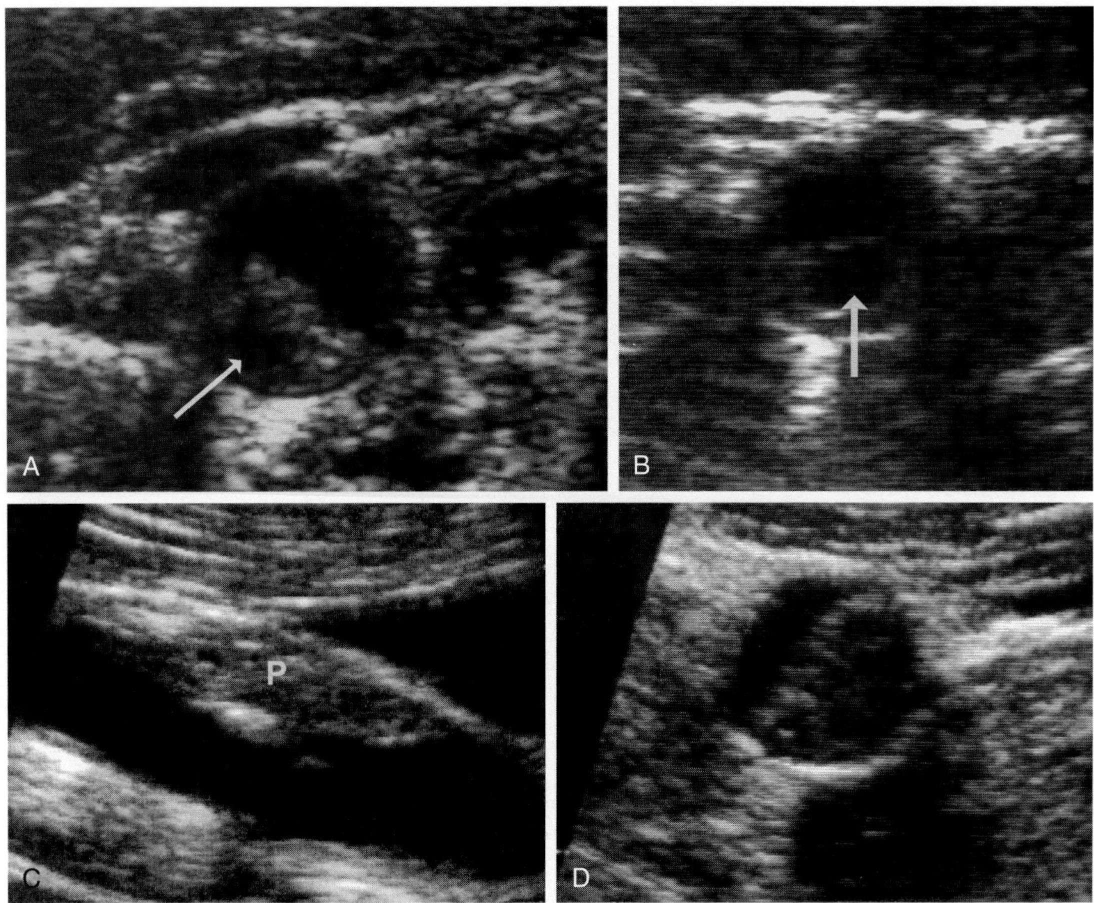

FIGURE 9–7 Heterogeneous plaque. *A* and *B,* Large focal hypoechoic areas are present (*arrows*), suggesting intraplaque hemorrhage. *C* and *D,* The plaque (P) is diffusely heterogeneous, with multiple areas of low echogenicity. A focal crypt with an overhanging edge is present in *C,* consistent with ulceration.

plaque calcification represents old areas of hemorrhage or necrosis, then why is there no association between calcification and present or past neurologic symptoms? Given how common plaque calcification is, it appears that the underlying causes of calcification, including hemorrhage, occur quite frequently and are usually silent. Fourth, it has been suggested that sonographic heterogeneity may correlate better with plaque size than with any specific histologic feature, such as hemorrhage.[13] This correlation stands to reason, considering that small plaques tend to be uncomplicated on histologic examination, whereas plaque enlargement is accompanied by a complicated histology. Finally, if ultrasound features of plaque appear to have clinical significance, then a longitudinal, randomized study is needed to determine whether removal of such plaque (endarterectomy) or medical therapy has any long-term beneficial effect. No such study has been conducted, and, to my knowledge, none is anticipated.

Considering all the uncertainty that surrounds plaque echo features and their clinical significance, I believe that *plaque homogeneity or heterogeneity should not be considered in deciding who is a candidate for endarterectomy.* You might ask whether we should give up on ultrasound plaque features, considering the previously discussed experimental results. Probably not, in my opinion. Improvements in ultrasound instrumentation may enhance our ability to characterize atherosclerotic plaque, and conclusive longitudinal studies might yet be conducted.

PLAQUE SURFACE FEATURES

It is well established that embolic occlusion of the intracranial carotid arteries is a

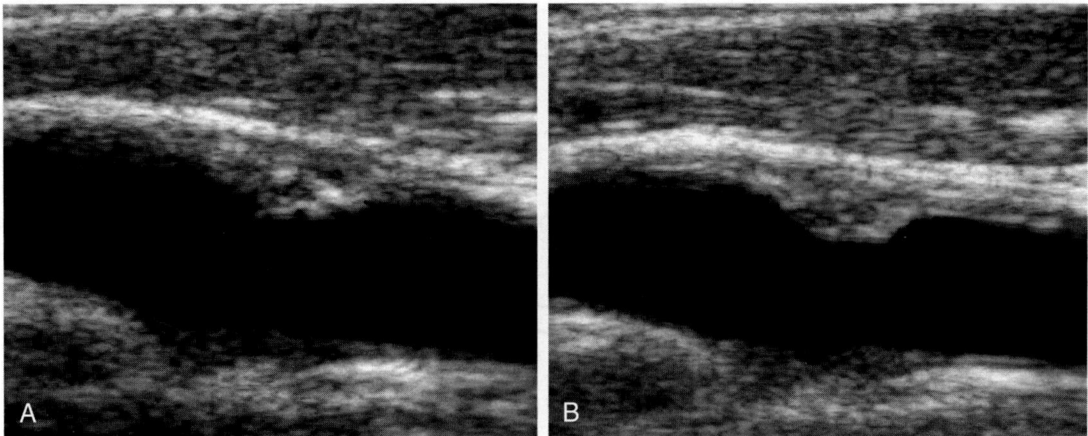

FIGURE 9–8 Spurious plaque ulceration. *A,* The plaque on the wall of the vessel nearest to the transducer appears to have an irregular surface. *B,* With slight adjustment of the image plane, the plaque is visualized better and clearly has a smooth surface.

primary cause of stroke, and that embolization per se is more important than carotid stenosis or occlusion.[30–32] It has further been established that denuded or ulcerated carotid plaque surfaces are common sources of cerebral emboli. Therefore, ultrasound assessment of plaque surface features has been of considerable research interest.[1, 14, 15, 30, 33–36]

Unfortunately, the performance of ultrasonography for plaque surface assessment has been disappointing. Only one histologically based series of meaningful size[14] has shown that duplex ultrasonography is effective for detecting ulcers (100% sensitivity and specificity). Other histologically verified studies[15, 33, 34, 37] have shown either no correlation or poor ultrasound results for ulcer detection (33 to 67% sensitivity and 31 to 84% specificity). It appears that these poor results are caused by the inability of ultrasonography to differentiate between ulcer craters and other plaque deformities, as illustrated in Figures 9–8 and 9–9. Even the angiographic depiction of plaque ulceration is unreliable, as indicated by the deletion of this parameter from the North American Symptomatic Carotid Endarterectomy Trial.[1]

In my opinion, duplex sonography is generally not useful for assessing gross surface characteristics of plaque, and surface features should *not* generally be considered as an indication for endarterectomy. Does that mean that I *never* diagnose plaque ulceration with ultrasonography? In fact, I do occasionally comment on the presence of an ulcer, but *only* when color-Doppler imaging clearly shows a large, sharply defined excavation of potential clinical importance (Fig. 9–10). Before I call something an ulcer, I must be convinced of the following: (1) the cavity is truly within the plaque; (2) the cavity is sharply marginated (perhaps with overhanging edges, as in Figs. 9–7*C* and 9–10); and (3) there is flow within the cavity. The

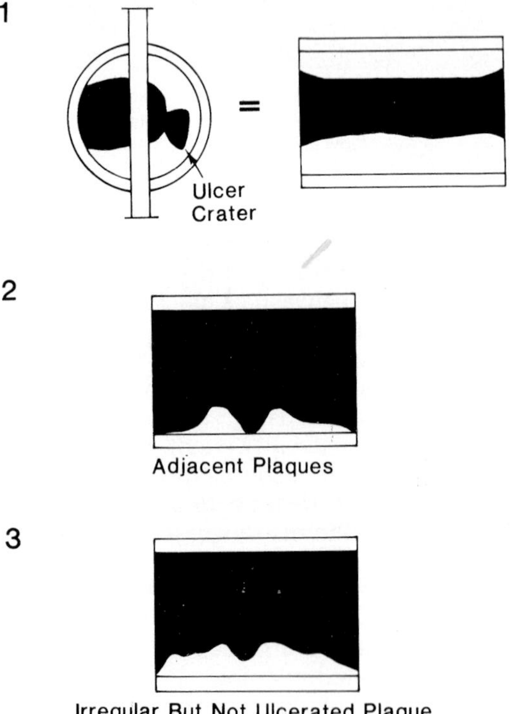

FIGURE 9–9 Sources of error in ulcer diagnosis: *1,* The image plane (*vertical bar*) does not include the ulcer. *2,* Adjacent plaques simulate ulceration. *3,* The plaque surface is irregular but not ulcerated.

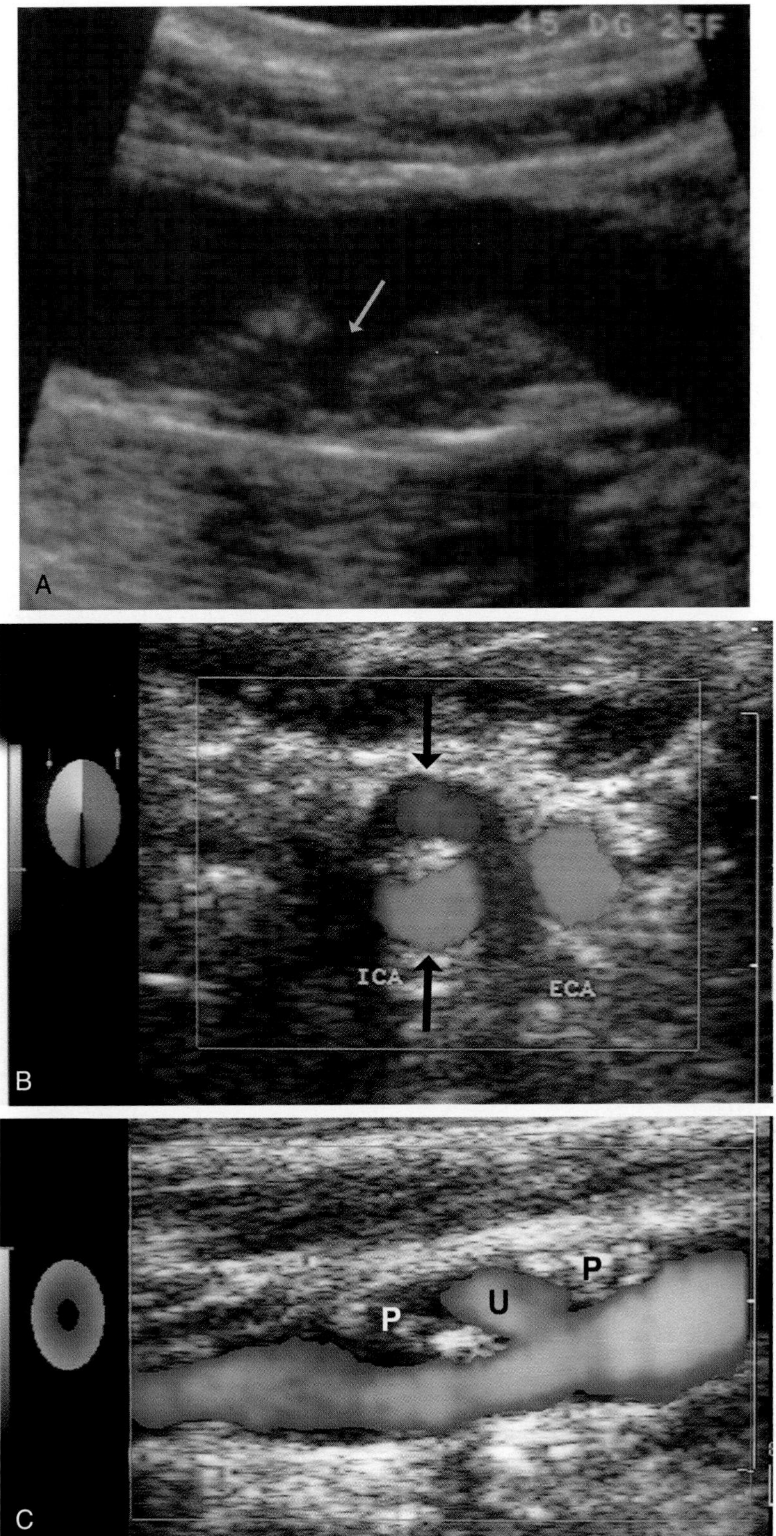

FIGURE 9–10 Large plaque ulcers. *A,* A discrete crypt (*arrow*) is clearly present within this plaque. *B,* A large ulcer creates a "pseudodissection" on this transverse image of an internal carotid artery (*arrows*). The blue area is the ulcer crater and the red area is the arterial lumen. ICA = internal carotid artery; ECA = external carotid artery. *C,* A power Doppler image in the same patient confirms the presence of a large ulcer (U). P = plaque.

first two features help to exclude a pseudoulcer caused by adjacent plaques, and the third feature excludes a focal hypoechoic region (e.g., plaque hemorrhage) that mimics an ulcer on casual observation.

PLAQUE SURVEILLANCE

A great deal of research is under way concerning medical therapy of atherosclerosis.[1–5, 7, 9–11] Such therapy includes lifestyle changes and the use of drugs that either prevent the development of atherosclerosis or decrease its severity. Sonography may play a role in these therapeutic efforts, because it is the only imaging modality (other than magnetic resonance imaging) that can examine plaque directly. Sonography has been proposed for three aspects of plaque evaluation: (1) early plaque detection; (2) characterization of plaque severity; and (3) assessment of the response of plaque to therapy. Ultimately, certain aspects of plaque composition may also be found to have therapeutic implications, because lipid and collagen content can be judged in a general way.

Ultrasound plaque staging and follow-up consist of precise measurement of plaque (see Fig. 9–1) at locations that are easily visualized, such as the carotid and femoral artery bifurcations. Careful measurement and hard copy documentation are required, as well as the use of image planes that can be reproduced from one examination to another. Although measuring plaque seems like a simple task, precision and reproducibility are significant issues.

REFERENCES

1. Streiffler JY, Benavente AJ, Fox AJ: The accuracy of angiographic detection of carotid plaque ulceration: Results from the NASCET study (Abstract). Stroke 22:149, 1991.
2. Pignoli P, Tremoli E, Poli A, et al: Intimal plus medial thickness of the arterial wall: A direct measurement with ultrasound imaging. Circulation 6:1399–1406, 1986.
3. Poli A, Tremoli E, Colombo A, et al: Ultrasonographic measurement of the common carotid arterial wall thickness in hypercholesterolemic patients. Atherosclerosis 70:253–261, 1988.
4. Riley WA, Barnes RW, Applegate WB, et al: Reproducibility of noninvasive ultrasonic measurement of carotid atherosclerosis. The Asymptomatic Carotid Artery Plaque Study. Stroke 23:1062–1068, 1992.
5. Bond MG, Wilmoth SK, Enevold GL, et al: Detection and monitoring of asymptomatic atherosclerosis in clinical trials. Am J Med 86:33–36, 1989.
6. Li R, Cai J, Tegeler C, et al: Reproducibility of extracranial carotid atherosclerotic lesions assessed by B-mode ultrasound: The atherosclerosis risk in communities study. Ultrasound Med Biol 22:791–799, 1996.
7. Salonen R, Seppanen K, Rauremaa R, Salonen JT: Prevalence of carotid atherosclerosis and serum cholesterol levels in eastern Finland. Arteriosclerosis 8:788–792, 1988.
8. Sutton-Tyrrell K, Wolfson SK, Thompson T, Kelsoey SF: Measurement variability in Duplex scan assessment of carotid atherosclerosis. Stroke 23:215–220, 1992.
9. Prati P, Vanuzzo D, Casaroli M, et al: Prevalence and determinants of carotid atherosclerosis in a general population. Stroke 23:1705–1711, 1992.
10. Gibbons GH, Dzau VJ: The emerging concept of vascular remodeling. N Engl J Med 330:1431–1438, 1994.
11. Ross R, Glomset JA: The pathogenesis of atherosclerosis (Part 1). N Engl J Med 295:369–377, 1976.
12. Ross R, Glomset JA: The pathogenesis of atherosclerosis (Part 2). N Engl J Med 295:420–425, 1976.
13. O'Leary D, Glagov S, Zarins C, Giddens D: Carotid artery disease. *In* Rifkin MD, Charboneau JW, Laing FC (eds): Ultrasound 1991: Special Course Syllabus, 77th Scientific Assembly and Annual Meeting. Oak Park, IL, RSNA Publications, 1991, pp 189–200.
14. O'Donnell TR Jr, Erodoes L, Mackey WC, et al: Correlation of B-mode ultrasound imaging and arteriography with pathologic findings at carotid endarterectomy. Arch Surg 120:443–449, 1985.
15. Lusby RJ, Ferrel LD, Ehrenfeld WK, et al: Carotid plaque hemorrhage. Arch Surg 117:1479–1487, 1981.
16. Reilly LM: Importance of carotid plaque morphology. *In* Bernstein EF (ed): Vascular Diagnosis, 4th ed. St. Louis, Mosby–Year Book, 1993, pp 333–340.
17. Bluth EI: Evaluation and characterization of carotid plaque. Semin Ultrasound CT MR 18:57–65, 1997.
18. Weinberger J, Marks SJ, Gaul JJ, et al: Atherosclerotic plaque at the carotid artery bifurcation: Correlation of ultrasonographic imaging with morphology. J Ultrasound Med 6:363–366, 1987.
19. Edwards JH, Kricheff II, Gorstein F, et al: Atherosclerotic subintimal hematoma of the carotid artery. Radiology 133:123–129, 1987.
20. Seeger JM, Klingman N: The relationship between carotid plaque composition and neurologic symptoms. J Surg Res 43:78–85, 1987.
21. Bassiouny HS, Sakaguchi Y, Mikucki SA, et al: Juxtalumenal location of plaque necrosis and neoformation in symptomatic carotid stenosis. J Vasc Surg 26:585–594, 1977.
22. Imparato AM, Riles TS, Gorstein F: The carotid bifurcation plaque: Pathologic findings associated with cerebral ischemia. Stroke 3:238–245, 1979.
23. Reilly M, Lusby RF, Highes L, et al: Carotid plaque histology using real time ultrasonography: Clinical and therapeutic implications. Arch Surg 120:1010–1012, 1985.
24. Bluth EI, Kay D, Merritt CRB, et al: Sonographic characterization of carotid plaque: Detection of hemorrhage. AJNR Am J Neuroradial 7:311–314, 1986.
25. Imparato AM, Riles TS, Mintzer K, et al: The importance of hemorrhage in the relationship between

gross morphologic characteristics and cerebral symptoms in 376 carotid artery plaques. Ann Surg 197:195–198, 1983.

26. Widder B, Paulat K, Hackspacher J, et al: Morphological characterization of carotid artery stenosis by ultrasound duplex scanning. Ultrasound Med Biol 16:349–354, 1990.
27. Ratiff DA, Gallagher PJ, Hames TK, et al: Characterization of carotid artery disease: Comparison of duplex scanning with histology. Ultrasound Med Biol 11:835–840, 1985.
28. Gray-Weale AC, Graham JC, Burnett JR, et al: Carotid artery atheroma: Comparison of preoperative B-mode ultrasound appearance with carotid endarterectomy specimen pathology. J Cardiovasc Surg 29: 676–681, 1988.
29. Wolverson MK, Bashiti HM, Peterson GJ: Ultrasonic tissue characterization of atheromatous plaques using a high resolution real time scanner. Ultrasound Med Biol 6:669–709, 1983.
30. Carr S, Farb A, Pearce WH, et al: Atherosclerosis plaque rupture in symptomatic carotid artery stenosis. J Vasc Surg 12:755–766, 1996.
31. Brown PB, Zwiebel WJ, Call CK: Degree of cervical carotid artery stenosis and hemispheric stroke: Duplex sonographic US findings. Radiology 170:541–543, 1989.
32. Carroll BA: Duplex sonography in patients with hemispheric stroke symptoms. J Ultrasound Med 8:535–539, 1989.
33. Bluth EI, McVay LV, Merritt CRB, Sullivan MA: The identification of ulcerative plaque with high resolution duplex sonographic carotid scanning. J Ultrasound Med 7:73–76, 1988.
34. O'Leary DH, Holen J, Ricotta JJ, et al: Carotid bifurcation disease: Prediction of ulceration with B-mode ultrasound. Radiology 162:523–525, 1987.
35. Hallam MJ, Reid JM, Cooperberg PL: Color-flow Doppler and conventional duplex scanning of the carotid bifurcation: Prospective, double-blinded, correlative study. Am J Radiol 153:1101–1105, May 1989.
36. Steinke W, Kloetzsch C, Hehherici M: Carotid artery disease assessed by color Doppler flow imaging: Correlation with standard Doppler sonography and angiography. Am J Radiol 154:1061–1068, 1990.
37. Sitzer M, Wolfram M, Jorg R, et al: Color-flow Doppler-assisted duplex imaging fails to detect ulceration in high-grade internal carotid artery stenosis. J Vasc Surg 24:461–465, 1996.

Chapter 10

Doppler Evaluation of Carotid Stenosis

■ *William J. Zwiebel, MD*

DOPPLER STENOSIS MEASUREMENT PRINCIPLES

At the outset, it is a good idea to review the basics of carotid artery stenosis measurement, even though this subject is also covered in Chapter 3. Although arterial stenoses can be visualized directly with color-flow ultrasonography, Doppler spectral analysis remains the mainstay of carotid stenosis assessment. Experience has shown that with color flow, it is frequently not possible to visualize the stenotic carotid artery with sufficient clarity to permit accurate stenosis measurement. Visualization problems are caused by vessel tortuosity, acoustic shadows generated by calcified plaque, and other factors.

There are three important areas to consider in Doppler evaluation of an arterial stenosis: the prestenotic region (or zone), the stenosis itself (or stenotic zone), and the poststenotic region (or zone). The most important Doppler measurements are made in the stenotic zone; however, prestenotic and poststenotic Doppler findings that are of diagnostic importance are considered as well.

Common Carotid Artery Pulsatility

The preponderance of clinically significant carotid obstructive lesions occur in the origin of the internal carotid artery (ICA), and for these lesions, the cervical part of the common carotid artery (CCA) represents the prestenotic zone. Less commonly, significant carotid stenosis occurs within the proximal CCA, usually at the origin. For these lesions, the cervical part of the CCA represents the postobstructive zone, so pulsatility changes in the CCA can be either preobstructive or postobstructive phenomena. Such changes may be important diagnostically; therefore, the assessment of CCA pulsatility is an essential part of every carotid ultrasound examination.[1–4]

Because most of the CCA flow goes to the brain, the normal CCA waveform has low-pulsatility (low-resistance) features, as shown in Figure 10–1. The brain likes to be continuously immersed in oxygenated blood, so it has a low-resistance circulation that provides continuous flow throughout systole and diastole. The low-resistance CCA pattern may be altered by severe proximal or distal obstruction.

If the distal CCA or ICA is severely blocked, CCA waveforms proximal to the blockage have high-pulsatility features, as seen in Figure 10–1. In addition, CCA waveform height (amplitude) may also be reduced because of an overall decrease in carotid artery flow. These abnormalities occur in the presence of severe stenosis and occlusion, and they may occur both with obstruction at the carotid bifurcation and within the cranium (e.g., the carotid siphon). Isolated external carotid artery (ECA) obstruction *does not* appreciably alter CCA waveforms, because the volume of flow in the ECA is relatively low, and the ECA is a high-resistance circulation to begin with.

Severe stenosis of the innominate artery or CCA proximal to the clavicle produces *damped* CCA waveforms in the neck. The CCA waveforms may also be low in amplitude if flow is substantially reduced by the obstruction.[3, 5] Damping is usually most evident in the CCA but may also be seen in the ECA and ICA waveforms, as shown in Figure 10–2. The recognition of CCA damping is of

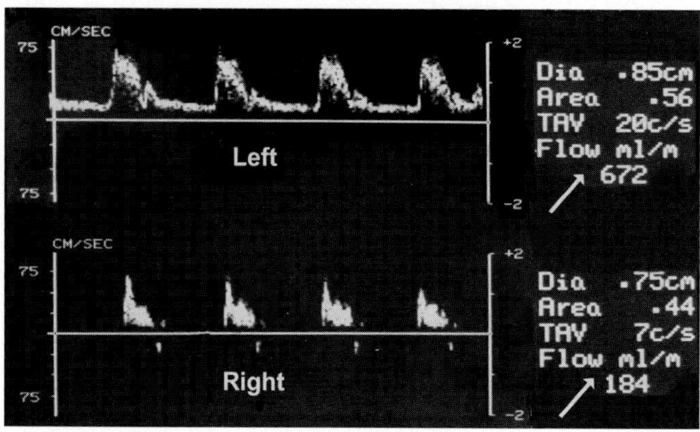

FIGURE 10–1 High common carotid artery (CCA) pulsatility. Virtually no flow is present during most of diastole in the right CCA (*bottom*), and the waveforms have a triphasic pattern. These findings indicate high-flow resistance. The volume flow is 184 mL/min (*arrow*), which is quite low. Normal CCA volume flow is about 450 mL/min. These flow change are due to right internal carotid artery occlusion (not shown). The left CCA (*top*) shows normal pulsatility features and high-volume flow (*arrow*, 672 mL/min) due to collateralization.

considerable importance, as it usually is the only ultrasound evidence of carotid stenosis below the clavicle.

Attempts have been made to quantify CCA waveform abnormalities by numerical pulsatility measurements,[4–11] but the simplest and most effective method of interpretation is visual—comparing the waveform shapes in the right and left CCAs. In healthy patients, the waveforms should be fairly symmetric and should exhibit low-pulsatility features. Discrepancies in waveform shape, as shown in Figures 10–1 and 10–2, are a "red flag" that should cause the examiner to pause and look for confirmatory evidence of proximal or distal obstruction. The asymmetric absence of CCA diastolic flow is a particularly significant finding that almost invariably indicates severe obstruction of the distal CCA or ICA.[6, 9]

Caution must be exercised in the visual interpretation of carotid waveforms because the overall status of the cardiovascular system may profoundly affect the CCA waveform shape. For no apparent reason, waveforms are sometimes slightly more pulsatile in one CCA than the other, and such minor discrepancies may be dismissed as physiologic. Severe pulsatility discrepancis, however, should be approached with caution, and if no apparent cause of such a discrepancy is found, another mode of examination such as magnetic resonance imaging should be considered to search for an obstructive lesion outside of the range of carotid ultrasonography (e.g., at the aortic arch.) Symmetric CCA waveform abnormality is less of a problem, because symmetric abnormality suggests physiologic effects. Hypertension or diminished arterial compliance from peripheral arterial disease, for example, can increase CCA pulsatility bilaterally.[10–13] Conversely, diminished cardiac output or severe aortic valve disease can produce symmetric damping of CCA waveforms.

Stenotic Zone

The stenotic zone is "the heart of the matter" in diagnosing carotid stenosis, and utmost care is required in measuring velocity changes in this zone. The flow velocity in the stenotic lumen is elevated in proportion to the degree of luminal narrowing, and this principle is the basis for Doppler stenosis assessment. By measuring the flow velocity with Doppler sonography, one can indirectly determine the severity of narrowing. The increase in stenotic zone velocity is small until the lumen diameter is reduced to about 50% of its original size. Thereafter, the velocity goes up rapidly as stenosis severity increases.

Three stenotic zone velocity measurements are key to carotid stenosis diagnosis: the peak systolic velocity (also called peak systole), the end diastolic velocity (also called end diastole), and the systolic velocity ratio, which is peak systole in the stenosis divided by peak systole in the ipsilateral CCA. Because of their importance, I call these velocity measurements the *cardinal Doppler parameters*. The use of these parameters is illustrated in Figures 10–3 to 10–6. Sonographers must be aware that the highest velocity in the stenotic lumen may be localized in a small area. *It is critical to search about the stenotic lumen with the sample volume for the highest velocity* (see Fig. 10–4), otherwise stenosis severity may be grossly underestimated.

Text continued on page 144

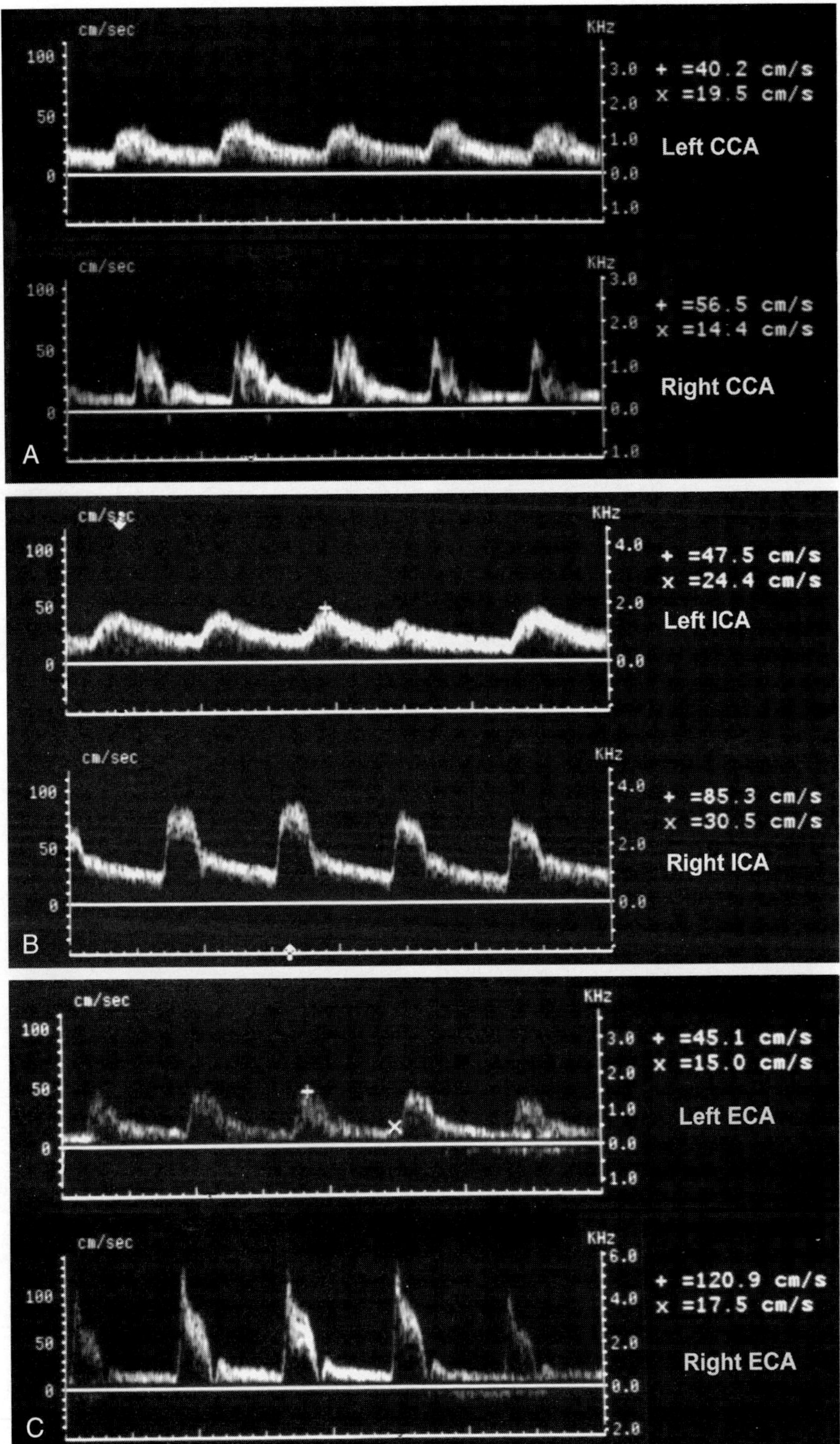

FIGURE 10–2 Damped carotid artery waveforms due to severe stenosis at the left common carotid artery (CCA) origin. *A,* The left CCA waveforms (*top*) are visibly damped in comparison to the right CCA (*bottom*). Peak systole (+) is lower on the left but end diastole (X) is higher, as compared with the right, indicating low-flow resistance on the left side due to ischemia. *B,* Damped, low-resistance flow changes are present in the left internal carotid artery (ICA) (*top*), as compared with the right ICA (*bottom*). *C,* Damped, low-resistance flow changes are also present in the left external carotid artery (ECA) (*top*), as compared with the right ECA (*bottom*).

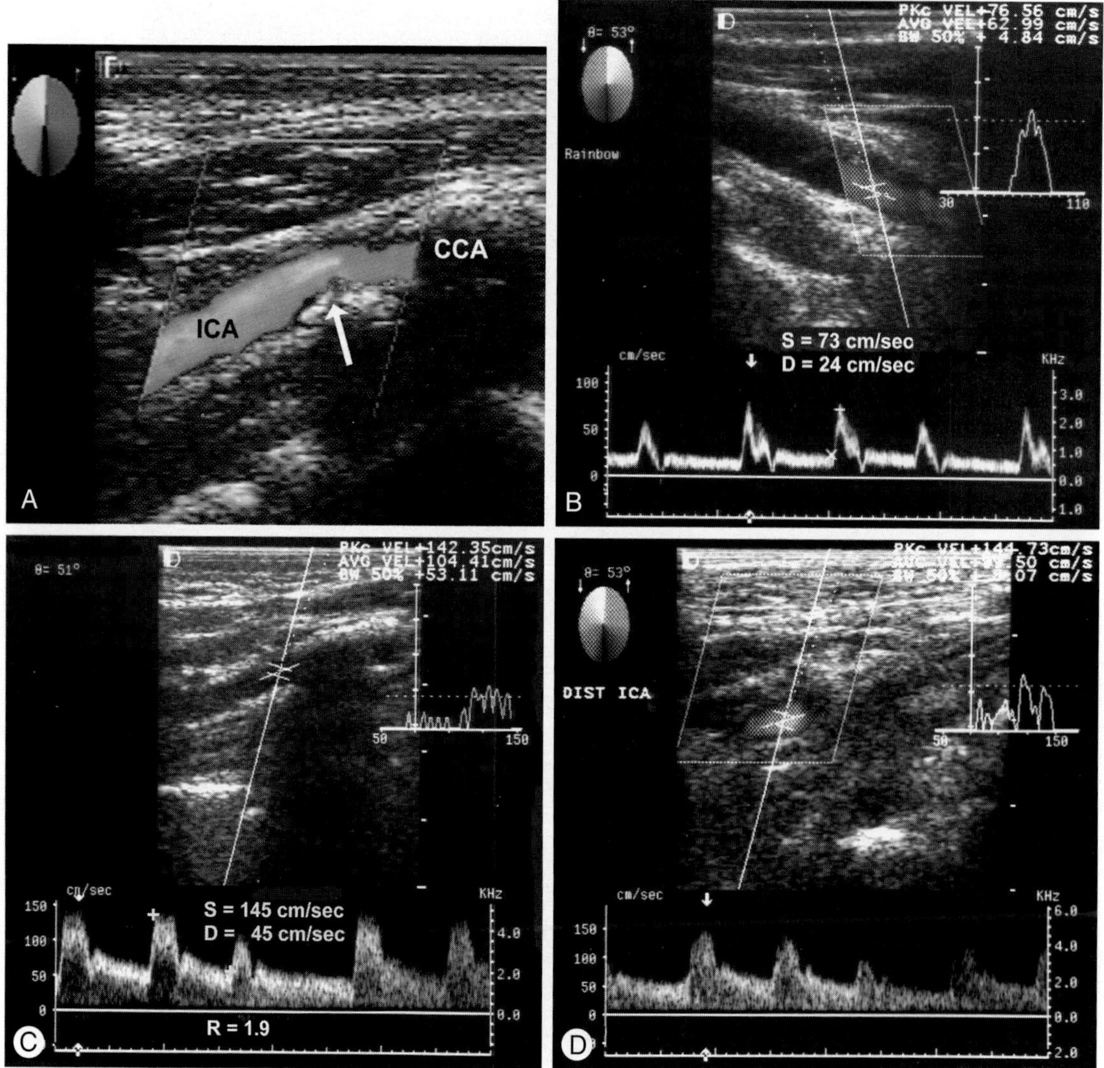

FIGURE 10–3 Mild internal carotid artery (ICA) stenosis. *A,* The color-Doppler image shows a large plaque (*arrow*) at the ICA origin and a color shift indicating elevated flow velocity. CCA = common carotid artery. *B,* CCA peak systole (S) and end diastole (D) are shown. *C,* Peak systole (S) in the ICA is 145 cm/sec, end diastole (D) is 45 cm/sec, and the systolic ratio (R) is 1.9. These values are consistent with relatively mild stenosis. *D,* Moderate poststenotic flow disturbance (spectral fill-in) is present.

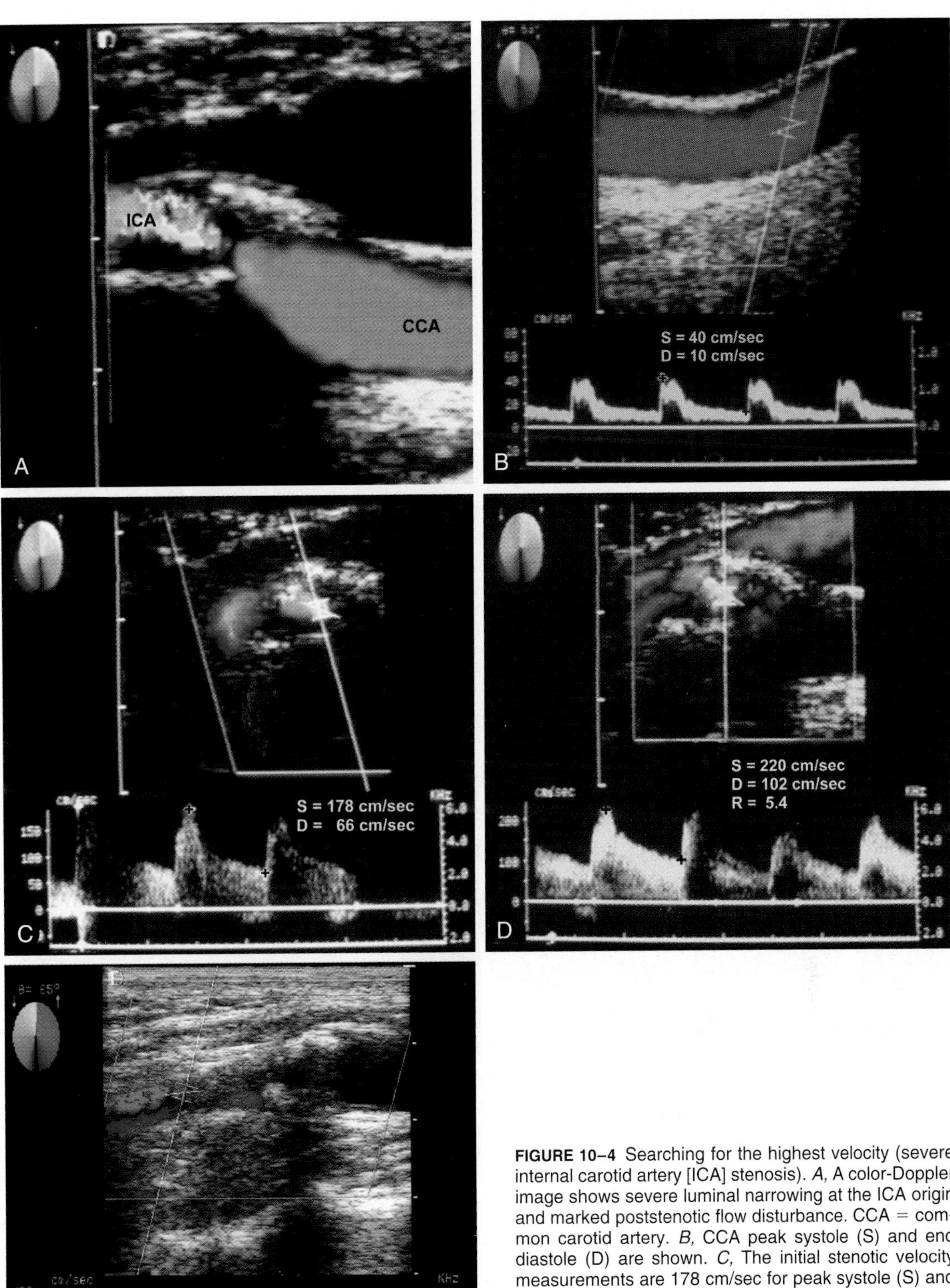

FIGURE 10–4 Searching for the highest velocity (severe internal carotid artery [ICA] stenosis). *A,* A color-Doppler image shows severe luminal narrowing at the ICA origin and marked poststenotic flow disturbance. CCA = common carotid artery. *B,* CCA peak systole (S) and end diastole (D) are shown. *C,* The initial stenotic velocity measurements are 178 cm/sec for peak systole (S) and 66 cm/sec for end diastole (D). *D,* The technologist searches further and identifies an area of even higher velocity with peak systole of 220 cm/sec, end diastole of 102 cm/sec, and a systolic velocity ratio (R) of 5.4. *E,* Severe poststenotic flow disturbance is evident, consistent with high-grade stenosis (simultaneous forward and reverse flow, poor definition of spectral border).

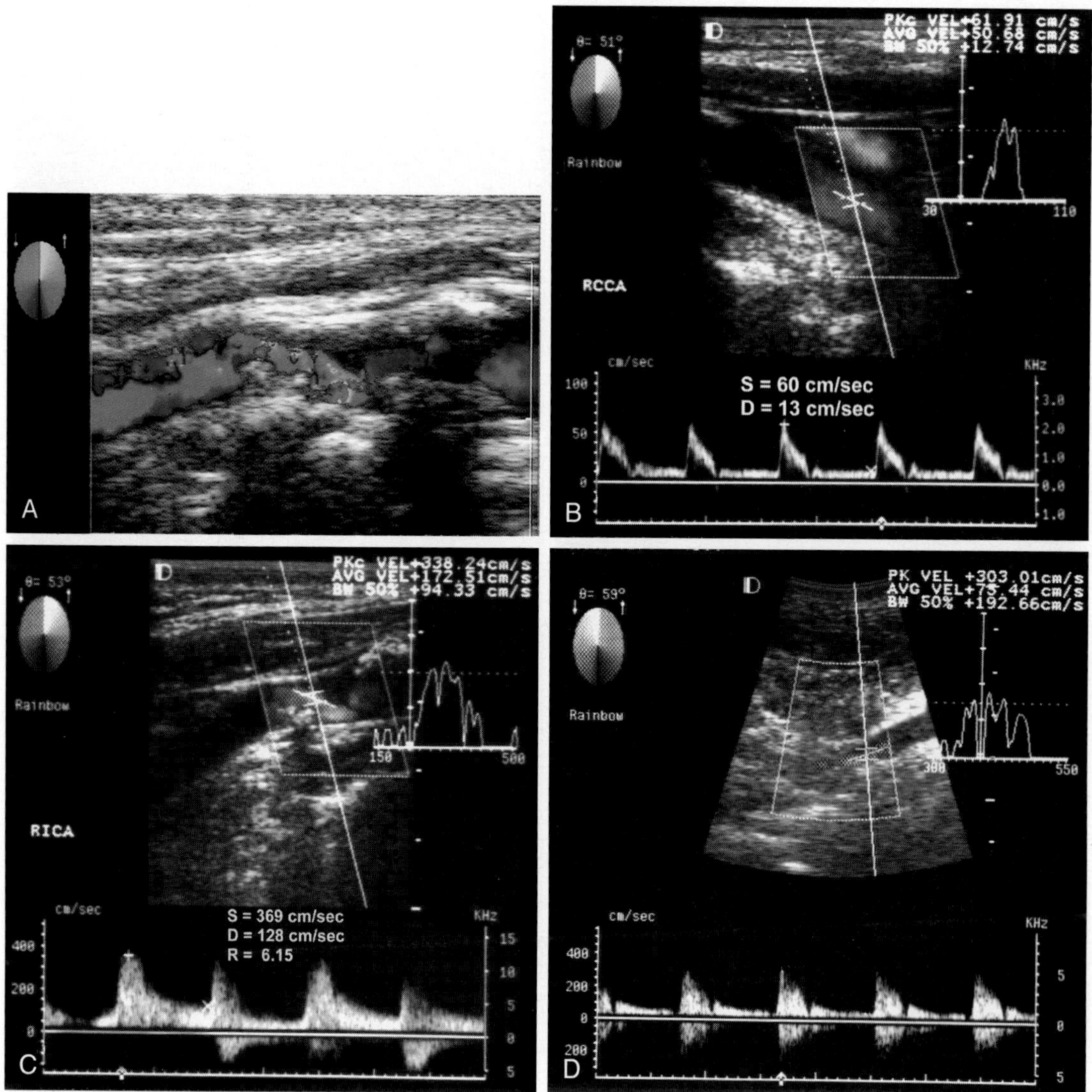

FIGURE 10–5 High velocities in severe internal carotid artery (ICA) stenosis. *A,* A color-Doppler image shows severe irregularity and narrowing of the ICA. *B,* Common carotid artery peak systole (S) and end diastole (D) are shown. Note the high-resistance flow pattern, with relatively little diastolic flow. *C,* Extreme high velocities and ratio are present in the stenosis. (Peak systole [S] is 369 cm/sec, end diastole [D] is 128 cm/sec, and the systolic velocity ratio [R] is 6.15.) *D,* Severe poststenotic flow disturbance is evident.

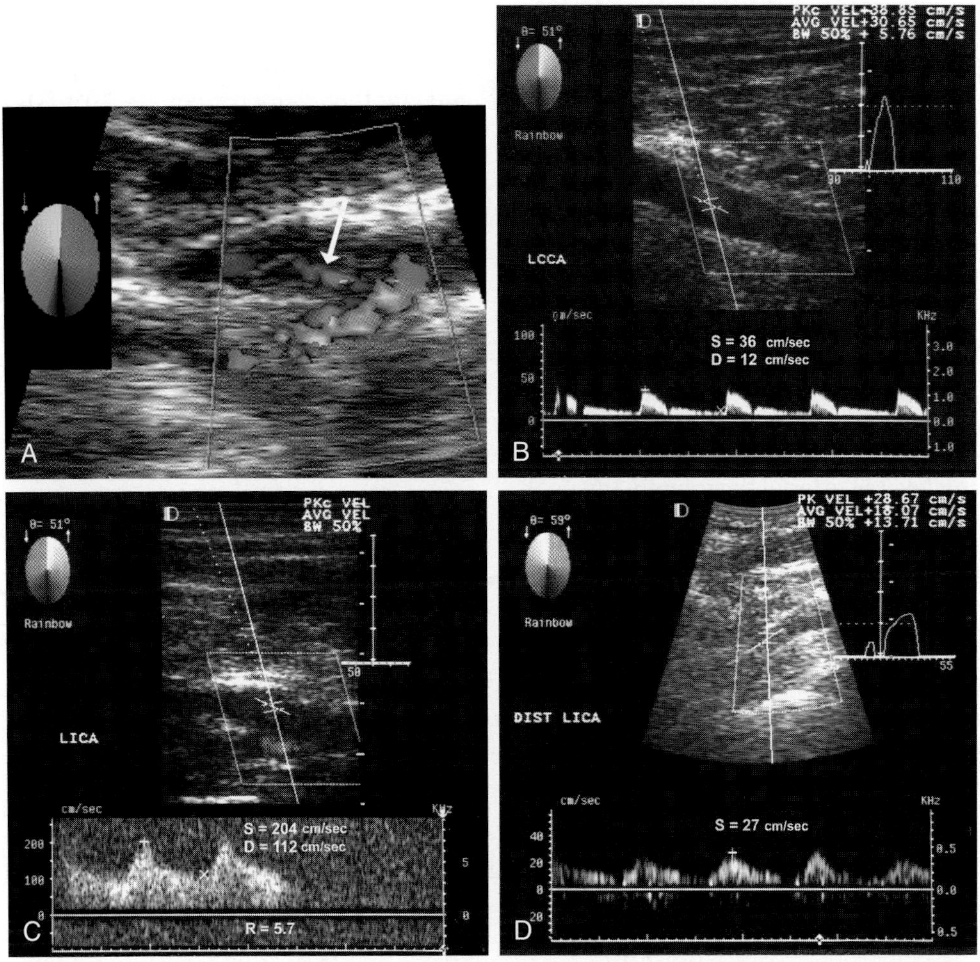

FIGURE 10–6 Severe internal carotid artery (ICA) stenosis with damped distal flow. *A,* A color-Doppler image shows virtual occlusion of the ICA with scattered areas of visible flow (*arrow*). *B,* Peak systole (S) and end diastole (D) are measured in the CCA. *C,* Flow signals could only be obtained in the ICA with high Doppler gain (hence the noise). Peak systole is 204 cm/sec, and end diastole is 112 cm/sec. *D,* ICA signals distal to the stenosis are severely damped (due to ischemia) with peak systole of only 27 cm/sec.

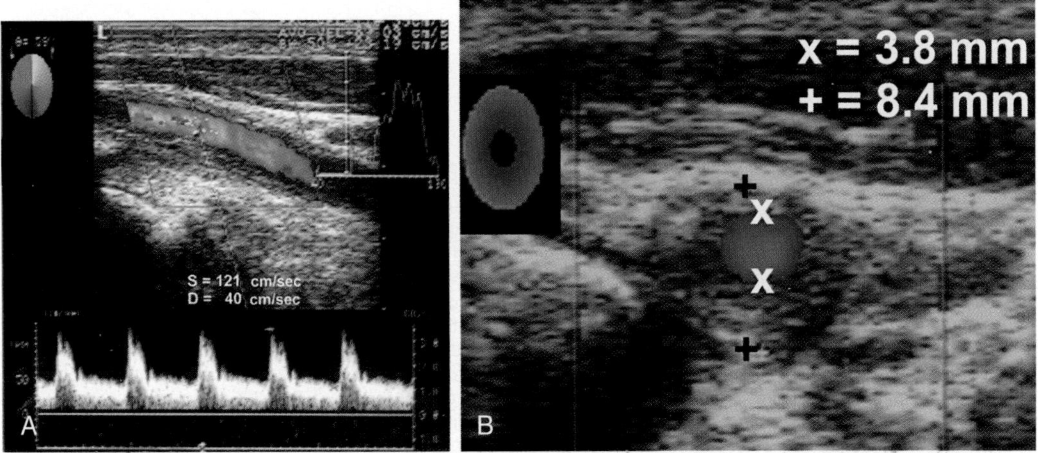

FIGURE 10–12 Common carotid artery (CCA) stenosis. (See p 152.) *A,* Visible narrowing is present in the CCA, and this generates mild velocity elevation. (Peak systole [S] 121 cm/sec, end diastole [D] 40 cm/sec.) *B,* Direct measurement shows 45% diameter reduction, consistent with the level of velocity elevation.

Peak Systolic Velocity

The best documented Doppler parameter for carotid stenosis is the stenotic zone peak systolic velocity. In theory, this parameter bears a well-defined relationship to the severity of luminal narrowing,[1, 12–14, 16, 17] as illustrated in Figure 10–7, although this relationship is less precise in a clinical setting. Please review Figure 10–7 before proceeding, and note in particular that peak systole drops off at high levels of stenosis. This may lead to false-positive diagnosis of carotid occlusion, as considered in Chapter 11.

At any level of arterial narrowing, the peak systolic velocity is affected by the length of the stenosis (i.e., the longer the stenosis, the lower the velocity) and by a host of physiologic factors that differ from one patient to another. Because of such differences, a *range* of velocities is encountered in a patient population at any level of carotid stenosis, as illustrated in Figure 10–8.[15] Because a range of velocities exists, a discrete cutoff point cannot be given to separate one level of stenosis from another. For instance, one cannot say with precision that a certain velocity equals a 60% stenosis and another velocity equals 70% stenosis. This issue is revisited later in this chapter.

End Diastolic Velocity

With arterial stenosis of less than 50% diameter reduction, the diastolic velocity remains normal[16, 18] because no appreciable pressure gradient is present across the stenosis during diastole. As a stenosis progresses beyond 50%, a pressure gradient across the stenosis is present in diastole, and diastolic velocities increase in proportion to the severity of the gradient (and lumen narrowing). The end diastolic velocity (see measurements illustrated in Figs. 10–4 to 10–6) rises rapidly as stenoses exceed 70% diameter reduction; therefore, this Doppler parameter is quite valuable for detecting high-grade carotid stenoses.

Systolic Velocity Ratio

I noted previously that physiologic factors, including blood pressure, cardiac output, pe-

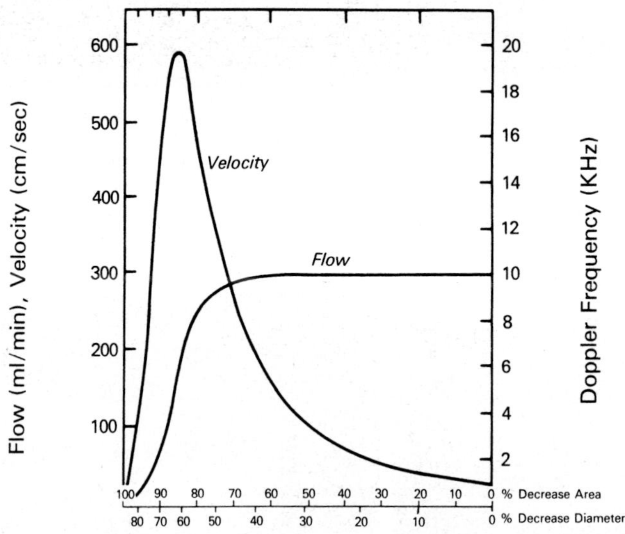

FIGURE 10–7 Relationship between peak systolic velocity and luminal narrowing (theoretical internal carotid artery with an original diameter of 5 mm). The scale at the bottom of the graft shows increasing stenosis severity *from right to left.* The peak velocity in the stenotic zone increases logarithmically as the lumen narrows until approximately 70% diameter reduction. Beyond this point, velocities decrease rapidly because of the effects of increased flow resistance. In severe stenoses, therefore, peak systolic velocity may be lower than expected (see Fig. 10–5). Volume flow, unlike velocity, remains stable until the lumen diameter is decreased by about 50 to 60%. Thereafter, the volume of blood flowing through the stenotic lumen decreases sharply. Note the relationship between percent diameter and area reduction, as shown at the base of the figure. A 50% diameter stenosis corresponds to about 75% area reduction, and 70% diameter stenosis equals about 90% area reduction. (Reprinted by permission of Elsevier Science, from Computer based pattern recognition of carotid artery Doppler signals for disease classification: Prospective validation by Langlois YE, Greene FM, Roederer GO, et al., Ultrasound in Medicine and Biology, Vol 10, pp 581–595, Copyright 1984 by World Federation of Ultrasound in Medicine and Biology.)

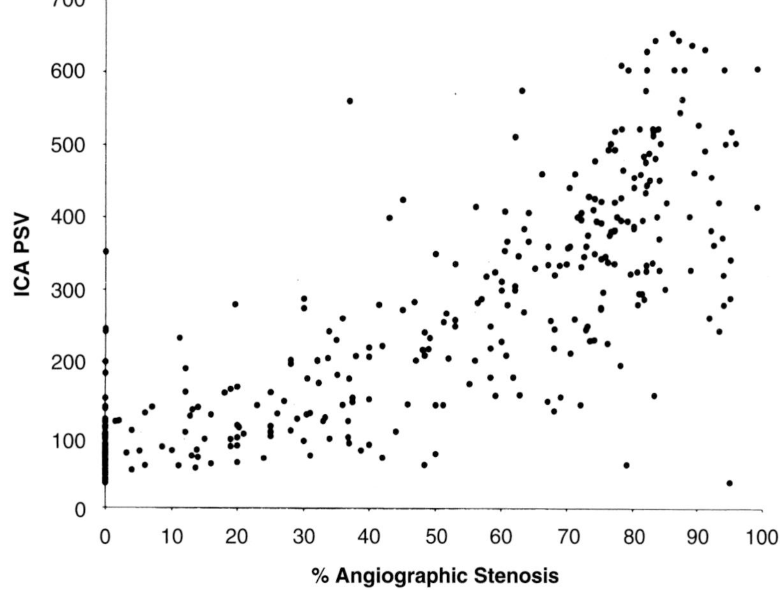

FIGURE 10–8 Distribution of data points for peak systolic velocity vs. internal carotid artery (ICA) stenosis. A graph of peak ICA velocity vs. percent of angiographic stenosis shows relative lack of concordance of data points. Graphs for the end diastolic velocity and the systolic velocity ratio from the same article (not shown) demonstrated similar wide variation. (From Moneta GL, Edwards JM, Papanicolaou G, et al: Screening for asymptomatic internal carotid artery stenosis: Duplex criteria for discriminating 60% to 99% stenosis. J Vasc Surg 21:989–994, 1995.)

ripheral resistance, and arterial compliance, may affect pulsatility in the carotid arteries, both in normal individuals and in patients with stenosis. These factors also affect stenotic zone velocity. For example, at the same level of carotid obstruction, stenotic zone velocity is likely to be higher in a hypertensive patient than in a normotensive individual. Conversely, diminished cardiac output may reduce stenotic zone velocity.[1, 12, 17, 18]

Systolic and diastolic velocities in the stenotic zone are also affected by collateralization. All velocity measurements in one carotid system may be increased when blood is shunted to that system in response to contralateral CCA or ICA obstruction. Such shunting of flow may artifactually increase stenotic zone velocity measurements, causing overestimation of stenosis severity.[19, 20] Conversely, a proximal CCA (or innominate artery) stenosis may reduce ipsilateral carotid flow and thereby decrease velocity measurements in an ipsilateral ICA stenosis. In this case, stenosis severity might be underestimated.

The systolic velocity ratio is recommended to avoid errors caused by physiologic factors or collateralization. As noted previously, this ratio is the peak systolic velocity in the stenotic ICA divided by the peak systolic velocity in the ipsilateral CCA (see Figs. 10–3 to 10–6). Several older Doppler studies and reports published after the North American Symptomatic Carotid Endarterectomy Trial (NASCET) suggest that ratio measurements are more accurate than peak systolic velocity measurements for evaluating ICA stenosis.[1, 20–22] This has not been substantiated by all authors;[23, 24] nonetheless, I feel that the systolic velocity ratio should be included in all carotid ultrasound studies, as is common practice in the United States. Bluth and colleagues[12] also suggest the use of the diastolic velocity ratio (ICA/CCA), but this ratio has not been widely reported on in the medical literature. Dhanjil and colleagues[25] advocate a ratio that compares ICA peak systole with the ipsilateral CCA end diastole. To my knowledge, this ratio has not been evaluated in other studies.

Poststenotic Zone

Although the stenotic zone Doppler findings are most important in measuring a carotid stenosis, valuable information can also be obtained in the poststenotic region. In this area, the high-velocity stream of blood from the stenotic lumen "spreads out" into a zone of relatively low velocity and pressure, producing a disorderly (nonlaminar) flow pattern that is manifested sonographically as *spectral broadening.* The severity of the poststenotic flow disturbance is roughly proportionate to the severity of luminal narrowing, and it has been postulated from the earliest days of Doppler sonography that the severity of the poststenotic flow disturbance might be used to measure carotid stenoses. A number of qualitative and quantitative schemes have been derived to relate spectral broadening[24–27] to the severity of carotid stenosis, but the clinical utility of these measurements is limited, and in clinical practice spectral broadening is evaluated visually (see Figs. 10–3 to 10–5). The three principal grades of spectral broadening are illustrated in Chapter 3, and readers unfamiliar with these grades should review this material. The following concepts are noteworthy concerning the assessment of spectral broadening in carotid stenosis.

1. Spectral broadening increases in proportion to the severity of carotid stenosis, but this relationship cannot be precisely quantified.
2. Fill-in of the spectral window (see Fig. 10–3*D*) suggests stenosis of more than 50% decrease in diameter, but this finding is not specific and can be seen with lesser degrees of luminal narrowing.[26–29]
3. Severely disturbed flow, characterized by high-amplitude, low-frequency Doppler signals, flow reversal, and poor definition of the spectral border (see Fig. 10–4*E*) is perhaps the most definitive form of spectral broadening and suggests carotid stenosis exceeding 70% diameter reduction.[26, 27]
4. In some cases, severe flow disturbance may be the only sign of carotid stenosis, for example, when the stenotic region is obscured by acoustic shadowing from calcified plaque and only the poststenotic region is visible.

DOPPLER STENOSIS PARAMETERS

Having reviewed the basic principles of stenosis assessment, I now direct your attention to the selection of parameters that identify clinically significant levels of carotid stenosis. This subject has undergone considerable revision since the mid-1980s, and for that reason, I begin with a brief historical review of the major carotid endarterectomy trials and their impact on carotid ultrasonography.

Carotid Endarterectomy Trials

The first successful carotid endarterectomy was reported in U.S. medical literature in 1956. During the 1960s, the popularity of this surgical procedure increased rapidly, and by the 1970s, carotid endarterectomy was frequently performed in the United States. The logic of preventing stroke by removing emboli-shedding carotid plaque seemed empirical, and indeed, some evidence of clinical effectiveness from endarterectomy trials existed. However, there was no definitive proof of effectiveness, based on unassailable data, even though thousands of carotid endarterectomies were performed annually in the United States (as well as in Europe). As might be expected, this situation led to considerable controversy, especially between neurologists (who favored medical therapy) and surgeons (who of course favored endarterectomy).

To determine, once and for all, whether carotid endarterectomy was an effective form of treatment, three large randomized studies were begun during the late 1980s, each of which compared carotid endarterectomy with conservative medical therapy. These studies were the North American Symptomatic Carotid Endarterectomy Trial (NASCET),[30] the European Carotid Endarterectomy Trial (ECET),[29] and the Asymptomatic Carotid Atherosclerosis Study (ACAS).[31] The end points for all three studies were reduction of hemispheric stroke and death. These trials clearly demonstrated that the long-term benefits of endarterectomy were significantly greater than medical treatment in patients with 60% or 70% ICA stenosis, whether symptomatic or asymptomatic. Endarterectomy was proven to decrease the risk of ipsilateral hemispheric stroke or death (from any cause) by 53 to 84% as compared with medical therapy. Furthermore, subsequent assessment of the data from the NASCET study suggests that the potential benefit of endarterectomy increases with the severity of stenosis.[33]

The three major endarterectomy trials were obviously a major turning point for carotid surgery. However, it is less well recognized that they were also a major turning point for carotid ultrasonography. First, they ensured the future of carotid ultrasound examinations, for it is reasonable to search for a carotid stenosis only if it is also reasonable to operate on the stenoses that are found. Second, the endarterectomy trials established 60% (ACAS) to 70% (NASCET) diameter reduction as *clinically significant* levels of ICA stenosis. The trials showed that endarterectomy was effective at or above these levels. More recently published data from the NASCET study showed modest stroke-reducing benefit for endarterectomy at 50% diameter ICA stenosis, but only when the patient's life expectancy was long and the rate of operative morbidity and mortality was low.[32] Third, the NASCET and ACAS results defined the preferred *method* for calculating ICA stenosis severity from arteriographic measurements. This definition had fundamental effects on ultrasound technique for reasons described in the next section. Finally, the carotid endarterectomy trials and subsequent studies brought out several important points regarding the accuracy of duplex ultrasound examination, as discussed later.

NASCET Stenosis Measurement

The method for measuring a carotid stenosis used in the NASCET study has become a standard for angiographic practice. As shown in Figure 10–9, this measurement technique compares the smallest ICA lumen size with the diameter of the distal tubular portion of the ICA. Two orthogonal angiographic views are obtained (anteroposterior and lateral), but *only the view showing the smallest lumen size is used. Neither the residual lumen size nor the stenoses percentage is averaged between the two views.*

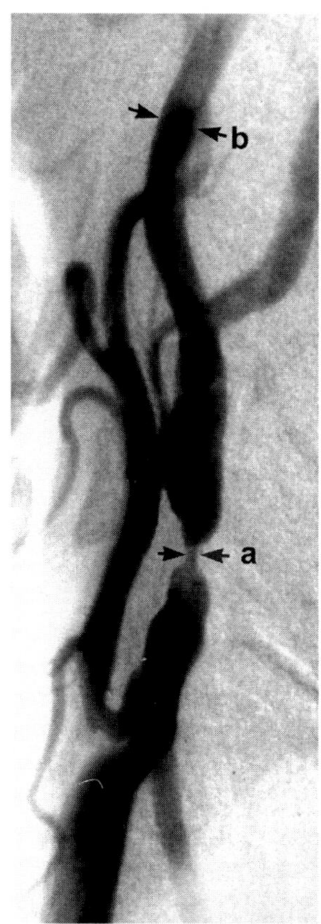

FIGURE 10–9 NASCET angiogram measurement protocol. The smallest residual internal carotid artery (ICA) diameter in the stenosis (a) is divided by the normal ICA diameter beyond the carotid bulb (b). Percent stenosis = a/b × 100. The smallest diameter in any radiographic projection is used. Values obtained in different projections are not averaged. NASCET = North American Symptomatic Carotid Endarterectomy Trial.

Before the NASCET study, Doppler parameters used to diagnose carotid stenoses were based on several different angiographic measurement techniques.[4, 34] In some series, the percent stenosis was calculated as shown in Figure 10–9. In other instances, however, the residual lumen diameter was compared with the bulbous portion of the ICA, which exaggerated the percent diameter reduction as compared with the NASCET method. In some of the older studies, stenosis measurements in orthogonal planes were averaged; in others, the smallest measurement was used. Finally, many of the older studies simply did not describe how the stenoses were measured! Because of these problems, Doppler velocity and frequency parameters used prior to the NASCET study, including those published in the previous edition of this text, may not be applicable to present concepts of carotid stenosis management, which are based on NASCET-style measurement. It has been necessary, therefore, to define new Doppler velocity parameters.

Doppler Parameters for 50%, 60%, and 70% ICA Stenosis

It would be really wonderful if Doppler velocity parameters were available that precisely defined specified levels of carotid stenosis. Unfortunately, this is not the case, as is seen in Figure 10–7, which shows the wide spread of velocities that were observed in one study at various levels of ICA stenosis.[15] Similar variation is seen in other major Doppler studies of carotid stenosis.[22, 31, 33] Furthermore, the preferred velocity cutoffs for 50%, 60%, or 70% stenosis published by various authors (Table 10–1) show that a wide range of velocity levels is used to identify ICA ste-

TABLE 10–1 DOPPLER PARAMETERS FOR INTERNAL CAROTID ARTERY STENOSIS

Reference	PSV	EDV	S Ratio	Sens (%)	Spec (%)
60% or Greater*					
Stanley et al[44]	>130			96	
		>40	—	89	
Burnham et al[41]	≥240			95	78
		≥110		86	95
			≥2.5	82	87
Moneta et al[15]	≥260			86	91
		≥70	—	90	84
Withers et al[36]	—	—	>3.0	77	95
70% or Greater*					
Hood et al[42]	>130			98	89
		>100	—	78	97
Neale et al[39]	≥270			96	86
		≥110	—	91	93
Faught et al[38]	>210			89	94
		>100	—	77	85
Moneta et al[22]	≥325			83	91
		—	≥4.0	91	87
Withers et al[36]	>225	—	—	88	97
Hunink et al[37]	>230	—	—	85	90

* North American Symptomatic Carotid Endarterectomy Trial (NASCET) measurement technique.
PSV = peak systolic velocity; EDV = end diastolic velocity; S Ratio = systolic velocity ratio; Sens = sensitivity; Spec = specificity.

nosis in clinical practice.[15, 22, 34–44] I have already indicated two potential causes for such variability: physiologic differences among patients and collateralization. In addition, there are at least three other potential causes: arteriographic measurement variability, sonographer variability, and Doppler instrument variability. Concerning arteriographic measurement variability, it should be noted that arteriography is a less-than-perfect "gold standard" against which to correlate Doppler velocity measurements.[34] Variability in the angiographic measurement of carotid stenoses contributes to the lack of precision in defining Doppler parameters. Second, wide variation in accuracy for carotid diagnosis has been noted among ultrasound departments.[33, 45, 46] Finally, wide variation *has* been found in velocity measurement accuracy among different ultrasound instruments and even among different transducers on the same instrument.[47–52] In vitro studies have shown as much as a 60% difference between Doppler ultrasound velocity measurements and true velocity (directly measured from flow rigs). Furthermore, velocity measurements may vary significantly when different Doppler angles are used on a single instrument. Velocity measurement inaccuracy appears to be greatest with inexpensive ultrasound instruments, but inaccuracy of potential clinical significance has also been found with more expensive devices.

The net result of the five sources of variability cited previously is lack of precision in identifying patients with clinically significant ICA stenosis, defined as 50, 60, or 70% diameter reduction. It has traditionally been stated that carotid ultrasonography is highly accurate, with sensitivity and specificity exceeding 90% for high-grade stenoses (e.g., 70% or greater diameter reduction).[48, 49, 53, 54] However, more recent studies suggest that ultrasonography may only be about 70% sensitive and specific for high-grade stenoses, if a broad spectrum of ultrasound departments is examined and if certain selection bias is eliminated.[34, 50] These new accuracy revelations have created considerable controversy, with some authors arguing that carotid ultrasonography is highly accurate and others arguing that it is only moderately accurate.[45, 46, 50] In spite of the controversial aspects of carotid stenosis measurement, a few things are clear:

1. Because of velocity measurement variability, it is not possible to publish a set of Doppler stenosis parameters that will be accurate in all ultrasound departments.
2. Each ultrasound department must, therefore, develop its own Doppler parameters

for identifying high-grade carotid stenoses.

3. Each ultrasound department must confirm the accuracy of carotid diagnosis internally, through correlation with surgical findings and other carotid imaging studies.
4. If different types of ultrasound equipment or transducers are used in one ultrasound department, it should be confirmed that the chosen Doppler parameters provide acceptable accuracy with all the equipment in use.
5. Ongoing assessment of diagnostic accuracy is strongly advised for every ultrasound department.

Developing Carotid Artery Stenosis Parameters

If each department must develop its own carotid artery velocity parameters, how does one go about the task? In essence, there are two approaches. The first is to use individual cutoff parameters to identify or exclude 50, 60, or 70% diameter stenosis. For example, a systolic velocity ratio of 4.0 or greater might be chosen to *identify* 70% or greater ICA stenosis, because of a high positive predictive value; a ratio of 2.5 or less might be chosen to *exclude* 60% stenosis because of a high negative predictive value. The second approach to the selection of Doppler stenosis criteria is to combine several parameters, such as the three cardinal parameters discussed previously. This is what my colleagues and I did in our ultrasound department. We chose two sets of values for peak systolic velocity, end diastolic velocity, and the systolic velocity ratio. When velocities meet or exceed one set of values, 60% or greater ICA stenosis is diagnosed. If they exceed the second set of values, 70% or greater ICA stenosis is diagnosed. We have confirmed, through angiographic correlation, that our sensitivity and specificity for 60 and 70% ICA stenosis exceeded 90% using the parameters we selected. As of this writing, we are assessing the feasibility of developing criteria for 50% ICA stenosis.

The first step for developing a set of Doppler stenosis parameters for your laboratory might be a review of the recent medical literature. The articles by Moneta and coworkers,[15, 22] Faught and colleagues,[38] and Winkelaar and associates[35] are suggested as starting points, because they present accuracy data for the cardinal velocity parameters in tabular form (see Moneta and coworkers data reproduced in Figs. 10–10 and 10–11). For example, in Figure 10–11, a peak systolic velocity of 325 cm/sec is 82.8% sensitive and 90.5% specific for 70% ICA narrowing. A peak systolic velocity of 210 cm/sec is considerably more sensitive (94.8%) but less specific (78.6%). The second step is to consider the velocity parameters that are preferred by various other authors.[47, 51] Unfortunately, this review can be quite confusing, because the parameters chosen by different authors vary widely and show considerable overlap between the 60% and 70% stenosis levels (see Table 10–1). The third and most important step is to review the historical data from your department. Choose a set of parameters from the literature and see how accurate they would have been if used on your patients through correlation with surgical or imaging findings. Fourth, adjust the parameters as needed to achieve a high level of accuracy. The final step is to conduct a prospective analysis of the accuracy of your department for the desired levels of stenosis. The process is summarized in Table 10–2.

It is noteworthy that Doppler parameters should be tailored to the clinical circumstances in which you practice. For instance, the vascular surgeons in our hospital prefer to emphasize specificity in selecting parameters for 50 or 60% ICA stenosis. This avoids false positives that might lead to questionably beneficial surgery.

I sincerely wish that I could publish a ready-made table of Doppler parameters for your use as I have done in previous editions. I am concerned, however, about whether such parameters would be accurate in your department in lieu of the variables (described previously) that have been recognized since publication of previous editions. It is necessary, therefore, for you to work out a series of Doppler parameters that are accurate for your department.

Which Parameter Is Best?

In the ultrasound literature, different authors state that one or another of the three major Doppler parameters (peak systole, end diastole, or systolic velocity ratio) is *the* most

	Sensitivity (%)	Specificity (%)	PPV (%)	NPV (%)	Accuracy (%)
ICA PSV > (cm/sec)					
100	99	44	60	98	69
150	96	67	71	95	80
200	93	76	76	93	84
220	91	83	82	92	87
260	86	91	88	88	88
300	78	95	93	84	87
350	60	97	94	74	80
400	43	98	96	67	73
ICA EDV > (cm/sec)					
30	99	20	50	95	55
40	95	65	69	94	78
70	90	84	82	91	87
90	84	90	87	87	87
120	74	94	91	82	85
140	62	95	91	75	80
170	35	97	92	65	69
200	22	98	90	61	64
ICA PSV/CCA PSV >					
2.0	98	67	71	97	81
2.5	96	77	78	96	86
2.8	94	82	82	95	88
3.2	92	86	85	93	89
3.5	89	89	87	91	89
4.0	82	93	91	86	88
4.5	72	95	92	80	94
5.5	51	97	93	71	76
6.6	37	98	95	65	71

FIGURE 10–10 Doppler parameters for 60% internal carotid artery (ICA) stenosis, as reported by Moneta and colleagues. Sensitivity, specificity, positive predictive value (PPV), negative predictive value (NPV), and accuracy are listed for predicting 60% ICA stenosis (NASCET/diameter), using peak systolic velocity, end diastolic velocity, and systolic ratio values. NASCET = North American Symptomatic Carotid Endarterectomy Trial; ICA PSV = internal carotid artery peak systolic velocity; ICA EDV = internal carotid artery end diastolic velocity; CCA PSV = common carotid artery peak systolic velocity. (From Moneta GL, Edwards JM, Papanicolaou G, et al: Screening for asymptomatic internal carotid artery stenosis: Duplex criteria for discriminating 60% to 99% stenosis. J Vasc Surg 21:989–994, 1995.)

accurate predictor of clinically significant ICA stenosis.[15, 22, 35–44] Unfortunately, there is no consistency in these proclamations. If I had to choose a favorite parameter, it would be the systolic velocity ratio, because a ratio compensates for patient-to-patient physiologic variability and may also compensate for instrument variability (assuming that velocity measurement accuracy is equal at all velocity levels).

A word of caution is in order concerning the systolic velocity ratio. The accuracy of this ratio depends on the accuracy with which the CCA velocity is measured. Inaccurate assignment of the Doppler angle or placement of the Doppler sample volume may artificially lower the CCA velocity, spuriously elevating the systolic velocity ratio. This error can cause significant misdiagnosis and could even lead to unnecessary carotid surgery in a department that relies heavily or solely on the systolic velocity ratio. Meyer and associates[47] noted in 1997 that the CCA velocity is not constant in normal individuals and increases as one moves proximally within the CCA from the carotid bifurcation. Because this increase is great enough to affect the systolic velocity ratio, they suggest that CCA measurements be made at a standard distance below the bifurcation. They do not state, however, what this distance should be.

What If the Parameters Do Not Agree?

From a diagnostic perspective, it is comforting when all three cardinal Doppler parameters are in agreement; that is, all three

	Sensitivity (%)	*Specificity (%)*	*PPV (%)*	*NPV (%)*	*Accuracy (%)*
ICA PSV > (cm/sec)					
140	98.3	61.9	54.3	98.7	73.4
190	96.6	72.2	61.5	97.8	79.9
210	94.8	78.6	67.1	97.1	83.7
230	93.1	81.0	69.2	96.2	84.8
250	91.4	82.5	70.7	95.4	85.3
265	89.7	84.9	73.2	94.7	86.4
280	84.5	86.5	74.2	92.4	85.9
295	84.5	88.1	76.6	92.5	87.0
325	82.8	90.5	80.0	91.9	88.0
345	70.7	92.9	82.0	87.3	85.9
375	65.5	96.0	88.4	85.8	86.4
400	51.7	96.8	88.2	81.3	82.6
440	41.4	98.4	92.3	78.5	80.4
ICA EDV > (cm/sec)					
30	94.8	65.1	55.6	96.5	74.5
50	93.1	77.0	65.1	96.0	82.1
70	93.1	80.2	68.4	96.2	84.2
90	86.2	83.3	70.4	92.9	84.2
110	82.8	85.7	72.7	91.5	84.8
130	75.9	90.5	78.6	89.1	85.9
140	72.4	90.5	77.8	87.7	84.8
145	65.5	92.1	79.2	85.3	83.7
150	58.6	92.9	79.1	83.0	82.1
155	50.0	95.2	82.9	80.5	81.0
165	41.4	95.2	80.0	77.9	78.3
200	24.1	97.6	82.4	73.7	74.5
ICA PSV/CCA PSV >					
2.0	96.6	64.3	55.4	97.6	74.5
2.5	96.6	73.0	62.2	97.9	80.4
3.0	96.6	78.6	67.5	98.0	84.2
3.6	93.1	82.5	71.1	96.3	85.9
3.8	91.4	84.9	73.6	95.5	87.0
4.0	91.4	86.5	75.7	95.6	88.0
4.2	89.7	87.3	76.5	94.8	88.0
4.4	86.2	88.1	76.9	93.3	87.5
4.6	79.3	89.7	78.0	90.4	86.4
4.7	75.9	89.7	77.2	89.0	85.3
5.0	69.0	90.5	76.9	86.4	83.7
5.5	60.3	92.9	79.5	83.6	82.6
6.0	53.4	92.9	77.5	81.3	80.4
7.0	46.6	96.0	84.4	79.6	80.4

FIGURE 10–11 Doppler parameters for 70% internal carotid artery (ICA) stenosis, as reported by Moneta and colleagues. Sensitivity, specificity, positive predictive value (PPV), negative predictive value (NPV), and accuracy in predicting 70% ICA stenosis (NASCET/diameter), using peak systolic velocity, end diastolic velocity, and systolic ratio values. NASCET = North American Symptomatic Carotid Endarterectomy Trial; ICA PSV = internal carotid artery peak systolic velocity; ICA EDV = internal carotid artery end diastolic velocity; CCA PSV = common carotid artery peak systolic velocity. (From Moneta GL, Edwards JM, Chitwood RW, et al: Correlation of North American Symptomatic Carotid Endarterectomy Trial (NASCET) angiographic definition of 70% to 99% internal carotid artery stenosis with duplex scanning. J Vasc Surg 17:152–159, 1993.)

TABLE 10-2 DEVELOPING CAROTID STENOSIS PARAMETERS

1. Review published parameters.
2. Select parameters that seem appropriate for your practice.
3. Test the parameters retrospectively through surgical or imaging correlation.
4. Adjust the parameters, if needed.
5. Test the parameters prospectively.

exceed the cutoff levels for 50, 60, or 70% stenosis. What about cases in which one or two parameters meet the cutoff level, but the others do not? When Doppler measurements do not correspond, the reader is strongly advised to scrutinize the technical adequacy of the carotid examination, especially with respect to the ICA/CCA ratio, as discussed earlier.

What About the Common and External Carotid Arteries?

Peak velocity values have been defined only for stenoses in the ICA. This is because the great majority of carotid stenoses are located in the ICA. Velocity parameters for the CCA and ECA have not been defined.

One can assume that the ICA parameters are approximately correct for the CCA, but physiologic differences exist between CCA and ICA flow, and these vessels are of substantially different size. It is not clear, therefore, that the ICA parameters carry over to the CCA. Fortunately, because the CCA is a straight tube, CCA stenoses often can be measured directly from cross-sectional images of the CCA, using gray-scale or color-Doppler techniques (Fig. 10–12 [see p 143]).

ECA stenoses usually cannot be visually evaluated because of vessel tortuosity, branching, and acoustic shadows, so the only alternative is Doppler evaluation. Few data exist with respect to Doppler parameters for ECA stenoses. One article notes that the ECA/CCA systolic velocity ratio is usually 2 or less for ECA stenoses of 50% diameter or less and that this ratio is usually 2 or more for ECA stenoses of 70% or greater.[55] But this article also shows that ECA flow velocity is highly variable and depends on the status of both the ipsilateral ICA and the contralateral carotid arteries. An ipsilateral ICA occlusion, for example, can easily raise the ECA/CCA ratio above 2 in the *absence* of ECA stenosis. Considering the variability in ECA flow, I continue to merely "guesstimate" ECA stenosis as minimal (less than 200 cm/sec), moderate (200 to 300 cm/sec), or severe (greater than 300 cm/sec).

Emboli Cause Stroke, so Why Measure Stenosis?

The majority of hemispheric strokes are caused by embolic occlusion of intracranial arteries, not by the hemodynamic effects of stenosis, so why focus on carotid stenosis? This focus is important because stenosis can be measured with reasonable accuracy, and because the association between stenosis and stroke risk has been clearly defined by the three major carotid endarterectomy studies. In measuring stenosis, we are indirectly estimating the volume of carotid plaque or the *plaque burden.* Big plaques cause high-grade stenosis. Big plaques also shed emboli, because they are often complicated by hemorrhage, necrosis, and ulceration. It makes sense, therefore, to base clinical decisions on stenosis severity, although it might be better to measure plaque volume directly, if that could be done accurately.

Stenosis Measurement: Image, Spectrum, or Both?

Unfortunately, the results of color-Doppler stenosis imaging have been disappointing, owing to vessel tortuosity and inability to clearly visualize the lumen on transverse images. In spite of these limitations, I feel that it is useful to assess the degree of stenosis visually, using the color-Doppler image, to avoid error. Doppler spectrum findings should be cross-checked with color-Doppler image assessment of stenosis severity. If one method suggests a high-grade stenosis and the other does not, the findings should be reviewed to resolve the discrepancy. In my ultrasound department, this practice has prevented diagnostic error in several instances of which I am aware.

Doppler velocity increases are reliably detected only in carotid stenoses that equal or exceed 50% decrease in diameter,[1, 2, 12, 56] so Doppler is unreliable for detecting lower levels of carotid stenosis. As an alternative, the color-Doppler image can be used to measure carotid stenoses of less than 50% diameter.

REFERENCES

1. Zwiebel WJ, Knighton R: Duplex examination of the carotid arteries. Semin Ultrasound CT MR 11:97–135, 1990.
2. Zwiebel WJ: Analysis of carotid doppler signals. *In* Zwiebel WJ (ed): Introduction to Vascular Ultrasonography, 2nd ed. Philadelphia, WB Saunders, 1986, pp 171–216.
3. Brunholzl CH, Von Reutern GM: Hemodynamic effects of innominate artery occlusive disease: Evaluation by Doppler ultrasound. Ultrasound Med Biol 15:201–204, 1989.
4. Planilo T, Pourcelot L, Pottier JM: Etude de la circumlation carotidienne par les methodes ultrasoniques et la thermographie. Rev Neurol (Paris) 126: 127–141, 1972.
5. Courbier R, Reggi M, Jausseran JM: Exploration of carotid arteries and vessels of the neck by Doppler techniques. *In* Dietrich EB (ed): Noninvasive Cardiovascular Diagnosis: Current Concepts. Baltimore, University Park Press, 1978, pp 61–73.
6. Rutherford RB, Kreutzer EW: Doppler ultrasound techniques in the assessment of extracranial arterial

occlusive disease. *In* Nicolaides AN, Yao JST (eds): Investigation of Vascular Disorders. New York, Churchill Livingstone, 1980, pp 139–154.

7. Archie JP: A simple, non-dimensional, normalized common carotid Doppler velocity wave-form index that identifies patients with carotid stenosis. Stroke 12:322–324, 1981.
8. Perry MO, Spradlin S: Analysis of carotid wave form. Cardiovasc Ultrasonography 3:223–226, 1984.
9. Breslau PJ, Fell F, Phillips DJ, et al: Evaluation of carotid bifurcation disease: The role of common carotid velocity wave form patterns. Arch Surg 117: 58–60, 1982.
10. Campbell WB, Skidmore R, Baird RN: Variability and reproducibility of arterial Doppler waveforms. Ultrasound Med Biol 10:601–606, 1984.
11. Baird RN, Gird DR, Clifford PC, et al: Upstream stenosis: Its diagnosis by Doppler signals from the femoral artery. Arch Surg 115:1316–1322, 1980.
12. Bluth EI, Wetzner SM, Stavros AT, et al: Carotid duplex sonography: A multicenter recommendation for standardized imaging and Doppler criteria. Radiographics 8:487–506, 1988.
13. Spencer MP: Techniques of Doppler examination. *In* Spencer MD, Reid JM (eds): Cerebrovascular Evaluation With Doppler Evaluation. The Hague, The Netherlands, Martinus Nijhoff, pp 77–80.
14. Douville Y, Johnston KW, Kassam M: Determination of the hemodynamic factors which influence carotid Doppler spectral broadening. Ultrasound Med Biol 11:417–423, 1985.
15. Moneta GL, Edwards JM, Papanicolaou G, et al: Screening for asymptomatic internal carotid artery stenosis: Duplex criteria for discriminating 60% to 99% stenosis. J Vasc Surg 21:989–994, 1995.
16. Langlois YE, Greene FM, Roederer GO, et al: Computer based pattern recognition of carotid artery Doppler signals for disease classification: Prospective validation. Ultrasound Med Biol 10:581–595, 1984.
17. Zwiebel WJ, Austin CW, Sackett JF, et al: Correlation of high-resolution, B-mode and continuous-wave Doppler sonography with arteriography in the diagnosis of carotid stenosis. Radiology 149:523–532, 1983.
18. Blackshear WM, Philips DJ, Chikos PM: Carotid artery velocity patterns in normal and stenotic vessels. Stroke 1:67–71, 1980.
19. Beckett WW, Davis PC, Hoffman JC: Duplex Doppler sonography of the carotid artery: False-positive results in an artery contralateral to an artery with marked stenosis. AJR Am J Roentgenol 155:1091–1095, 1990.
20. AbuRahma AF, Richmond BK, Robinson PA, et al: Effect of contralateral severe stenosis or carotid occlusion on duplex criteria of ipsilateral stenoses: Comparative study of various duplex parameters. J Vasc Surg 22:751–762, 1995.
21. Garth KE, Carroll BA, Summer EG: Duplex ultrasound scanning of the carotid arteries with velocity spectral analysis. Radiology 147:823–827, 1983.
22. Moneta GL, Edwards JM, Chitwood RW, et al: Correlation of North American Symptomatic Carotid Endarterectomy Trial (NASCET) angiographic definition of 70% to 99% internal carotid artery stenosis with duplex scanning. J Vasc Surg 17:152–159, 1993.
23. Keagy BA, Pharr WF, Thomas D, et al: A quantitative method for the evaluation of spectral analysis patterns in the carotid artery stenosis. Ultrasound Med Biol 8:625–630, 1982.
24. Kalman PG, Johnston KW, Auech P, et al: In vitro comparison of alternative methods for quantifying the severity of Doppler spectral broadening for the diagnosis of carotid arterial occlusive disease. Ultrasound Med Biol 11:435–440, 1985.
25. Dhanjil S, Jameel M, Nicolaides A, et al: Ratio of peak systolic velocity of internal carotid to end diastolic velocity of common carotid: New duplex criteria for grading internal carotid stenosis. J Vasc Tech 21:237–240, 1997.
26. Kassam M, Johnston KW, Cobbold RSC: Quantitative estimation of spectral broadening for the diagnosis of carotid arterial disease: Method and in vitro results. Ultrasound Med Biol 11:425–433, 1985.
27. Brown PM, Johnston KW, Kassam M, et al: A critical study of ultrasound Doppler spectral analysis for detection of carotid disease. Ultrasound Med Biol 8:515–523, 1982.
28. Knox RA, Philips DJ, Breslau PJ: Empirical findings relating volume size to diagnostic accuracy in pulsed Doppler cerebrovascular studies. J Clin Ultrasound 10:227–232, 1982.
29. MRC European Carotid Surgery Trial: Interim results for symptomatic patients with severe (70–90%) or with mild (0–29%) carotid stenosis. European Carotid Surgery Trialists' Collaborative Group. Lancet 337:1235–1243, 1991.
30. North American Symptomatic Carotid Endarterectomy Trial collaborators: Beneficial effect of carotid endarterectomy in symptomatic patients with high-grade carotid stenosis. N Engl J Med 325:445–453, 1991.
31. Executive Committee for the Asymptomatic Carotid Atherosclerosis Study: Endarterectomy for asymptomatic carotid artery stenosis. JAMA 273:1421–1428, 1995.
32. Barnett HJM, Taylor DW, Eliosziw M, et al: Benefit of carotid endarterectomy in patients with symptomatic moderate or severe stenosis. N Engl J Med 339:1415–1425, 1998.
33. Eliasziw M, Rankin RN, Fox AJ, et al: Accuracy and prognostic consequences of ultrasonography in identifying severe carotid artery stenosis. Stroke 26:1747–1752, 1995.
34. Toole JF, Castaldo JE: Accurate measurement of carotid stenosis. J Neuroimaging 4:222–230, 1994.
35. Winkelaar GB, Chen JC, Salvian AJ, et al: New duplex ultrasound criteria for managing symptomatic 50% or greater carotid stenosis. J Vasc Surg 29:986–994, 1999.
36. Withers CE, Gosink BB, Keightley AM: Duplex carotid sonography peak systolic velocity in quantifying internal carotid artery stenosis. J Ultrasound Med 9:345–349, 1990.
37. Hunink MGM, Polak JF, Barlan MM, O'Leary DH: Detection and quantification of carotid artery stenosis: Efficacy of various Doppler velocity parameters. AJR Am J Roentgenol 160:619–625, 1993.
38. Faught WE, Mattos MA, vanBemmelen PS, et al: Color-flow duplex scanning of carotid arteries: New velocity criteria based on receiver operator characteristic analysis for threshold stenoses used in the symptomatic and asymptomatic carotid trials. J Vasc Surg 19:818–828, 1994.
39. Neale ML, Chambers JL, Kelly AT, et al: Reappraisal of duplex criteria to assess significant carotid stenosis with special reference to report from the North

American Symptomatic Carotid Endarterectomy Trial and the European Carotid Surgery Trial. J Vasc Surg 20:642–649, 1994.
40. Carpenter JP, Lexa FJ, Davis JT: Determination of sixty percent or greater carotid artery stenosis by duplex Doppler ultrasonography. J Vasc Surg 22:697–705, 1995.
41. Burnham CB, Ligush J, Burnham SJ: Velocity criteria redefined for the 60% carotid stenosis. J Vasc Tech 10:5–11, 1996.
42. Hood DB, Mattos MA, Mansour A, et al: Prospective evaluation of new duplex criteria to identify 70% internal carotid artery stenosis. J Vasc Surg 23:254–262, 1996.
43. Suwanwela N, Can U, Furie KL, et al: Carotid Doppler ultrasound criteria for internal carotid artery stenosis based on residual lumen diameter calculated from en bloc carotid endarterectomy specimens. Stroke 27:1965–1969, 1996.
44. Stanley JM, Stevens SL, Freeman MB, Goldman MH: Accuracy of end-diastolic velocity for predicting hemodynamically significant internal carotid artery stenosis. J Vasc Tech 21:17–19, 1997.
45. Ackerman RH, Candia MR: Identifying clinically relevant carotid disease. Stroke 25:1–3, 1994.
46. Ringelstein EB: Skepticism toward carotid ultrasonography. A virtue, an attitude, or fanaticism? Stroke 26:1743–1746, 1995.
47. Meyer JI, Khalil RM, Obuchowski NA, Baus LK: Common carotid artery: Variability of Doppler US velocity measurements. Radiology 204:339–341, 1997.
48. Daigle RJ, Stavros AT, Lee RM: Overestimation of velocity and frequency values by multielement linear array Dopplers. J Vasc Tech 14:206–213, 1990.
49. Hoskins PR: Accuracy of maximum velocity estimates made using Doppler ultrasound systems. Br J Radiol 69:172–177, 1996.
50. Howard G, Chambless LE, Baker WH, et al: A multicenter validation study of Doppler ultrasound versus angiography. J Stroke Cerebrovasc Dis 1:166–173, 1991.
51. Scissons RP, Salles-Cunha S, Altenburg L, et al: Doppler peak systolic velocity measurements: Correction of angle-dependent errors. J Vasc Tech 21:233–236, 1997.
52. Fillinger MF, Baker RJ, Zwolak RM, et al: Carotid duplex criteria for a 60% or greater angiographic stenosis: Variation according to equipment. J Vasc Surg 24:856–864, 1996.
53. Howard G, Baker WH, Chambless LE, et al: An approach for the use of Doppler ultrasound as a screening tool for hemodynamically significant stenosis (despite heterogeneity of Doppler performance). Stroke 27:1951–1957, 1996.
54. Beach KW: The evaluation of velocity and frequency accuracy in ultrasound duplex scanners. J Vasc Tech 14:214–220, 1990.
55. Päivänsalo MJ, Siniluoto TMJ, Tikkakoski TA, et al: Duplex US of the external carotid artery. Acta Radiologica 37:41–43, 1996.
56. Erickson SJ, Mewissen MW, Foley WD, et al: Stenosis of the internal carotid artery: Assessment using color Doppler imaging compared with angiography. AJR Am J Roentgenol 152:1299–1305, 1989.

Chapter 11

Miscellaneous Carotid Subjects: Occlusion, Dissection, Endarterectomy, Carotid Body Tumor

■ *William J. Zwiebel, MD*

CAROTID OCCLUSION

Arterial occlusion is diagnosed with ultrasound through the following observations: (1) absence of arterial pulsations; (2) lumen filled with echogenic material; (3) absence of flow (color or spectral Doppler); and (4) small vessel size (chronic occlusion).[1–7] The typical findings of carotid occlusion are shown in Figures 11–1 and 11–2. At first glance, the diagnosis of occlusion appears to be an easy matter, but false-positive diagnoses may occur when the artery is obscured by acoustic shadowing, when image quality is poor, when Doppler signals are weak, and especially when the vessel is nearly occluded and only a "trickle" of flow is present. The latter problem is of considerable clinical importance, for an occluded vessel is irremediable, whereas a nearly occluded vessel may be treated with endarterectomy if the stenosis is localized and the distal vessel is of good caliber. A nearly occluded internal carotid artery (ICA) often produces the angiographic "string sign" (Fig. 11–3*A*). It is important to realize that the apparent small caliber of the arterial lumen implied by the "string" of contrast is an artifact. The string sign results from puddling of the slow moving contrast agent in the dependent (posterior) portion of the arterial lumen with the patient supine. The lumen, in fact, is widely patent, and the stenosis is localized at the proximal end of the string.

Differentiation between highly stenosed and occluded carotid arteries was a major problem for duplex ultrasound in the pre–color-flow days, but with technical diligence, stenosis and occlusion can be accurately differentiated using color-flow instruments (see Fig. 11–3*B, C*). The use of power Doppler imaging is particularly advocated because of its sensitivity to low flow rates. Recent articles[6,7] report close to 100% sensitivity and specificity in the diagnosis of near-occlusion of the ICA, but to attain this level of accuracy, several technical details must be followed. First, adjust the instrument to detect minimum flow velocity. The pulse repetition frequency should be as low as possible and the low-frequency filter should be minimized so that low-frequency signals are not excluded. Second, obtain the best possible view of the occluded vessel and scrutinize the lumen for any hint of flow. Remember that the view chosen should optimize the Doppler angle of the color-flow image. I generally prefer power Doppler, but color-Doppler instruments may work better in some cases, especially when movement artifacts are a problem. Third, if any hint of flow is detected, interrogate the color area with spectral Doppler imaging. The signals obtained may be very weak, so high Doppler gain settings often are needed. Do not mistake the highly damped arterial flow signals for venous flow (check the flow direction). Finally, look at the occluded vessel from several transducer approaches, including the transverse plane, before concluding that flow is absent.

Atherosclerosis is by far the most common cause of carotid artery occlusion, but fibromuscular dysplasia and arterial dissection (discussion follows) are additional causes. The ICA is most commonly occluded, but occlusion also may occur in the common (CCA) or external (ECA) carotid artery. The incidence of CCA occlusion is approximately one tenth of the incidence of ICA occlusion,[5] but this incidence is sufficiently large for the occasional diagnosis of CCA occlusion in a typical community-based vascular diagnosis facility. CCA occlusion is frequently accompanied by stroke or other neurologic events but may also be encountered in the absence of neurologic symptoms.[5] The ICA may remain patent in spite of CCA occlusion because collateral supply to the ICA may develop through the ECA branches. In this case, flow reverses in the collateral ECA branches and remains cephalad in the ICA (see Fig. 11–2).

CAROTID ARTERY DISSECTION

Arterial dissection refers to the entry of blood, under arterial pressure, into the wall of the artery, separating the layers of the wall and creating a false lumen.[8–11] For blood to enter the wall and cause dissection, there must, of course, be a rent in the intima. This rent can occur in response to violent trauma or in response to conditions that weaken the arterial wall, which are cited later. The location at which the wall layers separate varies. In some cases, only the intima is dissected from the wall, whereas in other cases, portions of the media or the media and adventitia may delaminate. Thus, the thickness of the membrane separating the true and false lumina varies. Dissection at the adventitial layer may permit pseudoaneurysm formation adjacent to the artery.

Arterial dissection produces a false lumen that may be blind ended or may reconnect with the true lumen at a site distal to the point of dissection. The false lumen may remain patent or may thrombose (occlude). The general consequences of carotid dissection are stenosis (the false lumen bulging into and narrowing the true lumen), occlusion (of the true and false lumen), and false aneurysm formation (when dissection extends to the serosal layer). Central nervous system consequences include stroke, ipsilateral blindness, cranial neuropathy, and subarachnoid hemorrhage.

Cervical carotid artery dissection occurs in three circumstances: (1) dissection may extend cephalad from the aortic arch into the CCA and even into the bifurcation branches; (2) the cervical carotid arteries may undergo dissection spontaneously; and (3) carotid dissection may occur in response to trauma.

Three to seven percent of aortic arch dissections are complicated by stroke or transient cerebral ischemia, usually because of acute CCA occlusion but also because of embolization.[12] Carotid artery extension is most common with ascending arch dissection (Stanford's type A). This type of dissection is usually related to elastic tissue degeneration, as seen with Marfan's or Ehlers-Danlos syndromes. Stanford's type B dissection, occurring distal to the aortic arch, is most common in the elderly and is usually due to smooth muscle degeneration associated with aging. Although ulceration of atherosclerotic plaque may lead to aortic dissection, this mechanism occurs uncommonly; therefore, aortic dissection should not generally be regarded as a consequence of atherosclerosis.

Spontaneous dissection originating in the carotid arteries usually occurs in the ICA but may also originate in or involve the CCA. Spontaneous dissection in the absence of underlying arterial wall pathology may not really be spontaneous and may, in fact, result from nonviolent trauma, such as unusually strenuous exercise or rapid neck motion. In some cases the predisposing trauma may be unrecognized by the patient. Factors contributing to spontaneous carotid dissection include hypertension, fibromuscular hyperplasia, and conditions that weaken the arterial wall, such as Marfan's syndrome, cystic medial necrosis, and Ehlers-Danlos syndrome.

Carotid dissection resulting from violent trauma most commonly originates with direct injury to the ICA, either from stretching of the artery across cervical spine structures or from direct arterial compression by cervical spine elements or the mandible.[11] Trauma causes a rent in the intima and an injury that weakens the underlying wall structure, permitting delamination. Serious neurologic consequences are more common with traumatic carotid dissection than with atraumatic dissection.[10]

Text continued on page 161

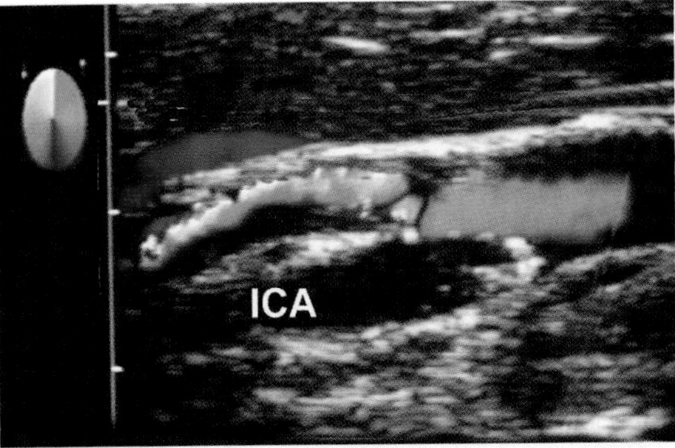

FIGURE 11–1 Internal carotid artery (ICA) occlusion. No flow is present in the ICA, and the vessel is filled with minimally echogenic material. These are typical features of carotid occlusion. The external carotid artery (upper vessel) is stenotic.

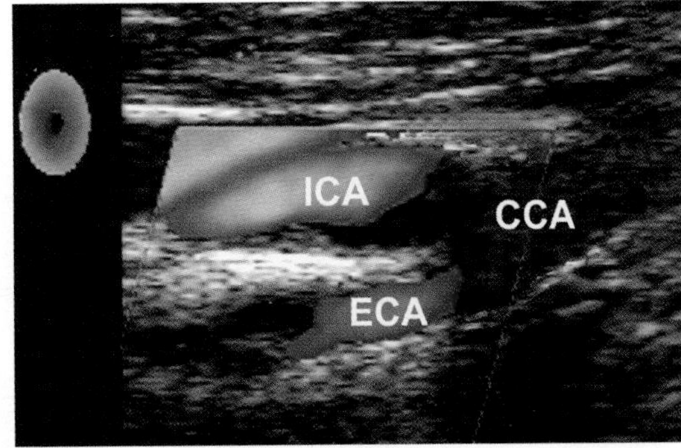

FIGURE 11–2 Common carotid artery (CCA) occlusion. This power Doppler image shows absence of flow in the CCA, yet both the internal (ICA) and the external (ECA) carotid arteries are patent. ICA flow is maintained by collateralization through the ECA.

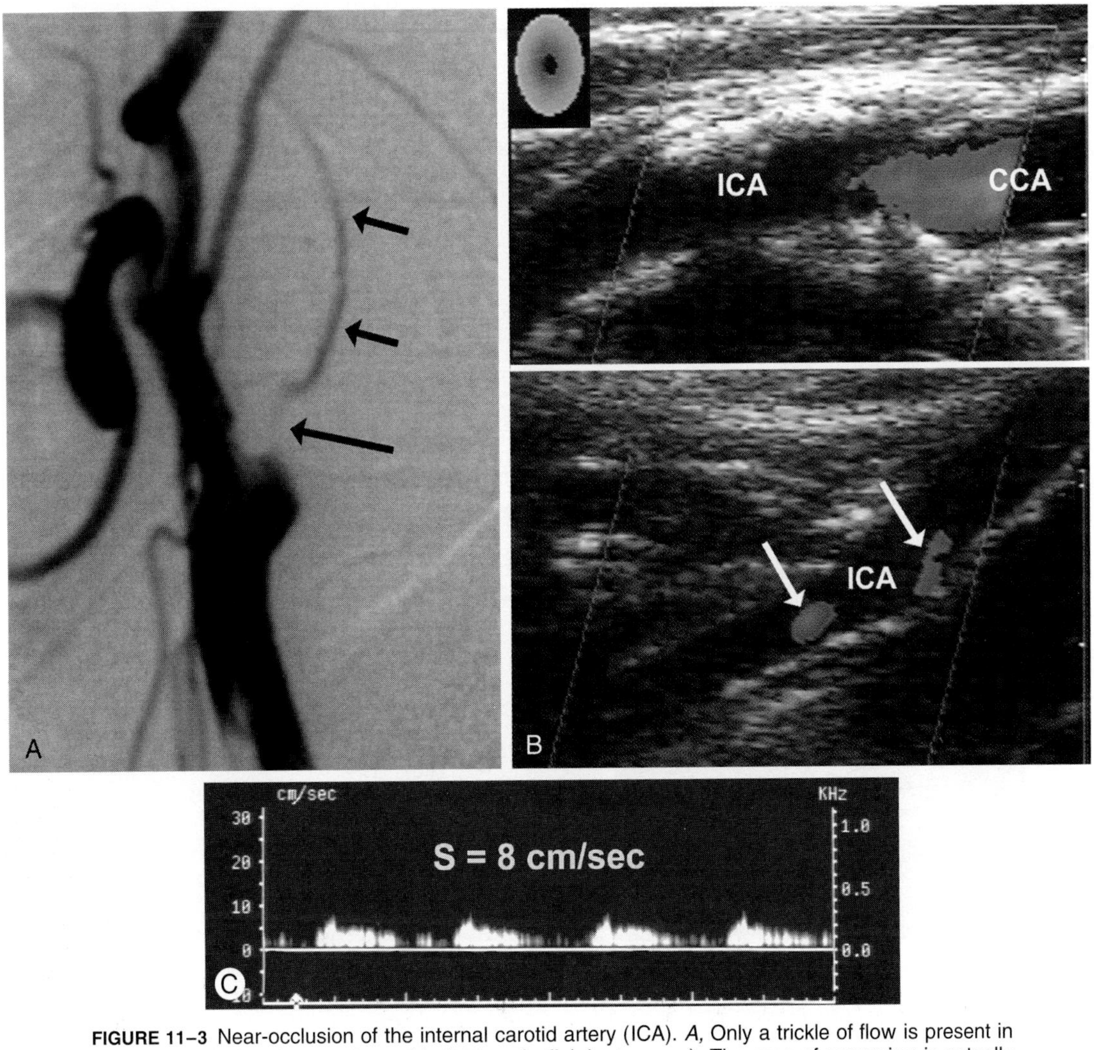

FIGURE 11–3 Near-occlusion of the internal carotid artery (ICA). *A,* Only a trickle of flow is present in the ICA, producing the arteriographic "string sign" (*short arrows*). The area of narrowing is actually confined to the ICA origin (*long arrow*), and the rest of the vessel is widely patent. The string results from puddling of the contrast agent against the posterior wall of the vessel with the patient supine. *B,* At first glance (*top*) it appears that the ICA is occluded, but with diligent scanning, flow is identified by focal areas of color (*bottom*). *C,* Doppler investigation of the areas of color shows markedly damped flow signals and low peak systolic velocity (S).

FIGURE 11–4 Carotid artery dissection. (See p 161.) *A,* A short-axis, color-Doppler image shows markedly disturbed flow in the common carotid artery (CCA). The cause is not apparent. IJV = internal jugular vein. *B,* Two frames from a video recording of the same vessel show a thin dissection membrane (*arrows*) that moves freely within the arterial lumen.

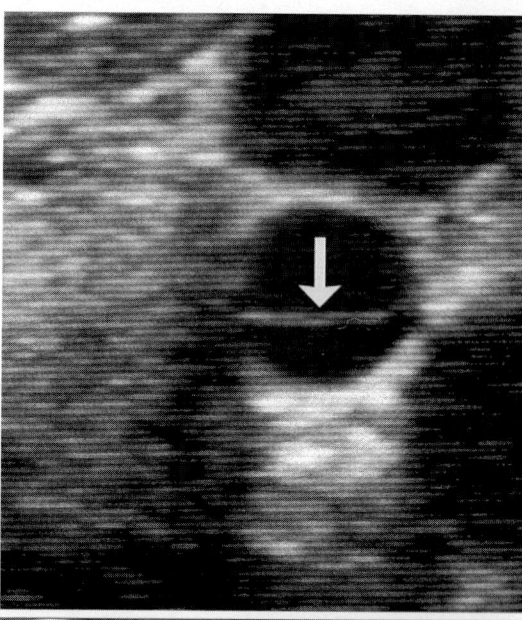

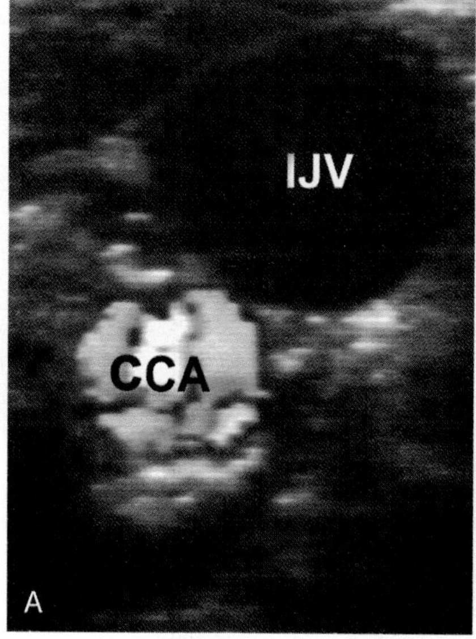

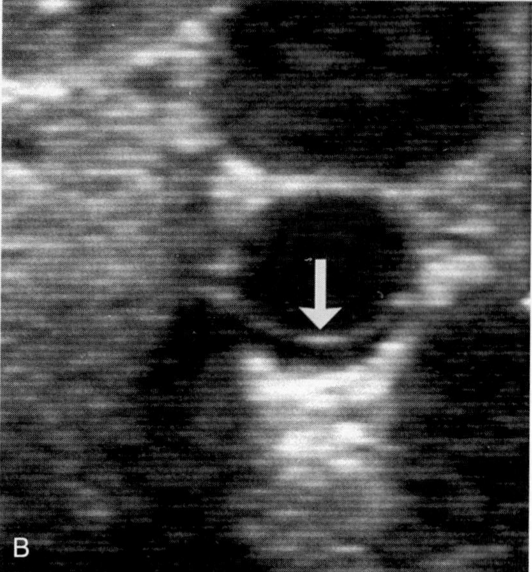

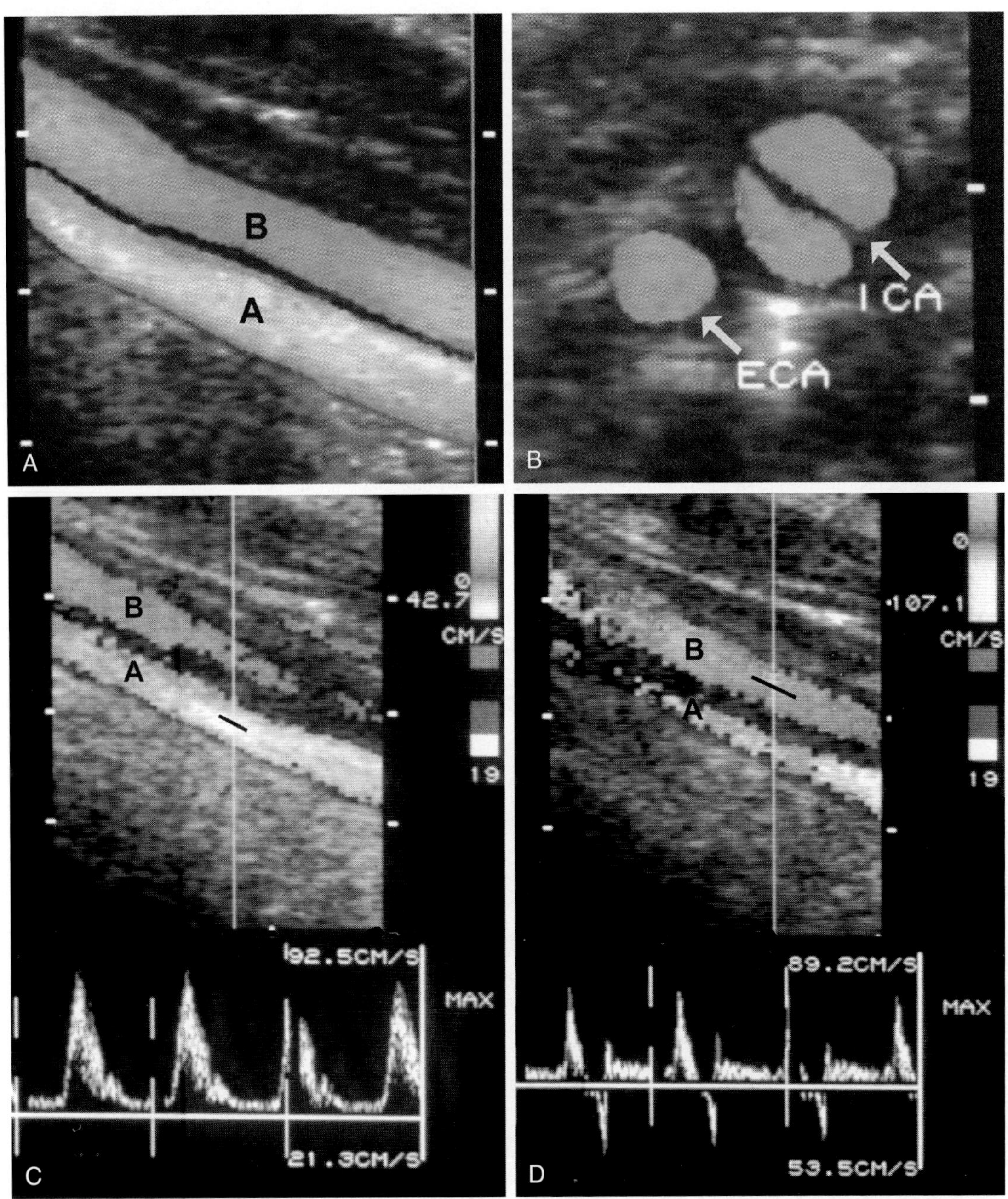

FIGURE 11–5 Carotid artery dissection. (See p 161.) *A,* A long-axis color-Doppler view shows that the common carotid artery is divided into two lumina, marked A and B, by a thick dissection membrane, which moved very little during each cardiac cycle. *B,* The dissection membrane extends into the internal carotid artery (ICA), as seen on this short-axis view. ECA = external carotid artery. *C,* Doppler waveforms in lumen A have continuous forward flow throughout the cardiac cycle. *D,* A to-and-fro flow pattern is present in lumen B.

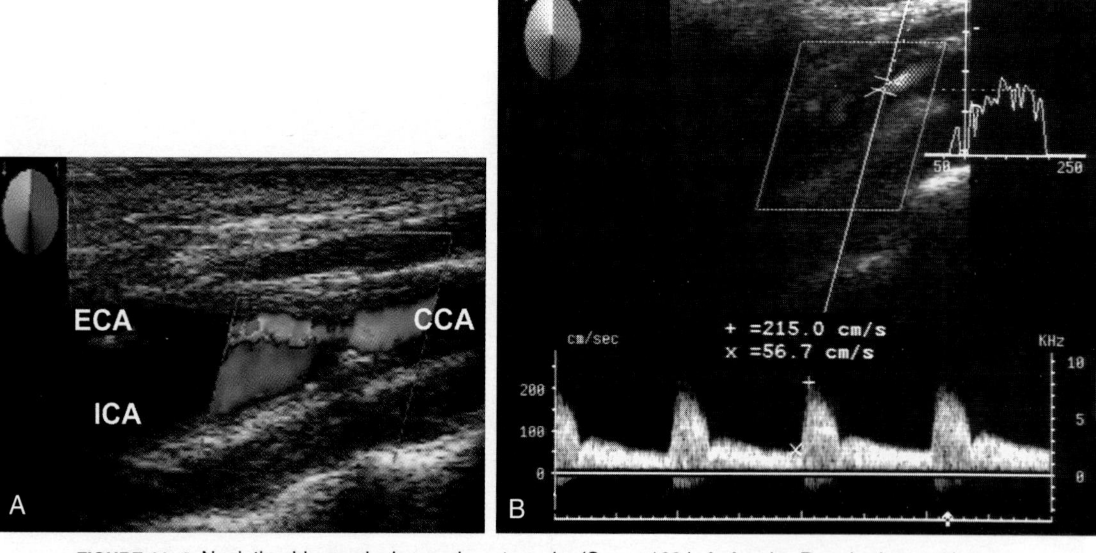

FIGURE 11–9 Neointimal hyperplasia causing stenosis. (See p 163.) *A,* A color-Doppler image shows substantial narrowing of the common carotid artery (CCA) and poststenotic flow disturbance at the site of an endarterectomy performed 12 months previously. ECA = external carotid artery; ICA = internal carotid artery. *B,* Doppler interrogation shows moderate velocity elevation in the stenotic area. Peak systole (+) is 215 cm/sec and end diastole (x) is 56.7 cm/sec.

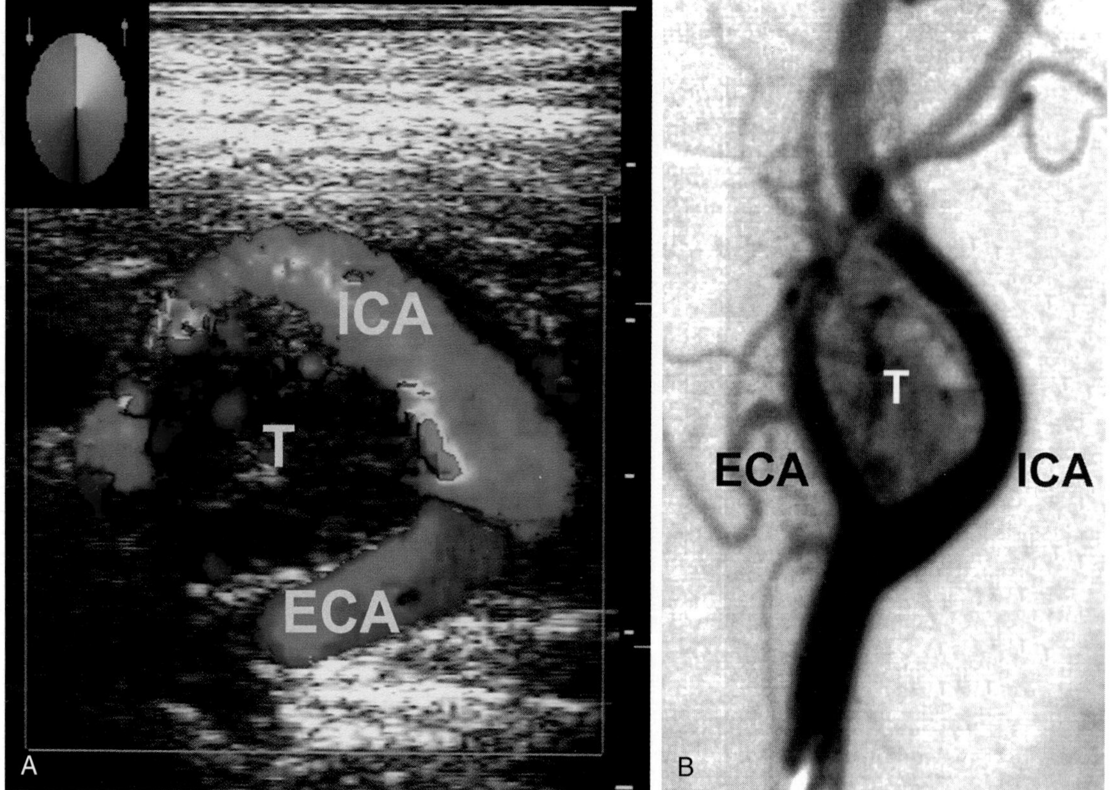

FIGURE 11–10 Carotid body tumor. (See p 164.) *A,* A longitudinal color-Doppler image shows a homogeneous, hypoechoic tumor (T), which splays the internal (ICA) and external (ECA) carotid artery branches. Blood flow (color areas) was easily detected in the tumor. *B,* Carotid arteriography in the lateral projection shows the highly vascular nature of the mass.

The duplex ultrasound findings associated with carotid dissection are dramatic when only the intima is delaminated from the rest of the wall. The loosened intima flutters back and forth in the flow stream with each cardiac cycle, generating severe flow disturbances, as shown in Figure 11–4 (see p 158). This dramatic appearance may not always occur, however. If the tissue between the lumina is thick, one may simply visualize a duplicated carotid lumen, as illustrated in Figure 11–5 (see p 159). In other cases the lumen may simply be narrowed, and the cause may be inapparent with casual examination. When carotid dissection is detected, the sonographer should try to obtain as much of the following information as possible: (1) the extent of dissection should be ascertained, which in turn may indicate whether dissection originated in the aortic arch, the CCA, or the ICA; (2) the presence, direction, and characteristics of flow in the true and false lumen should be documented; (3) if dissection causes stenosis, the degree of narrowing should be evaluated visually and with velocity measurement; and (4) the patency of the ECA and ICA should be determined, and Doppler waveform characteristics should be scrutinized in both vessels to determine the effects of dissection on the ICA circulation and to detect collateralization.

ENDARTERECTOMY WITHOUT ARTERIOGRAPHY

In the United States, it has become increasingly popular to perform carotid endarterectomy without preceding arteriography, relying instead on duplex ultrasound findings to indicate the severity of carotid stenosis.[13–20] Cranial computed tomography or magnetic resonance imaging is typically combined with carotid ultrasound to ensure the absence of significant intracranial pathology. The use of magnetic resonance imaging offers the additional advantage of vascular imaging to assess the status of the distal ICA, the vertebral system, and the major intracranial vessels.

The rationale for performing endarterectomy without preceding arteriography is as follows:

- Arteriography is expensive, especially if hospital admission is needed
- Arteriography conveys a slight risk (stroke 0.1 to 0.6%, death <0.1% [in the best of circumstances])
- Arteriography rarely affects the surgical plan (1% of cases according to Dawson and colleagues[15])
- Sufficient arteriographic information can be obtained with magnetic resonance imaging.

I generally agree with this approach, although I am also familiar with arguments that arteriography *is* necessary for endarterectomy planning.[14, 20] A cautious approach is advised, however, and certain conditions should be met before endarterectomy is performed without arteriography. First, and foremost, the accuracy of the ultrasound department must be known. Second, stenosis-producing atherosclerotic plaque should be localized to the carotid bifurcation. If atherosclerotic plaque appears severe and extensive, there is probably greater risk for extracranial stenotic lesions that might affect surgical planning, and magnetic resonance angiography or catheter arteriography should be considered. Third, ultrasound findings should be unequivocal. If the ultrasound examination is compromised or the findings are uncertain, arteriography should be considered. Even if the examination is of good quality, it is our policy to repeat the duplex ultrasound examination before surgery to confirm the findings. Fourth, if the ICA appears occluded and the patient is a surgical candidate, arteriography may be indicated to differentiate between occlusion and high-grade stenosis. Finally, if the patient is symptomatic, the symptoms should be hemispheric and ipsilateral to the carotid stenosis. Obviously, symptoms unrelated to carotid atherosclerosis are not cured with endarterectomy; furthermore, such symptoms may require further clinical evaluation.

ENDARTERECTOMY FOLLOW-UP

In most clinical centers it is routine to reexamine the carotid bifurcation at regular intervals after endarterectomy (e.g., 3 months, 6 months, 12 months, and annually thereafter). The purpose of such frequent examinations is to detect postsurgical complications, which generally fall into three categories.[21–25] Those complications occurring within the first month often are directly related to surgical problems, such as retained plaque, arterial clamp injury, or an intimal flap (from loosening of the cut edge of the intima at the margin of the endarterectomy). The first 2 years after surgery is the period when most (about 70%) of re-stenoses occur,[21] but it is important to realize that re-stenosis *does* occur later than 2 years after surgery.

The cause of re-stenosis varies with the postoperative time interval. Re-stenosis within the first 3 years results from neointimal hyperplasia (smooth muscle and fibrous overgrowth of the tissue layer that replaces the intima after surgery). After 3 years, the material causing re-stenosis is more apt to resemble atherosclerotic plaque, with abundant collagen, foam cells, and calcium deposits.[22] The histologic transition from early to late re-stenosis is a continuum, however, with an early neointimal hyperplasia appearance gradually giving way to a more atherosclerotic appearance in late-occurring re-stenosis. In general, the tissue causing re-

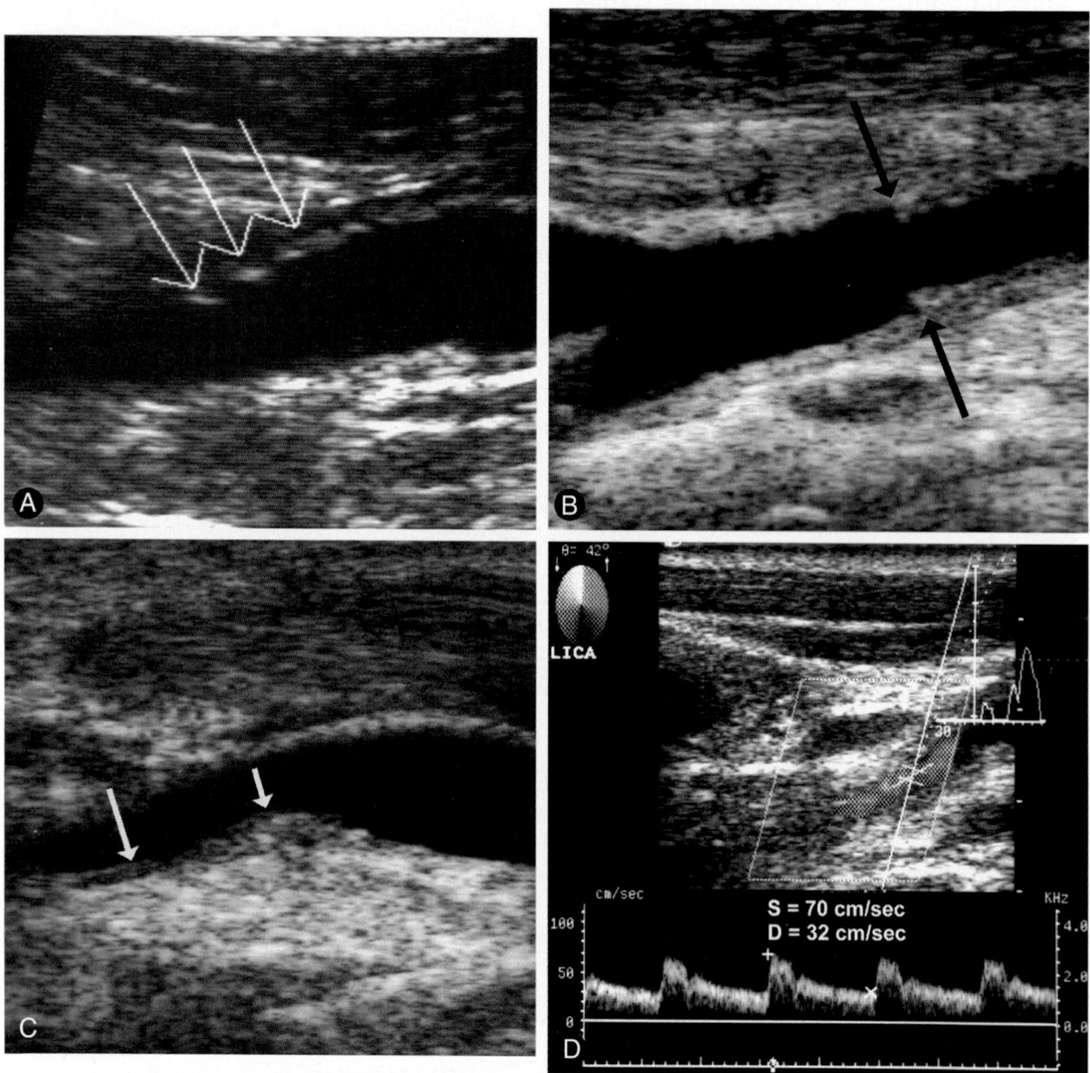

FIGURE 11–6 Postendarterectomy findings. *A,* A longitudinal view of the distal common and proximal internal carotid arteries shows bright reflections in the near wall representing sutures. *B,* The proximal end of the endarterectomy is clearly visible (*arrows*). Note the absence of the intimal reflection to the left of the arrow (cephalad). *C,* The distal end of the endarterectomy (*long arrow*) is well seen in the internal carotid artery. Note the resumption of the intimal line to the left of the arrow (cephalad). A localized area of neointimal hyperplasia is present (*small arrow*). *D,* The hyperplastic area prompted Doppler interrogation, revealing slight flow velocity elevation. S = peak systole; D = end diastole.

stenosis after endarterectomy is not prone to embolization. Most re-stenoses, therefore, are asymptomatic, and in these cases surgery is performed only to prevent carotid occlusion. Thus, for most postendarterectomy stenoses, surgery is not contemplated until the recurrent stenosis is very severe (usually 75 to 80% or greater diameter reduction). Because the tissue causing late re-stenosis resembles atherosclerotic plaque, symptoms are more commonly associated with late re-stenosis than with early re-stenosis.

The reported rate of clinically significant re-stenosis after endarterectomy is 9.8 to 23.2%.[22] This range is related, in part, to the definition of stenosis (e.g., 50 or 60% narrowing) and the duration of follow-up. In a large series reported by Mattos and colleagues[21] (409 carotid endarterectomies followed for as long as 16 years)[21], the overall re-stenosis rate (50% or greater diameter) was 10.5%. This seems to be a reliable number, as equivalent re-stenosis rates are common in other publications.[22] The incidence of high-grade obstruction (80% diameter or occlusion) was only 1.7% in the Mattos and colleagues series,[21] prompting these authors and others[25] to question the need for frequent sonographic follow-up in asymptomatic patients after endarterectomy.

As seen with ultrasound, the postendarterectomy carotid bifurcation (Fig. 11–6) normally shows absence of the intimal reflection, because the intima has been removed. A small amount of wall thickening (neointima) is usually apparent, and in some cases the sutures used to close the artery may produce focal bright reflections. The proximal and distal ends of the endarterectomy are marked by the absent intima, but it is often difficult to visualize the distal end of the endarterectomy (within the ICA), as image quality may not be satisfactory. Blood flow is laminar or only slightly disturbed at the endarterectomy site.

Abnormal postendarterectomy findings include flow disturbances, caused by an intimal flap or retained plaque; stenosis; and occlusion. Intimal flaps (Fig. 11–7) typically occur at the distal end of the endarterectomy, where the cut edge of the intima is subject to dislodgement by the cephalad flow stream. The elevated intima can cause tremendous flow disturbance and may ultimately lead to re-stenosis. Although the distal end of the endarterectomy often cannot be directly visualized on the gray-scale image, flow disturbances resulting from an intimal flap or distal

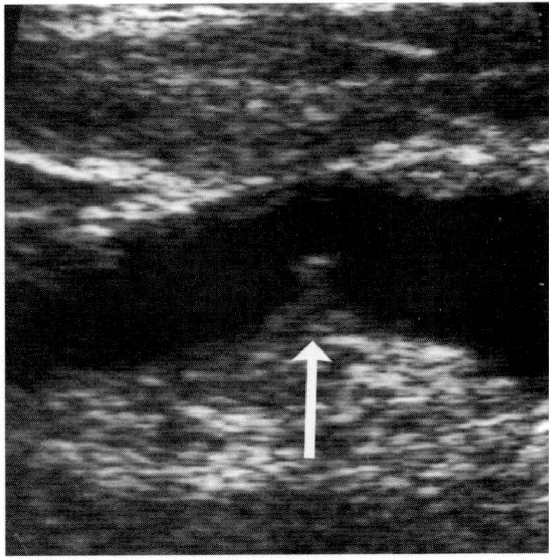

FIGURE 11–7 Distal endarterectomy defect. A localized band of tissue (*arrow*) projects into the internal carotid artery (ICA) lumen at the distal end of the endarterectomy. This produced a large amount of turbulence (not illustrated), prompting surgical correction. An intimal flap was found.

endarterectomy stenosis should be readily apparent, *as long as the sonographer is careful to examine the distal portion of the ICA.* Neointimal hyperplasia (Figs. 11–8 and 11–9 [see also p 160]) generally produces diffuse narrowing at the endarterectomy site, with proportionate elevation of flow velocity and poststenotic flow disturbance. The same velocity criteria are used for diagnosis of postoperative stenoses as are used preoperatively. Occlusion is diagnosed on the basis of findings described previously in this chapter.

CAROTID BODY TUMOR

The normal carotid body is a tiny ovoid structure 1 × 1.5 mm in size located in the adventitia of the carotid bifurcation. The function of the carotid body is not well understood, but it is a component of the autonomic nervous system that participates in the control of arterial pH, blood gas levels, and blood pressure.[11]

Carotid body tumors[11] are paragangliomas of relatively low malignant potential that arise in the carotid body. The most common presentation is a palpable neck mass, with headache. Neck pain is the second most common presentation. These are rare tumors, and because of their rarity, up to 25% are initially

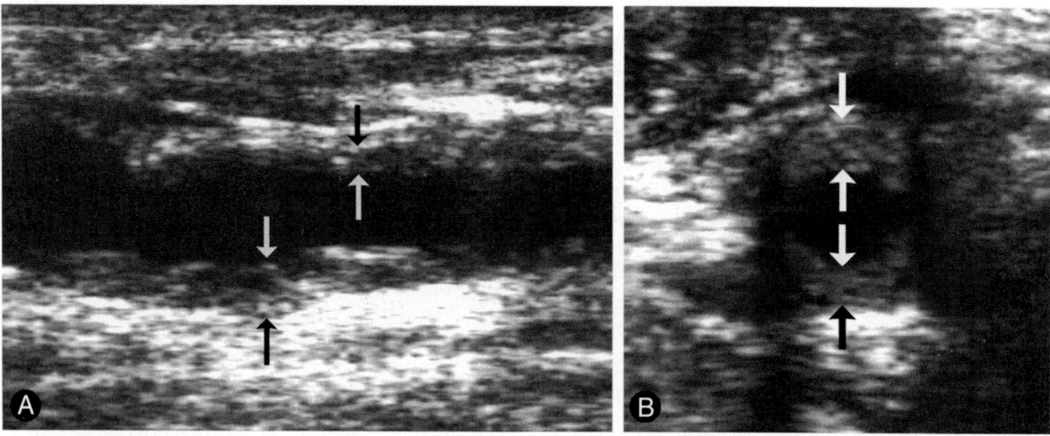

FIGURE 11–8 Neointimal hyperplasia. *A* and *B*, Long- and short-axis views, respectively, of the common carotid artery show considerable thickening of the arterial wall (*arrows*) at the site of an endarterectomy performed 18 months previously. Note that the hyperplastic tissue is homogeneous and medium in echogenicity, similar to fibrous plaque. The wall and surrounding tissues are quite attenuating, producing acoustic shadows on the short-axis view that obscure portions of the wall.

thought to be enlarged lymph nodes before surgical biopsy (which can lead to substantial hemorrhage of these highly vascular tumors).[11] Although the malignant potential of carotid body tumors is small, resection is standard therapy to prevent local adverse effects, such as laryngeal nerve palsy and invasion of the carotid arteries. Local recurrence occurs in 6% of cases and distant metastasis in 2% of cases.

On sonographic examination, carotid body tumors are highly vascular masses nestled within the "crotch" of the carotid bifurcation (Fig. 11–10 [see p 160]). In some cases the tumor may encase or surround the ECA or ICA, potentially complicating surgical excision. It is useful, therefore, to assess the relationship of the tumor to the bifurcation vessels. Ultrasound may also be used to follow the growth of small tumors if surgery is not anticipated. Arteriography is usually performed preoperatively, and the tumor may be embolized angiographically to reduce vascularity in anticipation of surgery.

REFERENCES

1. Middleton WD, Foley WD, Lawson TL: Color-flow Doppler imaging of carotid artery abnormalities. AJR Am J Roentgenol 150:419–425, 1988.
2. Erickson SJ, Middleton WD, Mewissen MW, et al: Color Doppler evaluation of arterial stenoses and occlusions involving the neck and thoracic inlet. Radiographics 9:389–406, 1989.
3. Hallam MJ, Reid JM, Cooperberg PL: Color-flow Doppler and conventional duplex scanning of the carotid bifurcation: Prospective, double-blinded correlative study. AJR Am J Roentgenol 152:1101–1105, 1989.
4. Steinke W, Kloetzsch C, Hennerici M: Carotid artery disease assessed by color Doppler flow imaging: Correlation with standard Doppler sonography and angiography. AJR Am J Roentgenol 154:1061–1068, 1998.
5. Chang YJ, Lin SK, Ryu SJ, Wai YY: Common carotid artery occlusion: Evaluation with duplex sonography. AJNR Am J Neuroradiol 16:1099–1105, 1995.
6. Lee DH, Gao FQ, Rankin RN, et al: Duplex and color Doppler flow sonography of occlusion and near occlusion of the carotid artery. AJNR Am J Neuroradiol 17:1267–1274, 1996.
7. Mattos MA, Hodgson KJ, Ramsey DE, et al: Identifying total carotid occlusion with colour flow duplex scanning. Eur J Vasc Surg 6:204–210, 1992.
8. Petro GR, Witwer GA, Cacayorin ED, et al: Spontaneous dissection of the cervical internal carotid artery: Correlation of arteriography, CT, and pathology. AJNR Am J Neuroradiol 148:393–398, 1987.
9. Hennerei M, Steinke W, Rautenberg W: High-resistance Doppler flow pattern in extracranial carotid dissection. Arch Neurol 46:670–672, 1989.
10. Provenzale JM: Dissection of the internal carotid and vertebral arteries: Imaging features. AJR Am J Roentgenol 165:1099–1104, 1995.
11. Cottrell ED, Smith LL: Management of uncommon lesions affecting the extracranial vessels. *In* Rutherford RB (ed): Vascular Surgery, Vol II. Philadelphia, WB Saunders, 1995, pp 1622–1636.
12. Walker PJ, Sarris GE, Miller DC: Peripheral vascular manifestations of acute aortic dissection. *In* Rutherford RB (ed): Vascular Surgery, Vol II. Philadelphia, WB Saunders, 1995, pp 1087–1102.
13. Summer DC, Russell JB, Miles RD: Are noninvasive tests sufficiently accurate to identify patients in need of carotid arteriography? Fifth Annual Meeting of the Midwestern Vascular Surgical Society, Chicago, IL, September 25–26, 1981.
14. Geuder JW, Lamparello PJ, Riles TS, et al: Is duplex scanning sufficient evaluation before carotid endarterectomy? J Vasc Surg 9:193–201, 1989.

15. Dawson DL, Zierler E, Strandness E, et al: The role of duplex scanning and arteriography before carotid endarterectomy: A prospective study. J Vasc Surg 18:673–683, 1993.
16. Moneta GL, Saxon RR, Taylor LM, Porter JM: Carotid imaging before carotid endarterectomy. Semin Vasc Surg 8:21–28, 1995.
17. Kuntz KM, Skillman JJ, Whittemore AD, Kent KC: Carotid endarterectomy in asymptomatic patients: Is contrast angiography necessary? A morbidity analysis. J Vasc Surg 22:706–716, 1995.
18. Muto PM, Welch HJ, Mackey WC, O'Donnell TF: Evaluation of carotid artery stenosis: Is duplex ultrasonography sufficient? J Vasc Surg 24:17–24, 1996.
19. Patel MR, Kuntz KM, Klufas RA, et al: Preoperative assessment of the carotid bifurcation. Stroke 26:1753–1758, 1995.
20. Howard G, Baker WH, Chambless LE, et al: An approach for the use of Doppler ultrasound as a screening tool for hemodynamically significant stenosis (despite heterogeneity of Doppler performance). Stroke 27:1951–1957, 1996.
21. Mattos MA, VanBemmelen PS, Barkmeier LD, et al: Routine surveillance after carotid endarterectomy: Does it affect clinical management? J Vasc Surg 17:819–831, 1993.
22. Chervu A: Recurrent carotid artery stenosis: Diagnosis, management, and prevention. Semin Vasc Surg 8:70–75, 1995.
23. O'Donnell TF, Rodriguez AA, Fortunato JE, et al: Management of recurrent carotid stenosis: Should asymptomatic lesions be treated surgically? J Vasc Surg 24:207–212, 1996.
24. Carballo RE, Towne JB, Seabrook GR, et al: An outcome analysis of carotid endarterectomy: The incidence and natural history of recurrent stenosis. J Vasc Surg 23:749–754, 1996.
25. Golledge J, Cuming R, Ellis M, et al: Clinical follow-up rather than duplex surveillance after carotid endarterectomy. J Vasc Surg 25:55–63, 1997.

Chapter 12

ULTRASOUND VERTEBRAL EXAMINATION

■ *William J. Zwiebel, MD*

Vertebral sonography is included in this text as a matter of completeness, even though I am not overly impressed with the utility of ultrasound vertebral artery (VA) examination. In our vascular diagnosis department, we principally examine the VAs in the course of carotid ultrasonography and then only to confirm that the VAs are patent and that the vertebral flow is cephalad in direction. Only rarely are the VAs the primary objective of ultrasound examination in our department, and we generally do not recommend ultrasonography as a primary method for vertebrobasilar examination. For most clinical issues concerning the vertebrobasilar system, we recommend magnetic resonance angiography.

In spite of this negative introduction, I believe that vascular ultrasound practitioners should have a basic understanding of vertebrobasilar anatomy, examination technique, and pathology that can be diagnosed with ultrasonography. Conveying this information is the goal of this chapter.

NATURE OF VERTEBROBASILAR DISEASE

The term *vertebrobasilar insufficiency* (VBI) is used when neurologic manifestations suggest insufficient blood flow in portions of the brain supplied by the VAs and basilar arteries (the brain stem, the cerebellum, and the posterior portion of the cerebral hemispheres).[1–6] If the symptoms are transitory, the condition may be called *transient vertebrobasilar ischemia.* If the neurologic signs or symptoms are permanent, the term *vertebrobasilar stroke* may be used. Unfortunately, VBI is not defined by a specific set of neurologic signs or symptoms, and similar neurologic dysfunction may occur with various other disorders, such as cardiac dysfunction, epilepsy, neoplasms, and migraine. To make matters more confusing, some of the neurologic symptoms of VBI may also occur with carotid insufficiency.

Atherosclerosis is clearly the primary cause of VBI, but the mechanism by which atherosclerosis generates VBI symptoms is unclear. Atherosclerotic stenosis or occlusion occurs primarily at the VA origin. The second most common site of atherosclerotic obstruction is intracranial, just beyond the C1 vertebral arch. Less commonly, and with increasing age, plaque develops more diffusely at the vertebral transverse foramen, in the intracranial segments of the VA and basilar artery, or in the intracranial branches of these vessels.[3] Although atherosclerosis is the underlying cause of VBI in many cases, the exact pathogenesis is varied and is often uncertain.[1–5] Potential causes of VBI include the following:

1. Embolization
2. Atherosclerotic obstruction of small intracranial branches
3. Vertebrobasilar occlusive disease, usually coupled with carotid artery occlusive disease (causing hypotension)
4. Vertebrobasilar ectasia (with shedding of clot)
5. Cardiac dysrhythmia (causing hypotension)
6. Artery-to-artery steal syndromes
7. Vertebral artery impingement (e.g., related to large cervical osteophytes)

Because the potential sources of VBI are varied, comprehensive imaging assessment of the vertebrobasilar circulation is required. Arteriography and magnetic resonance angiography are the only imaging procedures broadly recommended for comprehensive assessment of the vertebral basilar system. Duplex ultrasonography is severely limited for vertebral examination because of technical and anatomic problems discussed later. The combination of duplex sonography and transcranial Doppler imaging provides a better "picture" of the status of the vertebrobasilar system, but this picture is still quite limited as compared with magnetic resonance imaging or angiography.

ANATOMIC CONSIDERATIONS

The vertebrobasilar system has several anatomic features with which readers should be familiar (Fig. 12–1). First, the vertebrobasilar system is unique in that the two VAs unite (at the skull base) to form a common conduit, the basilar artery. This arrangement presents considerable opportunity for collateralization that generally ameliorates the effects of unilateral vertebral obstruction. Second, the multiple arterial anastomoses present in the circle of Willis (see Chapter 7) permit wide-ranging collateralization between the carotid and vertebrobasilar circulations. In the presence of carotid occlusive disease, the volume of blood carried by the VAs may increase markedly, affecting Doppler ultrasound findings. Third, the VAs are asymmetric in size in 73% of normal individuals,[5,6] and the VA on the left is larger (dominant) in about 80% of such cases.[7] Fourth, the VA origin is commonly tortuous in older individuals, limiting ultrasound visualization and producing confusing flow disturbances. The vertebral origin is also located deep to the clavicle, which limits ultrasound access, particularly on the left side. Fifth, the VAs pass through foramina (tunnels) in the transverse processes of C1 through C6. Direct ultrasound diagnosis is not possible in the segments lying within the foramina. Sixth, as each of the VAs exits from the transverse process of C1, it forms a prominent, posteriorly directed loop that is difficult to image with ultrasonography. Finally, a short segment of each VA lies within the skull, where it is inaccessible to ultrasound examination, although it may be examined with transcranial Doppler imaging. This segment is the second most common location for vertebral obstructive lesions.

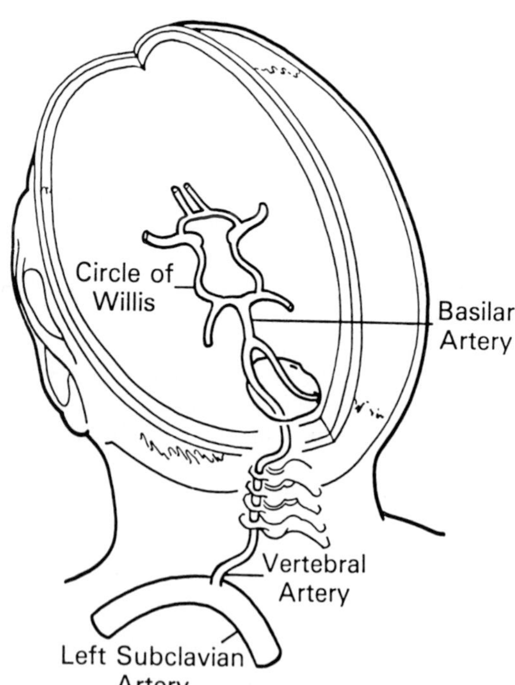

FIGURE 12–1 Vertebrobasilar anatomy. Note that the vertebral arteries pass through the transverse processes and unite at the base of the brain to form the basilar artery.

VERTEBRAL ULTRASOUND TECHNIQUE

The VAs[7–11] are examined with the patient in the same position as for a carotid study. Please note that only steps one through three are used routinely in our vascular diagnosis department. The remaining steps are used only in selected instances.

Step one: To find the VA, begin with an image of the common carotid artery and shift the image plane laterally until shadows are identified that represent the transverse processes of the cervical vertebra. Next, gently adjust the image plane until one segment (or more) of the VA is seen between the transverse processes (Fig. 12–2).

Step two: Note the direction of flow in the VA and confirm that flow is cephalad by comparing the vertebral and carotid flow directions.

Step three: Measure the diameter of a normal-appearing segment of the VA and record the waveform in that segment.

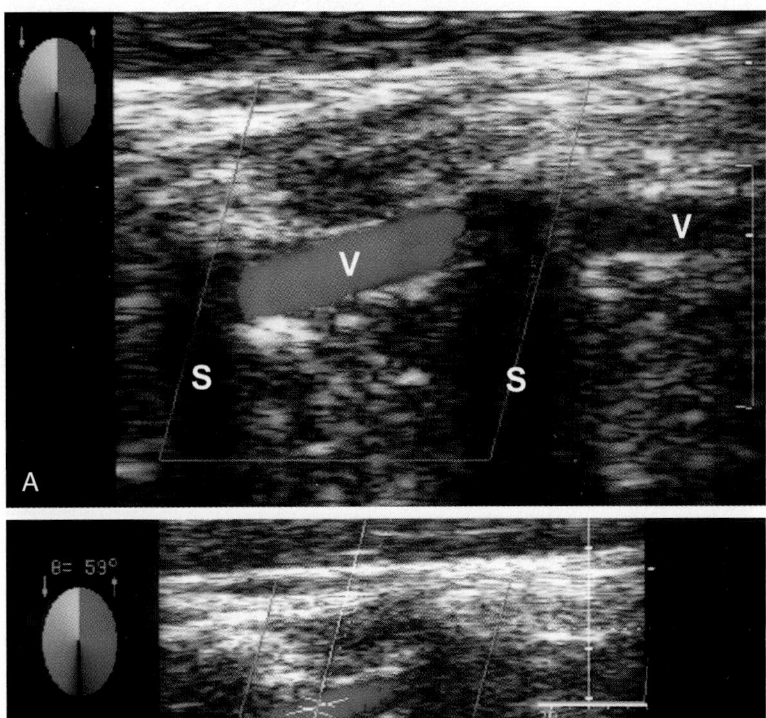

FIGURE 12–2 Normal vertebral artery. *A,* A segment of a vertebral artery (V) is seen in color between two transverse processes that cast acoustic shadows (S). *B,* Vertebral artery Doppler waveforms have low-resistance features and resemble internal carotid waveforms.

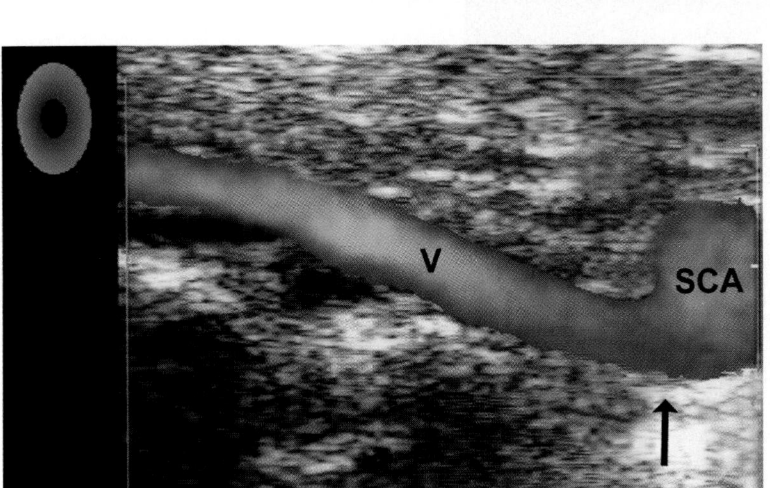

FIGURE 12–3 Normal vertebral artery origin. A longitudinal, power Doppler image shows the origin (*arrow*) of the vertebral artery (V) from the subclavian artery (SCA).

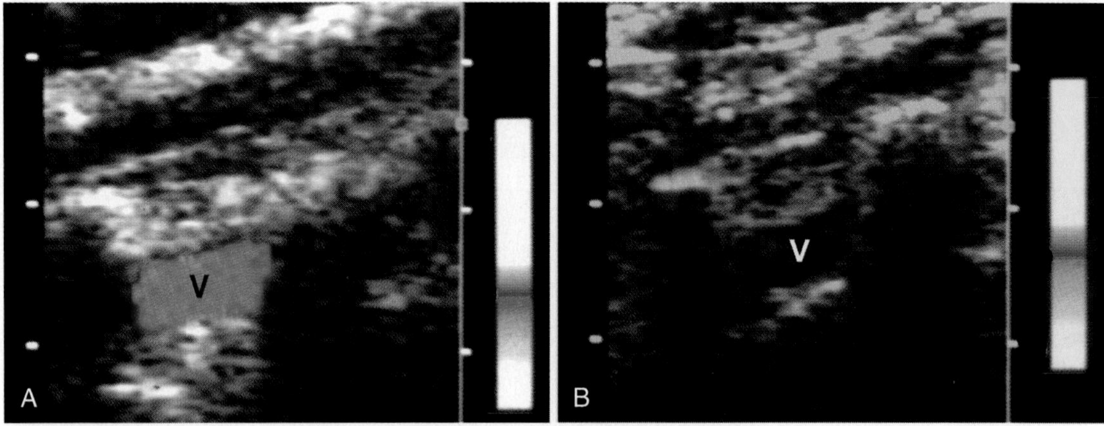

FIGURE 12–4 Absent vertebral artery flow. *A,* A color-Doppler image shows readily that flow is present in this vertebral artery (V). *B,* The contralateral vertebral artery (V) is visible, but no flow could be detected. Absence of flow in this case was confirmed angiographically.

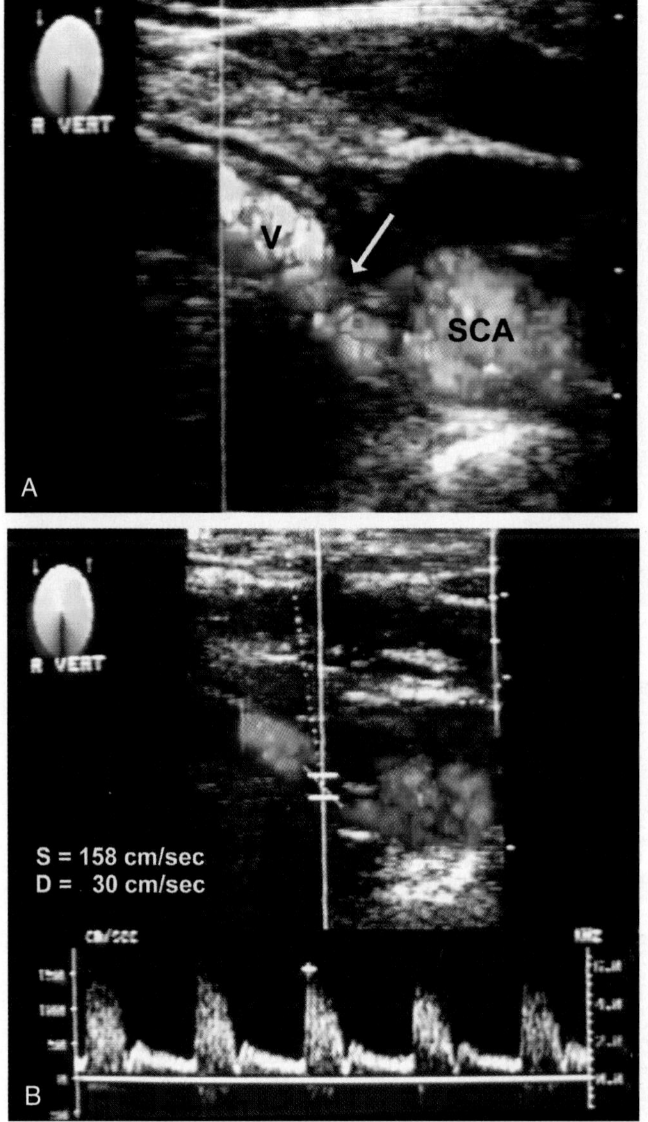

FIGURE 12–5 Vertebral artery origin stenosis. *A,* A color-Doppler image shows visible narrowing (*arrow*) of the origin of this vertebral artery (V), and marked poststenotic flow disturbance. SCA = subclavian artery. *B,* Doppler investigation of the stenosis indicates a peak systolic velocity of 158 cm/sec and end diastolic velocity of 30 cm/sec.

Step four: Trace the vertebral artery inferiorly to its origin at the subclavian artery (Fig. 12–3), and look for flow disturbances or high-velocity signals that may indicate stenosis. Below the C6 level, the VA does not pass through the transverse vertebral foramina, but it follows a generally straight course, except near its origin.

Step five: Survey cephalad along the visible length of the VA in the neck with color-Doppler imaging, tracing the course of the VA from one transverse foramen to the next. Watch for flow disturbances or elevated velocity suggestive of stenosis.

NORMAL VERTEBRAL ULTRASOUND FEATURES

On color-flow examination, the VA demonstrates cephalad flow throughout the cardiac cycle and a low-resistance flow pattern. Vertebral veins may occasionally be seen adjacent to the VA, but flow in these vessels is caudad (toward the heart) and nonpulsatile. These components of the vertebral venous plexus can usually be differentiated easily from the VA. The origin of a normal VA may be difficult to demonstrate clearly because of tortuosity of the proximal portion of the vessel. Furthermore, the origin may lie quite low, beneath the clavicle. The success rate for standard duplex (non–color-flow) visualization of the VA origin ranges from 82 to 90% on the right side and from 50 to 63% on the left side.[7–10] Color-Doppler imaging has made the visualization of the VA origin easier, and the VA origin can be seen regularly by an experienced sonographer. I am not aware, however, of recent statistics on the rate of successful VA origin visualization with color-Doppler imaging.

The mean VA diameter is 4 mm,[8] but VA size is variable, and the VAs are asymmetric in size in 73% of normal individuals.[5,6] Because of this variability, little diagnostic information is conveyed directly by vertebral caliber.

VA Doppler waveforms have low-resistance characteristics similar to those seen in the internal carotid artery (see Fig. 12–2). A large volume of cephalad flow is present throughout diastole and the systolic waveform is relatively broad. The waveform pattern is generally symmetric in the VAs, but systolic and diastolic velocities may differ considerably if the arteries are asymmetric in size. Normal peak systolic velocities range from 20 to 40 cm/sec, and systolic velocities lower than 10 cm/sec are potentially abnormal.[9] Higher velocities may be normal in the dominant VA of an asymmetric pair or with contralateral VA occlusion. Minor flow disturbances are common in normal VAs, regardless of the site of examination.[8,10] These disturbances should not be regarded as pathologic. Severe flow disturbances are abnormal, however, and suggest hemodynamically significant stenosis.

ABNORMAL VERTEBRAL ULTRASOUND FINDINGS

Potentially abnormal VA ultrasound findings may be categorized as follows:

1. Nonvisualization
2. Very small size
3. Absence of flow
4. Increased flow velocity
5. Decreased velocity
6. Abnormal flow direction

Each of these abnormalities are considered in turn.

Nonvisualization

Failure to identify a VA suggests that the vessel is occluded. Care must be taken, however, to avoid misdiagnosis caused by poor visualization or small size in an asymmetric pair. Even when visualization is good, I have occasionally misdiagnosed VA occlusion, only to have a small but otherwise normal vessel identified angiographically. Because of these experiences, I report VA occlusion in couched terms, such as "apparently occluded."

Small Size

As noted previously, VA size is variable, and large side-to-side differences may occur in normal individuals. In my experience, however, inordinately small VA diameter (2 mm or less) suggests obstruction (usually at the VA origin). It is a good idea, therefore, to examine the origin of a small VA for signs of stenosis.

Absent Flow

Absence of flow in a successfully imaged VA indicates occlusion of the vessel (Fig. 12–4). A false-positive diagnosis of occlusion may occur, however, in highly stenosed vessels with only a trickle of flow.[7, 9, 10, 12]

Focal Velocity Elevation

A focal velocity increase (significantly exceeding 40 cm/sec, peak systole) suggests a vertebral stenosis of at least 50% diameter reduction, especially when accompanied by severely disturbed flow downstream from the stenosis[7, 11] (Fig. 12–5). Velocity parameters defining specific levels of VA stenosis have not been defined as they have for carotid stenosis.

Decreased Velocity

Flow velocity may be reduced distal to a severe VA stenosis and the Doppler waveform may have a damped appearance (Fig. 12–6). These are typical ischemic findings, as discussed in Chapter 3. Reduced VA velocity may also be seen when a severe obstruction is *distal* to the site of Doppler examination (in either the VA or basilar artery).[9] In such cases, however, the waveforms are not damped and instead have a high-resistance pattern (sharp systolic peak and reduced or absent diastolic flow).

Abnormal Flow Direction

VA flow is cephalad in direction throughout the cardiac cycle, and any deviation from this pattern is abnormal. The vertebral-to-subclavian steal may cause vertebral flow reversal (Fig. 12–7) or a to-and-fro flow pattern. The vertebral-to-subclavian steal is caused by atherosclerotic stenosis or occlusion of a subclavian artery *proximal* to the ipsilateral VA origin, with resultant collateralization through the vertebral basilar system (Fig. 12–8). Subclavian stenosis and the subclavian steal have a distinctly left-sided predilection. About 85% of cases involve the left subclavian artery and only 15% involve the right subclavian or innominate artery.[13, 14] It has been found that the subclavian steal is almost always a harmless hemodynamic phenomenon. Subclavian steal uncommonly causes neurologic symptoms and rarely causes vertebrobasilar stroke (even in the presence of VA or carotid obstructive lesions).[13, 14] In spite of the innocuous nature of the vertebral-to-subclavian steal, sonographers should recognize and properly diagnose this condition, as it is an indication of subclavian artery insufficiency that may be clinically important.

The following three ultrasound findings may be seen with vertebral-to-subclavian steal: (1) vertebral flow is reversed throughout the cardiac cycle; (2) flow is bidirectional (forward in systole and reverse in diastole); or (3) flow is normal with the patient at rest. In the last two instances, the steal may be intensified and more clearly demonstrated by

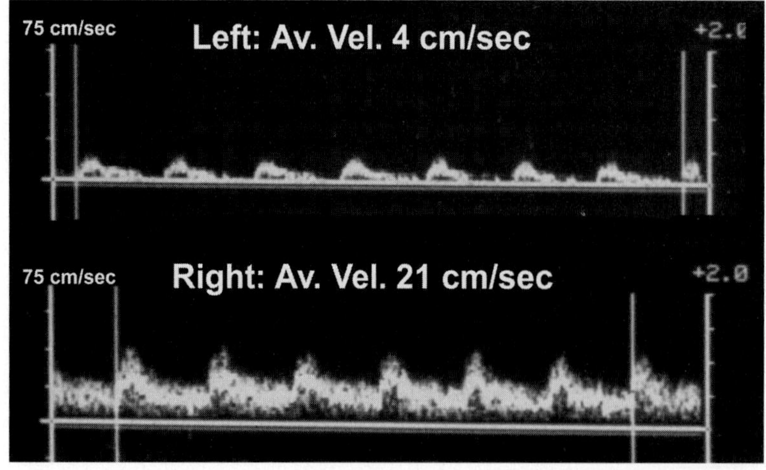

FIGURE 12–6 Damped vertebral artery flow signals. Doppler waveforms in the left vertebral artery (*top*) are markedly damped and of low amplitude, indicating stenosis at a location proximal to the transducer. The average velocity is 4 cm/sec. Flow signals are normal in the right vertebral artery (*bottom*), with an average velocity of 21 cm/sec.

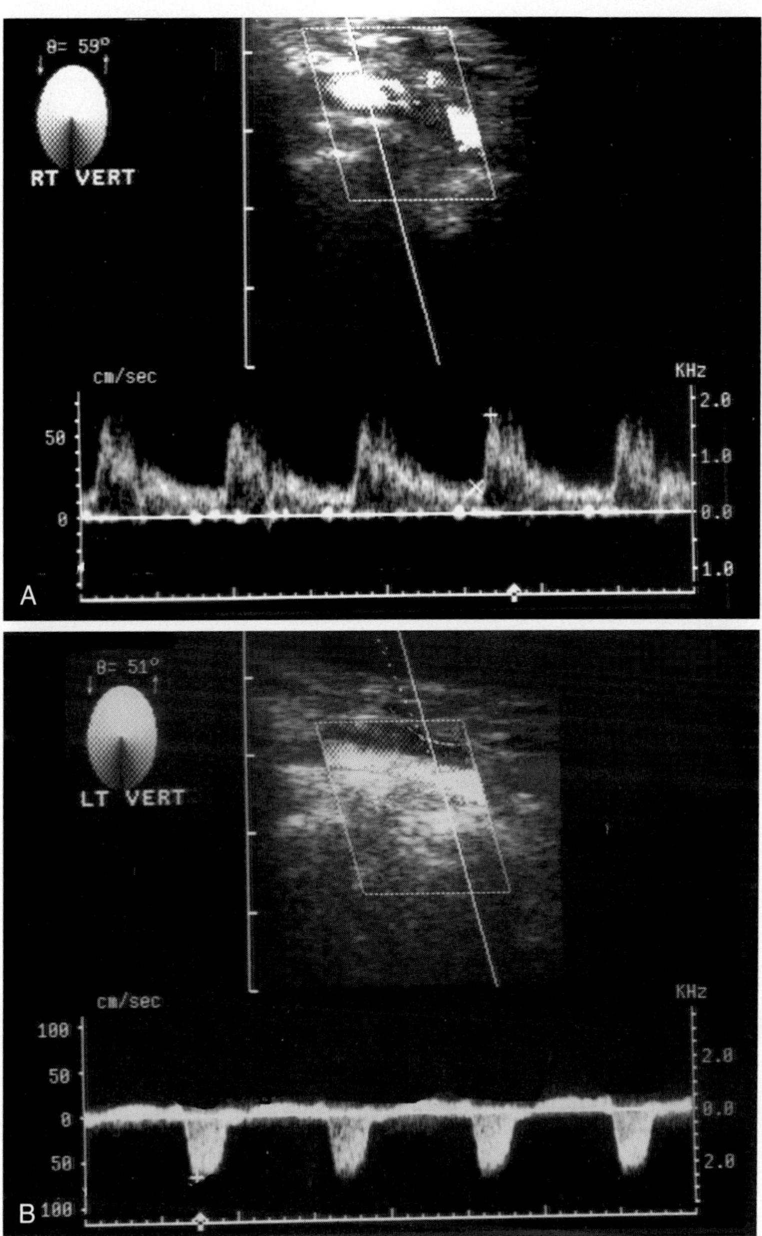

FIGURE 12–7 Vertebral-to-subclavian steal. *A,* Right vertebral artery flow signals are normal. *B,* Flow is reversed in the left vertebral artery.

Illustration continued on following page

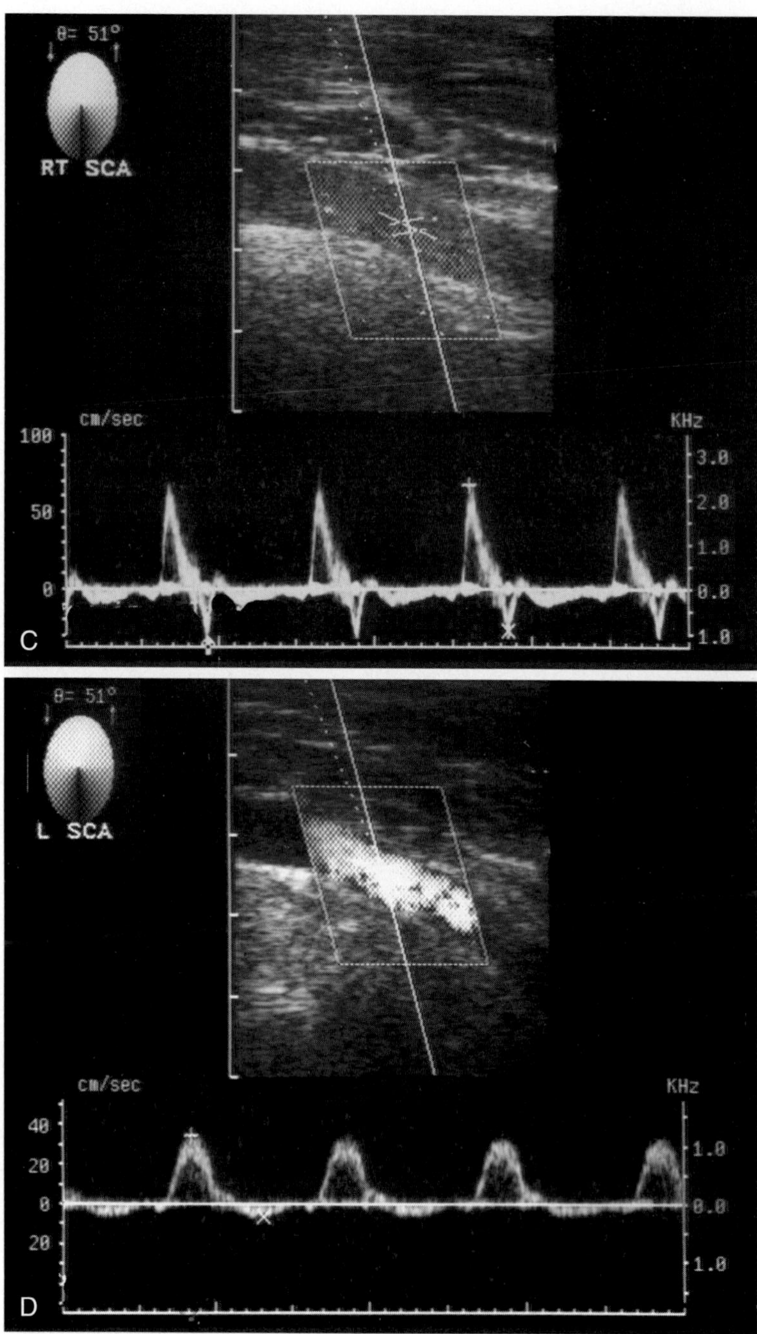

FIGURE 12–7 *Continued. C,* Right subclavian artery Doppler waveforms are normal (triphasic). *D,* Left subclavian artery waveforms are markedly damped because of subclavian occlusion.

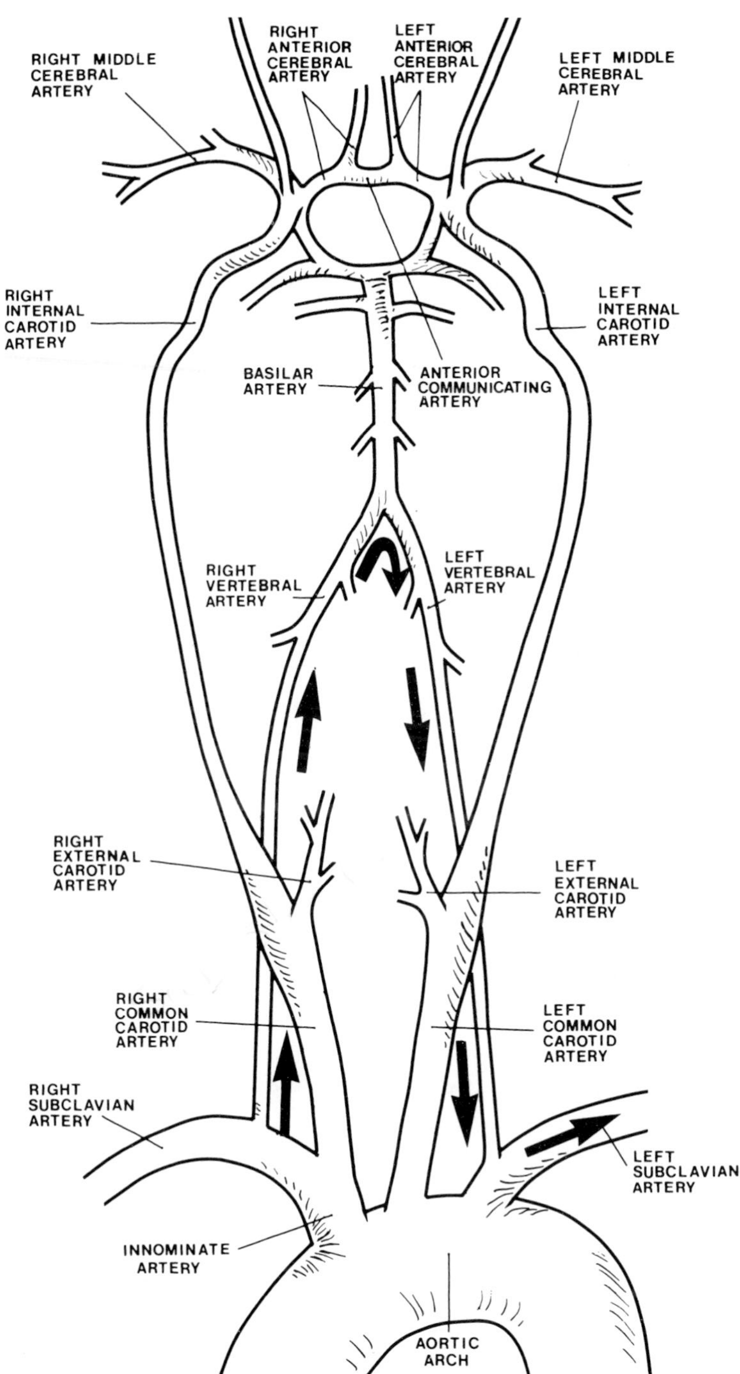

FIGURE 12–8 Illustration of the route of flow in the vertebral-to-subclavian steal.

inducing arm hyperemia with an inflated blood pressure cuff. The cuff is placed around the arm and inflated above systolic pressure for approximately 5 minutes. With deflation of the cuff, flow in the ipsilateral VA remains cephalad in direction in normal individuals. If subclavian steal is present, however, the vertebral waveform quickly inverts or becomes biphasic after pressure is released.

REFERENCES

1. Ausman JI, Shrontz CE, Pearce JE, et al: Vertebrobasilar insufficiency. A review. Arch Neurol 42:803–808, 1985.
2. White DN: Vertebral ultrasonography. *In* Zwiebel WJ (ed): Introduction to Vascular Ultrasonography, 2nd ed. Philadelphia, WB Saunders, 1986, pp 217–243.
3. Moossy J: Morphology, sites and epidemiology of cerebral atherosclerosis. *In* Millikan CH (ed): Cerebrovascular Disease. Baltimore, Williams & Wilkins, 1966, pp 1–22.
4. Crompton MR: Pathology of degenerative cerebral arterial disease. *In* Russell RW, Ross E (ed): Cerebral Arterial Disease. London, Churchill Livingstone, 1976, pp 40–56.
5. Meyer JS, Lobe C: Strokes Due to Vertebro-Basilar Disease. Springfield, IL, Charles C Thomas, p 137, 1965.
6. Stopford JSB: The arteries of the pons and medulla oblongata. J Anat 50:131–136, 1916.
7. Ackerstaff RGA, Grosveld WJHM, Eikelboom BC, Ludwig, JW: Ultrasonic duplex scanning of the prevertebral segment of the vertebral artery in patients with cerebral atherosclerosis. Eur J Vasc Surg 2:387–393, 1988.
8. Touboul PJ, Bousser MG, LaPlane D, Castaigne P: Duplex scanning of normal vertebral arteries. Stroke 17:921–923, 1986.
9. Bendick PJ, Glover JL: Hemodynamic evaluation of vertebral arteries by duplex ultrasound. Surg Clin North Am 70:235–244, 1990.
10. Jak JG, Hoeneveld H, van der Windt JM, et al: A six year evaluation of duplex scanning of the vertebral artery. A non-invasive technique compared with contrast angiography. J Vasc Tech 13:26–30, 1989.
11. Bendick PJ, Jackson VP: Evaluation of the vertebral arteries with duplex sonography. J Vasc Surg 3:523–530, 1986.
12. Visona A, Lusiani L, Castellani V, et al: The echo-Doppler (duplex) system for the detection of vertebral artery occlusive disease: Comparison with angiography. J Ultrasound Med 5:247–250, 1986.
13. Bornstein NM, Krajewski A, Norris JW: Basilar artery blood flow in subclavian steal. Can J Neurol Sci 15:417–419, 1988.
14. Bornstein NM, Norris JW: Subclavian steal: A harmless haemodynamic phenomenon? Lancet 2:303–305, 1986.

Chapter 13

TRANSCRANIAL DOPPLER SONOGRAPHY

■ *Shirley M. Otis, MD* ■ *E. Bernd Ringelstein, MD*

In 1965, Miyazaki and Kato[1] first reported the use of Doppler ultrasound for the assessment of extracranial cerebral vessels. Despite its rapid development in other fields, this technique was not applied to the intracranial vessels until 1982. At that time, Aaslid and colleagues[2] developed a transcranial Doppler (TCD) device with a pulsed sound emission of 2 MHz that could successfully penetrate the skull and accurately measure blood flow velocities in the basal vessels in the circle of Willis. Since that time there has been an amazingly rapid development of this technique, which has turned out to be a useful tool, with both clinical and research applications.

With the introduction of TCD, it became possible to record intracranial blood flow velocity directly, so TCD became an important noninvasive method for assessing cerebral hemodynamics and for evaluating intracranial cerebrovascular disease. The relationship remains unclear between the actual cerebral blood flow and the flow velocities measured by TCD within the basal cerebral arteries. This limitation can be overcome and is rather unimportant, however, because changes in blood flow velocity reflect *relative* changes in regional cerebral blood flow.[3,4] In addition to its noninvasive character and low cost, TCD offers these decisive advantages: relative changes in cerebral flow can be measured objectively, immediately, for as long as desired, and for as often as desired.[5] These factors make TCD an attractive monitoring tool, particularly during neurosurgical, vascular surgical, cardiac, and cerebrovascular procedures. During surgery of this type, immediate information about cerebral blood flow status allows adjustments to be made that can help reduce the incidence of post-procedure cerebral complications.[6–10] The abrupt or short-lasting effects of any external mechanical manipulation or functional stimulation of the intracranial circulation can be assessed in real time by TCD. TCD also permits the assessment of cerebral circulatory pathophysiology in acute stroke.[11–13] The established applications of TCD sonography in clinical and experimental settings are the following:

1. Detection of intracranial stenosis in the major basal arteries
2. Evaluation of hemodynamic effects of extracranial occlusive disease on intracranial blood flow (e.g., occlusions, subclavian steal)
3. Adjunct in inconclusive extracranial tests
4. Detection of arteriovenous malformations (AVMs) and identification of feeders
5. Intermittent monitoring and follow-up
    a. Monitoring vasospasm (subarachnoid hemorrhage and migraine)
    b. Monitoring spontaneous or therapeutically induced recanalization of occluded vessels
    c. Monitoring after occluding interventions (e.g., establishment of collateral pathways)
    d. Follow-up of occlusive disease during anticoagulative therapy
    e. Follow-up of feeders of AVMs during radiation therapy of aneurysms
6. Continuous monitoring during
    a. Neuroradiologic interventions (balloon occlusion and embolization)
    b. Acute pharmacologic trials of vasoactive drugs
    c. Carotid endarterectomy
    d. Cardiopulmonary bypass

   e. Increasing intracranial pressure
   f. Evolution of brain death

7. Functional tests
   a. Stimulation of cerebral vasomotor areas with carbon dioxide (CO_2) or other vasoactive drugs (assessing autoregulation)
   b. External stimulation of visual cortex
   c. Preoperative compression tests for evaluation of collateralizing capability of circle of Willis

This is not a complete list, because the applications of this rapidly developing technology are still evolving.

EXAMINATION TECHNIQUES

General Prerequisites

Two prerequisites must be fulfilled before performing a TCD examination: (1) the status of the extracranial arteries must be known completely, and (2) the patient must be resting comfortably to avoid major fluctuations of P_{CO_2} and movement artifacts. In addition, two main anatomic considerations must be dealt with by the examiner: (1) the number and accessibility of the ultrasonic "windows" or foramina within the skull that can be penetrated with the ultrasonic beam are often limited or not easily identified; and (2) the arteries at the base of the skull vary greatly in respect to size, course, development, and site of access.[13–19]

The transmission of ultrasound through the cranium is a significant problem that has been extensively studied.[20, 21] Transmission of ultrasound depends on the skull structure, which consists of the three layers of bone. Each layer influences ultrasound transmission in different ways. The middle layer (diploe) has the most significant effect in terms of attenuation and scattering of the sound beam. The outer and inner layers, made of cortical bone, generally cause refraction of the beam. The temporal region is an attractive area for ultrasound evaluation because of the essential absence of bony spicula. Grolimund[22] has performed a number of in vitro experiments to determine the effects of the skull bone on Doppler ultrasound. His experiments have shown that a wide range of energy loss occurs in different skull samples because power loss depends on skull thickness, which varies greatly from one location to another and among individuals. In no case was the power measured behind the skull greater than 35% of the transmitted power. It was further shown that the skull has the effect of an acoustic lens and that refraction of the beam depends more on the variation of bone thickness than on the angle of insonation. These data suggested that it is advantageous to use ultrasound lenses with relatively long focal lengths to improve Doppler sensitivity, particularly at depths of 5 to 10 cm.

Transcranial Doppler Devices

For transcranial applications, the primary design consideration is an excellent signal-to-noise ratio. This is one reason why available transcranial instruments have a lower bandwidth, and, therefore, a larger and less defined sample volume than most other pulsed Doppler instruments. Commercial systems are available that use a 2-MHz, pulsed, range-gated Doppler device with good directional resolution. The following are additional instrument requirements: (1) transmitting powers between 10 and 100 mW/cm/sec, (2) adjustable Doppler gate depth, (3) pulse repetition frequency up to 20 kHz, (4) focusing of the ultrasonic beam at a distance of 40 to 60 mm, and (5) online time-average velocity and peak systolic velocity derived from spectral analysis of the ultrasonic signals.[23]

Many instruments are currently available that meet the mentioned requirements, including the first commercially produced transcranial Doppler device, the TCD-64R,* and the Transpect transcranial Doppler.† Both systems include a special 2-MHz transducer for continuous monitoring, which can be attached to the patient's head by a headband or helmet. As a result of advances in technology, transcranial color-coded duplex sonography (TCCD) is also available and performs with a variety of capable machines using a color-Doppler system that is equipped usually with 2.0- to 2.5-MHz phased array transducers (Fig. 13–1). This diagnostic method allows noninvasive imaging of not only intracranial vascular structures but also parenchymal anatomy.[24, 25]

---

*Eden Medical Electronics, Überlingen, Germany.
†Medasonics, Mountain View, CA.

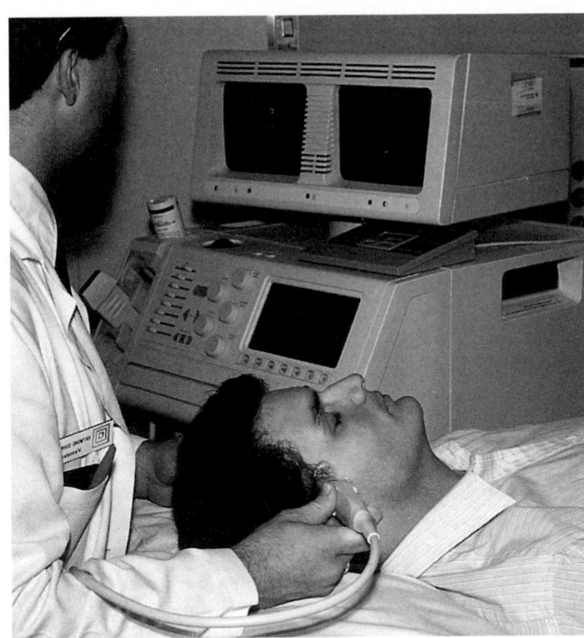

FIGURE 13–1 One (ATL UM9) of a variety of capable machines with a 2.0- to 2.5-MHz phased array transducer used in duplex transcranial Doppler–color imaging. (Courtesy of ATL Ultrasound, Bothell, WA).

Ultrasonic Windows

Four different TCD approaches have been described to insonate the intracranial arteries (Fig. 13–2): the transtemporal, transorbital, suboccipital, and submandibular approaches.[26]

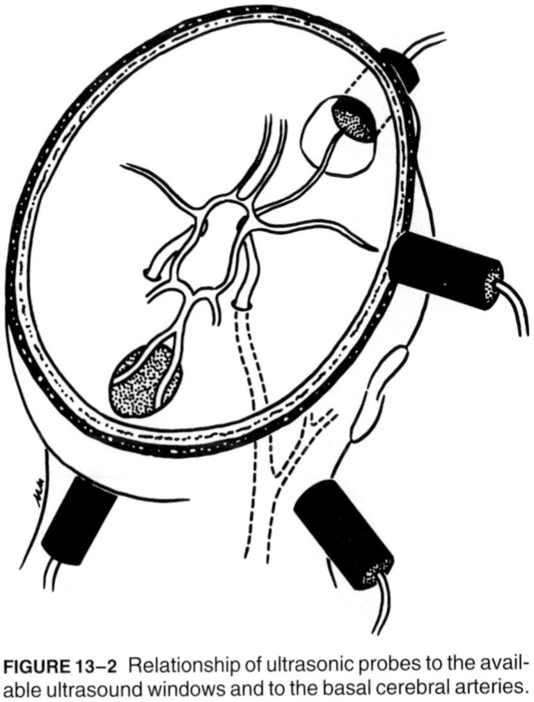

FIGURE 13–2 Relationship of ultrasonic probes to the available ultrasound windows and to the basal cerebral arteries.

Transtemporal Approach

The probe is placed on the temporal aspect of the head, cephalad to the zygomatic arch, and immediately anterior and slightly superior to the tragus of the ear conch (Fig. 13–3, position *1*). This is usually the most promising examination site. A more posterior win-

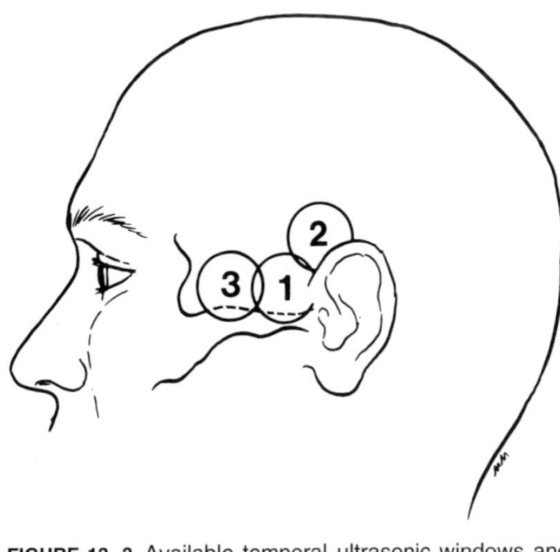

FIGURE 13–3 Available temporal ultrasonic windows and probe placement. *1,* Preauricular position. *2,* Posterior window. *3,* Anterior window. The probe should first be placed in the preauricular region to identify the middle cerebral artery. Very subtle meander-like movements of the probe should be performed in each position. If position 1 is not successful, position 2 should be tried next, before position 3 is chosen.

dow immediately cephalad and slightly dorsal to the first one (Fig. 13–3, position *2*) may be more appropriate in a minority of cases, especially for insonation of the P2 segment of the posterior cerebral arteries (PCAs). In some patients a more frontally located temporal ultrasonic window may be present (Fig. 13–3, position *3*). By using these transtemporal approaches, the beam can be angulated anteriorly or posteriorly relative to the corresponding probe positions on the opposite side of the head. The *anterior* orientation of the beam allows for the insonation of the M_1 and M_2 segments of the middle cerebral arteries (MCAs), the C_1 segment of the carotid siphon (CS), the A_1 segment of the anterior cerebral artery (ACA), and often the anterior communicating artery (Fig. 13–4*A*). The *posteriorly* angulated beam insonates the P_1 and P_2 segments of the PCA, the top of the basilar artery (BA), and the posterior communicating arteries (Fig. 13–4*B*). The nomenclature system used for describing the segment of the basal* cerebral arteries is illustrated in Figure 13–4*C*.

Transorbital Approach

Components of the anterior cerebral circulation may be evaluated by placing the transducer against the closed eyelid. From this position, the ophthalmic artery can be insonated at depths of 45 to 50 mm, whereas the C_3 segment (anterior knee of the CS) is normally met at insonation depths of 60 to 65 mm (Fig. 13–5*A*). At slightly greater insonation depths of 70 to 75 mm, the C_2 segment shows flow away from the probe (downward deflection), and the C_4 segment shows flow toward the probe (upward deflection). These flow directions apply only when the beam is nearly sagittal (slight medial obliquity) and enters the skull through the supraorbital or infraorbital fissures. Using a strongly oblique approach, with the probe at the superior outer quadrant of the eyelids and angulated medially, the ultrasound beam penetrates the optic canal and is aimed at the contralateral ACA and supraclinoidal CS, and may even hit the proximal MCA. Typical insonation depths and velocities are shown in Figure 13–5*B*.

Suboccipital Approach

The suboccipital approach is essential for screening the vertebral artery (VA) and the BA throughout their entire length. The probe is placed exactly between the posterior margin of the foramen magnum and the palpable spinous process of the first cervical vertebra, with the beam aimed at the bridge of the nose (Fig. 13–6*A*).[2] The insonation depth is set at 65 mm, and the right and left VAs are tracked individually from this point toward the foramen magnum, using progressively smaller insonation depths (from 50 down to 35 mm). As the depth decreases, the sound beam is angled more and more sharply toward the side of the head. The extradural part of the VA on the posterior arch of the atlas can also be screened. Flow is toward the transducer in this segment. The BA can be tracked cephalad from the point at which the VAs unite. The superior end of the BA is reached at a depth of approximately 95 to 125 mm. Flow

*The term *basal* as used here refers to all the large vessels at the base of the brain. This term should not be confused with basilar artery, which is a specific vessel.

FIGURE 13–4 Position of the probe in the temporal region to insonate the anterior and posterior parts of the circle of Willis. *A,* Line XX′ indicates a frontal plane that runs through the regular placement of the probe on either side and, simultaneously, perpendicular to the sagittal midline of the skull. Z′ indicates the site of the intracranial ICA bifurcation. The X′Z′ distance is 63 ± 5 mm. The angle μ is the angle with which the probe is aimed more anteriorly in the MCA and ACA segments. This angle was found to be 6 ± 1.1 degrees. *B,* The angle ω indicates the angle with which the beam is directed more posteriorly to insonate the top of the BA (T) and the P_1 segments (P′) on both sides. This angle was found to be 4.6 ± 1.2 degrees. The BA bifurcation could be insonated at depths of 78 ± 5 mm, corresponding to the distance XT or X′T, respectively. Y indicates the fictional point at which the pathway of the beam then transits the contralateral skull—that is, approximately 2 to 3 cm behind the external acoustic meatus. The P_2 segments (P) can also be insonated if the beam is directed even more posteriorly and slightly caudally (line X′P). W lies approximately 5 cm behind the contralateral external acoustic meatus. *C,* Basal cerebral arteries of the circle of Willis. OA = ophthalmic artery; CS = carotid siphon (C_1–C_3); ICA = internal carotid artery; ACA = anterior cerebral artery (A_1, A_2); ACoA = anterior communicating artery; MCA = middle cerebral artery (M_1, M_2); PCA = posterior cerebral artery (P_1, P_2); PCoA = posterior communicating artery; BA = basilar artery; VA = vertebral artery.

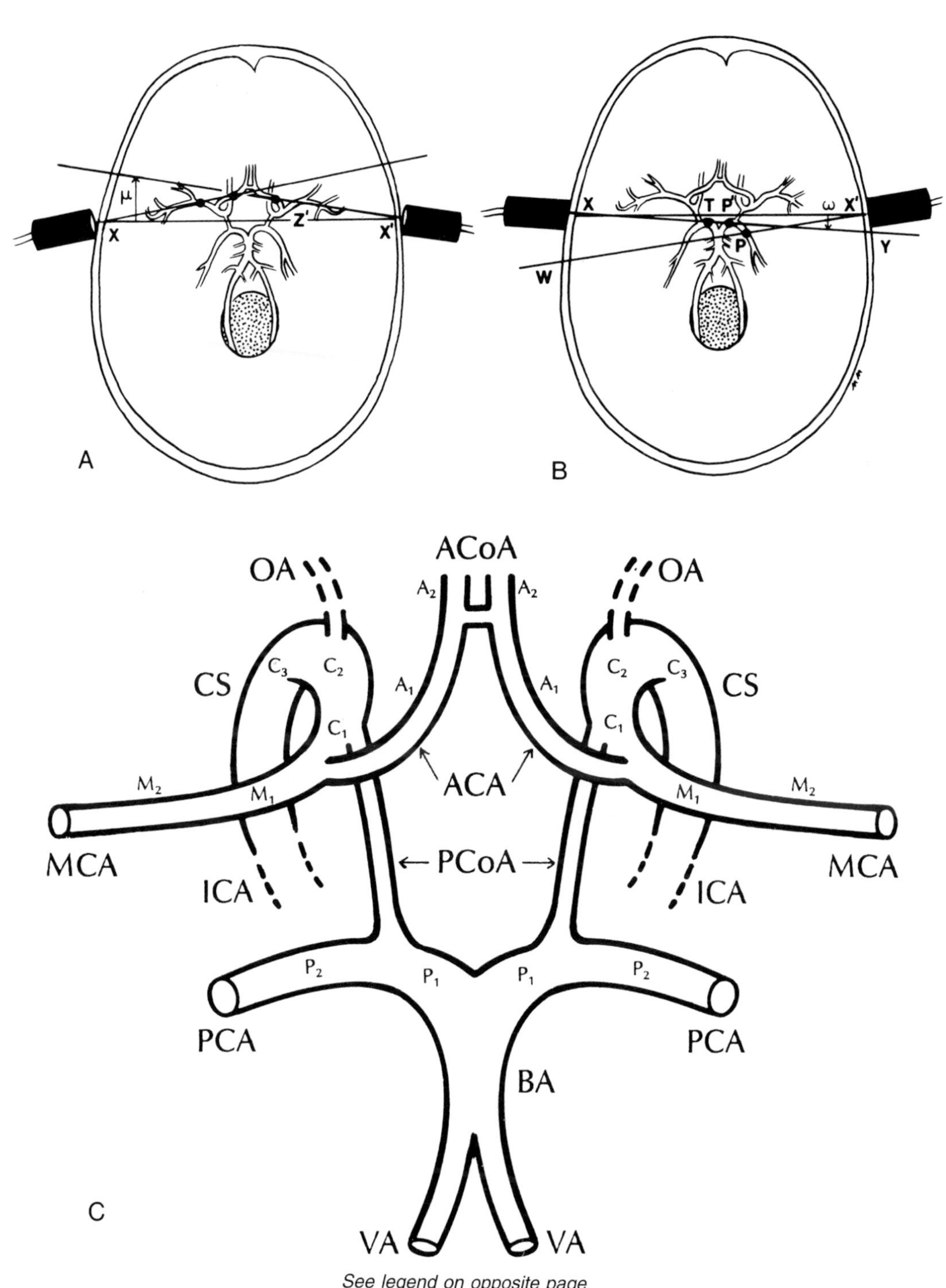

See legend on opposite page

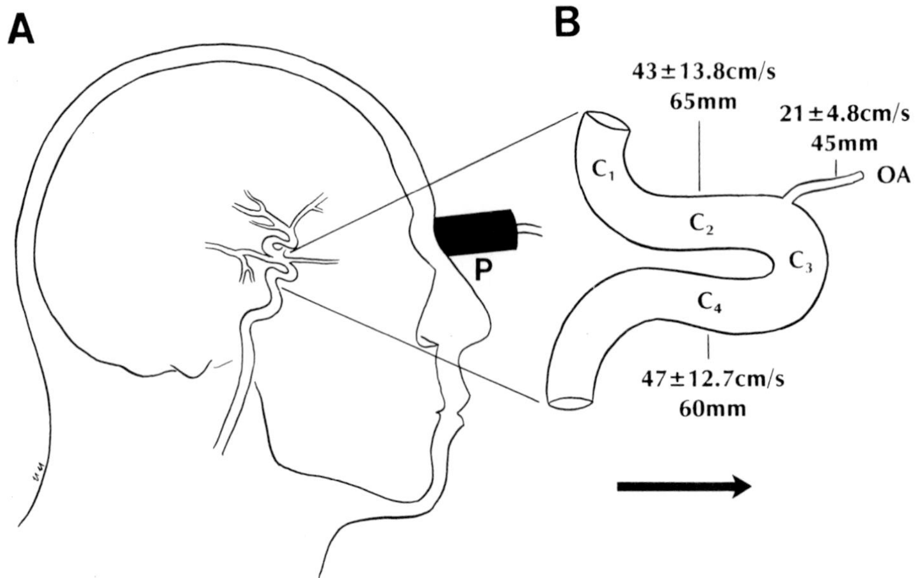

FIGURE 13–5 Insonation of the ophthalmic artery and carotid siphon by the transorbital approach. *A,* Probe (P) location and relationship to the ophthalmic artery and carotid siphon. *B,* Representative insonation depths and normal flow values within various segments of the carotid siphon (C_1—C_4) and ophthalmic artery (OA).

in the VAs is normally directed away from the probe. Typical insonation depths and flow velocities are shown in Figure 13–6*B*.

Submandibular Approach

The submandibular approach completes the examination in that the retromandibular and more distal extradural parts (C5 to C6 segments) of the internal carotid artery (ICA) can be evaluated (Fig. 13–7*A*). This particular examination is a useful complement to extracranial studies, because it facilitates the detection of ICA dissection and chronic ICA occlusion with abundant collateralization through the external carotid artery. With the transducer positioned as shown in Figure 13–7*A,* the beam is directed slightly medially and posteriorly. The ICA can regularly be tracked to a depth of 80 to 85 mm, to where it bends medioanteriorly to form the CS. Typical insonation depths and flow velocities are shown in Figure 13–7*B*.

Diagnostic Approach

The Basic Examination

In general, it is most convenient to start with a transtemporal approach, to identify the MCA on either side at an insonation depth of 50 to 55 mm, and then to track the ipsilateral arterial network, step by step, in various directions. Proof of traceability of the MCA is necessary for its unequivocal identification. This is also true for other arteries at the base of the brain. *Traceability* refers to the fact that the MCA (and usually other arteries) can be tracked in incremental steps from a more shallow insonation depth (35 mm) to deeper sites (55 mm) without changes in the character of the flow profile and flow direction. When tracking the MCA medially (65 to 70 mm), an abrupt change in flow direction (away from rather than toward the probe) indicates insonation of the A1 segment of the ACA. Flow signals *toward* the probe at this depth usually emanate from the CS at its junction with the MCA (Fig. 13–8*A*). Typical insonation depths and flow velocities are shown in Figure 13–8*B*.

By angulating the beam more posteriorly from a transtemporal approach, the P1 segment of the PCA can be picked up most readily at an insonation depth of 65 to 70 mm. The PCA can then be tracked to the BA (75 mm) and from there to the contralateral PCA (80 to 85 mm) (see Fig. 13–4*B*). The two criteria of traceability (i.e., the display of bilateral blood flow at the junction with the BA and the change of flow direction

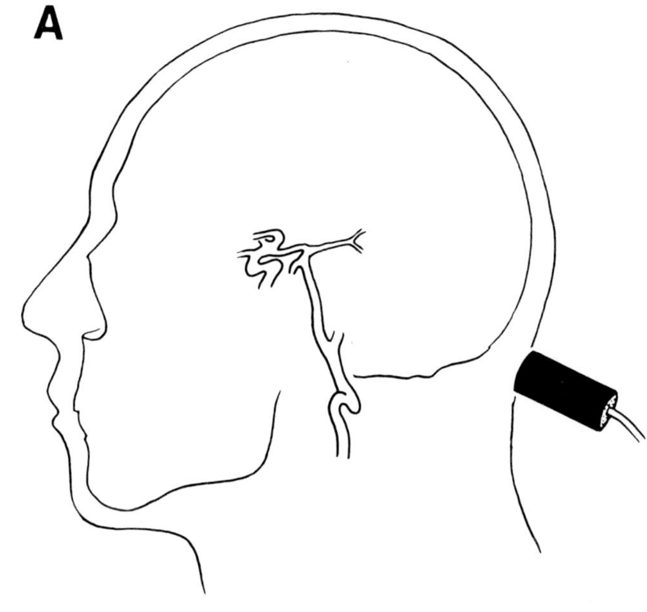

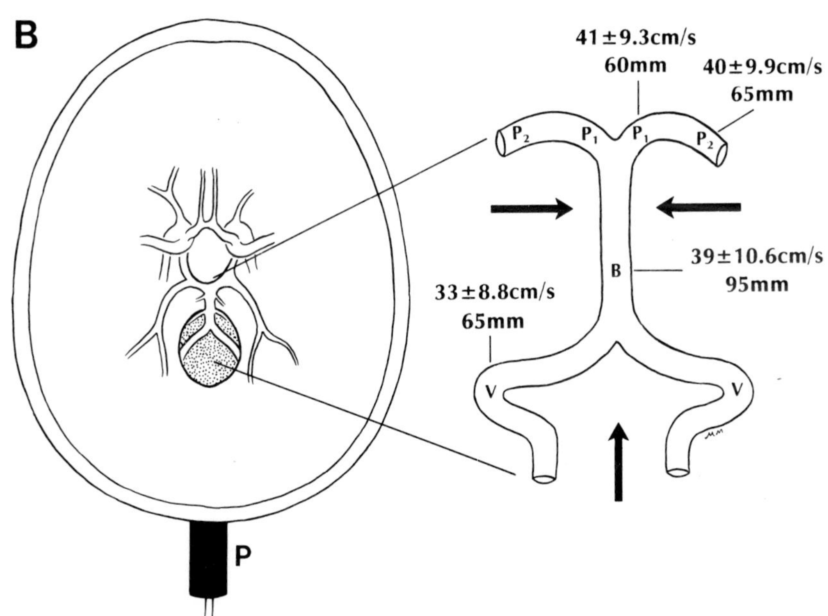

FIGURE 13–6 *A,* Transcranial Doppler examination of the vertebral system by the suboccipital approach. *B,* Representative insonation and normal flow values within the distal vertebral arteries (V) and the basilar trunk (B). The P_1 and P_2 velocities are measured transtemporally. P = probe.

within the contralateral PCA) are very important features for identifying the PCAs without compression tests.

After the completion of the examination from both temporal windows, additional information may be obtained through the orbital, suboccipital, or mandibular pathways. The vessels that are accessible from these sites, as well as the techniques for identifying these vessels, are described previously. A protocol for TCD examination is presented in Table 13–1.

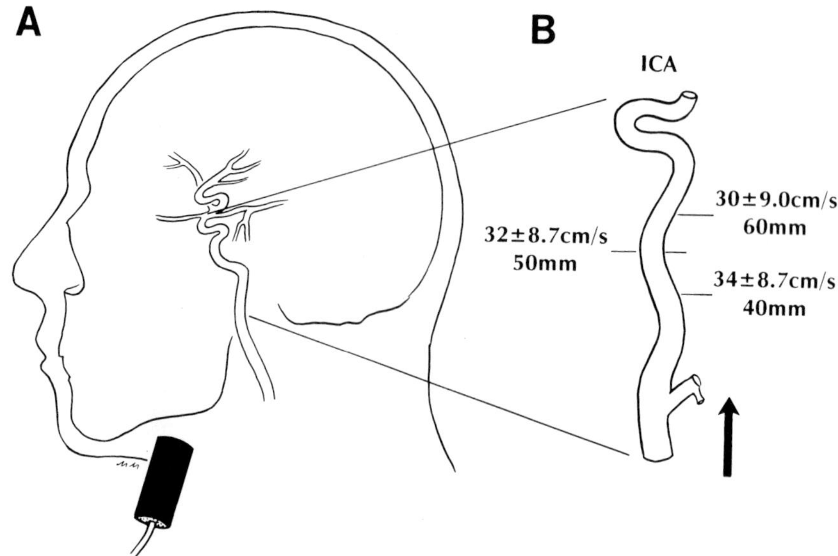

FIGURE 13–7 *A,* Transcranial Doppler examination of the petrous portion of the internal carotid artery (ICA) by the submandibular approach. The ICA can be traced from depths of 25 to 80 mm corresponding to the C5 segment of the ICA. *B,* Representative insonation depths and normal flow values within the distal intracranial ICA.

Transcranial Color-Coded Duplex Sonography

Because of the variability and complexity of the vessels that comprise the circle of Willis, hand-held TCD devices are subject to problems of vessel identification and documentation; furthermore, TCD does not provide morphologic information about the basal vessels. Further technical challenges are presented with the tranducer-to-artery angle and the spatial relationship between intracranial arteries. A combination of these problems leads to the most common inherent pitfall associated with TCD imaging, that

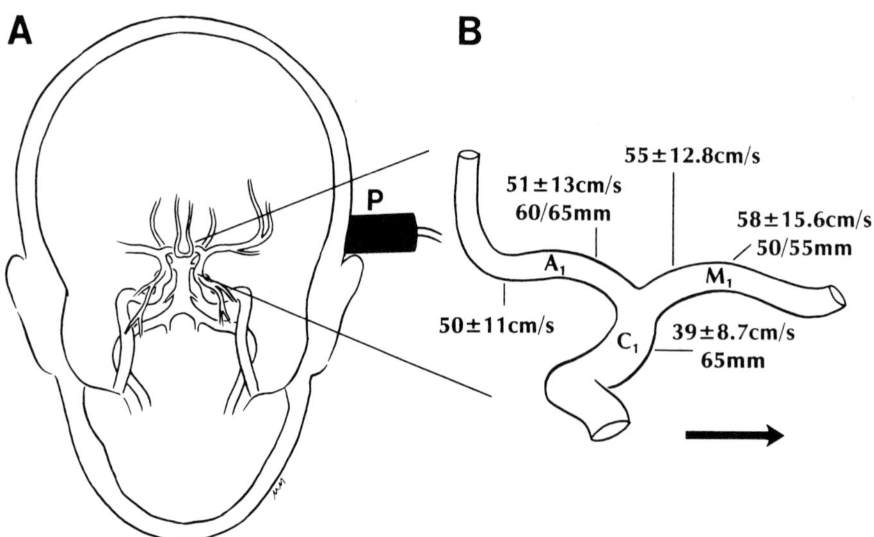

FIGURE 13–8 Transtemporal probe (P) placement and its relationship to the middle cerebral artery (MCA). *A,* The beam axis is in line with the C_1, M_1, and A_1 segments of the cerebral vasculature. *B,* Representative insonation depths and normal flow values within the MCA, the anterior cerebral artery, and the internal carotid artery bifurcation.

TABLE 13–1 TRANSCRANIAL DOPPLER PROTOCOL: IDENTIFICATION CRITERIA AND NORMAL FLOW VELOCITIES

Position of Probe	Arterial Segment	Insonation Depth: *Range (mm)*	Insonation Depth: *Reference Depth (mm)*	Normal Flow Velocity (Mean ± SD) (cm/sec)	Main Features for Identification of Vessel Segment
Transtemporal	MCA	30–60	50	55 ± 12	M_1: Insonation depth 50 mm; traceability forward and backward; flow toward probe; slightly anterior angulation of beam
	M_1	45–60	50	55 ± 12	
	ACA	60–75	70	50 ± 11	Insonation depth; flow away from probe; traceability slightly anterior angulation of beam; for clear-cut differentiation from carotid siphon, use compression tests
	C_1 (C_2) (carotid siphon transtemporal approach)	60–70	65	39 ± 9	Insonation depth; relatively low flow velocity compared to M_1 segment; slightly anterior and caudal angulation of beam; flow toward probe
	P_1 (posterior cerebral artery)	60 (55)–75	70	39 ± 10	Insonation depth; flow toward probe (ipsilateral P_1); traceability to top of basilar and contralateral P_1; slightly posterior and caudal angulation of beam; relatively low flow velocity compared with M_1 segment; compression test necessary for unequivocal differentiation from MCA branches
	P_1 and P_1' (top of basilar)	70–80	75	40 ± 10	Insonation depth; bidirectional flow; traceability backward and forward; angulation of beam
	P_2 (PCA) (probe placed in position *2,* in Fig. 13–8*A*)	60–65	65	40 ± 10	Flow away from probe; placement of probe; posterior angulation of probe; modulation by opening and closing eyes
Suboccipital	Extradural distal vertebral artery	40–55	50	34 ± 8	Suboccipital placement of probe; insonation depth; strongly lateral angulation of beam; flow toward probe
	Intradural distal vertebral artery	60–95 (100)	70	38 ± 10	Insonation depth

Table continued on following page

TABLE 13–1 TRANSCRANIAL DOPPLER PROTOCOL: IDENTIFICATION CRITERIA AND NORMAL FLOW VELOCITIES *Continued*

Position of Probe	Arterial Segment	Insonation Depth: *Range (mm)*	Insonation Depth: *Reference Depth (mm)*	Normal Flow Velocity (Mean ± SD) (cm/sec)	Main Features for Identification of Vessel Segment
					Beam aimed at bridge of nose or slightly laterally; traceability forward and backward; compression tests at common carotid or vertebral arteries sometimes necessary
	Basilar trunk	70 (65)–115 (120)	95 (100, if possible)	41 ± 10	Insonation depth; flow away from probe; often slight increase of flow velocity compared to vertebral artery; traceability of vertebrobasilar axis; compression tests
Ophthalmic	C_2 (carotid siphon, transorbital approach)	65–80	70	41 ± 11	Sagittal or slightly oblique angulation of beam; flow away from beam; flow away from probe; insonation depth
	C_3 (carotid siphon, transorbital approach)	65 (60)	65 (bidirectional, not measured)	—	Bidirectional signal; sagittal angulation of beam; insonation depth
	C_4 and distal part of C_5 (carotid siphon, transorbital approach)	65–80 (85)	70	47 ± 14	Sagittal or slightly oblique and caudal angulation of beam; flow toward probe; insonation depth
	Ophthalmic artery	35–55	45	21 ± 5	Insonation depth; flow toward probe
	Contralateral A1 (ACA) (transorbital approach, ancillary approach if lack of temporal window)	75–80	Not defined	Measurements in a few cases only	Strongly oblique angulation of beam through optic canal; flow toward probe; compression test necessary for differentiation from carotid siphon and MCA
Submandibular	C_6 and retromandibular segment of ICA (extradural ICA; submandibular)	35–80 (85)	60	30 ± 9	Flow away from probe; medial angulation of beam; insonation depth

MCA = middle cerebral artery; ACA = anterior cerebral artery; PCA = posterior cerebral artery.

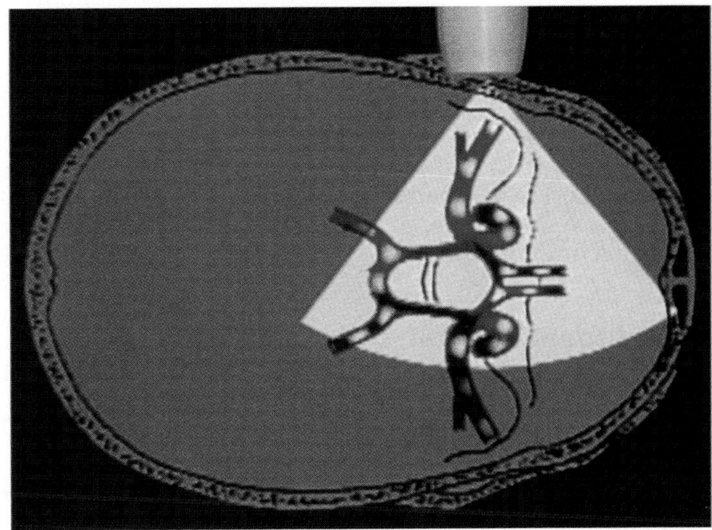

FIGURE 13–9 Vascular imaging requires unique orientations to the intracranial vasculature. Schematic diagram of the circle of Willis insonated from the transtemporal approach. (Courtesy of ATL Ultrasound, Bothell, WA.)

is, the misidentification of intracranial arteries. Technical advances have enabled clinicians to penetrate the available ultrasound windows and skull foramina with B-mode imaging.[24, 25, 27–30]

TCCD is an emerging diagnostic method allowing noninvasive imaging of intracranial vascular structures (Fig. 13–9). This visual imaging allows a real-time morphologic view of the arteries under investigation, permitting exact localization of the pulse wave sample volume (Fig. 13–10). Because vascular lesions represent the primary application for TCD examination, the addition of the morphologic information allows more rapid identification of the vessels in question and shortens examination time. This technique has evolved rapidly over the last several years and includes not only vascular imaging but also imaging of the brain parenchyma. Parenchymal imaging, however, has a number of technical limitations, and its current resolution remains inferior to that of conventional computed tomography and magnetic resonance imaging.[29] Because of the bone limitations of the skull to ultrasound, vascular imaging requires unique orientations to the intracranial vasculature, and thus significant experience is required to become proficient in the technique. However, the advantages of imaging make this well worth the time and effort. TCCD has a potentially important fu-

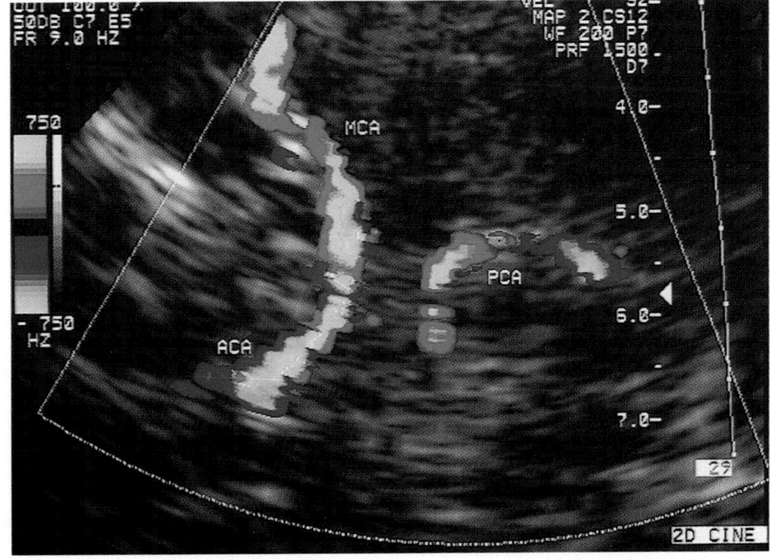

FIGURE 13–10 Transcranial color-Doppler image of the circle of Willis from the transtemporal window (MCA, ACA, PCA). MCA = middle cerebral artery; ACA = anterior cerebral artery; PCA = posterior cerebral artery.

ture in monitoring intracranial artery stenosis. The single most important advantage of this method over standard TCD is its ability to image an artery and ascertain specifically that there is no color-flow signal, adding to the certainty of arterial occlusion diagnosis. This, of course, has particular significance when interventional measures are being contemplated and monitored.

Vessel Identification

The primary TCD parameters for identifying the cerebral arteries are the following:

1. Insonation depth
2. Direction of blood flow at insonation depth
3. Flow velocity (mean flow velocity and systolic or diastolic peak flow velocity)
4. Probe position (e.g., temporal, orbital, suboccipital, and submandibular)
5. Direction of the ultrasonic beam (e.g., posterior, anterior, caudad, cephalad)
6. Traceability of vessels
7. Response to carotid compression[26]

In many individuals (particularly the elderly), and in those with pathologic conditions, compression tests may be necessary to identify certain arterial segments unequivocally.[14, 31, 32] Compression tests during TCD examinations can be performed on the common carotid arteries, low in the neck (with two fingers) (Fig. 13–11*A*), or on the vertebral arteries at the mastoid slope (Fig. 13–11*B*). A low risk of creating an embolism from plaques in the carotid arteries is thought to exist, provided that compression is performed by an experienced investigator and that the condition of the carotid arteries has been assessed with B-mode ultrasound imaging.[33, 34] Compression maneuvers are generally not necessary for arterial identification, but they are extremely valuable in assessing collateral pathways. The possible effects of compression maneuvers on intracranial flow are illustrated in Figure 13–12 and listed in Table 13–2. Responses include no reaction, increased flow velocity, decreased flow velocity, reversal of flow, alternating flow direction (to and fro), and cessation of flow.

Flow Velocity Measurements

The mean flow velocities and standard deviations of various vessel segments at different insonation depths are shown in Tables 13–3 and 13–4.[35] Normal flow velocity values in adults show little variation among different investigators (Table 13–5).[10, 14, 31, 36–40] The highest velocities are almost always found in the MCA or the ACA. The PCAs and BAs have lower Doppler shifts than the MCA in normal subjects. The same pattern has not been noted, however, in cerebral blood flow studies, with flow measured in centimeters per second. Two explanations have been of-

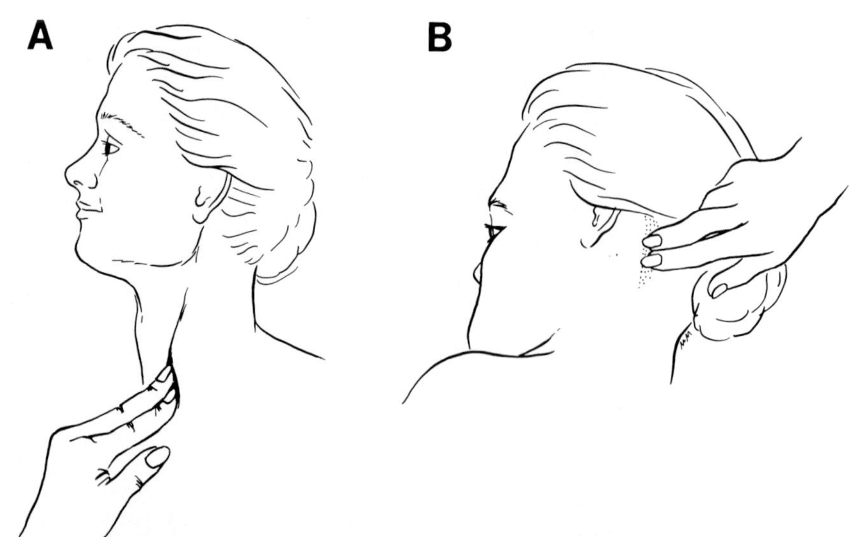

FIGURE 13–11 Compression tests. *A,* Compression of the common carotid artery low in the neck. *B,* Compression of the vertebral artery at the mastoid slope.

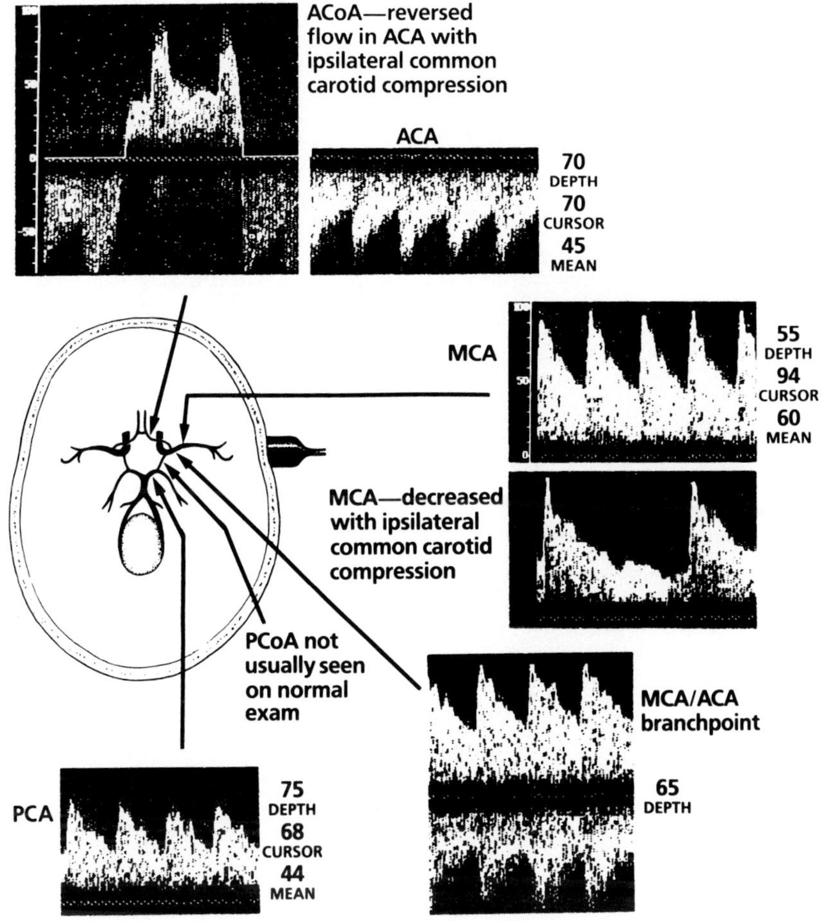

FIGURE 13–12 Transcranial Doppler examination of the intracranial arteries, showing their normal locations and the effects of common carotid artery compressive maneuvers. ACoA = anterior communicating artery; ACA = anterior cerebral artery; MCA = middle cerebral artery; PCoA = posterior communicating artery; PCA = posterior cerebral artery. (From Otis S, Ringelstein EB: Transcranial Doppler sonography. *In* Bernstein ED [ed]: Noninvasive Diagnostic Techniques in Vascular Disease. St. Louis, CV Mosby, 1990, p 71.)

fered for this discrepancy between velocity and volume flow: the measurement sites may be different[41] or, more probably, different velocities occur as a compensatory mechanism to keep volume flow constant in vessels of different sizes.[18] Thus, velocities are slower in large vessels and faster in small vessels. Flow velocities in the basal cerebral arteries decrease consistently with increasing age (see Tables 13–3 and 13–4).[36, 37, 42] This finding, which correlates well with age-related changes in cerebral blood flow,[43, 44] underlines the validity and sensitivity of TCD velocity data as a semiquantitative estimate of cerebral blood flow. This correlation between velocity and blood flow is particularly true if *serial* measurements are made on the *same* individual.

Functional Reserve Testing

TCD is an ideal functional test for detecting rapid changes in cerebral perfusion, because the technique provides excellent resolution of flow velocity changes occurring over time. Functional tests are predominantly aimed at the evaluation of the reserve mechanism of the cerebral vasculature, using various stimuli such as hypocapnia or hypercapnia, increased or reduced systemic arterial pressure, and hypoxia. The response of cerebral circulation to CO_2 has been demonstrated by many.[44, 45]

Blood flow velocity is measured with the subject supine and instructed to rest comfortably. While the subject is breathing room air and relaxing, a mask is placed on the face to

TABLE 13–2 EFFECTS OF COMMON CAROTID ARTERY COMPRESSION TESTS ON VARIOUS VESSEL SEGMENTS AND THEIR FUNCTIONAL INTERPRETATION

Insonated Vessel Segment	Findings at Rest	Effect of Ipsilateral CCA Compression Test	Effect of Contralateral CCA Compression Test	Functional Meaning of Compression Test
MCA (M_1/M_2)	Normal flow velocity; flow toward probe	↓ or ↓ ↓ or [STOP]	⦸ or [↓]	Confirmation of vessel identity
ACA (=A_1)	Normal flow velocity; flow away from probe	[↓ ↓] or [STOP] ⤵ or ⤵ with D	[⦸] or ↑ or ↑ ↑ with or without D	Confirmation of vessel identity; presence or absence of potential anterior collateral pathway
ACoA	(1) No signal available; (2) indistinguishable from contralateral ACA; (3) indistinguishable from ipsilateral ACA	(1) [↑ ↑ with D and flow toward probe]; (2) ⦸ or ↑ or ↑ ↑; (3) see ACA	(1) ↑ ↑ with D and flow away from the probe; (2) [↓ ↓] or [STOP] or ⤹ or ⤵ with D; (3) ⦸ or ↑ or ↑ ↑	(1) Confirmation of existence of ACoA; (2, 3) see ACA
PCA (P_1)	Normal flow signal; flow toward probe	⦸ or ↑ or ↑ ↑	⦸ or ↑	Confirmation of vessel identity; presence or absence or potential posterior collateral pathway
PCA (P_2)	Normal flow signal; flow away from probe	⦸ or ↓, or ↓ ↓ or [STOP] if ICA supplied	⦸ or [↓]	Confirmation of vessel identity and type of PCA supply; differentiation of basilar and/or ICA blood supply
PCoA (transtemporal or transorbital approach)	(1) No signal available; (2) indistinguishable from PCA or MCA branches without compression maneuvers; (3) alternating flow	(1) in nonembryonal type: ⤵ with D or ↑ ↑ with D; with flow toward probe in vicinity of PCA; with flow toward probe during transorbital insonation; (2) in embryonal type; ↓ or ↓ ↓ ↶⤵ or ⤵	(No reactions observed so far)	Confirmation of existence of PCoA; differentiation of posterior and anterior collateral pathways; differentiation of basilar or ICA blood supply
DVA	Normal flow signal away from probe	⦸ or ↑	⦸ or ↑	Confirmation of existence of posterior collateral pathway
BA	Normal flow signal away from probe	⦸ or ↑ or [↑ ↑]	⦸ or ↑ or [↑ ↑]	Confirmation of existence of posterior collateral pathway; conclusive differention from carotid vascular tree within large insonation depths
ICA, C_2–C_4 segments of siphon (transorbital approach)	Normal flow toward probe, away from probe, or bidirectional	STOP or ↓ ↓ and/or [↑ ↑ with D]	⦸ or ↑	Exclusion of silent ICA occlusion; analysis of potential collateral pathways
ICA–C_1 (transtemporal approach)	(1) Low-frequency flow toward the probe; or (2) indistinguishable from MCA (M1)	STOP or ↓ ↓	⦸ or ↑	(1, 2) Analysis of potential collateral pathways; (2) differentiation from MCA often possible

ICA = internal carotid artery; MCA = middle cerebral artery; ACoA = anterior communicating artery; PCA = posterior cerebral artery; PCoA = posterior communicating artery; P1 = precommunicating part of PCA; P2 = postcommunicating part of PCA; BA = basilar artery; DVA = distal vertebral artery; CCA = common carotid artery; D = local distortion of blood flow caused by "relative stenosis"; ⦸ = no effect; ↑ = slight increase of flow velocity; ↑ ↑ = strong increase in flow velocity; ↶⤵ = alternating flow direction; ⤵ = reversal of flow direction; ↓ = slight decrease in flow velocity; ↓ ↓ = strong decrease in flow velocity; [ ] = very rare event.

Modified from Ringelstein EB: A practical guide to transcranial Doppler sonography. *In* Weinberger J (ed): Noninvasive Imaging of Cerebral Vascular Disease. New York, AR Liss, 1989.

TABLE 13-3 NORMAL VALUES OF MEAN BLOOD VELOCITY FOR ARTERIES* (TRANSTEMPORAL APPROACH)

	Mean Blood Velocity (cm/sec)		
Age (years)	*MCA (M1)*	*ACA (A1)*	*PCA (P1)*
10–29	70 ± 16.4	61 ± 14.7	55 ± 9.0
30–49	57 ± 11.2	48 ± 7.1	42 ± 8.9
50–59	51 ± 9.7	46 ± 9.4	39 ± 9.9
60–70	41 ± 7.0	38 ± 5.6	36 ± 7.9
Insonated depth (mm)	50–55	60–65	60–65

*Measurements for the middle (MCA), anterior (ACA), and posterior (PCA) cerebral arteries according to age.

TABLE 13-4 NORMAL VALUES OF MEAN BLOOD VELOCITY FOR ARTERIES* (SUBOCCIPITAL APPROACH)

	Mean Blood Velocity (cm/sec)		
Age (years)	*PCA (P_1)*	*BA*	*VA*
10–29	54 ± 8.0	46 ± 11	45 ± 9.8
30–49	40 ± 8.5	38 ± 8.6	34 ± 8.2
50–59	39 ± 10.1	32 ± 7.0	37 ± 10.0
60–70	35 ± 11.1	32 ± 6.7	35 ± 7.0
Insonated depth (mm)	60–65	85–90	60–65

*Measurements for the posterior cerebral (PCA), basilar (BA), and vertebral (VA) arteries according to age.

allow acclimation to the test situation. The TCD transducer is placed over one temporal plane and the MCA is recorded at a depth of 50 to 55 mm, depending on the optimization and stability of the signal. The end tidal CO_2 volume percentage (CO_2 vol%) is recorded by an infrared CO_2 analyzer while the subject breathes room air (normocapnia); breathes air with CO_2 concentrations of 2, 3, 4, and 5%; and undergoes various intensities of hyperventilation.

During changing CO_2 concentrations, the relationship between flow velocity and volume flow within a large cerebral artery is linear, provided that the CO_2 level does not directly affect the diameter of the large proximal arterial segments.[46, 47] The CO_2 dilatory effect is mainly restricted to the peripheral arterial vascular bed, in particular the small cortical vessels.[44] Thus, intraindividual changes in flow velocity during TCD examination directly reflect changes in volume flow.[48] Velocities measured from the MCA with changing CO_2 concentrations show a bi-asymptotic S-shaped curve (Fig. 13–13).

Intactness of vasomotor reserve implies that a drop in perfusion pressure can be counterbalanced by vasodilatation of cortical arterioles to maintain sufficient cortical blood supply. The vasomotor reserve may become exhausted if the resistance vessels of brain areas with low perfusion pressure are already maximally dilated.[4, 48–50] In this state, the resistance vessels are refractory to any further vasodilatory stimuli, and hypercapnia cannot increase blood flow. This condition may be critical, because ischemic brain injury can occur if the perfusion pressure is further reduced for any reason. CO_2 reactivity allows the reaction of cerebral arteries in different pathologic situations to be studied and the cerebral vascular reserve to be measured. These tests are useful in evaluating the hemodynamic impact of extracranial occlusive carotid disease and other conditions of reduced cerebral perfusion, such as migraine hypoxia, high-altitude exposure, blunt head trauma, and acute embolic stroke.[51] Quantification is usually possible for any alteration of brain vasculature or brain injury in which vasodilatation may play a pathogenic role.[48]

The pulsatility index, as defined by Gosling, has been found to be a sensitive index of diastolic runoff—that is, with increased peripheral vasodilatation, diastolic runoff is expected to increase and pulsatility index to

TABLE 13-5 MEAN BLOOD FLOW VELOCTIY VALUES FOR ARTERIES*

		Mean Blood Flow Velocity (cm/sec)			
Source	Reference No.	*MCA*	*ACA*	*PCA*	*BA*
Aaslid et al	14	62 ± 12	51 ± 12	44 ± 11	48 (mean)
DeWitt and Wechsler	38	62 ± 12	52 ± 12	42 ± 10	42 ± 10
Grolimund and Seiler	39	47 ± 15	49 ± 15	37 ± 10	—
Harders	37	65 ± 17	50 ± 13	40 ± 9	39 ± 9
Hennerici et al	36	58 ± 12	53 ± 10	37 ± 10	36 ± 12
Lindegaard et al	31	67 ± 7	48 ± 5	42 ± 6	—
Ringelstein et al	10	55 ± 12	50 ± 11	39 ± 10	41 ± 10
Russo et al	40	65 ± 13	48 ± 20	35 ± 18	45 ± 10

Measurements for the middle cerebral (MCA), anterior cerebral (ACA), posterior cerebral (PCA), and basilar (BA) arteries.

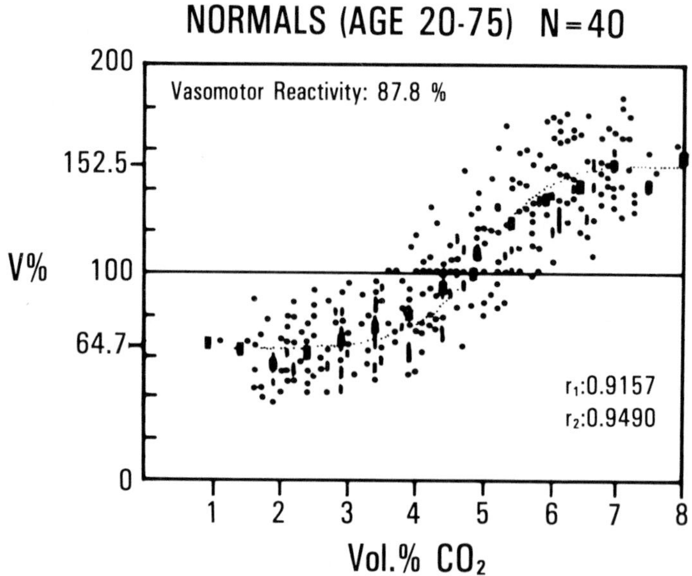

FIGURE 13–13 Vasomotor reactivity in 40 normal individuals (ages 20 to 75 years). Blood flow velocity changes are shown during CO_2-induced hypercapnia (*upper curve*) and hypocapnia (*lower curve*). The average change was 87.8% (52.5% and 35.3% hypercapnia and hypocapnia, respectively). (From Ringelstein EB, Sievers C, Ecker S, et al. Noninvasive assessment of CO_2-induced cerebral vasomotor response in normal individuals and patients with internal carotid artery occlusions. Stroke 19:964, 1988. Copyright © American Heart Association.)

decrease.[52] The pulsatility transmission index studied by Lindegaard and colleagues[31] in carotid stenosis is thought to be a more sensitive indicator of vasodilatation than flow velocity, presumably because it reflects a combination of reduced partial pressure (decreased MCA flow) and lowered cerebrovascular resistance. The usefulness of these parameters has not been proved, however, and they appear to be poor discriminators of patients at risk for low-flow infarctions.[53]

DIAGNOSTIC PARAMETERS FOR SPECIFIC CLINICAL APPLICATIONS

Intracranial Stenosis and Occlusion

Duplex ultrasound has been widely accepted as an accurate, noninvasive method for the diagnosis of extracranial carotid disease. TCD represents an extension of the use of Doppler techniques to the intracranial arteries. The detection of CS stenosis using TCD was first reported in 1986 by Spencer,[54] who used similar criteria to those used for carotid bifurcation disease.[13] Since then, a number of authors have reported similar findings for the CS[55–58] and have extended TCD applications to other brain arteries. The most obvious clinical advantage of TCD is the rapid screening of the acute stroke patient for intracranial high-grade stenosis or occlusion. Normal TCD findings in stroke patients have considerable clinical impact.

STENOSIS. The following are typical features of circumscribed stenosis of a large basal cerebral artery: (1) increased flow velocity; (2) disturbed flow (spectral broadening, and enhanced systolic and low-frequency echo components); and (3) covibration phenomena (vibration of vessel wall and surrounding soft tissue).[58] As an extracranial disease, mild stenosis increases peak velocity with little change in the rest of the Doppler pattern, whereas moderate or severe stenosis leads to a greater increase in peak velocity with spectral broadening, increased diastolic velocity, and turbulent flow. A poststenotic drop in peak velocity is usually demonstrated as well (Fig. 13–14).

Other conditions are difficult to distinguish from intracranial stenosis. Increased velocity and turbulence are seen in intracranial arteries that are providing collateral

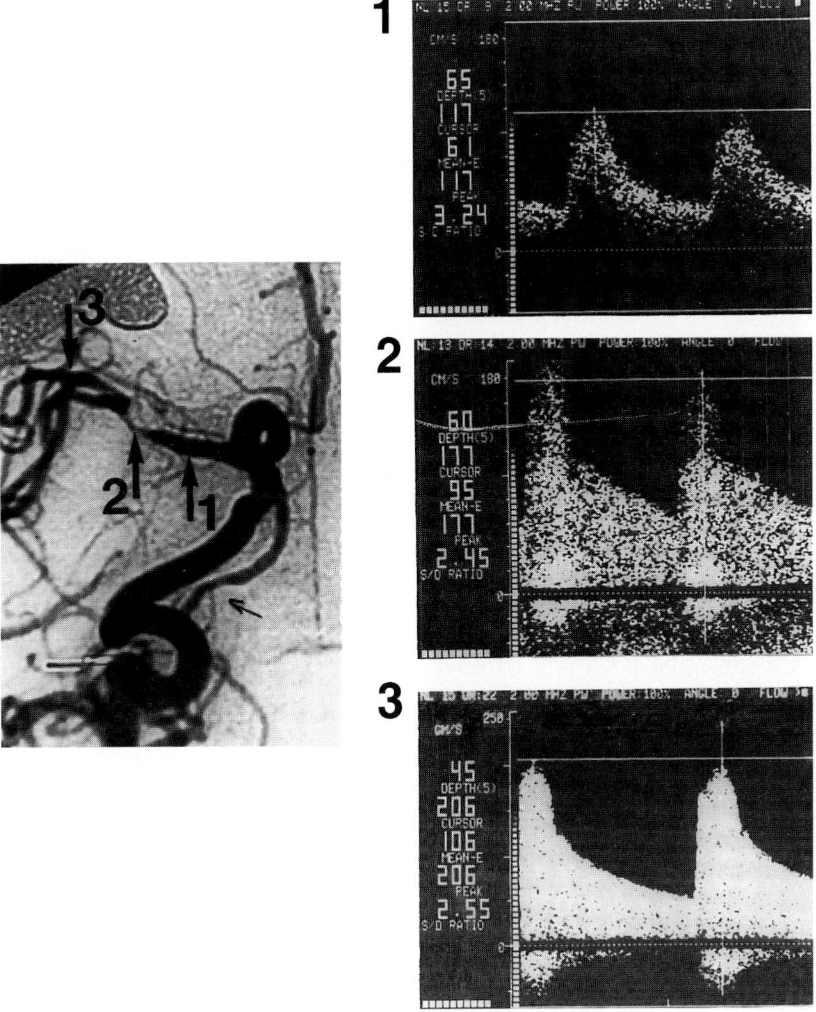

FIGURE 13–14 Middle cerebral artery stenosis and associated transcranial Doppler changes: (*1*) normal proximal flow; (*2*) increased systolic and diastolic peak velocity and spectral broadening (turbulent flow) at the center of the stenosis; (*3*) distal turbulent flow.

flow.[52] Increased velocity also occurs in intracranial arteries supplying AVMs.[31, 55, 59, 60] In such cases, the velocity increases are generally seen *throughout* the course of the involved arteries, which distinguishes these conditions from *localized* areas of increased velocity resulting from stenosis.

Vasospasm and stenosis can be differentiated sonographically because vasospasm is usually more generalized than atherosclerosis, often occurs bilaterally in several arterial distributions, and changes progressively over time.[61] It can be helpful to follow vasospasm patients with daily examinations.

OCCLUSION. Basal cerebral artery occlusion can be detected by three observations: (1) the absence of arterial signals at an expected depth; (2) the presence of signals in vessels that communicate with the occluded artery; and (3) altered flow in communicating vessels, indicating collateralization. For example, occlusion of the MCA is diagnosed from the lack of an MCA signal in the presence of flow signals from other vessels (i.e., the PCA, the ACA, or the distal CS). This combination of findings also confirms that the temporal window is satisfactory. An inadequate temporal window is a potential cause of false-positive diagnosis of MCA occlusion. Dislocation of the MCA as a result of cerebral hematoma or tumor must also be excluded by computed tomography, because such displacement may cause an absence of the MCA flow signal at the site at which it is regularly expected to occur. Patients with acute infarcts with MCA occlusion may demonstrate recanalization when followed serially.[62, 63]

PITFALLS AND DIAGNOSTIC ACCURACY. Noninvasive demonstration of intracranial arterial stenosis and occlusion is a valuable clinical tool, but various errors can occur: (1) misinterpretation of hyperdynamic collateral channels as stenosis, (2) displacement of arteries because of a space-occupying lesion, (3) misinterpretation of physiologic variables in the circle of Willis, (4) misdiagnosis of vasospasm as stenosis, and (5) misinterpretation of reactive hyperemia as stenosis.

With experience, many of these problems can be alleviated. Little information is available, however, concerning the sensitivity and specificity of TCD in the detection of intracranial lesions. A major problem has been marked variation in the sensitivity and specificity of TCD from one arterial segment to another. This means that accuracy parameters have to be calculated separately for the CS and the various segments in the MCA, ACA, and PCA, and particularly for the VA and BA. Investigators have reported success in detecting stenosis in both the MCA and VA-BA systems.[12, 18, 55–57] but accuracy in the VA-BA system remains a particular problem. Difficulties with VA-BA diagnosis result from the following: (1) the course and site of the arteries are unpredictable, (2) often the junction of the VAs cannot be reliably identified, (3) absence of the VA flow signal on one side may not represent disease, (4) an occlusion of one VA does not necessarily produce intracranial flow abnormalities,[19] (5) distal segmental occlusion of the BA and "top of the basilar" occlusion does not necessarily lead to flow abnormalities in the VAs, and (6) the signal-to-noise ratio is low at the depth required for VA insonation (90 mm).

Assessment of the Effects of Extracranial Occlusive Disease

The next important clinical application of TCD involves the hemodynamic effects of extracranial vascular disease on the intracranial circulation.

CAROTID STENOSIS OR OCCLUSION. The identification of collateral flow in patients with extracranial carotid disease is now possible with TCD.[12, 14, 19] The course and number of functional collaterals are variable and until recently could be assessed only with angiography. In addition to identifying collateral routes, the potential for collateral circulation in the circle of Willis can be assessed with TCD. The patency of the circle of Willis can be tested by recording the blood velocity and flow direction changes that occur in the basal cerebral arteries in response to common carotid compression.

Significant changes occur in the intracranial circulation because of extracranial flow-limiting disease. The MCA velocity decreases ipsilateral to severe carotid stenosis or occlusion, and the pulsatility index generally decreases as a result of vasodilatation in the distal arterial circulation ipsilateral to the obstruction.[31, 55, 64] Increased velocities and turbulence may be encountered in collateral arteries, and these findings are accentuated during contralateral common carotid compression. The presence of a functional anterior communicating artery is indicated by increased velocity in the ACA contralateral to the ICA stenosis and reversal of flow in the ipsilateral ACA. Similar findings are shown in the PCA, revealing functional collateral flow from the posterior circulation to the MCA and ACA through the posterior communicating artery. Increased flow velocity has also been recorded in the BA in patients with severe bilateral carotid disease, with collateral flow being supplied to both hemispheres from the posterior circulation. Correlation of TCD findings with angiography is good,[12] but depending on the pressure of the contrast injection,[31] angiography may not demonstrate functional reversal of flow. Many believe that TCD provides a more accurate indication of functional collateral flow than angiography.

Evaluation of hemodynamic disturbances within the carotid artery–MCA pathway is of particular interest in patients with subtotal ICA obstruction, both unilateral and bilateral. Although the predominant mechanism of stroke is thromboembolism rather than a low-flow effect, a small subgroup of patients experiences transient ischemic attacks (TIAs), permanent stroke, or progressive ischemic eye disease caused by critically reduced blood flow.[65–67] This subgroup of patients may benefit from recanalization surgery, including external carotid–internal carotid bypass. The identification of these individuals is based on the detection of an exhausted cerebral vascular reserve, which can be done through TCD assessment of the CO_2 responsiveness of the cerebral arteries. This technique is a reliable indicator of the collateral reserve capacity in patients with severe carotid artery disease.[3, 20, 49, 68] TCD evaluation of the flow velocity within the MCA can easily be used to measure the CO_2 reactivity of the peripheral cerebral vasculature.[3, 4, 69] The vasomotor reserve may be dramatically reduced in patients with unilateral or bilateral ICA occlusion, and a reduction to less than 34% is strongly associated with low-flow ischemic brain or eye symptoms (low-flow infarction), positional TIAs, and chronic ischemic eye disease. (Compare the 34% figure with the normal 86 ± 16% change in flow velocity shown in Fig. 13–13.)

VERTEBROBASILAR SYSTEM. The subclavian steal mechanism is the classic paradigm for studying hemodynamic disturbances in the human vertebrobasilar system. Rapid flow changes caused by any type of VA blood flow restriction can be measured directly within the BA. Under resting conditions, blood flow within the BA is almost never critically impaired, even if the steal is continuous. If the contralateral feeding VA is also diseased, however, BA blood flow may become reduced, may demonstrate a to-and-fro pattern, or may even be reversed. During hyperemia testing of the stealing arm, flow velocity and direction of flow within the basilar trunk may become less or more affected (Fig. 13–15). BA blood flow is very resistant to any critical changes resulting from the subclavian steal mechanism. Actually the subclavian steal is a benign condition, and even in symptomatic patients most vertebrobasilar symptoms are caused by cerebral microangiopathy rather than large artery flow disturbance.[12, 70] In rare cases, TCD has convincingly identified individuals who might benefit from arterial recanalization.[18]

Transcranial Doppler Monitoring of Cerebral Vasospasm

The major clinical application of TCD is detection and monitoring of vasospasm caused by subarachnoid hemorrhage.[14, 61, 71] The importance of this application is well recognized. Spasm of cerebral arteries is a complication of subarachnoid hemorrhage, which is a significant cause of morbidity and

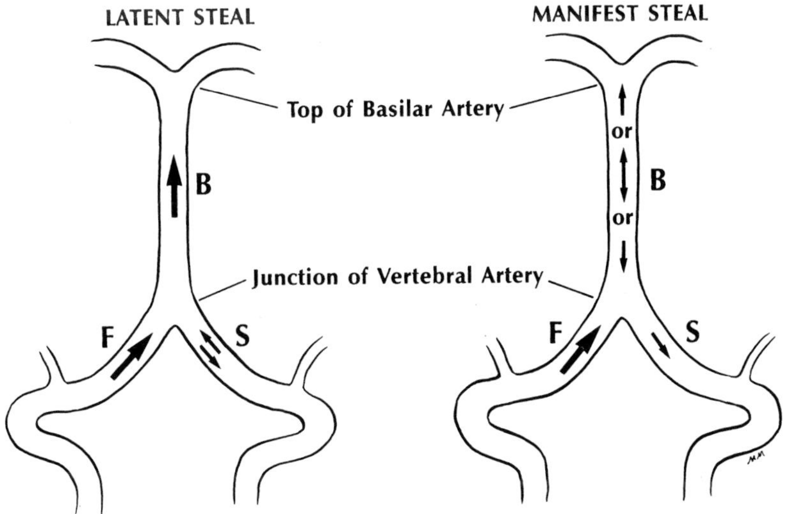

FIGURE 13–15 Schematic representation of flow conditions in various vertebrobasilar vessel segments in patients with subclavian steal mechanism. With latent steal, flow in the feeding vertebral artery (F) is increased during brachial hyperemia and is normal in the basilar trunk (B). By contrast, the blood column shows an alternating flow direction in the stealing vertebral artery (S). During manifest steal, blood flow in S is continuously reversed. This causes unaffected, alternating, or reverse blood flow within the basilar trunk. During transcranial Doppler examination, each of the three vessel segments can be clearly differentiated by means of its characteristic flow changes during brachial hyperemia.

mortality. Angiography is generally performed to localize an aneurysm before surgery, and it is helpful in assessing vasospasm, but angiography cannot be performed repeatedly to monitor vasospasm. TCD allows for the noninvasive detection and continuous monitoring of vasospasm. There is a close correlation between increased flow velocities within the spastic basal arteries (MCA, PCA, ACA) and the severity of the subarachnoid hemorrhage.[6, 37, 72, 73] This correlation is valid with respect to the size and extent of the subarachnoid clot, the clinical state of the patient, and the angiographically documented severity of spasm (if the Doppler shift is greater than 3 kHz or 120 cm/sec). The side with the more severe flow changes during TCD corresponds to the predominant location of the blood clot and the presumed site of the aneurysm. A steep increase in flow velocity (greater than 20 cm/sec/day) within the first few days after the bleed is associated with a poor prognosis. Usually, an MCA velocity exceeding 200 cm/sec in patients with vasospasm is associated with a critical reduction in cerebral blood flow (Table 13–6). The time course of the development of vasospasm is also of clinical interest. In general, vasospasm occurs from 4 to 14 days following subarachnoid hemorrhage, but a TCD-detectable increase in velocity often precedes the onset of symptoms by hours to days. This ability to detect vasospasm before symptoms appear allows prophylactic treatment to be instituted. TCD is becoming an important technique in the diagnosis, monitoring, and treatment of vasospasm, and the transcranial information is being used to determine the timing of operation and to assess the effect of new medical treatments.[72]

Intraoperative Monitoring

Another evolving and ostensibly important application of TCD is intraoperative monitoring. The unique advantages of TCD in comparison with other relative cerebral blood flow measurement techniques are its complete noninvasiveness and its potential for detecting rapid alterations of blood supply on a real-time basis. Although TCD records only the mean flow velocity of the blood column within the basal cerebral arteries, this parameter closely reflects the true volume flow when measured simultaneously and individually.[12, 51] In the past, alterations of the cerebral circulation could not be detected except by repeated angiography or blood flow measurements, which had to be performed in an offline fashion. These examinations are not monitoring techniques in the strict sense, because the data must be stored for later interpretation. Because of a suitable method for monitoring relative cerebral blood flow during invasive procedures was not available, electrophysiologic parameters were monitored instead, but these provided information only about abnormal metabolism that occurred *secondary* to reduced cerebral perfusion.

In contrast, TCD monitoring delivers direct, immediate information regarding cerebral perfusion, thus anticipating potential hazards or allowing rapid modification of therapy. TCD monitoring has been used during carotid endarterectomy, open heart surgery with cardiopulmonary bypass, and intensive care therapy.[12, 74–76] Continuous monitoring in these situations can be accomplished by the use of permanent temporal probes placed on the patient's head and fixed with bands or helmet-like constructions. So far, however, most of these devices have been plagued with artifactual signals, and hand-held positioning of the probe remains the method of choice. In most studies, the M_1 segment of the MCA is insonated at a depth of 50 to 55 mm. TCD monitoring can be performed either with repeated examinations at

TABLE 13–6 CLINICAL RELEVANCE OF INCREASED MIDDLE CEREBRAL ARTERY FLOW VELOCITIES AFTER SUBARACHNOID HEMORRHAGE

Middle Cerebral Artery Flow Velocity	Time-Averaged Peak Velocity (mean; cm/sec)	Clinical Consequences
Normal or nonspecifically increased	≤80	Should be observed further
Subcritically accelerated	>80–120	Moderate vasospasm; preventive therapy indicated
Critically accelerated	>120–140	Severe vasospasm; consequent treatment necessary
Highly critical flow acceleration	>140	Severe vasospasm; delayed ischemic deficit highly probable

Modified from Harders A: Neurosurgical Applications of Transcranial Doppler Sonography. New York, Springer-Verlag, 1986.

extremely short invervals or continuously over a longer period.

Most experience with TCD monitoring has been accumulated during carotid endarterectomy.[11, 51, 74, 75, 77, 78] The stump pressure measured during carotid artery clamping correlates linearly with MCA velocity (Fig. 13–16). It has been shown that MCA flow is affected far less during intraoperative clamping of the carotid artery than expected, raising the possibility that shunts are inserted too often. An MCA velocity of more than 10 cm/sec during clamping has been associated with adequate collateral circulation.[79] An MCA velocity reduction of 65% or less from preclamp values has also been found consistent with adequate collateral flow.[51] The effects of preoperative manual compression of the common carotid artery on MCA blood flow are also predictive of intraoperative events during cross-clamping of the exposed carotid bifurcation. A close relationship between preoperative and intraoperative MCA flow velocity reduction is evident.[74]

Preliminary experience with combined somatosensory evoked potential (SEP) monitoring and TCD velocity monitoring of the MCA during carotid endarterectomy has shown that a velocity reduction of at least 65% is necessary to alter the somatosensory evoked cortical response.[74] In our experience, even the absence of any measurable MCA flow, however, does not necessarily lead to SEP changes. These findings suggest that most postoperative neurologic deficits associated with carotid endarterectomy are secondary to acute thrombosis and surgery-related embolism, rather than hypoperfusion. The hemodynamic effects of carotid bifurcation plaque removal on MCA velocity can be measured. It has been shown that the average MCA velocity is only slightly increased postoperatively, again indicating that removal of a stenosis is only rarely of hemodynamic importance.

TCD monitoring during open heart surgery has revealed a number of disturbances in cerebral blood flow that result from extracorporeal bypass (a pumping technique that severely alters blood flow physiology).[7–9, 76] Brain damage and perioperative stroke may occur during extracorporeal bypass. TCD measurements have thrown considerable doubt on the theory that such injury is caused by critical *hypoperfusion.* On the contrary, accidental cerebral *hyperperfusion* may play a more decisive role, as well as air microemboli and loss of cerebral autoregulation. Preoperatively, TCD may identify patients at high risk for ischemic encephalopathy, with the help of the CO_2 inhalation test for assessing the autoregulatory capacity of the brain.

Intensive Care Unit Monitoring

TCD monitoring during intensive care therapy is a broad and as yet unexplored field. Monitoring may be informative and possibly beneficial for the patient's outcome in subarachnoid hemorrhage with vasospasm, as mentioned previously, and also in high- and low-pressure hydrocephalus, increased in-

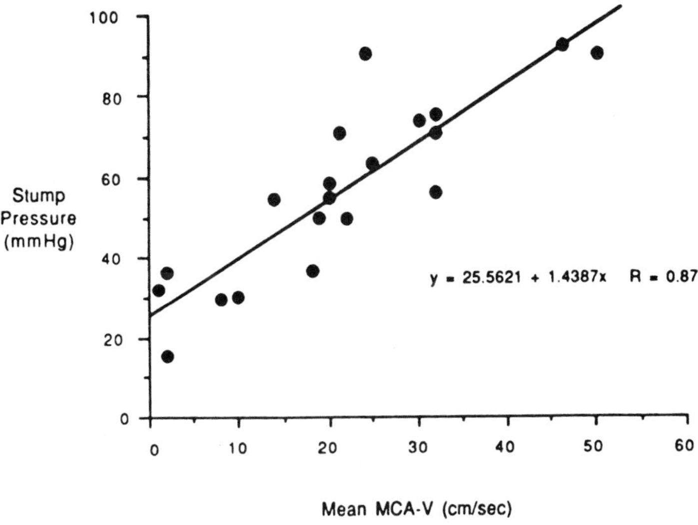

FIGURE 13–16 Middle cerebral artery blood flow velocity during carotid clamping, revealing a linear correlation with measurement of stump pressure (From Schneider PA, Rossman ME, Torem S, et al: Transcranial Doppler [TCD] in the management of extracranial cerebrovascular disease: Implications in diagnosis and monitoring. J Vasc Surg 7:227, 1988.)

tracranial pressure, low-flow states associated with extracranial occlusive disease, myocardial failure or valvular disease, and impending brain death.[51] TCD monitoring may provide further information about the pathophysiology of various abnormal conditions that affect intensive care patients and ultimately may be helpful for therapy. Hyperperfusion and hypoperfusion phenomena following blunt injury of the head provides exciting possibilities for TCD monitoring.[51] CO_2 reactivity may influence prognosis, in that strict cerebral blood flow control may lead to a reduction in cerebral injury. Aaslid and Lindegaard[80] have identified a new parameter from the ultrasound flow profiles that is highly indicative of cerebral perfusion pressure, and thus of the momentary intracranial pressure. If the relevance of this parameter can be verified, it may benefit large groups of intensive care patients with elevated intracranial pressure, from whatever cause, and perhaps may lead to the development of more effective therapeutic regimens for this life-threatening condition.

Brain Death

The accurate diagnosis of brain death has become more important in view of the ethical issues that surround the transplantation of kidneys or other organs. Determination of brain death is based on three parameters: (1) clinical criteria; (2) electroencephalographic criteria; and (3) angiographic demonstration of absent intracranial circulation.[81] The arrest of intracranial flow results in a characteristic reflux phenomenon in the basal cerebral arteries during late systole. This to-and-fro movement is easily noted in the TCD flow velocity waveform (Fig. 13–17).[51, 80, 82] Depending on the cardiac output, flow profiles may be sharp or pulsatile, or they may be dampened with sluggish acceleration and even more sluggish deceleration. TCD monitoring may, in the future, replace more invasive methods for demonstrating cerebral circulatory arrest.

Arteriovenous Malformations and Fistulae

Although an AVM is a developmental abnormality, the arteries and veins involved in supplying blood to the AVM are essentially normal and are the usual arteries supplying the region of the brain where the AVM is located. These arteries, which exclusively or partially feed AVMs, can unequivocally be identified with TCD by means of their significant flow abnormalities—that is, increased flow velocity, reduced pulsatility, and reduced responsiveness to CO_2.[41, 59] These abnormalities permit localization of the AVM and evaluation of its hemodynamic state. Flow velocities as high as 280 cm/sec can be measured in arteries feeding an AVM. Severe reduction of pulsatility is indicated by a diastolic-to-systolic ratio greater than 0.74 or a resistivity index less than 0.27.[59] Obviously, a striking hemispheric difference of flow velocities is evident on side-to-side comparison. Under CO_2 stimulation, pure AVM feeders either display no changes in flow velocity or show only a slight increase of diastolic flow velocity. These vessels are totally unresponsive to hypocapnia. Arteries that contribute only slightly to AVM flow may not be

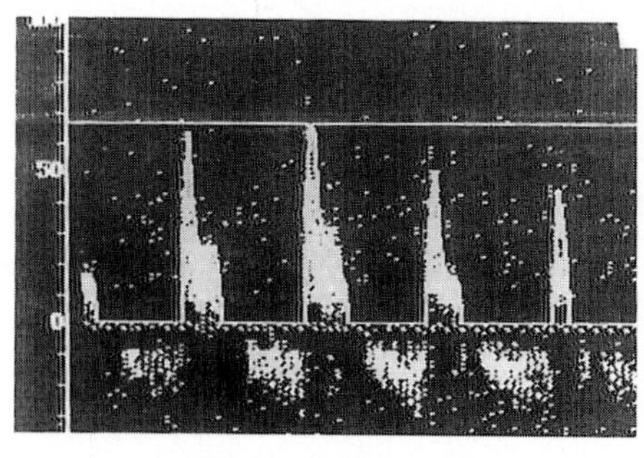

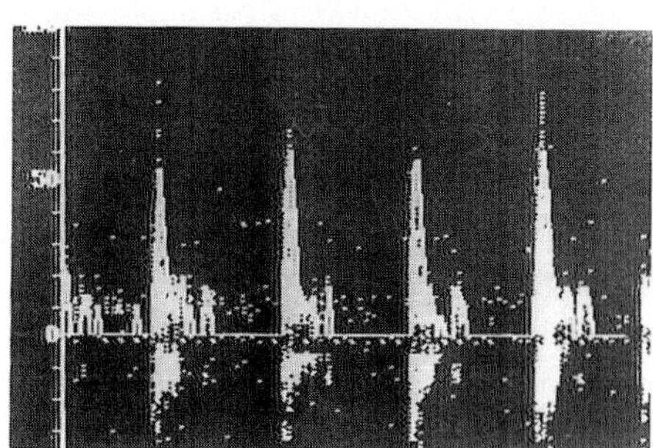

FIGURE 13–17 Brain death transcranial Doppler changes noted in the left middle cerebral and extracranial common carotid arteries. The characteristic reflux phenomenon seen during late systole is demonstrated.

identified by velocity and pulsatility change but show decreased responsiveness to CO_2. A positive linear relationship exists among mean flow velocity and both the diameter of the feeder and the volume of the malformation. A negative linear relationship exists between flow velocity and the length of the feeder. Draining veins associated with vascular malformation can be identified by pulsatile flow near the angioma and by complete lack of flow alteration during the Valsalva maneuver.

TCD re-examination may be particularly helpful after AVM intervention to detect residual feeders and to identify severe flow changes related to bleeding. In successfully treated AVMs, flow velocities in the feeders were found to decrease dramatically to below-normal levels and then to return gradually to levels characteristic of normal cerebral arteries.[83]

In addition to AVMs, other types of intracranial arteriovenous shunts can be detected with TCD, such as CS–cavernous sinus fistulae or dural fistulae. These arteriovenous shunts are detected by very high flow velocities and severe flow disturbances at the fistula site, or by arterialized flow in veins that drain the fistula.[61]

CONCLUSION

TCD, an ultrasound technique that measures physiologic parameters of blood flow in the major intracranial arteries, has tremendous potential, and this is becoming more apparent as investigators from different backgrounds become familiar with its use. The TCD instrument is inexpensive and portable; the technique is noninvasive and is therefore risk free. Because of the lack of risk, the procedure may be performed repeatedly over time to follow physiologic changes that result from pathologic conditions such as vasospasm, or to monitor variations in cerebral blood flow during surgery.

As attractive as these features are, however, TCD is burdened with several inherent difficulties. The accuracy of the procedure depends on the knowledge, skill, and experience of the technician and interpreter. In addition, they must be intimately familiar with the anatomy and physiology of the cerebral arteries. Finally, proper interpretation of TCD studies requires correlation of TCD information with that obtained from carotid sonography and with the patient's clinical information.

In a 1990 position statement, the American Academy of Neurology[84] declared that TCD was an established method for the following: (1) detecting severe stenosis in the major basal intracranial arteries; (2) assessing patterns and extent of collateral circulation in patients with known stenosis or occlusion of the cerebral vessels; (3) evaluating and following vasoconstriction from any cause; (4) detecting AVMs and assessing their supply arteries and flow patterns; and (5) assessing patients with suspected brain death. In addition, TCD can be used for intraoperative monitoring and for investigating the natural progression of cerebrovascular disease.

Potential future uses of TCD include the assessment of intracranial pressure in intensive care patients, the assessment of migraine, and the evaluation of children with vasculopathies (e.g., sickle cell disease, neurofibromatosis).

REFERENCES

1. Miyazaki M, Kato K: Measurement of cerebral blood flow by ultrasonic Doppler technique. Jpn Circ J 29:375, 1965.
2. Aaslid R, Markwalder T-M, Norris H: Noninvasive transcranial Doppler ultrasound recording of flow velocity in basal cerebral arteries. J Neurosurg 57:769, 1982.
3. Ringelstein EB, Otis SM, Schneider PA: Noninvasive assessment of CO_2-induced cerebral vasomotor reactivity. Comparison with rCBF findings during 133-xenon inhalation measurement. J Cereb Blood Flow Metab 1:161, 1989.
4. Ringelstein EB, Sievers C, Ecker S, et al: Noninvasive assessment of CO_2-induced cerebral vasomotor response in normal individuals and patients with internal carotid artery occlusions. Stroke 19:963, 1988.
5. Aaslid R: Visually evoked dynamic blood flow response of the human cerebral circulation. Stroke 18:771, 1987.
6. Harders A: Monitoring of hemodynamic changes related to vasospasm in the circle of Willis after aneurysm surgery. *In* Aaslid R (ed): Transcranial Doppler Sonography. New York, Springer-Verlag, 1986, p 132.
7. Lundar T, Lindegaard K, Froysaker T: Cerebral perfusion during nonpulsatile cardiopulmonary bypass. Ann Thorac Surg 40:144, 1985.
8. Lundar T, Lindegaard K, Froysaker T: Dissociation between cerebral autoregulation and carbon dioxide reactivity during nonpulsatile cardiopulmonary bypass. Ann Thorac Surg 40:582, 1985.
9. Lundar T, Lindegaard K, Froysaker T: Cerebral carbon dioxide reactivity during nonpulsatile cardiopulmonary bypass. Ann Thorac Surg 41:525, 1986.
10. Ringelstein EB, Otis SM, Kahlscheuer B, et al: Transcranial Doppler sonography. Anatomical landmarks and normal velocity values. Ultrasound Med Biol 16:745–761, 1990.

11. Edelmann M, Nielen C, Richert F, et al: TCD monitoring of middle cerebral artery blood flow velocity during carotid endarterectomy. Further experiences. Presented at the First International Conference on Transcranial Doppler Sonography, Rome, Italy, May 1986.
12. Ringelstein EB: A practical guide to transcranial Doppler sonography. *In* Weinberger J (ed): Noninvasive Imaging of Cerebral Vascular Disease. New York, AR Liss, 1989, p 75.
13. Spencer MP, Whisler D: Transorbital Doppler diagnosis of intracranial arterial stenosis. Stroke 17:916, 1986.
14. Aaslid R, Markwalder TM, Nornes H: Noninvasive transcranial Doppler ultrasound recording of flow velocity in the basal cerebral arteries. J Neurosurg 57:769, 1982.
15. Arnolds B, von Reutern GM: Transcranial Doppler sonography: Examination technique and normal reference values. Ultrasound Med Biol 12:115, 1986.
16. Gilsbach J, Harders A: Comparison of intraoperative and transcranial Doppler. *In* Aaslid R (ed): Transcranial Doppler Sonography. New York, Springer-Verlag, 1986, p 106.
17. Ries F, Solymosi L, Horn R, et al: Evaluation of the hemodynamic effect of extra- and intracranial cerebrovascular lesions by 3-D transcranial Doppler scanning. J Cardiovasc Ultrasonogr 7:78, 1988.
18. Ringelstein EB: Transcranial Doppler sonography. *In* Poeck K, Ringelstein EB, Hacke W (eds): New Trends in Diagnosis and Management of Stroke. New York, Springer-Verlag, 1987, pp 3–28.
19. Ringelstein EB, Holling A: Analysis of the circle of Willis by TCD: Program development, validation and clinical impact. Presented at the Second International Conference on Transcranial Doppler Sonography. Salzburg, Austria, November 27–30, 1988.
20. Gibbs JM, Wise RJS, Leenders KL, Jones T: Evaluation of cerebral perfusion reserve in patients with carotid artery occlusion. Lancet 1:310–314, 1984.
21. White DN, Curry GR, Stevenson RJ: The acoustic characteristics of the skull. Ultrasound Med Biol 4:225, 1978.
22. Grolimund P: Transmission of ultrasound through the temporal bone. *In* Aaslid R (ed): Transcranial Doppler Sonography. New York, Springer-Verlag, 1986, p 10.
23. Aaslid R (ed): Transcranial Doppler Sonography. New York, Springer-Verlag, 1986, p 29.
24. Bogdahn U, Becker G, Winkler J, et al: Transcranial color-coded real-time sonography in adults. Stroke 21:1680–1688, 1990.
25. Tsuchiya T, Yasaka M, Yamaguchi T, et al: Imaging of the basal cerebral arteries and measurement of blood velocity in adults by using transcranial real-time color flow Doppler sonography. AJNR Am J Neuroradiol 12:497–502, 1991.
26. Aaslid R (ed): Transcranial Doppler Sonography. New York, Springer-Verlag, 1986, p 39.
27. Becker G, Bogdahn U: Transcranial color-coded real-time sonography in adults. *In* Babikian V, Wechsler L (eds) Transcranial Doppler Ultrasonography. St. Louis, Mosby–Year Book, 1993.
28. Schöning M, Buchholz R, Walter J: Comparative study of transcranial color duplex sonography and transcranial Doppler sonography in adults. J Neurosurg 78:776–784, 1993.
29. Bogdahn U, Becker G: Transcranial color Doppler imaging. *In* Tegeler C, Babikian V, Gomez C (eds): Neurosonology 19:214–220, Mosby 1996.
30. Katz ML, Smalley KJ, Comerota AJ: Transcranial Doppler: Prospective evaluation of hand-held vs. mapping technique. J Vasc Surg 14:69, 1990.
31. Lindegaard R, Bakke SJ, Grolimund P: Assessment of intracranial hemodynamics in carotid artery disease by transcranial Doppler ultrasound. J Neurosurg 63:890, 1985.
32. Padayachee TS, Kirkham FJ, Lewis RR, et al: Transcranial measurement of blood velocities in the basal cerebral arteries using pulsed Doppler ultrasound: A method of assessing the circle of Willis. Ultrasound Med Biol 12:5, 1986.
33. Silverstein A, Doniger D, Bender MB: Manual compression of the carotid vessels, carotid sinus hypersensitivity, and carotid artery occlusions. Ann Intern Med 52:172, 1960.
34. Webster JE, Gurdjian FJ: Observation upon response to digital carotid artery compression. Neurology 7:757, 1957.
35. Otis S, Ringelstein EB: Transcranial Doppler sonography. *In* Bernstein ED (ed): Noninvasive Diagnostic Techniques in Vascular Disease. St. Louis, CV Mosby, 1990, p 59.
36. Hennerici M, Rautenberg W, Sitzer G, et al: Transcranial Doppler ultrasound for the assessment of intracranial arterial flow velocity—Part I. Examination technique and normal values. Surg Neurol 27:439, 1987.
37. Harders A: Neurosurgical Applications of Transcranial Doppler Sonography. New York, Springer-Verlag, 1986, p 24.
38. Dewitt LD, Wechsler H: Transcranial Doppler. Stroke 19:915, 1988.
39. Grolimund P, Seiler RW: Age dependence of the flow velocity in the basal arteries—a transcranial Doppler ultrasound study. Ultrasound Med Biol 14:191, 1988.
40. Russo G, Profeta G, Acampora S, et al: Transcranial Doppler ultrasound examination technique and normal reference values. J Neurosurg Sci 30:97, 1986.
41. Frackowiak RSJ, Lenzi GL, Jones T: Quantitative measurements of cerebral blood flow and oxygen metabolism in man using 15-oxygen and positron emission tomography. Theory, procedure and normal values. J Comput Assist Tomogr 4:727, 1980.
42. Padayachee TS, Kontis S, Gosling RG: Changes in middle cerebral artery Doppler parameters with age in normal subjects. Presented at the First International Congress on Transcranial Doppler Sonography, Rome, Italy, May 1986.
43. Kennedy C, Sokoloff L: An adaptation of the nitrous oxide method to the study of the cerebral circulation in children: Normal values for cerebral blood flow and cerebral metabolic rate in childhood. J Clin Invest 36:1130, 1957.
44. Kety SS: Human cerebral blood flow and oxygen consumption as related to aging. J Chronic Dis 3:478, 1956.
45. Harper AM, Glass HI: Effect of alterations in the arterial carbon dioxide tension on the blood flow through the cerebral cortex at normal and low arterial blood pressures. J Neurol Neurosurg Psychiatry 28:449, 1966.
46. Kety SS, Schmidt CF: The effects of altered tensions of carbon dioxide and oxygen on cerebral blood flow and oxygen consumption of normal young men. J Clin Invest 27:484, 1948.
47. Huber P, Handa J: Effect of contrast material, hypercapnia, hyperventilation, hypertonic glucose and

papaverine on the diameter of the cerebral arteries—angiographic determination in man. Invest Radiol 2:17, 1987.
48. Markwalder TM, Grolimund P, Seiler RW, et al: Dependency of blood flow velocity in the middle cerebral artery on end-tidal carbon dioxide partial pressure—a transcranial ultrasound Doppler study. J Cereb Blood Flow Metab 4:368, 1984.
49. Bishop CFR, Powell S, Insall M, et al: The effect of internal carotid artery occlusion on middle cerebral artery blood flow at rest and response to hypercapnia. Lancet 1:710, 1986.
50. Bullock R, Mandelow AD, Bone I, et al: Cerebral blood flow and CO_2 responsiveness as an indicator of collateral reserve capacity in patients with carotid arterial disease. Br J Surg 72:348, 1985.
51. Ringelstein EB: Transcranial Doppler monitoring. *In* Aaslid R (ed): Transcranial Doppler Sonography. New York, Springer-Verlag, 1986, p 145.
52. Gosling RG, King DH: Processing arterial Doppler signals for clinical data. *In* De Vlieger M (ed): Handbook of Clinical Ultrasound. New York, John Wiley & Sons, 1978.
53. Ley-Pozo J, Willmes K, Ringelstein EB: Relationship between pulsatility indices of Doppler flow signals and CO_2-reactivity within the middle cerebral artery in extracranial occlusive disease. Ultrasound Med Biol 16:763, 1990.
54. Spencer MP: Intracranial carotid artery diagnosis with transorbital pulsed wave (PW) and continuous wave (CW) Doppler ultrasound. Presented at the First International Conference on Transcranial Doppler Sonography, Rome, Italy, May 1986.
55. Hennerici M, Rautenberg W, Schwartz A: Transcranial ultrasound for the assessment of intracranial arterial flow velocity—Part II. Surg Neurol 27:523, 1987.
56. Kirkham FJ, Levin SD, Neville BGR: Bedside diagnosis of stenosis of the middle cerebral artery. Lancet 1:797, 1986.
57. Niederkorn R, Neumayer K: Transcranial Doppler sonography: A new approach in the noninvasive diagnosis of intracranial brain artery disease. Eur Neurol 26:65, 1987.
58. Ringelstein EB, Zeumer H, Korbmacher G, et al: Transkranielle Doppler-sonographie der hirnversorgenden Arterien: Atraumatische Diagnostik von Stenosen und Verschluessen des Carotissiphons und der A. cerebri media. Nervenarzt 56:296, 1985.
59. Hassler W: Hemodynamic aspects of cerebral angiomas. Acta Neurochir [Suppl 37] (Wien):38, 1986.
60. Schwartz A, Hennerici M: Noninvasive transcranial Doppler ultrasound in intracranial angiomas. Neurology 36:626, 1986.
61. Aaslid R, Huber P, Nornes H: Evaluation of cerebrovascular spasm with transcranial Doppler ultrasound. J Neurosurg 60:37, 1984.
62. Del Zoppo GJ, Otis SM: Thrombolytic therapy in acute stroke. *In* Comerota AJ (ed): Thrombolytic Therapy. New York, Grune & Stratton, 1988, p 189.
63. Del Zoppo GJ, Zeumer H, Harker LA: Thrombolytic therapy in acute stroke: Possibilities and hazards. Stroke 17:595, 1986.
64. Wechsler LR, Sekhar LN, Luyckx K, et al: The effects of endarterectomy on the intracranial circulation studied by transcranial Doppler. Neurology 37 (Suppl I3):317, 1987.
65. Caplan LR, Sergay S: Positional cerebral ischemia. J Neurol Neurosurg Psychiatry 39:385, 1976.
66. Carter JE: Chronic ocular ischemia and carotid vascular disease. Stroke 16:721, 1985.
67. Ringelstein EB, Zeumer H, Angelou D: The pathogenesis of strokes from internal carotid artery occlusion: Diagnostic and therapeutic implications. Stroke 14:867, 1983.
68. Norrving B, Nilsson B, Risberg J: rCBF in patients with carotid occlusion—resting and hypercapnic flow related to collateral pattern. Stroke 13:155, 1982.
69. Widder B, Paulat K, Haskspacher J, et al: Transcranial Doppler CO_2 test for the detection of hemodynamically critical carotid artery stenoses and occlusions. Eur Arch Psychiatry Neurol Sci 236:162, 1986.
70. Ringelstein EB, Busker M, Buchner H: Evaluation of hemodynamic effects of subclavian steal mechanism on basilar artery blood flow with the help of transcranial Doppler sonography. Presented at the First International Conference on Doppler Sonography, Rome, Italy, May 1986.
71. Aaslid R, Nornes H: Musical murmurs in human cerebral arteries after subarachnoid hemorrhage. J Neurosurg 60:32, 1984.
72. Harders A, Gilsbach JM: Time course of blood velocity changes related to vasospasm in the circle of Willis measured by transcranial Doppler ultrasound. J Neurosurg 66:718, 1987.
73. Seiler RW, Grolimund P, Aaslid R, et al: Cerebral vasospasm evaluated by transcranial ultrasound correlated with clinical grade and CT-visualized subarachnoid hemorrhage. J Neurosurg 64:594, 1986.
74. Edelmann M, Ringelstein EB, Richert F: Transcranial Doppler sonography for monitoring of the middle cerebral blood flow velocity during carotid endarterectomy. Rev Bras Angiol Clin Vasc 16:96, 1986.
75. Schneider PA, Rossman ME, Otis SM, et al: Transcranial Doppler monitoring during carotid arterial surgery. Surg Forum 38:333, 1987.
76. von Reutern GM, Hetzel A, Birnbaum D, et al: Transcranial Doppler ultrasonography during cardiopulmonary bypass in patients with severe carotid stenosis or occlusion. Stroke 19:674, 1989.
77. Burmeister W, Fischer T, Maurer PC: Transcranial Doppler investigations of collateralization capacity of basal cerebral arteries in patients with extracranial carotid stenoses before and after operative treatment. Second International Symposium on Intracranial Hemodynamics: Transcranial Doppler and Cerebral Blood Flow. San Diego, February 15–18, 1988.
78. Schneider PA, Rossman ME, Torem S, et al: Transcranial Doppler (TCD) in the management of extracranial cerebrovascular disease: Implications in diagnosis and monitoring. J Vasc Surg 7:223, 1988.
79. Padayachee TS, Gosling RG, Bishop CC, et al: Monitoring middle cerebral artery blood velocity during carotid endarterectomy. Br J Surg 73:98, 1986.
80. Aaslid R, Lindegaard KF: Cerebral hemodynamics. *In* Aaslid R (ed): Transcranial Doppler Sonography. New York, Springer-Verlag, 1986, p 60.
81. Black PM: Brain death. Medical progress. N Engl J Med 299:338, 1978.
82. Lewis RR, Padayachee TS, Beasley MG: Investigation of brain death with Doppler-shift ultrasound. J R Soc Med 76:308, 1983.
83. Harders A: Neurosurgical Applications of Transcranial Doppler Sonography. New York, Springer-Verlag, 1986, p 35.
84. Caplan H, Brass H, DeWitt L, et al: Transcranial Doppler ultrasound: Present status. J Ultrasound Med 40:696, 1990.

SECTION 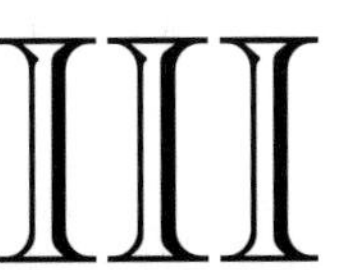

EXTREMITY ARTERIES

Chapter 14

The Role of Noninvasive Procedures in the Management of Extremity Arterial Disease

D. Eugene Strandness, Jr., MD

Almost all the diseases that affect the arterial supply to the limbs interfere with tissue perfusion by obstruction of the involved segment. Thus, the degree to which the disease produces symptoms or signs depends on both the location and extent of arterial involvement. If the available collateral circulation is adequate and is given time to respond to the occlusive event, lower limb survival can be expected. However, it is uncommon for the patient to be entirely free of symptoms in most cases of acute and chronic arterial occlusion.

It is important to recognize that the clinical manifestations of arterial obstruction are the same, regardless of the cause. It then becomes mandatory in approaching a patient with suspected arterial disease to establish that a stenosis or occlusion is indeed present and to proceed to identify not only the sites of involvement but the nature of the underlying disease.

Atherosclerosis is the most common cause of chronic occlusive disease in the Western world. The term used to describe this entity is *arteriosclerosis obliterans* (ASO). Lagging far behind in regard to prevalence is *thromboangiitis obliterans* (TAO). In this country, TAO accounts for less than 1% of all chronic vascular diseases involving large and medium-sized arteries.

To apply noninvasive diagnostic tests properly, it is essential to have an understanding of the more common disease entities and their clinical expression. If results of these tests are to be used intelligently, it must be understood that they complement the usual diagnostic work-up. In this chapter, some of these considerations are reviewed.

PATHOLOGY AND SITES OF INVOLVEMENT

It is important both from a clinical standpoint and with regard to noninvasive testing procedures to review the important relationship between pathology and sites of involvement. The atherosclerotic plaque, in its evolution, undergoes a series of complex changes that have yet to be defined precisely. The precursor of the far-advanced lesion—the complicated plaque—is the fibrous plaque. As it enlarges from its subintimal position, the fibrous plaque initially retains its smooth endothelial covering. At variable points in time, however, the plaque undergoes significant changes in content and surface characteristics. The advanced, complicated plaque develops a breakdown in its surface covering, with subsequent ulceration. The degenerating plaque contains fibrous tissue, fat, and calcium and produces varying degrees of hemorrhage, which occurs randomly within the lesion. Most plaques with clinical sequelae are of the complicated type. Although atherosclerosis is a widely distributed disease, specific sites of predilection tend to give it a segmental localization.

In the lower extremity, the most common site of involvement in both diabetic and nondiabetic patients is the superficial femoral artery in the adductor canal. Disease localized in this segment produces minimal to moderate claudication, because the collateral potential through the profunda femoris and geniculate arteries is usually high. Isolated disease in this region is rarely the cause of far-advanced ischemia and limb loss, because the occlusion that occurs secondary to atherosclerosis is usually gradual.

The aortoiliac segment is the second most common site for arterial occlusive lesions. For reasons that are poorly understood, involvement of this segment is more common in the nondiabetic patient than in the diabetic patient. Disease in this region often produces serious claudication, even though the collateral circulation is sufficient to maintain resting blood flow at normal levels. Because the occlusions are proximal to the profunda femoris artery, collateral inflow is severely limited and the entire limb becomes ischemic with exercise.

A remarkably silent area for arterial occlusive disease is the region below the knee. The tibial and peroneal arteries have extensive intercommunicating collateral channels, which can provide adequate blood flow to the foot until all three arteries are involved. Diabetic patients have a greater prevalence of atherosclerotic involvement of these vessels than nondiabetics.

Advanced ischemia severe enough to lead to limb loss is almost always the result of occlusion involving multiple arterial segments, because the resistance to flow offered by more than one system of collaterals is additive, resulting in a marked decrease in perfusion pressure and flow to the foot.

The pathogenesis of TAO is not well understood, but it probably starts as a panangiitis of both the artery and vein, which leads to thrombosis of the involved segments. This process, which is in some way related to the use of tobacco, starts in smaller arteries such as the palmar and plantar vessels. The involvement appears to progress in a proximal direction but does not usually have any skip areas. Progression without skip areas prevents the available collateral arteries from developing and supplying the foot or hand. The very severe ischemia and pain that result reflect this phenomenon.

CLINICAL PRESENTATION

It is convenient to subdivide patients' presenting ischemic symptoms into two categories, symptoms with exercise and symptoms at rest. This separation is important in understanding the underlying cause and types of noninvasive procedures that might be carried out to evaluate the physiologic impact of the underlying disorder.

Those symptoms that occur with exercise are referred to as *intermittent claudication.* Pain develops in a muscle group in response to exercise and is relieved by rest. The most common sites of such pain are the calf, thigh, hip, and buttock. The site of arterial involvement responsible for the symptoms is always proximal to the muscle group in which the pain develops. It must be recognized, however, that it does not necessarily follow that all muscles distal to the occluded segment develop pain with exercise. For example, although it is known that both calf and thigh pain can develop with iliac artery occlusion, only calf pain may be experienced. This probably occurs because the more distal muscle groups first become ischemic, limiting exertion before the more proximal muscle groups become symptomatic.

The claudication that develops in patients with TAO is uniquely located in the foot, producing what is commonly referred to as *instep claudication.* This symptom occurs very rarely in ASO and is probably a reflection of the more distal arterial involvement observed with TAO.

Symptoms at rest occur with multisegment disease and indicate far-advanced ischemia. Limb loss is usually inevitable unless something can be done to increase the blood supply to the part. The pain, which is often severe and unrelenting, involves the distal foot and toes. Early rest pain characteristically occurs only at night. In the case of lower extremity ischemia, the patient finds that placing the foot in a dependent position may alleviate the discomfort.

Vascular disease of the upper extremity is less common than that involving the lower limbs. Arteriosclerosis, when it develops, is almost always confined to the first part of the subclavian artery. In contrast to the lower limbs, in which chronic arterial occlusion regularly produces symptoms, subclavian artery occlusion is almost always silent.

Subclavian stenosis is usually discovered when a difference in the systolic blood pressure is noted between the two arms, generally 30 mm Hg or greater. When the patient develops claudication of an arm it is similar to that which occurs in the leg—that is, pain in the exercising muscle group brought on by exercise and relieved by rest. The lack of symptoms with subclavian stenosis is undoubtedly a result of the fact that the vertebral artery, which becomes a major source of collateral blood flow, can provide enough blood to meet the normal exercise needs of the arms. The sparing of the arteries distal to the origin of the subclavian from atherosclerosis remains a mystery, because all the risk factors that appear to be important seem to have little effect here. The one exception to this rule occurs in patients with chronic renal failure who have been undergoing dialysis. In this setting, it is common to see upper extremity occlusive lesions at sites other than the subclavian artery. Medial calcification is also commonly seen in this setting, but it has no relationship to the intimal lesions of arteriosclerosis.

The most common vascular disorders seen in the upper extremity relate to the development of cold sensitivity. When this occurs, it is important to determine whether the symptoms and signs are caused by primary Raynaud's disease or by some often serious underlying disorder, such as scleroderma. When cold sensitivity is secondary to an underlying disease, it is classified as secondary Raynaud's phenomenon. With the secondary condition, occlusions of the digital and, on occasion, the palmar arteries are common. In contrast, digital artery occlusions never occur in patients with primary Raynaud's disease. The vascular laboratory can be helpful in these patients by documenting the status of the digital and palmar arteries and by noting the digital blood pressure response to cooling.

The vascular laboratory is frequently requested to carry out studies of the thoracic outlet to document compression of the subclavian artery with the arm in certain positions. This test is usually requested for those patients who present with numbness, tingling, and, occasionally, pain with their arms in certain positions. It is relatively simple to do this, but the problem that always remains is whether vascular compression alone is responsible for the patients' complaints. In fact, most patients with thoracic outlet syndrome who do in fact have true compression as the cause of their symptoms have it on the basis of compression of the trunks of the brachial plexus.

The one entity that is definitely related to compression of the subclavian artery occurs when the patient has a cervical rib and an associated fibrous band that attaches to the back of the first rib. This band compresses the artery, and when this occurs, intimal damage with ulceration can occur, resulting in embolization to the hand and distal arm.

The diagnosis and degree of disability from arterial occlusive disease can usually be assessed by a complete medical history and physical examination. It is at this point that the physician must decide if it is necessary to proceed with arteriography. Until the development of ultrasonic duplex scanning, it was not possible to isolate the sites of involvement precisely by noninvasive means. This capability is now available, from the level of the abdominal aorta to the popliteal artery behind the knee, and the information obtained is extremely useful in planning therapy.

Because diabetes is such an important factor for the development of arterial occlusive disease, it is important to keep in mind that the noninvasive procedures used to study the disease may have to be different. In addition to the differences in the localization of the disease, the patient with type 2 diabetes also has a high occurrence of medial calcification. Although this process is not one that narrows the artery, it does make the measurement of the ankle/brachial index (ABI) difficult. For this reason, it has been recommended that the assessment of arterial disease in patients with diabetes include the measurement of the toe systolic pressure index (TSPI). Although ultrasound is used to measure the ankle systolic pressure, this is not possible at the level of the toe. For this test, it is necessary to use photoplethysmography or the mercury strain gauge method.[1]

PRACTICAL PROBLEMS

It is now clear that the medical history and physical examination are not adequate alone to provide an initial evaluation of a patient with or suspected of having peripheral arterial disease. Although there is no doubt that the decision to intervene by either endovascular or surgical means is based on patient presentation, some simple testing in the clinic is mandatory.

Although much of this book is devoted to the more sophisticated aspects of ultrasound testing, the use of the continuous wave Doppler (CWD) to measure the ankle systolic pressure must become a part of daily practice. However, common errors that are seen must be mentioned. Whenever one wishes to measure the ABI (ankle systolic pressure divided by brachial systolic pressure), it is mandatory that the arm pressure also be measured with the CWD. If this is done properly, the normal value for the ABI is 1.0 or greater. In practice any value above 0.90 is considered normal. The variability in the measurement is ±0.15.[2] A normal value for the TSPI is greater than 0.60, with a variability of ±0.17.[1] The information provided is verification of the diagnosis of arterial occlusive disease and an estimate of its severity. For example, in general an ABI more than 0.50 is seen with single-segment disease. If it is lower than 0.50, multisegment disease is often present. These same measurements must be repeated at the time of each visit.

If the use of noninvasive tests in this patient population is to be recommended, it is necessary to address the potential and real shortcomings of the traditional approach. Are there situations in which the overall evaluation can be improved by some relatively simple and straightforward testing procedures?

Is the Diagnosis Correct?

The diagnosis of intermittent claudication in the lower extremities is usually straightforward, but there are situations in which the clinical presentation may not satisfy the usually accepted criteria. More attention has been devoted to the pseudoclaudication syndromes that may produce symptoms similar to those observed with chronic arterial occlusion. These include such diseases as herniated nucleus pulposus, degenerative joint disease, spinal canal stenosis, and spinal cord tumors. These disorders may be suspected by noting that the walk-pain-rest cycle varies from day to day. With true claudication, this relationship is relatively constant from day to day. In addition, the pain of pseudoclaudication may occur while the patient is standing—something never observed with arterial disease.

Although the distinction between true claudication and pseudoclaudication may be suspected on clinical grounds, the ankle blood pressure response to exercise can be very helpful. As discussed in Chapter 16, patients with claudication secondary to arterial disease *always* have a decrease in their ankle systolic pressure when exercised to the point of pain. It is easy to verify this and to direct the patient for further work-up and therapy.[3]

In the upper extremity, the diagnosis of arterial occlusion is simple. However, when a patient with suspected cold sensitivity appears, it is often difficult to be sure if the diagnosis is correct. The vascular laboratory can be of great assistance in documenting the effects of cold exposure. In addition, demonstrating that cold sensitivity is associated with the presence of occlusive lesions in the digital and palmar arteries is certain evidence that an underlying and often serious disease is present.

Where Is the Disease Located?

Although the level at which the pulses can be palpated is useful in estimating the most proximal level of arterial occlusion, further information is desirable because it can have important therapeutic implications. Determining the level of occlusion is possible without arteriography by using a combination of noninvasive tests at the time of the patient's first visit. These include the measurement of segmental pressure gradients, screening of all large and medium-sized arteries with an ultrasonic duplex scanner, and waveform analysis of signals obtained from regions of suspected disease.

Although the presence or absence of pulses and the ABI are helpful in estimating the level of the occlusive disease, more information is necessary if some form of intervention is required. Once the decision is made to intervene, the next step for those with the available equipment is to survey the arterial system to document the exact sites of involvement. Ultrasonic duplex scanning can be used for this purpose. As is noted in this book, there is adequate validation to show that this is a reasonable and accurate approach to use.[4]

It is now possible to both localize the disease and estimate its hemodynamic significance. This information is of great value to both the arteriographer and the surgeon who is participating in the direct care of the patient.

Although indirect tests provide information about the segmental localization of vascular disorders, it has become apparent that more information can be obtained by the use of duplex scanning. With increasing experience, it is clear that not only can the sites of narrowing and occlusion be identified, but also their hemodynamic significance can be ascertained. Thus, with noninvasive techniques, it is now feasible to determine in many cases the type of therapy that can be used. This capability has great advantages, because a therapeutic approach can be planned before arteriography has been carried out. The patient can be counseled immediately about diagnostic and therapeutic options. The radiologist can plan contrast studies based on the duplex findings. In addition, the ability to plan therapy on the basis of noninvasive tests can result in a saving of time and better planning, if transluminal angioplasty is contemplated.

To What Extent Is the Patient Disabled?

Physicians traditionally use city blocks as a frame of reference in documenting the disability produced by lower extremity arterial occlusion. This is at best a crude estimate, because the length of city blocks varies, even within the same community. Furthermore, claudication is influenced by a number of factors, such as walking speed, grade, and walking patterns. Although using city blocks as the index of disability is acceptable to some physicians, a more objective assessment is possible with exercise testing. Use of the treadmill permits not only measurement of the physiologic response, but also the detection of other problems, such as shortness of breath and angina, which affect both walking time and subsequent therapeutic decisions. Treadmill testing remains an important part of the work-up of the patient when the cause of exercise-induced pain is not clear.[3] Healthy subjects with moderate workload do not show decreased ankle systolic pressure after exercise. However, the patient with occlusive arterial disease sustains a fall in ankle pressure with a delay in the recovery time. If the ankle systolic pressure falls by more than 20% from baseline and requires greater than 3 minutes to recover, the test result is abnormal. The more severe the claudication, the greater the fall in pressure and the longer the recovery time.

Another problem that is being encountered with increasing frequency is the problem of pseudoclaudication. As the patients age, the ravages of degenerative joint disease, spinal stenosis, and herniated nucleus pulposus become more of a problem. From a diagnostic standpoint these disorders can lead to the development of limb pain with walking. Although this can often be separated from true claudication on the basis of the history alone, treadmill exercise can sometimes be of great assistance in determining the underlying cause.

Because atherosclerosis that involves the peripheral arteries can also affect the coronary circulation, it is important that this area of the circulation not be ignored in the examination of patients with peripheral arterial disease. The development of angina pectoris or shortness of breath during a treadmill test for claudication should alert the physician to the fact that further investigation of the underlying cause is mandatory.

Is Collateral Artery Function Stable?

Documentation of improvement in limb perfusion or worsening secondary to disease progression is extremely difficult unless the change is dramatic. Furthermore, the patient is often seen relatively soon after the event that led to the arterial occlusion. It is generally unwise at the time of the initial visit to proceed with a more vigorous work-up, because collateral artery flow may develop further and result in marked improvement in the patient's status. This maturation of collateral circulation can now be determined objectively by repetitive measurements of ankle blood pressure and by assessment of the response to treadmill exercise.

It is now clear that collateral artery function after episodes of arterial occlusion can be assessed indirectly by the measurement of the ABI and TSPI. This is because as collateral circulation improves, the diameter of the midzone arteries increases. This decreases their resistance to blood flow, resulting in better flow and a higher ankle and toe systolic blood pressure. Conversely, if new disease develops that further blocks existing collateral pathways, the ankle and toe systolic pressures fall.[2, 3]

What Is the Potential for Limb Loss?

One of the major roles of the physician is to provide complete information to the patient about the potential for limb loss. If the patient has ischemia at rest, this is not difficult to assess, but frequently this is not the case. The measurement of ankle or digit pressure is extremely useful in providing a clue that the circulation is precarious and that the patient should not only be followed more closely but also be cautioned to watch for trouble signs indicating rapid deterioration of the circulation. If the perfusion pressure is low, frequent evaluations become increasingly important.

Has Arterial Surgery Been Successful?

The correction of arterial perfusion problems by direct arterial surgery is commonplace. In practice, verification of the immediate result is by the return of pulses. The long-term assessment of surgical success relies on patient testimony and retention of peripheral pulses.

Noninvasive tests have come to occupy an important place in this area for a number of reasons: (1) pulses may not always return particularly early, and some independent method of verification is desirable; (2) detection of failure, particularly in the first 24 hours, may be difficult on clinical grounds alone; and (3) it is now known that problems within an arterial reconstruction may be detected during follow-up, before the patient becomes symptomatic and the graft occluded. Therefore, it is possible to salvage arterial reconstructions at a stage when a simple procedure may be used to correct the defect.

Standard indirect tests are used at the patient's bedside in the hospital to document the early results. If there is a suspected problem, a duplex scan can be done to assess the reconstruction itself. After discharge, the schedule for monitoring the results depends on the nature of the reconstruction. The one area of reconstruction in which there is now nearly universal agreement applies to vein bypass grafts. It is now established that a surveillance program, particularly during the first year, is necessary.[5, 6] Duplex scanning of the graft should be done at the time of discharge or 1 to 2 weeks after discharge. The follow-up schedule is then at a minimum of every 3 months during the first year and semiannually thereafter. By using such a schedule, it is possible to detect problems within the graft that can be repaired before graft occlusion occurs. By this type of monitoring, it is possible to keep the secondary patency rates in the range of 90% at 3 years.

REFERENCES

1. Orchard TJ, Strandness DE Jr: Assessment of peripheral vascular disease in diabetes. Circulation 88:819–828, 1993.
2. Baker JD, Dix D: Variability of Doppler ankle pressure with arterial occlusive disease: An evaluation of ankle index and brachial-ankle pressure gradient. Surgery 89:134–137, 1981.
3. Strandness DE Jr: Exercise testing in the evaluation of patients undergoing direct arterial surgery. J Cardiovasc Surg 11:192–200, 1970.
4. Edwards JM, Coldwell DM, Goldman ML, Strandness DE Jr: The role of duplex scanning in the selection of patients for transluminal angioplasty. J Vasc Surg 13:69–74, 1991.
5. Caps MT, Bergelin RO, Cantwell-Gab K, Strandness DE Jr: Vein graft lesions: Time of onset and rate of progression. J Vasc Surg 22:466–475, 1995.
6. Idu MM, Blankenstein JD, de Gier P, et al: Impact of color-flow duplex surveillance program on infrainguinal vein graft patency: A five year experience. J Vasc Surg 17:42–53, 1993.

Chapter 15

ARTERIAL ANATOMY OF THE EXTREMITIES

■ *Gregory M. Keck, MD* ■ *William J. Zwiebel, MD*

The evaluation of arterial disease of the extremities requires knowledge of vascular anatomy. This chapter provides this basic information for the upper and lower extremities. Normal anatomy, common variants, and major collateral routes[1–6] are illustrated, primarily by representative arteriograms.

In this text, the following terms are used to describe extremity anatomy. The *arm* is the portion of the upper extremity between the shoulder and elbow. The *forearm* is the portion between the elbow and wrist. The *thigh* is the portion of the lower extremity between the hip and knee, and the *leg* is the portion between the knee and ankle.

UPPER EXTREMITY

Normal Features

The normal arterial anatomy of the upper extremity is depicted in Figure 15–1. Figures 15–2 through 15–5 are detailed arteriographic views of specific regions of the upper extremity arterial tree, beginning at the aorta and extending to the digits. These figures should be reviewed carefully, because their legends provide the bulk of the anatomic information.

Anatomic Variants

Many anatomic variants can occur in the arterial tree of the upper extremities. The more commonly encountered are presented in Table 15–1.[1–3] Familiarity with these variants can prevent confusion and error during duplex examination. An example of an upper extremity anatomic variant is presented in Figure 15–6.

Collateral Routes

Many of the tributaries seen in Figures 15–1 to 15–6 may serve as collaterals when the main arterial trunks of the upper extremity are blocked.

The following is a summary of the more common collateral routes[2]:

1. Obstruction of the proximal subclavian or brachiocephalic arteries
   a. From cranial and/or neck arteries to the subclavian artery distal to the obstruction (e.g., subclavian steal phenomenon)
   b. From pelvic, abdominal wall, and thoracic wall arteries to the subclavian artery distal to the obstruction
2. Obstruction of the distal subclavian or axillary arteries
   a. From the thoracic wall or shoulder region to the axillary artery distal to the obstruction
3. Obstruction of the brachial artery or its branch vessels
   a. From the distal arm to the proximal forearm
   b. From the midarm to the distal arm and/or forearm
   c. Retrograde filling from the palmar arches of the hand (Fig. 15–7)

Figure 15–7 shows an example of collateralization in response to radial artery occlusion.

Text continued on page 217

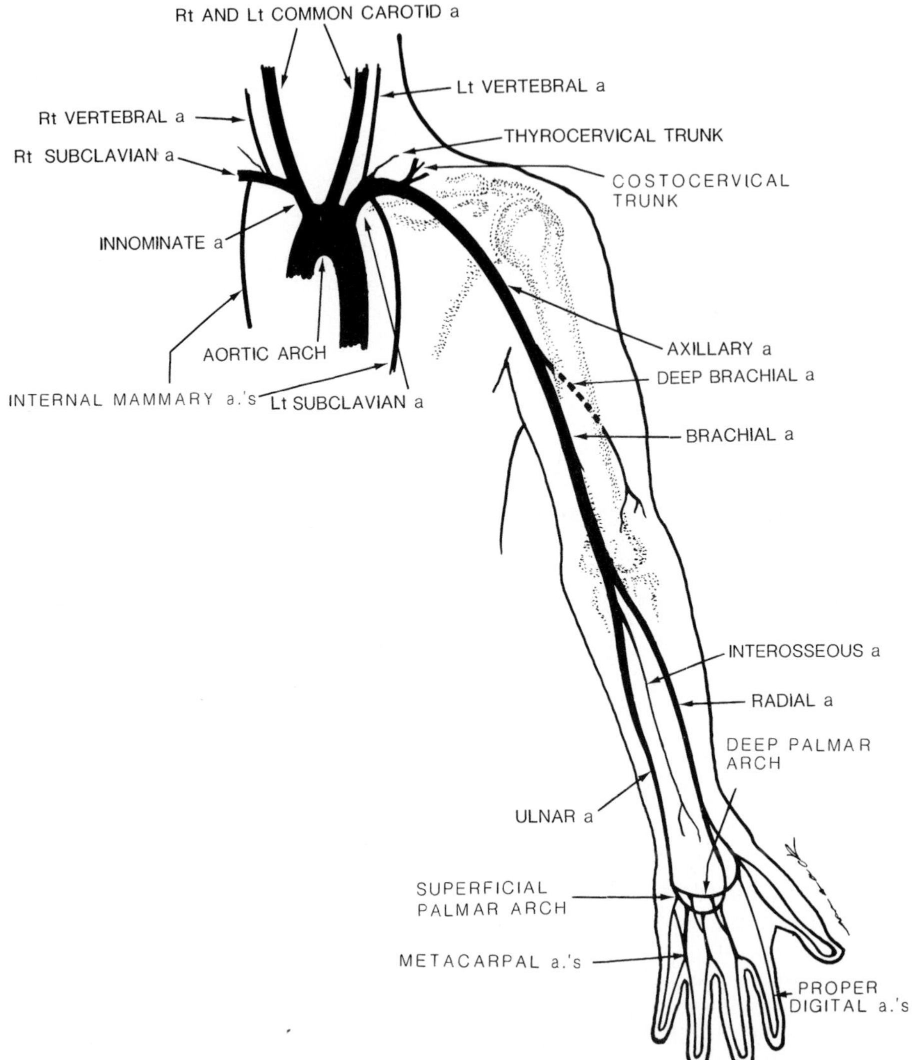

FIGURE 15–1 Arterial anatomy of the upper extremity. Note that the internal mammary arteries, which are tributaries of the subclavian arteries, are used commonly for coronary artery bypass. The deep palmar arch arises from the radial artery and the superficial palmar arch arises from the ulnar artery. These arches may or may not communicate with each other.

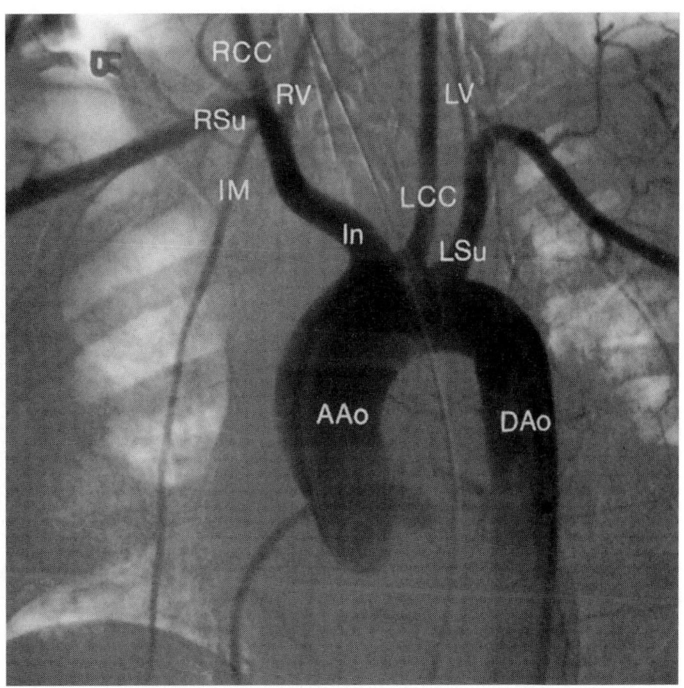

FIGURE 15–2 The aortic arch connects the ascending aorta (AAo) with the descending aorta (DAo). Three great vessels originate from the aortic arch; the innominate artery (In) originates on the right side of the arch, followed by the left common carotid artery (LCC) and the left subclavian artery (LSu). The innominate artery divides into the right common carotid artery (RCC) and the right subclavian artery (RSu). The right and left vertebral arteries (RV, LV) originate from the subclavian arteries, even though this is not apparent on the right side of this illustration. The internal mammary artery (IM) also arises from the subclavian artery.

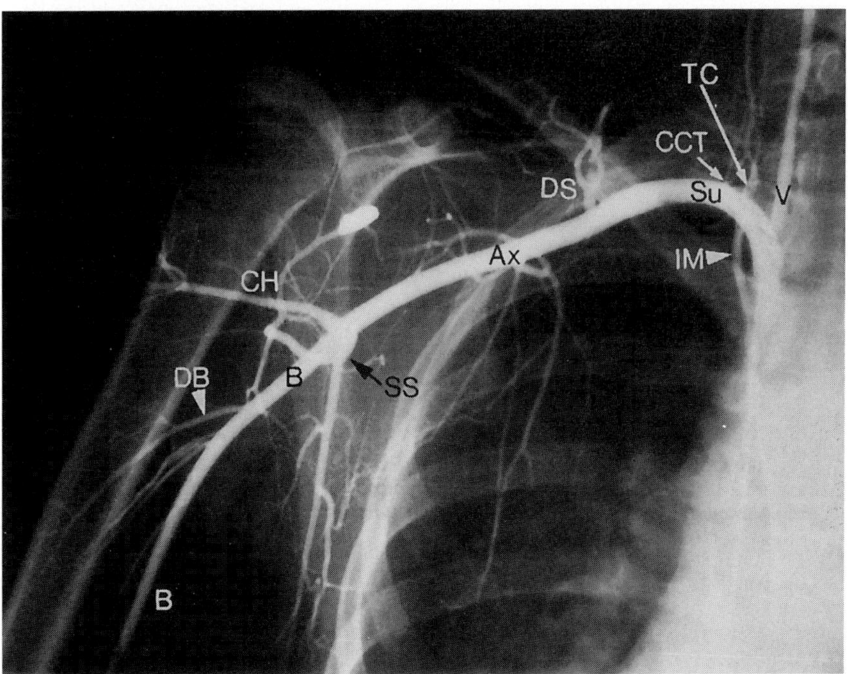

FIGURE 15–3 The subclavian artery (Su) becomes the axillary artery (Ax) at the lateral margin of the first rib. The axillary artery, in turn, becomes the brachial artery (B) after crossing the inferolateral margin of the teres major muscle.[3] The thyrocervical (TC) and costocervical (CCT) trunks are noteworthy branches of the subclavian artery, because they may be mistaken for the vertebral artery (V) during duplex examination. The multiple branches that supply the scapular musculature serve as collaterals when the subclavian or innominate arteries are obstructed. IM = internal mammary artery; DS = dorsal scapular artery; CH = circumflex humeral artery; DB = deep brachial artery; SS = subscapular artery.

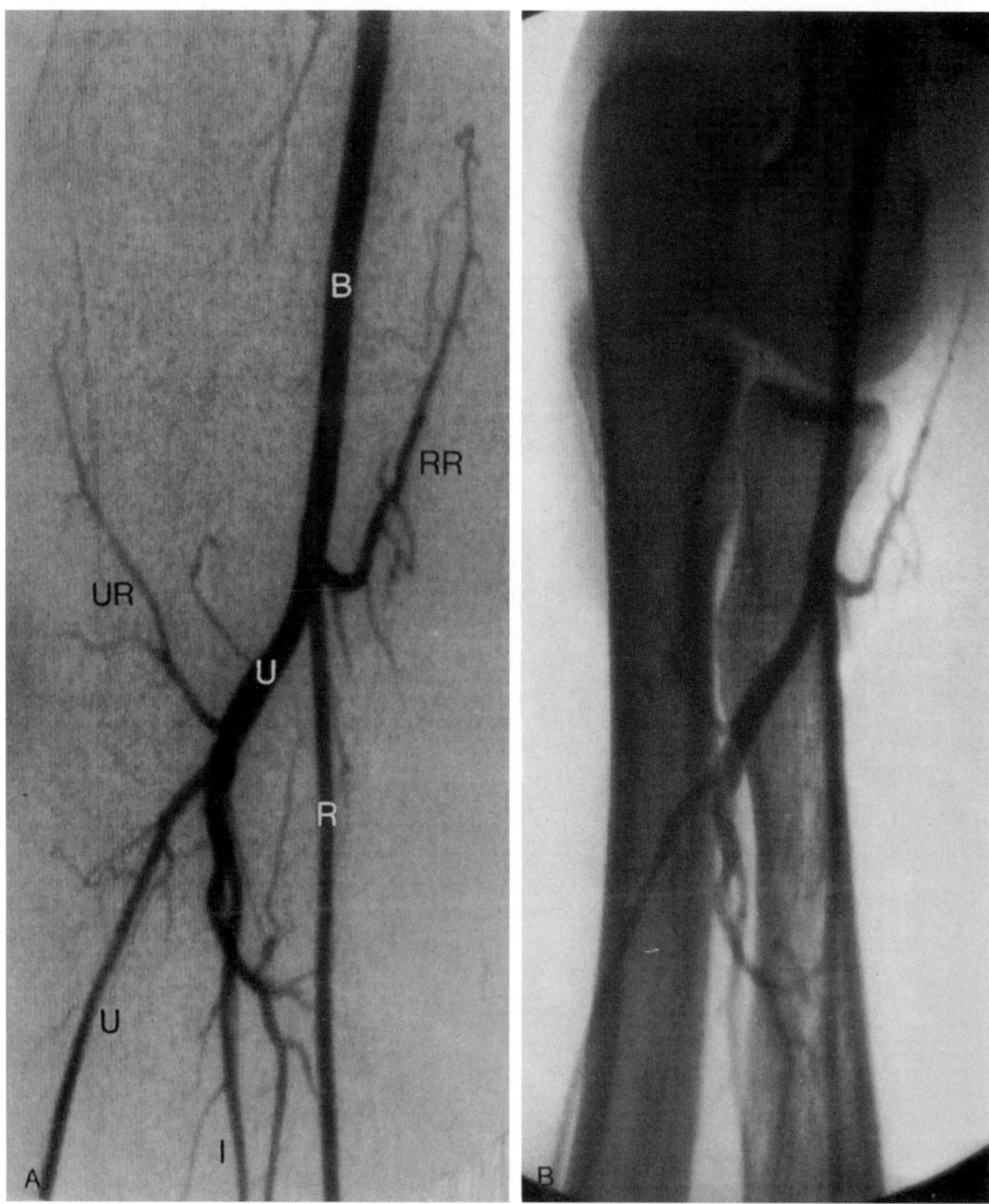

FIGURE 15–4 Arterial anatomy (*A*) and osseous landmarks (*B*) at the elbow. The brachial artery (B) divides at the elbow, forming the radial (R) and ulnar (U) arteries. The interosseous artery (I) is a branch of the ulnar artery, which in some individuals continues to the wrist. RR = recurrent radial artery; UR = ulnar recurrent artery.

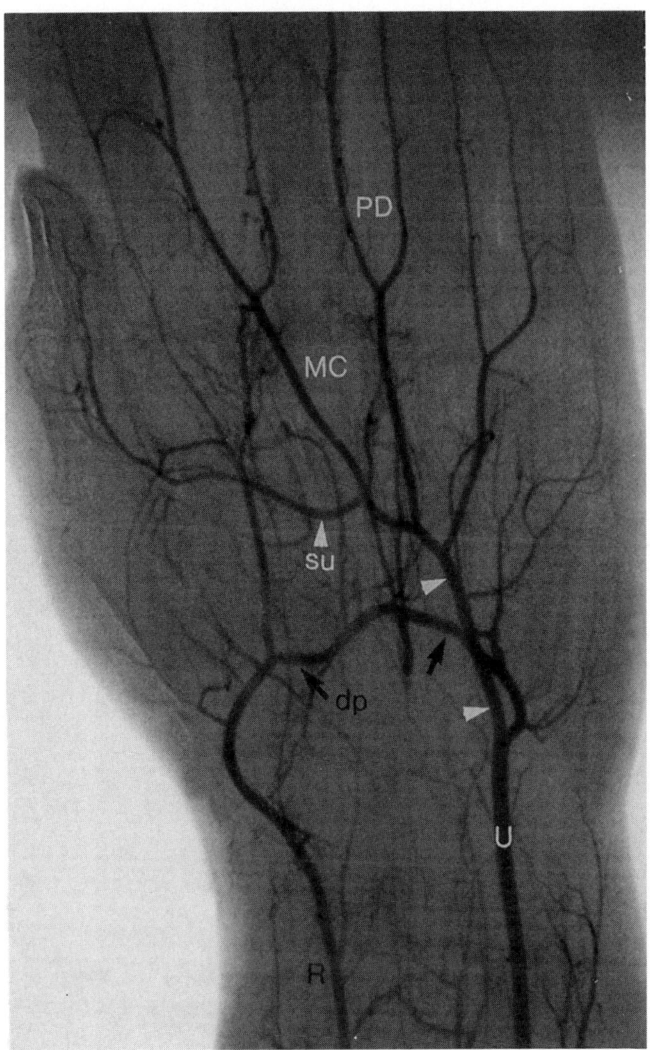

FIGURE 15–5 The radial artery (R) terminates in the deep palmar arch (dp, *black arrows*). The ulnar artery (U) terminates in the superficial palmar arch (su, *white arrowheads*). Communicating vessels usually connect the deep and superficial arches, as shown here. The metacarpal (MC) (also called the common palmar digital artery or dorsal metacarpal artery) and proper palmar digital (PD) arteries are branches of the superficial and deep arches.

TABLE 15–1 ARTERIAL VARIANTS OF THE UPPER EXTREMITY

Structure	Variant	Frequency of Occurrence in the Population (%)
Aortic arch and great vessels	Common origin of the right brachiocephalic and left common carotid arteries	22
	Left vertebral artery origin directly from the aorta	4–6
	Common origin of both common carotid arteries	<1
Arm and forearm	Radial artery origin from the axillary artery	1–3
	Early division of the brachial artery: 1. High origin of the radial artery (Fig. 15–6) 2. Accessory (duplicated) brachial artery	19
	Ulnar artery origin from the brachial or axillary artery	2–3
	Low origin (5–7 cm below elbow joint) of ulnar artery	<1
	Persistent median artery	2–4

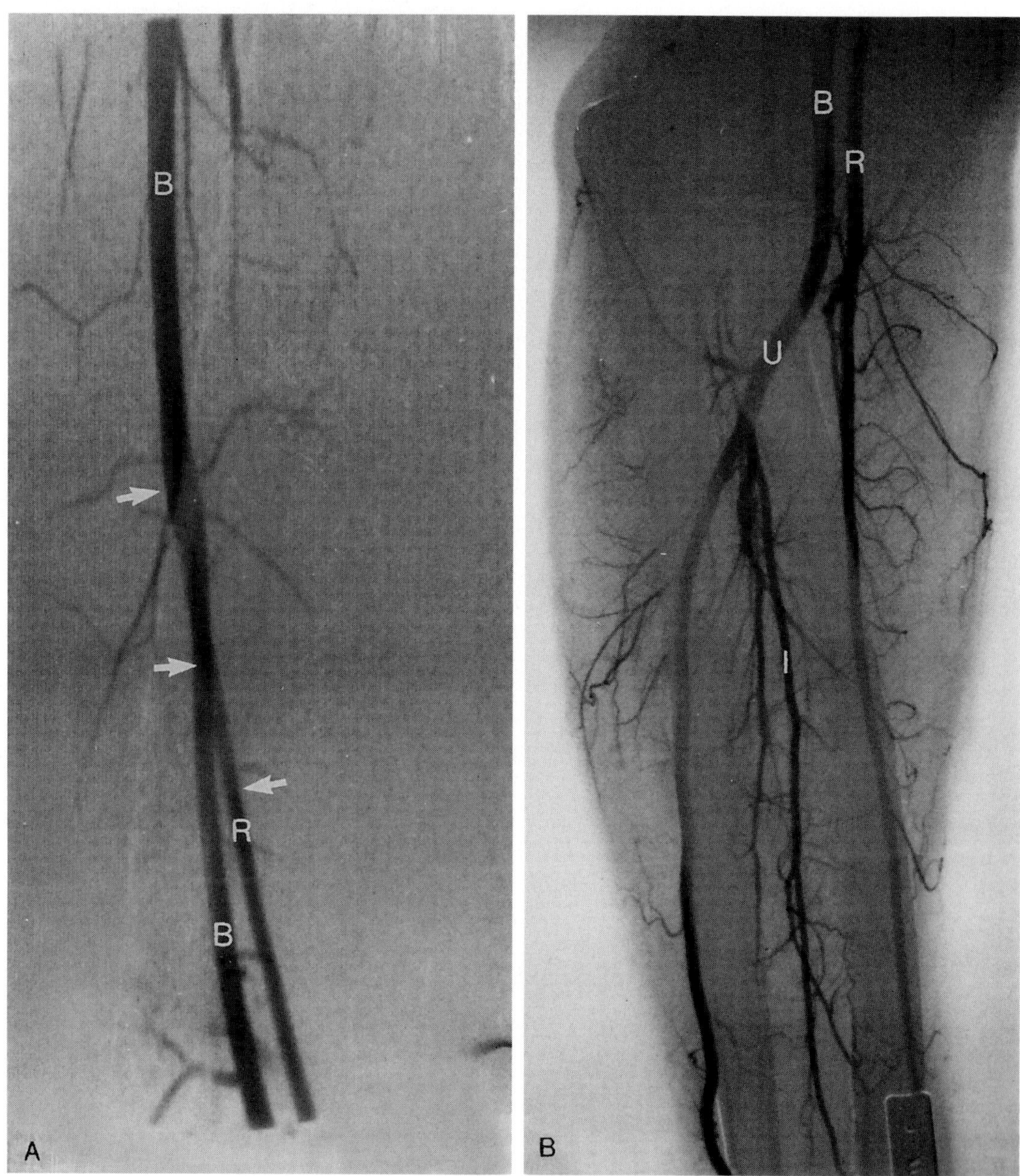

FIGURE 15–6 High origin of the radial artery. Arteriograms of the arm (*A*) and forearm (*B*) demonstrate a high origin of the radial artery (R, *arrows*) at the level of the midhumerus. B = brachial artery; U = ulnar artery; I = interosseous artery.

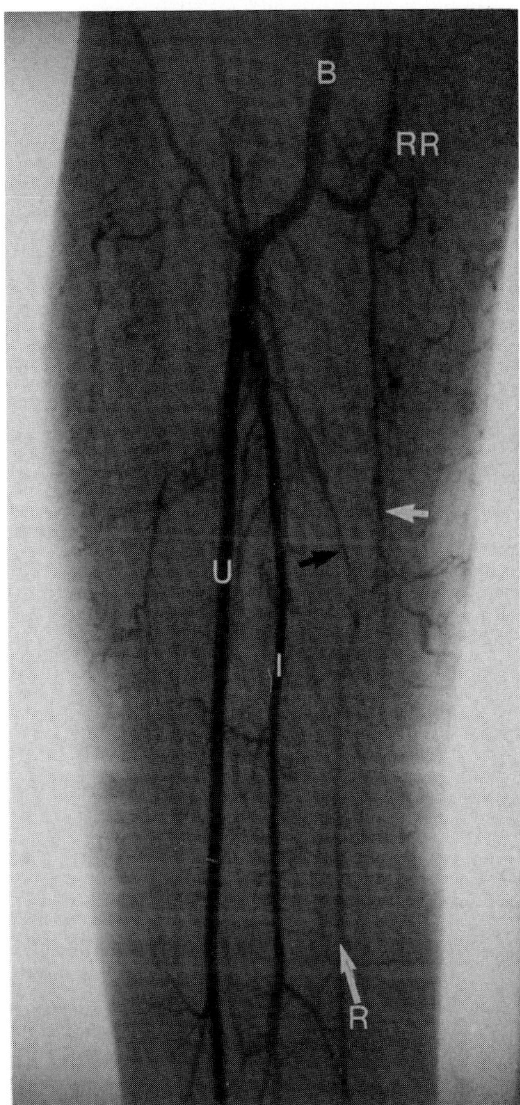

FIGURE 15–7 Collateral circulation in radial artery occlusion. The distal portion of the radial artery (R, *large arrow*) is primarily filled in a retrograde manner from the superficial and deep palmar arches (not shown). Antegrade collateral supply also is provided by the recurrent radial artery (RR, *small white arrow*) and by the interosseous artery (I, *small black arrow*). B = brachial artery; U = ulnar artery.

LOWER EXTREMITY

Normal Anatomy

The lower extremity arterial tree begins at the aortic bifurcation; therefore, the lower extremity arterial anatomy presented here will begin at this point and extend to the foot (for details concerning abdominal vascular anatomy, see Chapter 26). The major arteries of the lower extremity are illustrated in Figure 15–8. Figures 15–9 through 15–13 are angiographic depictions of the regional arterial anatomy of the lower extremity.

Anatomic Variants

The arterial anatomy of the lower extremity is fairly constant. Anatomic variations that may be encountered occasionally are presented in Table 15–2.[4] The statistics included in the table indicate the relative infrequency of these variations.

Collateral Routes

Multiple variations are possible in the collateral routes that circumvent lower extrem-

Text continued on page 227

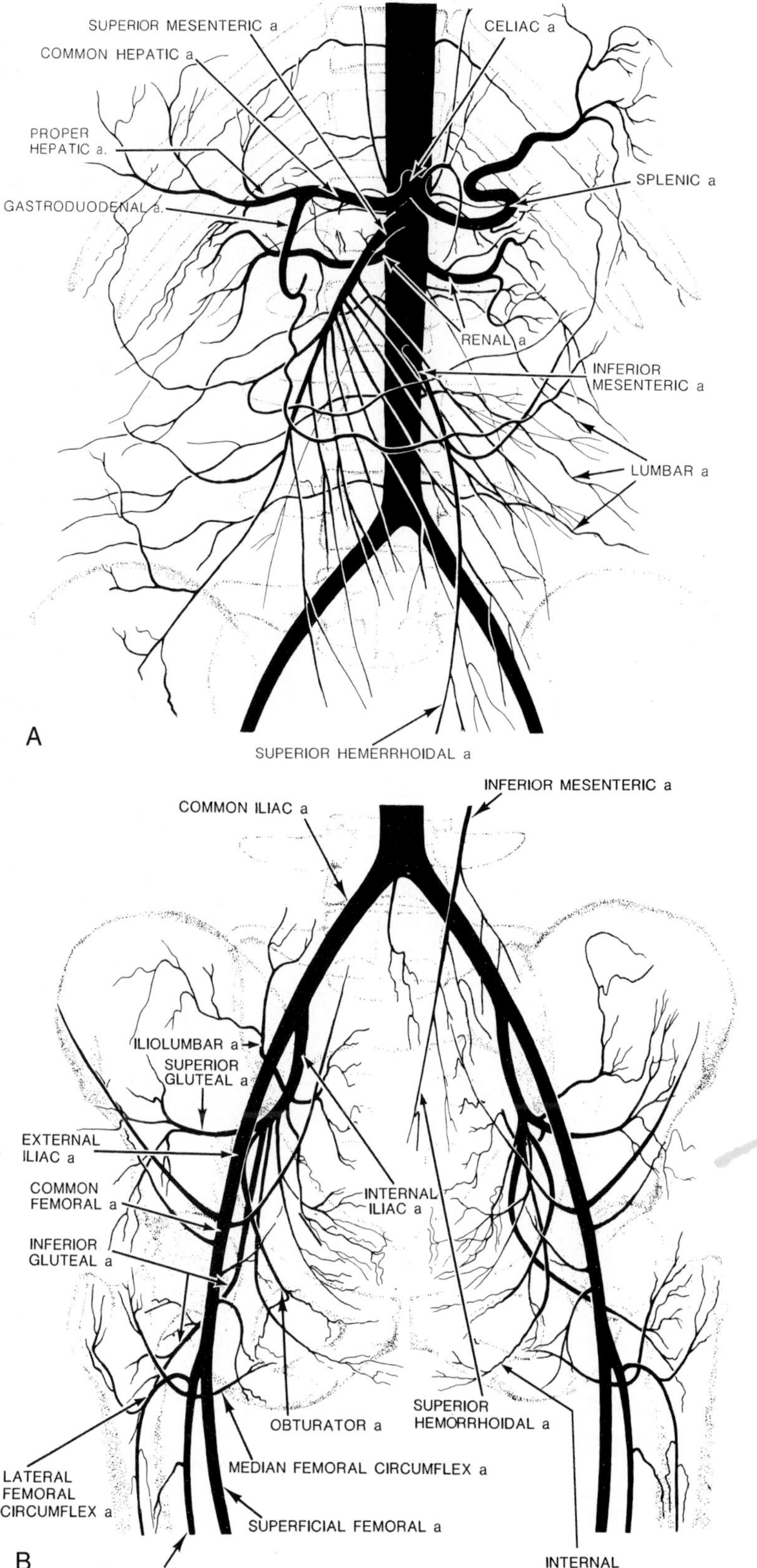

FIGURE 15–8 Arterial anatomy of the abdomen (*A*), pelvis (*B*), and lower extremity (*C*).

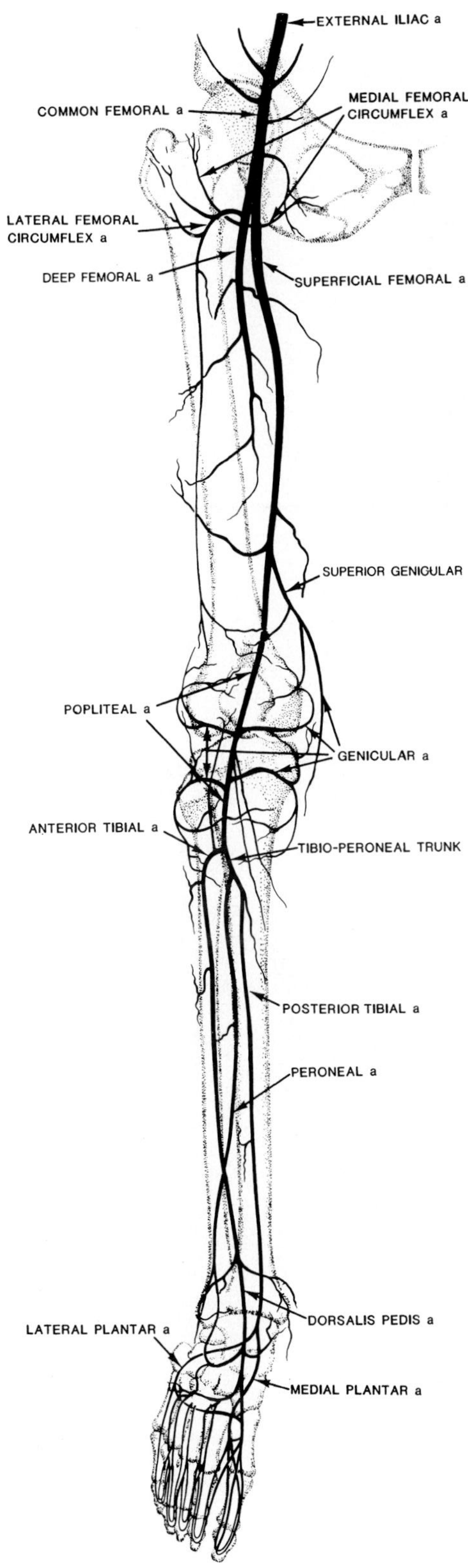

FIGURE 15–8 *Continued*

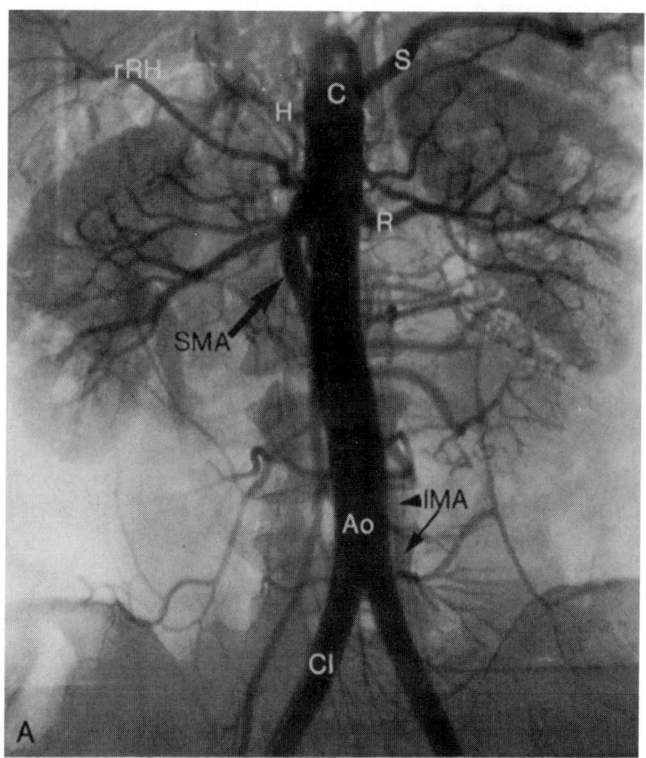

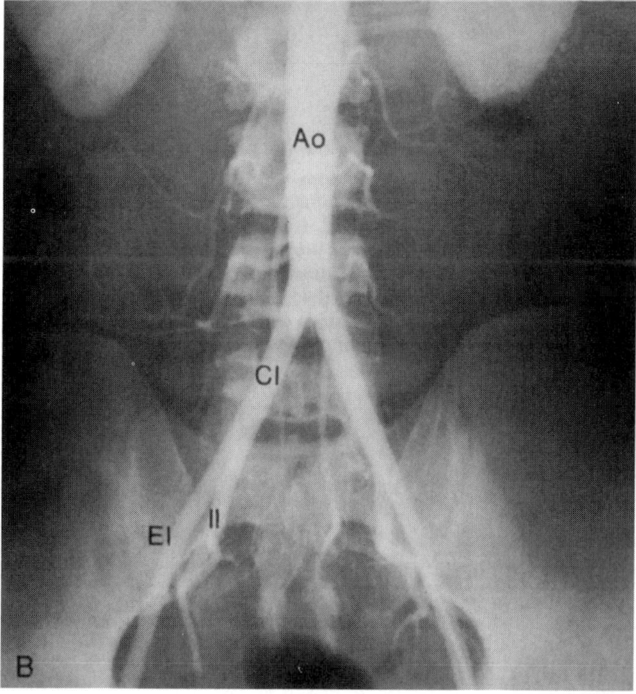

FIGURE 15–9 *A,* The abdominal aorta (Ao) terminates at its bifurcation into the common iliac arteries (CI) at the L4 vertebral level (S, splenic artery; H, hepatic artery; rRH, replaced right hepatic artery; R, left renal artery; SMA, superior mesenteric artery; IMA, inferior mesenteric artery). *B,* The common iliac arteries divide at the lumbosacral junction into the internal (II) and external iliac (EI) arteries. The internal iliac artery (also called the hypogastric artery) supplies the pelvic viscera and musculature. The branches of this artery become important collateral routes, as seen in other figures. The external iliac artery is continuous with the common femoral artery at the inguinal ligament, as shown in Figure 15–10.

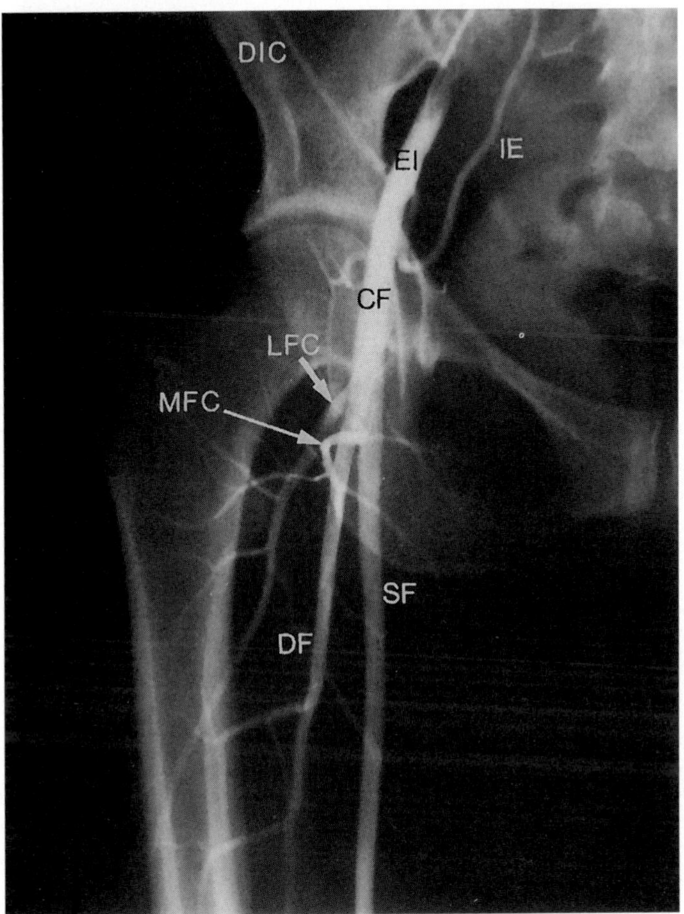

FIGURE 15–10 The external iliac artery (EI) is continuous with the common femoral artery (CF), which is a short segment (about 4 cm long). The common femoral artery bifurcates, forming the superficial (SF) and deep (DF) femoral arteries. A prominent branch, called the lateral femoral circumflex artery (LFC), arises dorsally, just before the common femoral artery divides. The superficial femoral artery (SF) continues throughout the thigh without major branches. The deep femoral artery (DF), also called the profunda femoris artery, has multiple muscular branches. The proximal muscular branches communicate with the pelvic arteries, and the distal branches communicate with tributaries of the popliteal artery at the knee. Thus, the deep femoral artery is an important collateral route, both for iliac and superficial femoral artery occlusion. IE = inferior epigastric artery; DIC = deep iliac circumflex artery; MFC = medial femoral circumflex artery.

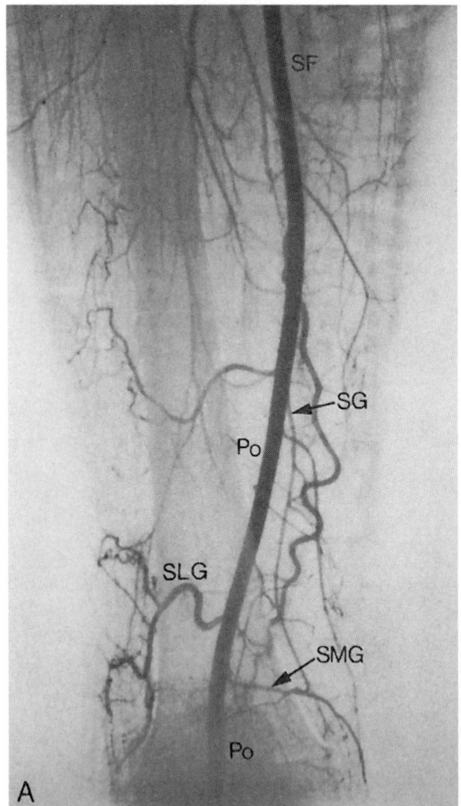

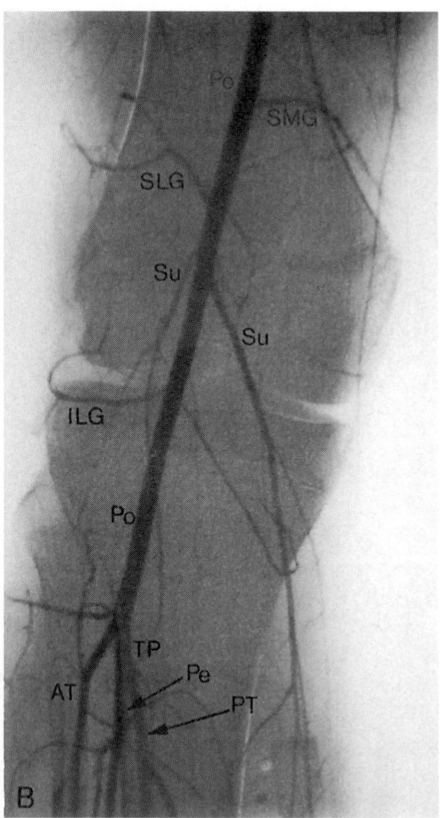

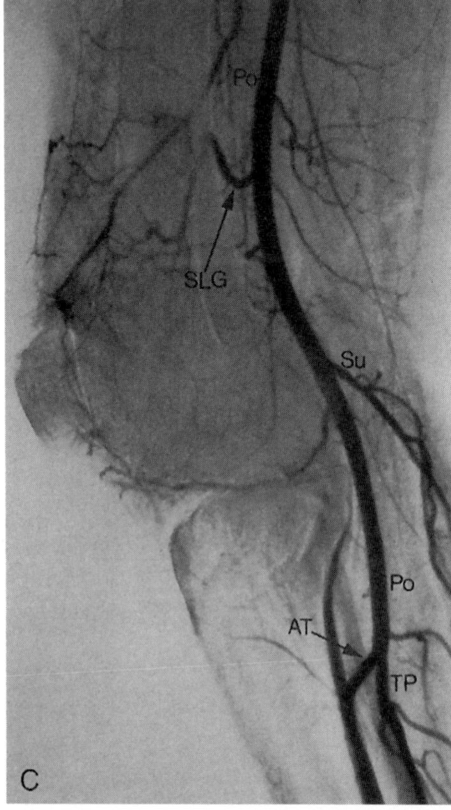

FIGURE 15–11 Anteroposterior (*A, B*) and lateral (*C*) views of the superficial femoral and popliteal arteries. In the distal portion of the thigh, the superficial femoral artery (SF) enters the adductor canal and becomes the popliteal artery (Po). This junction is also marked by the supreme genicular artery (SG). The popliteal artery passes behind the knee and ends, in most individuals, by bifurcating into the anterior tibial artery (AT) and the tibioperoneal trunk (TP). The genicular and sural arteries are important collateral routes for both superficial femoral and popliteal arterial obstruction. SG = supreme genicular artery; SLG = superior lateral genicular artery; ILG = inferior lateral genicular artery; SMG = superior medial genicular artery; Su = sural artery; Pe = peroneal artery; PT = posterior tibial artery.

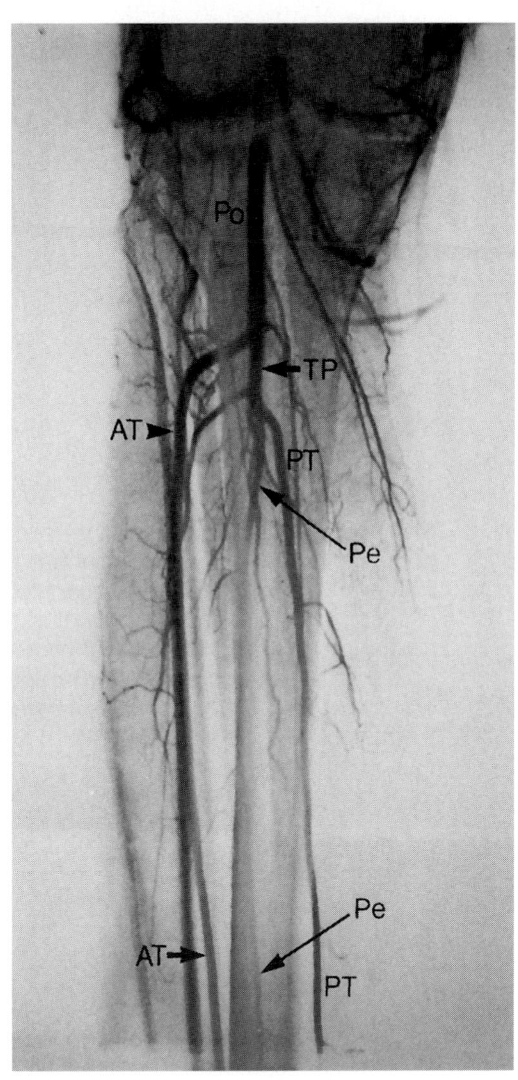

FIGURE 15–12 The anterior tibial artery (AT) courses anterolaterally from its origin and passes through the interosseous membrane. It then courses along the anterolateral aspect of the leg to the foot. The tibioperoneal trunk (TP) is of variable length, and usually bifurcates into the peroneal (Pe) and posterior tibial (PT) arteries. The peroneal artery, also seen in Figure 15–11*B,* extends down the leg to just above the ankle. The posterior tibial artery continues along a posteromedial course to the foot. Po = popliteal artery.

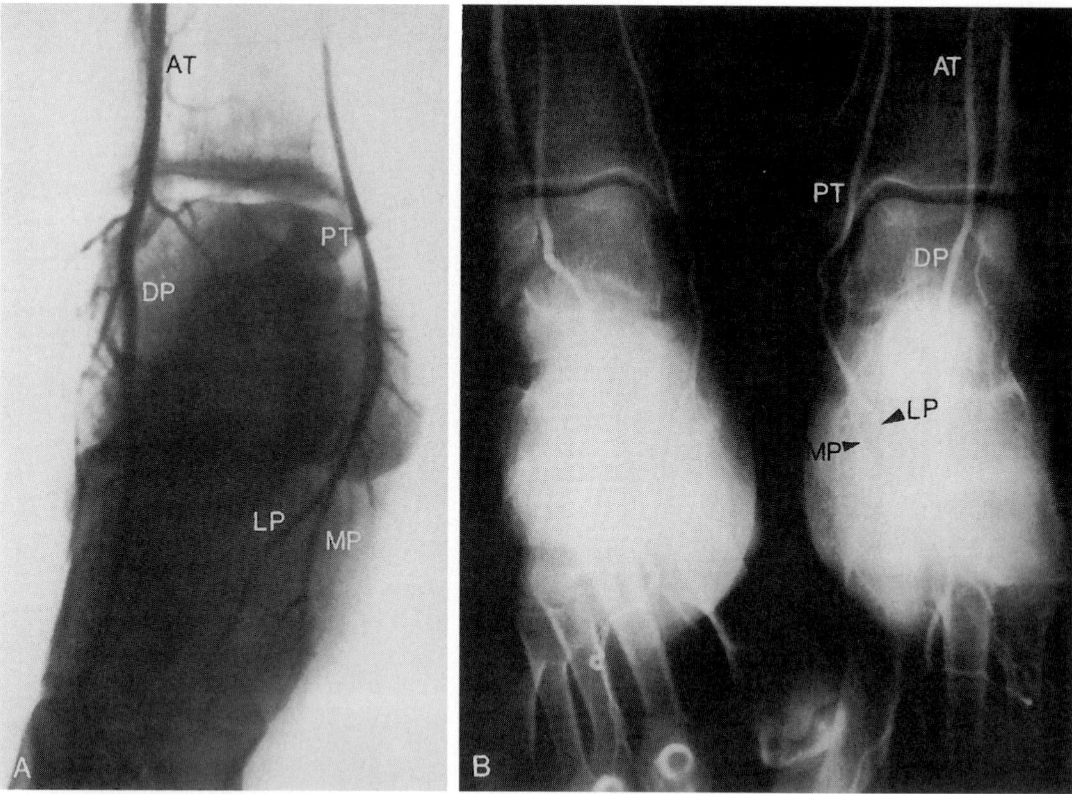

FIGURE 15–13 Oblique view of the right foot (*A*) and anteroposterior views of both feet (*B*). The anterior tibial artery (AT) courses onto the dorsum of the foot, where it becomes the dorsalis pedis artery (DP). The posterior tibial artery (PT) passes behind the medial malleolus and shortly thereafter bifurcates, forming the medial plantar (MP) and lateral plantar (LP) arteries. The plantar arch of the foot is formed by the union of the lateral plantar artery with the plantar metatarsal branch (not shown) of the dorsalis pedis artery. The plantar arch gives rise to the metatarsal and digital branches.

TABLE 15–2 ARTERIAL VARIANTS OF THE LOWER EXTREMITY

Variant	Frequency of Occurrence in the Population (%)
Duplication of the superficial femoral artery	Rare
High bifurcation of the popliteal artery	~4
High bifurcation of the popliteal artery, with the peroneal arising from the anterior tibial artery	~2
Normal level bifurcation of the popliteal artery, with the peroneal arising from the anterior tibial artery	Rare
Absent posterior tibial artery; may have distal reconstitution at the level of the ankle by way of the peroneal artery	1–5
Hypoplasia or aplasia of the anterior tibial artery with resultant absence of dorsalis pedis pulse	4–12
Anomalous location of the dorsalis pedis artery	8

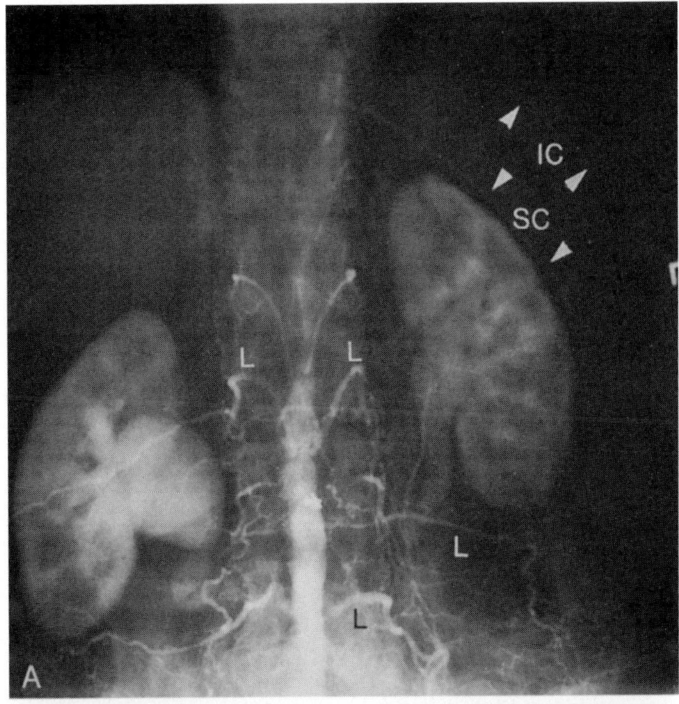

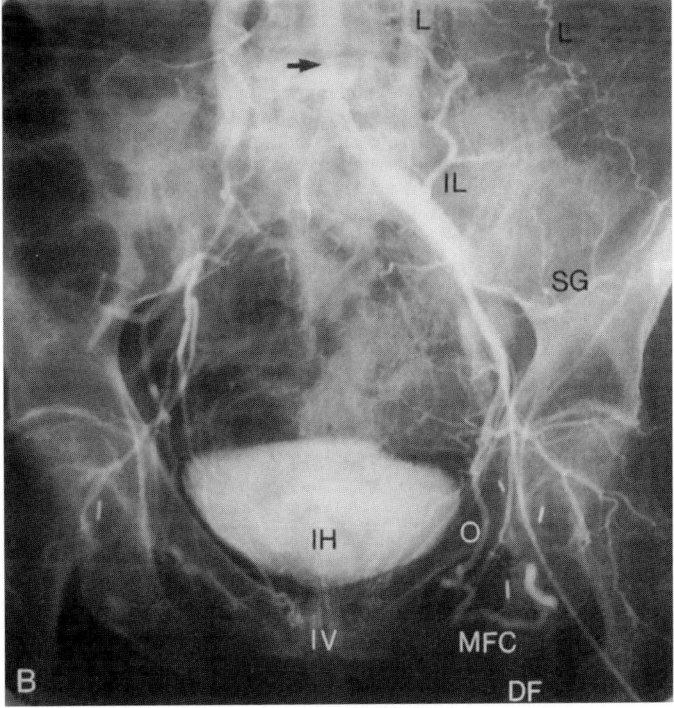

FIGURE 15–14 Aortic and iliac obstruction—superior (*A*) and inferior (*B*) segments. The site of a severe aortic stenosis is indicated by the *black arrow* in *B.* The right common iliac artery is occluded and the left external iliac artery is severely stenotic. The following collateral routes are apparent: (1) lumbar arteries (L) → to the iliolumbar (IL) and superior gluteal (SG) arteries; (2) intercostal (IC) and subcostal (SC) arteries (*arrowheads,* poorly opacified) → to the superior gluteal artery (SG); (3) obturator internis artery (O) → to the median femoral circumflex artery (MFC) and deep femoral artery (DF), circumventing the left external iliac obstruction; (4) inferior hemorrhoidal (IH) and inferior vesicle (IV) branches across the pelvis from the left to the right internal iliac system (circumventing the right common iliac occlusion).

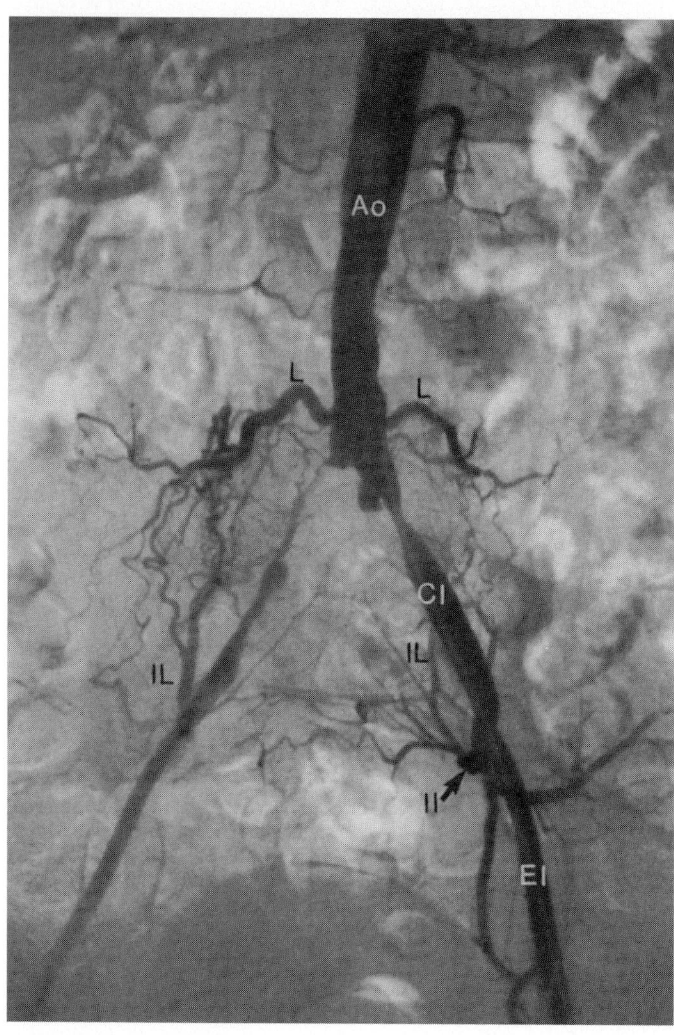

FIGURE 15–15 Right common iliac artery occlusion and left common iliac artery (CI) stenosis are circumvented by lumbar (L) collaterals, which communicate with iliolumbar (IL) branches of the internal iliac artery (II). The internal iliac artery, in turn, restores flow to the external iliac (EI) artery. Ao = aorta.

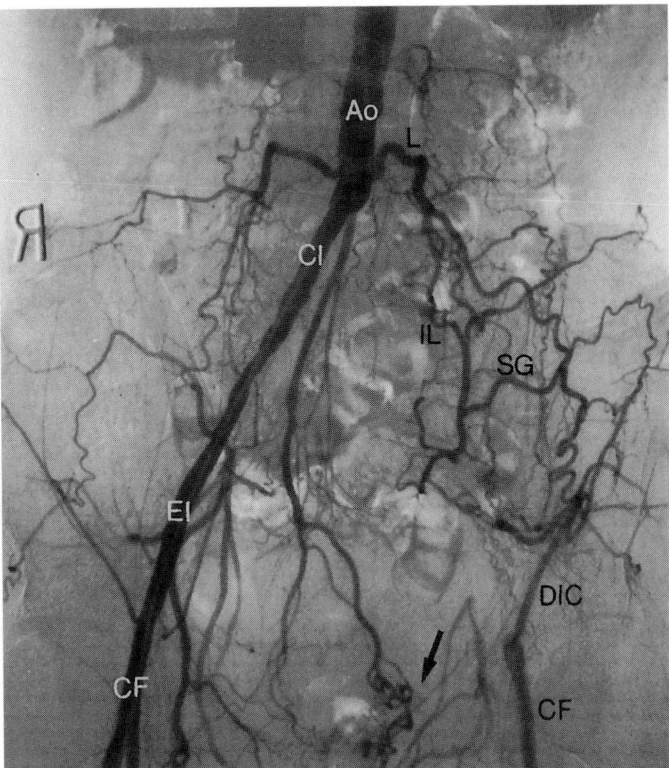

FIGURE 15–16 Hemorrhoidal collaterals (*arrow*) are of particular interest in this illustration. These branches of the inferior mesenteric artery illustrate the potential for collateralization from arteries that supply the gut. Prominent lumbar (L) → to gluteal (IL, SG) collaterals are evident on the left side. Ao = aorta; CI = common iliac artery; EI = external iliac artery; CF = common femoral artery; IL = iliolumbar artery; SG = superior gluteal artery; DIC = deep iliac circumflex artery.

ity arterial obstruction. The following is an outline of the more common collateral pathways.[4, 5]

1. Distal aorta or bilateral common iliac artery obstruction
   a. From thoracic and abdominal wall arteries to pelvic arteries distal to the obstruction
   b. From arteries of the bowel to pelvic arteries distal to the obstruction
   c. From lumbar arteries to pelvic arteries distal to the obstruction
2. Unilateral common iliac artery obstruction
   a. From contralateral iliac and/or femoral arteries to arteries of the pelvis or thigh distal to the obstruction
   b. Pathways as just mentioned, with supply to the ipsilateral pelvic arteries
3. External iliac and common femoral artery obstruction
   a. Collaterals arising primarily from ipsilateral pelvic arteries or contralateral pelvic and/or femoral arteries to supply arteries of the proximal thigh distal to the obstruction
   b. Previously mentioned pathways also possibly involved in varying degrees
4. Deep femoral artery obstruction
   a. Proximal ipsilateral pelvic arteries, contralateral pelvic arteries, and/or contralateral femoral arteries to the deep femoral artery distal to the obstruction
   b. The distal superficial femoral or popliteal arteries to the distal deep femoral artery
5. Superficial femoral or popliteal artery obstruction
   a. From the deep femoral artery to the distal superficial femoral artery or to the popliteal artery
   b. From the distal superficial femoral artery to the popliteal artery or to the proximal trifurcation vessels in the calf
   c. From the proximal to distal popliteal artery and/or popliteal artery to trifurcation vessels
6. Obstruction of trifurcation arteries
   a. From patent proximal calf branches to distal arteries in the lower leg or ankle
   b. From distal peroneal branches to distal anterior or posterior tibial arteries

It is important for vascular laboratory personnel to be familiar, in general terms, with these more commonly seen collateral path-

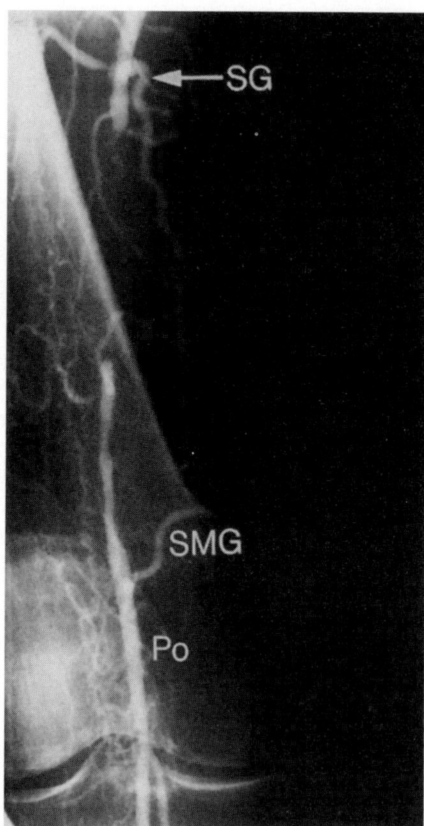

FIGURE 15–17 Occlusion of the proximal popliteal artery (Po) is circumvented by genicular collaterals (supreme genicular, SG → to superior medial genicular, SMG).

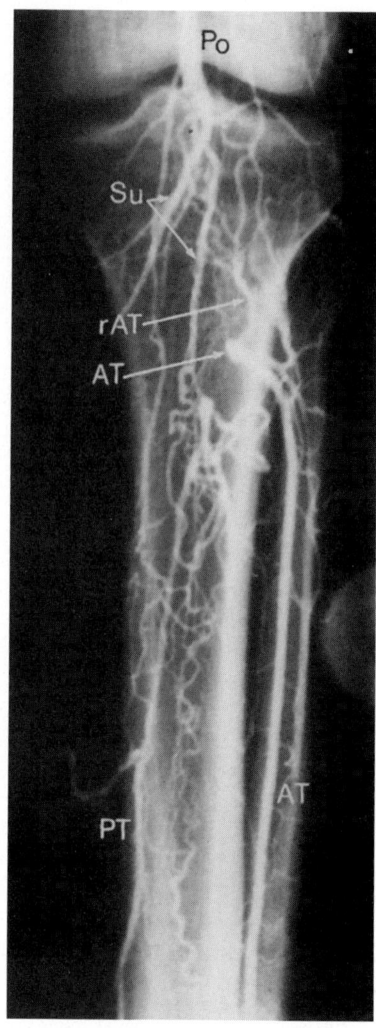

FIGURE 15–18 Distal popliteal (Po) artery occlusion is circumvented as follows: (1) sural (Su) and small muscular branches → to the recurrent anterior tibial artery (rAT), which supplies the anterior tibial artery (AT); (2) sural (Su) and small muscular branches → to the posterior tibial artery (PT).

ways. They are illustrated in Figures 15–14 to 15–18.

REFERENCES

1. Kadir S: Arteriography of the thoracic aorta. *In* Kadir S (ed): Diagnostic Angiography. Philadelphia, WB Saunders, 1986, pp 124–171.
2. Kadir S: Arteriography of the upper extremities. *In* Kadir S (ed): Diagnostic Angiography. Philadelphia, WB Saunders, 1986, pp 172–206.
3. Rose SC, Kadir S: Arterial anatomy of the upper extremity. *In* Kadir S: Atlas of Normal and Variant Angiographic Anatomy. Philadelphia, WB Saunders, 1991, pp 55–95.
4. Kadir S: Arteriography of the lower extremities. *In* Kadir S (ed): Diagnostic Angiography. Philadelphia, WB Saunders, 1986, pp 254–307.
5. Stieghorst MF, Crummy AB: Lower extremity arterial anatomy and collateral routs. *In* Zwiebel WJ (ed): Introduction to Vascular Ultrasonography, 2nd ed. Orlando, FL, Grune & Stratton, 1986, pp 278–303.
6. Muller RF, Figley MM, Rogoff SM, DeWeese JA: Arteries of the Abdomen, Pelvis and Lower Extremity. Rochester, NY, Eastman Kodak.

Chapter 16

Nonimaging Physiologic Tests for Assessment of Lower Extremity Arterial Disease

■ *R. Eugene Zierler, MD* ■ *D. Eugene Strandness, Jr., MD*

As indicated in Chapter 14, the basic purpose of lower extremity noninvasive testing is to document both the presence and severity of arterial disease. The importance of such documentation has been underscored by the study of Marinelli and colleagues,[1] in which 458 diabetic patients were evaluated prospectively for lower extremity arterial insufficiency. Arterial occlusive disease was documented by objective testing in 31% of patients who gave no history of claudication and in 21% with a normal physical examination.

Contrast arteriography may also be used to document lower extremity arterial disease. This technique is the standard method for preoperative assessment, and the precise anatomic information provided is essential in planning reconstructive arterial operations. There are certain limitations with arteriography, however, particularly in estimating the hemodynamic significance of stenoses. Single-plane views may underestimate the severity of disease whenever plaques do not produce concentric narrowing. The addition of multiple views may improve accuracy to some extent, but even then the problem of interpretation is considerable.[2–5] Furthermore, the presence of occlusive disease at multiple levels may make it difficult to predict which segment is most responsible for ischemic symptoms.[6, 7]

The limitations of contrast arteriography, together with the inherent invasiveness of this procedure, have stimulated the development of noninvasive physiologic methods for studying the arterial circulation of the lower extremities. Among the many devices and techniques that have been described,[8] those that employ Doppler ultrasound have been most widely applied and thoroughly evaluated. This chapter reviews Doppler and plethysmographic approaches to the evaluation of lower extremity arterial disease. The techniques described do not produce images of the arteries; hence, they are described as nonimaging or indirect methods. These techniques should not be confused with duplex sonography, which produces images of blood vessels. Duplex sonography of the lower extremities is discussed in Chapter 18.

INSTRUMENTATION

Doppler Flowmeters

The transmitting frequency of Doppler ultrasonic instruments used for peripheral arterial studies is in the range of 2 to 10 MHz. Because the depth in tissue to which the ultrasound beam penetrates is inversely proportional to the transmitting frequency, lower frequencies are best suited for examining deeply located vessels, such as those in the thigh. The Doppler effect refers to the shift in frequency that occurs when sound is reflected from a moving object. The Doppler shift in vascular diagnosis varies from a few hundred to several thousand cycles per second, and this signal can be amplified to provide an audible signal with a pitch (or frequency) that is directly proportional to blood velocity.

The simplest Doppler instruments used in peripheral vascular diagnosis are pocket-sized units with the audio output presented through earphones or a small loudspeaker. These are satisfactory for a rapid bedside arterial or venous examination. For more elaborate studies, a direction-sensing Doppler flowmeter (directional Doppler) is necessary to separate the forward- and reverse-flow components normally present in peripheral arteries.[9] The direction of flow may be indicated through stereo headphones, by deflections on a pair of meters, or as an analogue waveform on a strip chart recorder.

Pocket-sized Doppler devices and many directional instruments operate in the continuous wave mode. Because these instruments provide no information regarding distance from the ultrasound source, Doppler shifts resulting from motion in superimposed vessels are summed in the audible or analogue output. However, arterial and venous signals are easily distinguished by their different flow characteristics: venous flow produces low-frequency signals that vary with respiration, whereas arterial flow is associated with relatively high-frequency signals having pulsatile components that correspond to the cardiac cycle. Failure to obtain a Doppler signal from an artery usually indicates occlusion; however, extremely low flow rates (<2 cm/sec) do not produce a detectable Doppler shift.[10]

With pulsed wave ultrasound, it is possible to detect flow at discrete points along the sound beam.[11] This technique eliminates the problem of superimposed signals and permits characterization of flow patterns at specific sites in the arterial lumen. Pulsed wave Doppler devices have been employed in two imaging systems: the ultrasonic arteriograph for flow visualization[12] and the duplex scanner, which combines B-mode imaging and Doppler flow detection.[13, 14] These devices have been used extensively in the detection of carotid artery stenosis. Duplex scanning with spectral analysis of pulsed Doppler signals has also been used to assess abdominal and extremity arteries.[15–19] A more detailed discussion of basic principles and instrumentation in Doppler ultrasound is given in Chapter 2.

Plethysmographs

Plethysmographic techniques all rely on the measurement of volume changes in the extremities. Because these changes are primarily a result of alterations in blood volume, plethysmographic measurements can be used to assess blood flow parameters such as arterial pulsations and limb blood pressure. Most plethysmographs used in the noninvasive vascular laboratory measure volume indirectly, based on changes in limb circumference, electrical impedance, or reflectivity of infrared light.

The air-filled plethysmograph uses pneumatic cuffs that are placed around the limb being studied and inflated to a pressure in the range of 10 to 65 mm Hg.[20] This instrument is considered to be "segmental" because it measures only those volume changes in the limb segments surrounded by the cuffs. Enlargement of the enclosed limb segment with each arterial pulse compresses the air in the cuff, and the resulting increase in cuff pressure is recorded by a pressure transducer. Although the frequency response of air-filled plethysmographs is low (8 to 20 Hz), this method generally provides accurate volume pulse waveforms.

Strain-gauge plethysmography uses small silicone rubber tubes filled with mercury or a liquid-metal alloy.[21] This gauge is wrapped around the limb being studied and, as the encircled segment expands or contracts, the length of the strain gauge changes. Because the electrical resistance of the liquid-metal alloy in the gauge is proportional to its length, changes in limb circumference result in corresponding changes in the voltage drop across the gauge. Assuming that the limb resembles a cylinder, changes in limb circumference can be used to calculate changes in limb volume.[22] Thus, changes in gauge length or resistance are related to variations in volume. The high-frequency response of strain-gauge plethysmographs (up to 100 Hz) makes them particularly well suited for accurate recording of volume pulses in the limbs.[23] However, because they are also more sensitive and difficult to use in the clinical setting, this approach has not been used as widely as the other plethysmographic techniques.

Impedance plethysmography is based on the principle that the resistive impedance of a body segment is inversely proportional to its total fluid content. Therefore, changes in the blood volume of a limb are reflected by changes in electrical impedance.[23] The instrumentation usually includes four electrodes, an outer pair to send a weak current through the limb and an inner pair to sense the voltage drop. Impedance plethysmographs are relatively simple to operate and the results are easy to interpret. Impedance plethysmography has been one of the most popular methods for the noninvasive diagnosis of lower extremity deep vein thrombosis.

The sensor of the photoelectric plethysmograph contains an infrared light–emitting diode and a phototransistor. When this sensor is placed on the limb, the infrared light is transmitted into the superficial layers of the skin and the reflected portion is received by the phototransistor. The resulting signal is proportional to the quantity of red blood cells in the cutaneous circulation.[23] Although the photoelectric method does not measure actual volume changes, and is therefore not a true plethysmographic technique, the pulse waveforms obtained closely resemble those acquired with strain-gauge instruments. Photoelectric plethysmographs are frequently used in the vascular laboratory to detect blood flow when the application of Doppler or other plethysmographic techniques is especially difficult. For example, this technique can be used to detect arterial pulsations in the terminal portions of the digits.

Recording Devices

The indirect lower extremity arterial evaluation is based primarily on the noninvasive measurement of systolic blood pressures, the audible characteristics of arterial Doppler signals, and analogue waveforms derived from the Doppler signal. Although it is not usually necessary, the Doppler signals may be recorded on audiotape for subsequent analysis and review.

A simple device for generating an analogue waveform on a strip chart recorder is the zero crossing detector described in Chapter 2. Although this instrument is subject to errors and artifacts related to signal-to-noise ratio, amplitude dependency, and transient response,[24] it provides a graphic representation of the Doppler signal suitable for qualitative interpretation. Spectral analysis, as discussed in Chapter 3, is an alternative method for Doppler signal processing that overcomes the inherent limitations of the analogue waveform. This technique is usually considered part of duplex scanning.

Essential Equipment for Indirect Arterial Testing

The following is a brief description of the equipment needed for indirect lower extremity testing:

1. The qualitative assessment of arterial flow patterns requires a direction-sensing Doppler and a strip chart recorder coupled with a zero crossing detector.
2. The measurement of segmental systolic blood pressures in the extremities requires pneumatic cuffs of appropriate size, a manometer to measure cuff pressure, and a means for detecting distal flow. Any continuous wave Doppler or plethysmographic device can be used as a flow detector. The photoelectric plethysmograph is particularly valuable in situations in which low flow or arterial wall calcification makes Doppler flow detection difficult.

   A standard mercury or aneroid manometer is used to measure cuff pressure. Although cuff inflation can be accomplished manually, the examination is facilitated by using a rapid cuff inflator with a built-in manometer and an external air source.

   Cuff width is an important consideration in measurement of limb blood pressure.[25] To minimize cuff artifact, the cuff width should be at least 50% greater than the diameter of the limb in which pressure is being measured. The use of smaller cuffs results in the recording of falsely high pressures. Some laboratories use large cuffs, 18 to 20 cm wide, for the thigh and smaller, 12-cm-wide cuffs around the calf and ankle. The large thigh cuff allows only a single pressure measurement above the knee. An alternative method uses four 11-cm-wide cuffs placed at high-thigh (HT), above-knee (AK), below-knee (BK), and ankle levels. If the cuff artifact is properly accounted for, this technique can provide useful information on the distribution of occlusive arterial lesions in the lower extremity.[10, 26]
3. An electronic treadmill is required for exercise testing of patients with symptoms of lower limb claudication. One standard protocol uses a speed of 2 mph on a 12% grade; however, the speed and grade can be varied according to the individual limitations of each patient.[27]
4. The vascular laboratory should be kept warm enough to ensure the comfort of pa-

tients who must lie or walk with their limbs exposed during noninvasive testing. Cold-induced vasospasm may make arterial flow signals difficult to detect in patients with arterial occlusive disease. To avoid this problem, electric blankets are useful for keeping patients warm on the examining table.

METHODS FOR INDIRECT ARTERIAL TESTING AND THEIR PHYSIOLOGIC BASIS

Measurement of Arterial Pressure

In the arterial circulation, peak systolic pressure is amplified as the pulse wave progresses down the lower limb.[28] This amplification is a result of reflected waves originating from the relatively high peripheral resistance and differences in compliance between the central and peripheral arteries. Thus, the systolic pressure measured at the ankle is normally higher than that in the upper arm. However, the diastolic and mean pressures gradually decrease as the pulse wave moves distally.

Diastolic pressure in the lower limb is reduced only in the presence of severe proximal stenosis, but the peak systolic pressure decreases with lesser degrees of disease.[29] Therefore, determination of systolic blood pressure is most reliable for diagnosis of arterial narrowing. Normally, the mean pressure drop along the main arteries of the limb is minimal. The term *critical stenosis* has been used to describe the degree of narrowing that produces a significant drop in distal pressure or flow.[30] In the resting state, distal pressure is reduced by stenoses that decrease luminal diameter by about 50% or more. Because the critical stenosis value is flow dependent, lesser degrees of narrowing may be detected by increasing flow with exercise or reactive hyperemia.

It should be emphasized that blood pressure and flow are not necessarily altered to the same extent by arterial occlusive disease. Resting calf blood flow in patients with intermittent claudication seldom differs significantly from that measured in normal individuals.[31] Normal flow can be maintained distal to stenoses by a compensatory decrease in peripheral resistance, which results in a lowered peripheral pressure.

Ankle Pressure

The systolic pressure at any level of the lower extremity can be measured by positioning a pneumatic cuff at the desired site. Any patent artery distal to the cuff that is accessible to Doppler ultrasound can be used for flow detection, but the posterior tibial (PT) and dorsalis pedis (DP) arteries are usually most convenient. When the cuff is inflated to above systolic pressure, the arterial flow signal disappears. As cuff pressure is gradually lowered to slightly below systolic pressure, the flow signal reappears, and the pressure at which flow resumes is recorded as the systolic pressure. It is important to recognize that the level of pressure measurement is determined by cuff position and not by the site of Doppler flow detection.

Measurement of ankle systolic pressure is the most valuable physiologic test for assessing the arterial circulation in the lower limb. If the pressure measured by a cuff placed just above the malleoli is less than that of the upper arm, proximal occlusive disease in the arteries to the lower limb is invariably present.[21, 32, 33] In addition, the degree of reduction in ankle systolic pressure is proportional to the severity of arterial obstruction.[33] Patients with severe arterial occlusive disease and ischemic rest pain usually have ankle systolic pressures below 40 mm Hg. Occlusive lesions in the small arteries distal to the ankle cannot be detected by this method.

Ankle Pressure Index

Because the ankle systolic pressure varies with the central aortic pressure, it is desirable to compare each ankle pressure measurement with the simultaneous aortic pressure. The brachial systolic pressure measured by an upper arm cuff is essentially equal to central aortic pressure, assuming the subclavian and axillary arteries are not obstructed. The ratio of ankle systolic pressure to brachial systolic pressure is called the ankle pressure index. The use of this index compensates for variation in central perfusion pressure and allows direct comparison of serial tests.[32]

In the absence of proximal arterial occlusive disease, the ankle pressure index is always greater than 1, with a mean value of 1.11 ± 0.10.[34] Although the ankle pressure index does not discriminate among occlusions at various levels, in general, limbs with single-level occlusions have indexes greater than 0.5 and limbs with lesions at multiple levels have indexes less than 0.5.[33]

The ankle pressure index provides a general guide to the degree of functional disability in the lower extremity. In limbs with intermittent claudication, the ankle pressure index ranges from about 0.2 to 1.0, with a mean value of 0.59 ± 0.15.[34] This rather wide range is explained by differing levels of physical activity and pain tolerance among individuals. The ankle pressure index in limbs with ischemic rest pain ranges from 0 to 0.65, with a mean of 0.26 ± 0.13. Limbs with impending gangrene tend to have the lowest ankle pressures, with a mean ankle pressure index of 0.05 ± 0.08. Many limbs with impending gangrene or ischemic ulceration have absent Doppler flow signals at the ankle level. Although the ankle pressure index reflects the overall severity of arterial occlusive disease in the lower extremity, it is clear that there is considerable overlap among values from patients with different clinical presentations. Therefore, the ankle pressure index must be combined with other clinical information to determine the functional status of each patient.

Segmental Pressures in the Lower Extremity

The ankle pressure index cannot determine the location of proximal arterial lesions, nor does it indicate the relative significance of lesions at multiple levels. Some of this information may be obtained by measuring systolic pressure at various levels in patients with limbs exhibiting an abnormal ankle pressure.[21] In the procedure described here, four pneumatic cuffs, 83 cm long and 11 cm wide, with 41-cm-long inflatable bladders, are used on each leg. The cuffs are applied at HT, AK, BK, and ankle levels. Systolic pressure is determined at each level using the Doppler technique outlined previously. The Doppler probe can be placed over the PT or DP arteries for all measurements (Fig. 16–1).

The systolic pressure in the proximal thigh, as measured by the cuff method, normally exceeds brachial systolic pressure by 30 to 40 mm Hg. Direct intra-arterial pressure measurements have shown that the actual pressures in the brachial and common femoral arteries are identical[35]; however, the use of a relatively small cuff on the thigh results in a significant cuff artifact. The ratio of HT systolic pressure to brachial systolic pressure (thigh pressure index) is normally greater than 1.2.[36] An index between 0.8 and 1.2 suggests aortoiliac stenosis, whereas an index less than 0.8 is consistent with complete iliac occlusion. Although the thigh pressure index usually reflects iliac inflow to the common femoral artery, the combination of superficial femoral occlusion and profunda femoris stenosis may also result in reduced HT pressure.

The difference in systolic pressure between any two adjacent levels in the leg should be

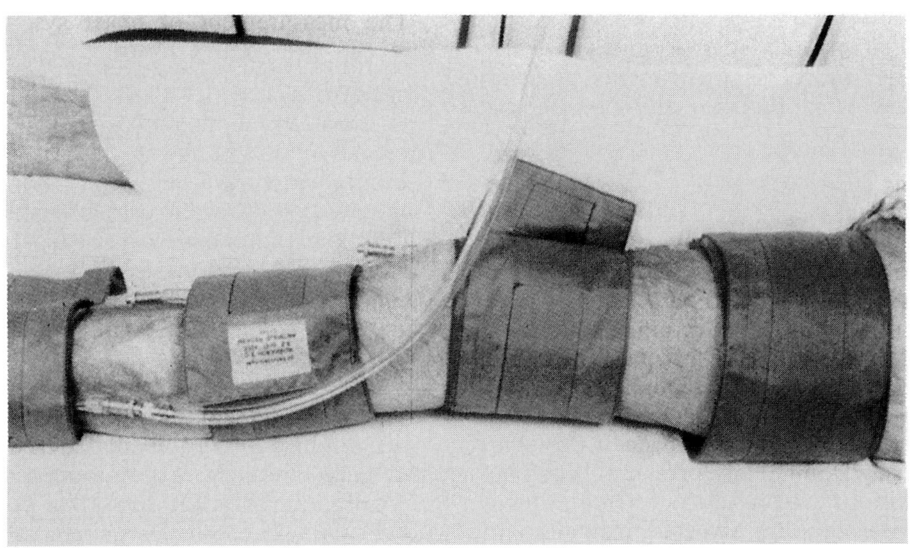

FIGURE 16–1 Cuffs are applied at high-thigh, above-knee, below-knee, and ankle levels for measurement of segmental pressures.

less than 20 mm Hg in normal individuals.[21] Gradients in excess of 20 mm Hg usually indicate significant occlusive disease in the intervening arterial segment: an HT-AK gradient reflects superficial femoral disease; an AK-BK gradient reflects popliteal disease; and a BK-ankle gradient reflects disease in the tibial and peroneal arteries.[10] In addition to vertical gradients down a single leg, the horizontal gradients between corresponding segments of the two legs may also suggest the presence of occlusive lesions. The systolic pressures measured at the same level in both legs normally should not differ by more than 20 mm Hg.

Toe Pressure

Measurement of toe pressure can be used to identify obstructive disease involving the pedal arch and digital arteries that does not produce changes in the ankle systolic pressure. Toe pressure is also valuable when the ankle pressure is found to be spuriously high because of proximal arterial calcification. Because of the smaller size and lower flow rates of digital arteries, flow detection by Doppler methods is usually difficult. In this situation, a photoelectric plethysmograph is especially useful.

The ratio of toe systolic pressure to brachial systolic pressure (toe pressure index) ranges from 0.80 to 0.90 in normal individuals.[37] The mean toe pressure index is 0.35 ± 0.15 in patients with intermittent claudication and 0.11 ± 0.10 in patients with rest pain or ischemic ulceration.[38] There appears to be no significant difference in mean toe pressure indexes between diabetic and nondiabetic patients.

Exercise and Reactive Hyperemia Testing

Lower extremity exercise and reactive hyperemia both increase limb blood flow by causing vasodilatation of peripheral resistance vessels. In limbs with normal arteries, this increased flow occurs with little or no decrease in ankle systolic pressure. When occlusive lesions are present in the main lower limb arteries, blood is diverted through high-resistance collateral pathways. Although the collateral circulation may provide adequate flow to the resting extremity with only a modest reduction in ankle pressure, the capability of collateral vessels to increase flow during exercise is limited. Pressure gradients, which are minimal at rest, may be accentuated when flow rates are increased by exercise. Thus, stress testing provides a method for detecting less severe degrees of arterial disease.

Treadmill Exercise

Standard treadmill exercise at 2 mph on a 12% grade is the simplest way to stress the lower limb circulation.[27] Treadmill testing is advantageous because it simulates the activity that produces the patient's symptoms and determines the degree of disability under controlled physiologic conditions. It also permits an assessment of nonvascular factors that may affect performance, such as musculoskeletal or cardiopulmonary disease. The ability to perform treadmill exercise is limited, however, by patient effort, motivation, and pain tolerance.

Walking on the treadmill is continued for 5 minutes or until symptoms occur and the patient is forced to stop. The walking time and nature of any symptoms are recorded, and the ankle and arm systolic pressures are measured before and immediately after exercise. Two components of the response to exercise are evaluated: (1) the magnitude of the immediate decrease in ankle systolic pressure; and (2) the time for recovery to resting pressure. Changes in both these parameters are proportional to the severity of arterial occlusive disease.

A normal response to exercise is a slight increase or no change in the ankle systolic pressure compared with the resting value (Fig. 16–2). If the ankle pressure is decreased immediately after exercise, the test is considered positive, and repeated measurements are taken at 1- to 2-minute intervals for up to 10 minutes, or until the pressure returns to pre-exercise levels. When a patient is forced to stop walking because of symptomatic arterial occlusive disease, the ankle systolic pressure in the affected limb is usually less than 60 mm Hg. If symptoms occur without a significant fall in the ankle pressure, a nonvascular cause of leg pain must be considered.

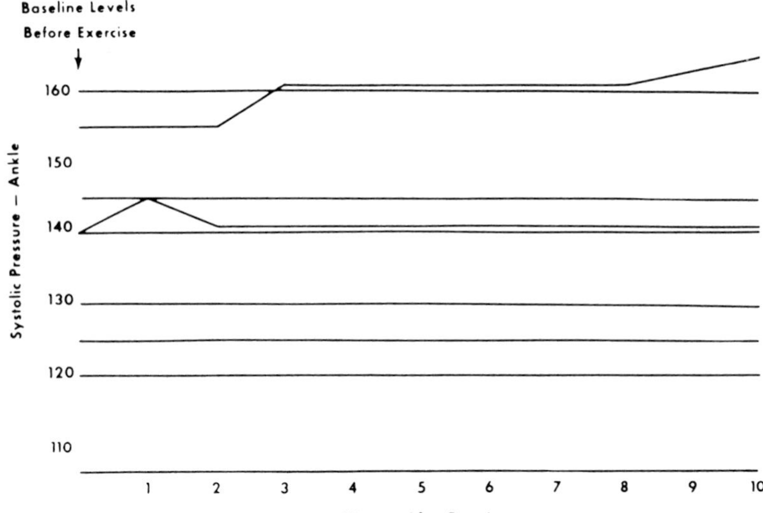

FIGURE 16–2 Ankle systolic pressure values are shown for eight normal subjects after walking on the treadmill for 5 minutes at 2 mph on a 12% grade. In each case the ankle pressure either remained at the pre-exercise level or increased slightly. (From Strandness DE: Abnormal exercise responses after successful reconstructive arterial surgery. Surgery 59:326, 1966.)

The postexercise ankle pressure changes in patients with symptomatic arterial disease can be divided into three groups.[33] Ankle pressures that fall to low or unrecordable levels immediately after exercise and then rise toward resting values in 2 to 6 minutes suggest occlusion or stenosis at a single level, such as the superficial femoral artery. When ankle pressures remain decreased or unrecordable for up to 12 minutes, lesions involving multiple arterial levels are almost always present. Rarely, this pattern may occur with an isolated iliac artery occlusion. In patients with ischemic rest pain, postexercise ankle pressures may remain unrecordable for 15 minutes or more.

Reactive Hyperemia Testing

Reactive hyperemia testing is an alternate method for stressing the peripheral circulation.[39] Inflating a pneumatic cuff at thigh level to suprasystolic pressure for 3 to 5 minutes produces ischemia and vasodilatation distal to the cuff. The changes in ankle pressure that occur on release of cuff occlusion are similar to those observed in the treadmill test. However, although normal limbs do not show a drop in ankle systolic pressure after treadmill exercise, a transient drop does occur with reactive hyperemia.[40] This decrease in ankle pressure is in the range of 17 to 34%.[40] In patients with arterial disease, there is a good correlation between the maximum pressure drop with reactive hyperemia and the maximum pressure drop after treadmill exercise. There may be considerable overlap in the ankle pressure response to reactive hyperemia among normal subjects and patients with arterial disease.[41] Patients with single-level arterial disease show less than a 50% drop in ankle pressure with reactive hyperemia, whereas patients with multiple-level arterial disease show a pressure drop greater than 50%.[40] Reactive hyperemia testing is useful for those patients who cannot walk on the treadmill because of amputations or other physical disabilities. Treadmill exercise is generally preferred over reactive hyperemia testing, because the former produces a physiologic stress that reproduces a patient's ischemic symptoms.

Doppler Signal Waveform Analysis

Qualitative analysis of the arterial flow pattern can be performed by simply listening to the Doppler audio output. An experienced examiner learns to recognize the high-pitched, harsh character and the changes in phasic components of the Doppler signal that are associated with stenoses. A graphic display of the velocity waveform permits more objective analysis. The previously dsecribed zero crossing detector is a convenient method for generating analogue waveforms on a strip chart recorder, and the output of this device closely resembles that of an electromagnetic flowmeter (Fig. 16–3).

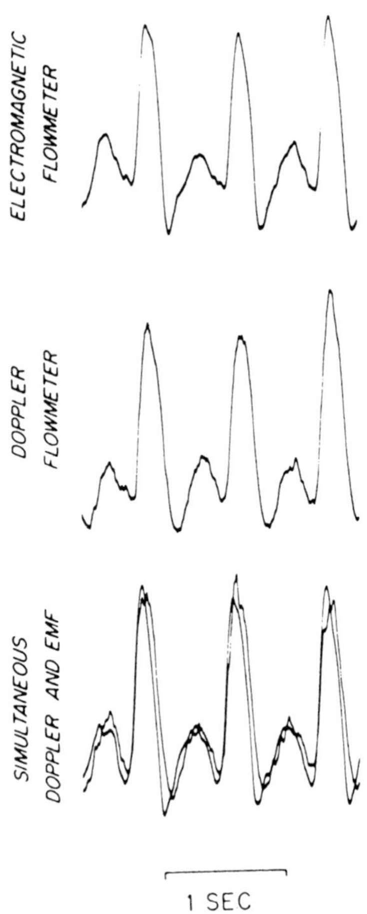

FIGURE 16–3 Comparison of electromagnetic and Doppler flow tracings obtained from the carotid artery of a dog shows their similarity. (From Strandness DE, Sumner DS: Hemodynamics for Surgeons. New York, Grune & Stratton, 1975, p 41.)

The Arterial Analogue Waveform

The flow pattern in the main arteries of the lower extremity normally has three components or phases during each cardiac cycle. The first phase has the highest Doppler frequency and is the large, forward velocity peak produced by cardiac systole. This is followed by a second, brief phase of flow reversal in early diastole and a third, low-frequency phase of forward flow in late diastole (Fig. 16–4). This triphasic flow pattern is modified by various factors, one of the most important being peripheral vascular resistance. For example, body heating, which causes vasodilatation and decreased resistance, abolishes the second phase of flow reversal; the opposite occurs on exposure to cold.

When a waveform is obtained from an arterial site *distal* to a stenosis or occlusion, a single, forward velocity component is observed, with flow remaining above the zero line throughout the cardiac cycle. The peak systolic frequency is lower than normal, and the waveform becomes flat and rounded (see Fig. 16–4). These changes result from decreased velocity of flow and from the compensatory fall in peripheral resistance that occurs in limbs with arterial occlusive disease.

If the Doppler probe is placed *directly over* a stenotic lesion, the signal has an abnormally high peak systolic frequency. This reflects the increased flow velocity in the stenotic segment. The character of Doppler signals obtained *proximal* to an arterial obstruction depends on the capability of the collateral circulation. If there are well-developed collaterals between the Doppler probe and the point of obstruction, the waveform may be normal. The flow signal obtained immediately proximal to an obstruction, when there is no collateral outflow, has

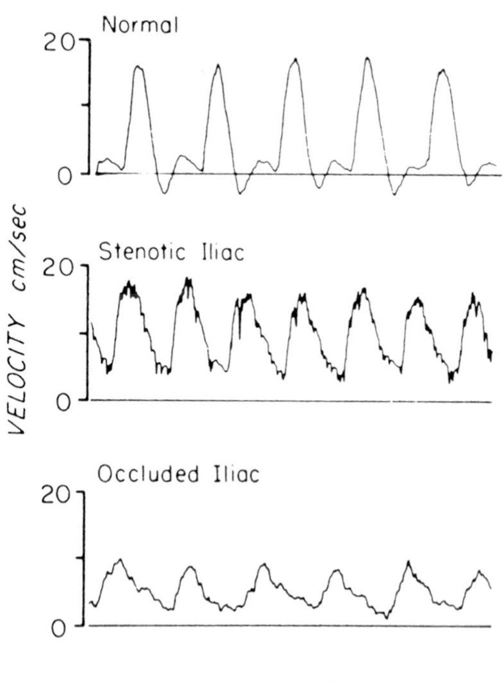

FIGURE 16–4 Velocity patterns obtained with a directional Doppler flowmeter from the femoral artery of a normal subject, a patient with a stenotic external iliac artery, and a patient with an occluded common iliac artery. The triphasic pattern in the normal artery includes a brief phase of flow reversal. Flow velocity is proportional to Doppler frequency. (From Strandness DE, Sumner DS: Hemodynamics for Surgeons. New York, Grune & Stratton, 1975, p 257.)

a harsh quality and has been described as a "thumping" sound.[42] Failure to obtain a flow signal over a vessel indicates occlusion or, rarely, a flow velocity too low to produce a detectable Doppler frequency shift.

Parameters Derived From the Velocity Waveform

Because the magnitude of the Doppler shift is directly proportional to the cosine of the beam-to-vessel angle, θ, as discussed in Chapter 2, a direct quantitative analysis of the velocity waveform requires a value for this angle. Accurate measurement of the beam-to-vessel angle is difficult with simple, hand-held Doppler equipment; however, quantitative data can still be obtained by using ratios of Doppler shifts that are independent of the beam-to-vessel angle.

One such ratio is the pulsatility index (PI), which is calculated by dividing the peak-to-peak frequency difference by the mean frequency (Fig. 16–5). Measurements for calculating PI can be based on either analogue waveforms or the output of a spectrum analyzer. The use of analogue waveforms has been criticized on the grounds that they may contain errors and artifacts.[24] Nonetheless, there is a close correlation between reduction in PI and the severity of arterial occlusive disease as assessed by arteriography and ankle pressure measurement.[43] The PI of the normal common femoral artery has a mean value of 6.7. More distally, the PI increases to 8 in the popliteal and 14.1 in the PT artery.[44] These values decrease in the presence of proximal occlusive lesions. In a study that compared common femoral artery PI with intra-arterial pressure measurement, a PI value greater than or equal to 4 was highly predictive of a hemodynamically normal aortoiliac segment.[45] The predictive value of a PI less than 4 depended on the condition of the superficial femoral artery. When the superficial femoral artery was patent, a PI less than 4 indicated a hemodynamically significant aortoiliac lesion, but a low PI value with an occluded superficial femoral artery was not diagnostic.

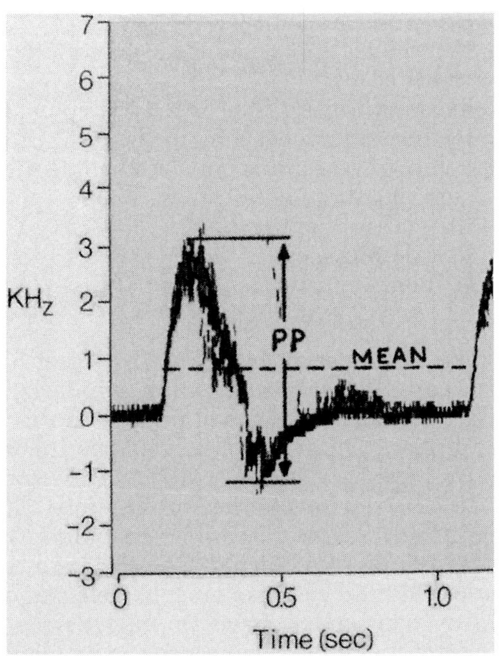

FIGURE 16–5 The pulsatility index (PI) is calculated by dividing the peak-to-peak frequency difference (PP) by the mean frequency. The waveform was produced by a spectrum analyzer. (From Knox RA, Strandness DE: Ultrasound techniques for evaluation of lower extremity arterial occlusion. Semin Ultrasound 2:271, 1981.)

Another approach to velocity waveform analysis is the Laplace transform (LT) method.[46, 47] For LT analysis, the waveform shape is expressed mathematically by a curve-fitting technique, and a damping coefficient that indicates lumen size is calculated. A comparison of common femoral artery PI and LT damping values indicated that the LT method was more sensitive in the detection of iliac artery stenoses.[46] Furthermore, the LT damping results were not affected by the presence or absence of occlusive disease in the superficial femoral artery. Thus, LT damping would be a more useful diagnostic test than PI in patients with multiple-level arterial occlusive disease.

A summary of the measurements and indexes used in lower extremity arterial diagnosis is given in Table 16–1.

Plethysmographic Assessment of Arterial Flow

Pulse Plethysmography

The soft tissues of the extremities expand and contract as blood moves through them with each cardiac cycle. By using a plethysmograph, these changes can be detected as a volume pulse (Fig. 16–6). Tissue volume initially increases during systole when arte-

TABLE 16–1 SUMMARY OF MEASUREMENTS AND INDEXES FOR THE LOWER EXTREMITY

Parameter	Value
Ankle systolic pressure	Normally exceeds brachial systolic pressure
Ankle pressure index	Normally > 1
High-thigh systolic pressure	Normally 30–40 mm Hg > brachial systolic pressure
Thigh pressure index	Normally > 1.2
Segmental pressure gradients	Normally <20 mm Hg between adjacent levels on the same leg or the same levels on the two legs
Toe systolic pressure	Normally 80–90% of brachial systolic pressure
Treadmill exercise test	Normal walking time 5 min without symptoms or drop in ankle systolic pressure (2 mph, 12% grade)

rial inflow exceeds venous outflow. The volume of the part decreases during diastole as inflow diminishes and outflow predominates. There is often a brief period of retrograde flow in the peripheral arteries during early diastole, and this flow reversal produces the dicrotic notch on the downslope of the volume pulse.

Although segmental plethysmography of the limbs can be performed with either air-filled or strain-gauge instruments, the air-filled method has been most popular.[20] As shown in Figure 16–7, the normal volume pulse rises rapidly to a sharp peak during systole and falls more slowly in diastole. The downslope of the normal volume pulse is bowed toward the baseline and includes the dicrotic notch mentioned earlier. With proximal arterial occlusive disease, one of the earliest changes in the volume pulse is loss of the dicrotic notch. When the proximal disease is more severe, the systolic rise becomes slower, the peak is delayed with a flat or rounded shape, and the downslope is bowed away from the baseline (see Fig. 16–7). Because segmental pressure measurements are more easily obtained than segmental plethysmographic measurements, the latter are not widely used in the routine noninvasive evaluation of the extremities. Segmental volume pulses may be valuable, however, when pressure measurements are artifactually elevated because of medial calcification.

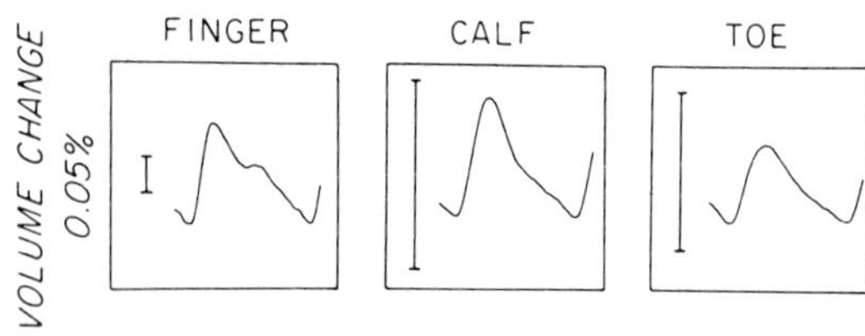

FIGURE 16–6 Normal plethysmographic volume pulses. Vertical bars indicate a 0.05% volume change. The dicrotic notch can be seen best on the downslope of the finger volume pulse. (From Strandness DE, Sumner DS: Hemodynamics for Surgeons. New York, Grune & Stratton, 1975, p 227.)

LOWER EXTREMITY ARTERIAL EXAMINATION

The sequence of noninvasive tests used in the routine lower extremity arterial examination can be summarized as follows:

1. Measurement of ankle pressures (DP and PT) and brachial pressures at rest
2. Calculation of ankle pressure indexes
3. Segmental pressure gradients, if ankle pressures are abnormal
4. Common femoral artery velocity waveforms at rest
5. Treadmill exercise or reactive hyperemia testing with repeat common femoral artery velocity waveforms and serial ankle pressure measurements
6. Special studies
   a. Toe pressure
   b. Plethysmography
   c. Duplex scanning

The examination begins with a brief history and physical examination emphasizing the symptoms and signs of peripheral vascular disease. The status of palpable peripheral pulses, the location of bruits, and the presence of ischemic skin lesions are noted. If a significant degree of cardiac or pulmonary disease is present, the patient's ability to perform treadmill exercise must be determined.

Any continuous wave Doppler device is satisfactory for measuring ankle or segmental limb pressures. Initially, ankle systolic pressure should be measured in both the DP and PT arteries (Fig. 16–8). Bilateral brachial pressures are also measured using the same Doppler technique. The ankle pressure index

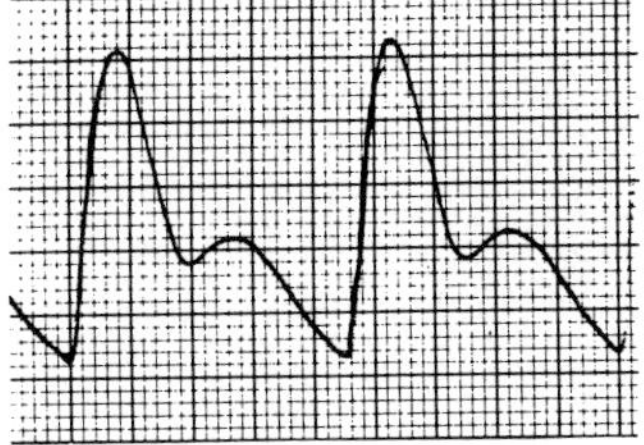

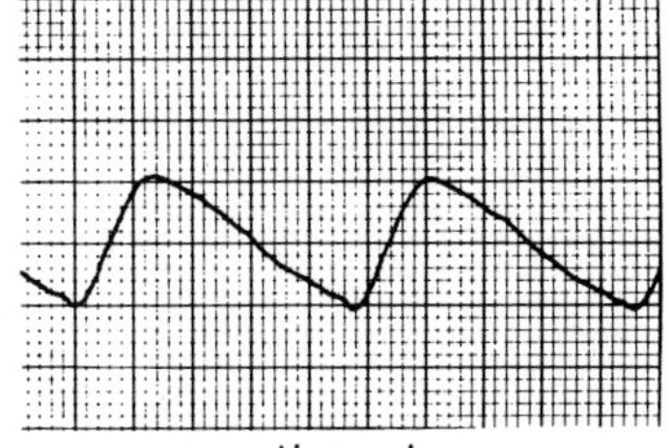

FIGURE 16–7 Normal and abnormal lower extremity volume pulse waveforms.

for each leg is calculated by dividing the highest ankle pressure by the highest brachial pressure. When the ankle pressure index is normal, measurement of segmental pressure gradients is not necessary. In limbs with severe arterial disease and no detectable flow signals at the ankle, thigh pressures can often be obtained by using the popliteal artery flow signal.

Analogue waveforms are usually recorded with a direction-sensing continuous wave Doppler and a strip chart recorder incorporating a zero crossing detector. The Doppler angle is adjusted by visual inspection of the waveform to minimize noise and artifact. Although waveforms can be obtained from any site with a Doppler signal, only the common femoral artery waveform is routinely recorded in most cases. This waveform is helpful in detecting proximal aortoiliac occlusive lesions. It is valuable to record the common femoral artery waveforms both before and immediately after treadmill exercise or reactive hyperemia testing, because some less severe lesions are apparent only at increased flow rates.

Stress testing with treadmill exercise or reactive hyperemia can be tolerated by most patients who do not have ischemic rest pain. As previously stated, the treadmill test is preferred because it is a more physiologic form of stress. The speed and grade of the electronic treadmill can be varied to suit the individual patient, but the standard test is done at 2 mph and a 12% grade. It is convenient to have the patient wear ankle cuffs and an arm cuff while walking on the treadmill (Fig. 16–9). Immediately after cessation of exercise, the patient returns to the examining table and ankle and arm pressures are measured. Serial ankle pressure measurements are then made at about 1-minute intervals for up to 10 minutes, or until they return to pre-exercise values. An automatic cuff inflator facilitates

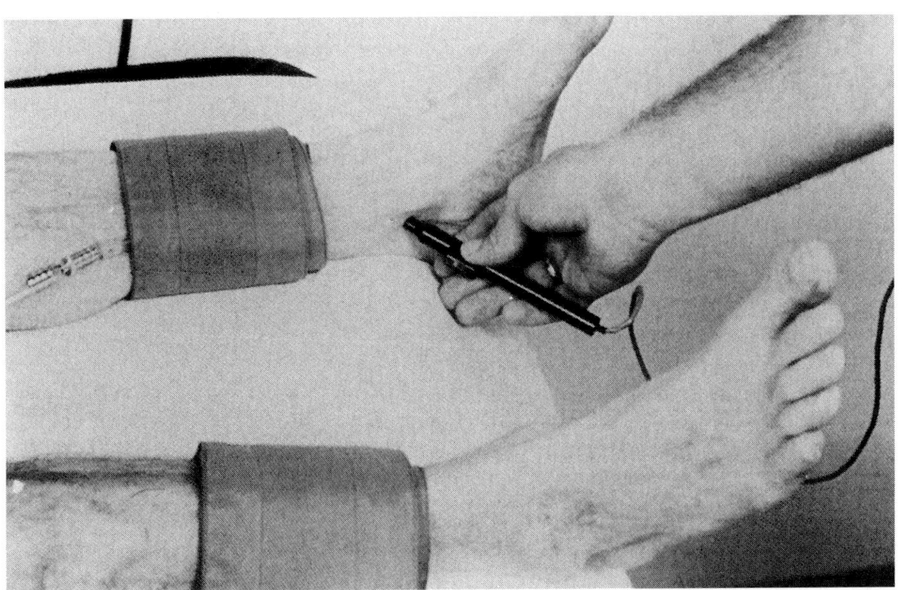

FIGURE 16–8 To measure ankle systolic pressures, the Doppler probe is positioned over the left posterior tibial artery.

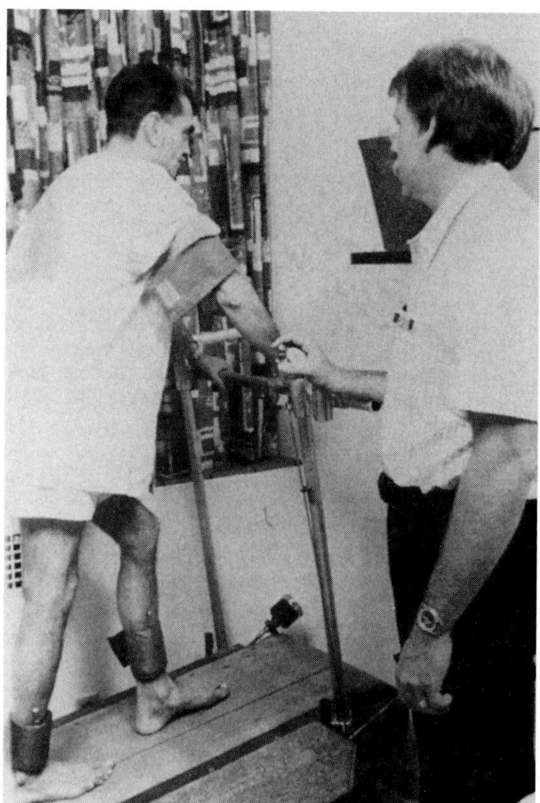

FIGURE 16–9 Ankle cuffs and one arm cuff are in place to facilitate postexercise pressure measurements in the treadmill stress test.

this rapid sequence of measurements. A form for recording the noninvasive test results is shown in Figure 16–10.

Additional studies, such as plethysmography or measurement of toe pressures, are of value only in selected clinical circumstances. Toe pressures can be used to detect occlusive lesions between the level of the ankle and the digital arteries. Duplex scanning is indicated when detailed information on the location and severity of lesions is desired without resorting to arteriography. Duplex methods are described in detail in Chapter 18.

SOURCES OF ERROR

Technical and Physiologic Variability

The variability in measurements of arterial pressure results from biologic and technical factors. The ankle pressure index and other ratios that relate peripheral and central arterial pressures compensate for changes in central pressure, thus avoiding a major source of biologic variation. Because of variability related to technique, changes in ankle pressure index must be 0.15 or greater to be considered significant.[48]

Incompressible Vessels

Accurate measurements of arterial pressure using pneumatic cuffs require that cuff pressure be transmitted through the arterial wall to the flow stream. The presence of medial calcification in the arterial wall results in varying degrees of incompressibility and recording of falsely high pressures.[21] Occasionally, it may be impossible to eliminate the distal flow signal, even with maximal cuff inflation pressures. When this situation is encountered, the main arteries are usually patent, because collateral vessels are more easily obliterated by the cuff.

Diabetic patients are particularly prone to medial calcification, and artifactual elevation of leg pressures must always be considered in this group. In approximately 5 to 10% of diabetic patients, ankle pressures cannot be measured because of incompressible vessels.[49] In these patients, toe pressure measurement is a more reliable method for assessing the severity of arterial occlusive disease, because the digital vessels are not affected by medial calcification.

Cuff Artifact

As previously mentioned, cuff width should be at least 50% greater than limb diameter for accurate pressure measurement. The use of smaller cuffs results in falsely elevated pressure readings, particularly in obese patients. In most patients, the magnitude of the cuff artifact can be anticipated, and relatively narrow thigh cuffs can be successfully used to measure segmental pressure gradients.

In theory, the pressure obtained with a pneumatic cuff on the proximal thigh should reflect the status of the aortoiliac segment. When the proximal thigh pressure is measured with a relatively narrow cuff, the sys-

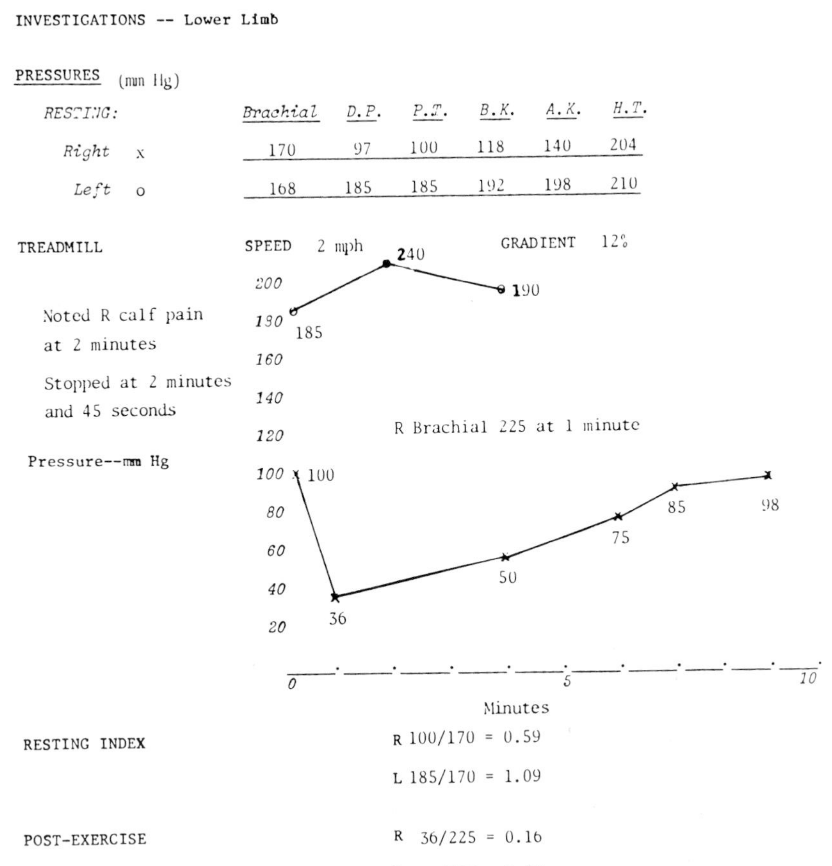

VETERANS ADMINISTRATION MEDICAL CENTER
Peripheral Vascular Service

INVESTIGATIONS -- Lower Limb

PRESSURES (mm Hg)

RESTING:	*Brachial*	*D.P.*	*P.T.*	*B.K.*	*A.K.*	*H.T.*
Right x	170	97	100	118	140	204
Left o	168	185	185	192	198	210

TREADMILL SPEED 2 mph GRADIENT 12%

Noted R calf pain at 2 minutes

Stopped at 2 minutes and 45 seconds

Pressure--mm Hg

RESTING INDEX
R 100/170 = 0.59
L 185/170 = 1.09

POST-EXERCISE
R 36/225 = 0.16
L 240/225 = 1.07

REACTIVE HYPEREMIA

FIGURE 16–10 Form for recording test results. D.P. and P.T. refer to the ankle pressures obtained with the Doppler probe over the dorsalis pedis and posterior tibial arteries, respectively. B.K. = below-knee; A.K. = above-knee; H.T. = high-thigh.

tolic pressure normally exceeds the brachial systolic pressure by a cuff artifact of 30 to 40 mm Hg, and the thigh pressure index is greater than 1.2.[36] Patients with decreased thigh pressure indexes would be expected to have significant aortoiliac disease; however, the presence of superficial femoral and profunda femoris artery disease can also result in a decreased thigh pressure index, even when the aortoiliac segment is hemodynamically normal. The main problem with this indirect assessment of aortoiliac or inflow disease is with the practical difficulty of measuring proximal thigh pressures accurately. When this situation is suspected, other methods such as segmental plethysmography, common femoral artery Doppler waveform analysis, or duplex scanning should be used.

Other Sources of Error

In limbs with severe arterial occlusive disease and low flow rates, Doppler signals may be unobtainable, even when the arteries are patent. Plethysmographic techniques may provide useful information in these cases. When very weak Doppler signals are detected, it may be difficult to distinguish between arterial and venous flow. A direction-sensing Doppler device is useful in this situation. In addition, venous signals are augmented with distal limb compression, whereas arterial signals either remain the same or diminish.

The pressure gradients between adjacent limb segments may be increased in markedly hypertensive patients. On the other extreme, segmental pressure gradients may be decreased when cardiac output is low.[50] When the collateral vessels bypassing an arterial obstruction are unusually large and efficient, the corresponding segmental gradient may be normal. If this is the case, a significant gradient should become apparent after treadmill exercise.

Arterial occlusive lesions distal to the ankle are not detected by the routine lower extremity evaluation, because the ankle is the most distal site of pressure measurement. Lesions involving the plantar or digital arteries, such as vasculitis and microembolism, may be identified by toe pressure measurement and digital plethysmography.

CLINICAL APPLICATIONS OF NONINVASIVE ARTERIAL TESTING

The goals of the lower extremity arterial evaluation are to confirm the diagnosis of arterial occlusive disease, indicate the location of any obstructing lesions, and quantify the resulting degree of disability. Various conditions produce signs and symptoms in the legs that may be confused with arterial occlusive disease (e.g., claudication, rest pain). These include the following: osteoarthritis (hip, knee); neurospinal disease (lumbar disk, spinal stenosis); nocturnal muscle cramps; peripheral neuropathy (diabetes mellitis); reflex sympathetic dystrophy (causalgia); deep vein thrombosis (venous claudication); cellulitis; and trauma. Furthermore, it is not unusual for a single patient to have multiple causes for leg pain, and it may be difficult to determine which is most responsible for a patient's symptoms. The measurements of arterial pressure and flow patterns described in this chapter can be applied to both the initial evaluation and subsequent follow-up of patients with arterial occlusive disease.

Initial Evaluation

In the evaluation of any patient with signs or symptoms that suggest arterial occlusive disease, two questions must be answered: (1) Is arterial occlusion present? (2) Is arterial occlusion causing the patient's symptoms? For the lower extremity, recording of ankle pressure indexes, segmental pressure gradients, Doppler velocity waveforms, and the response to treadmill exercise or reactive hyperemia answer these questions in most patients.

The finding of a normal ankle pressure index at rest and a normal response to treadmill exercise essentially rules out any significant lower extremity arterial occlusive disease. Some patients have a decreased ankle pressure index at rest and symptoms during treadmill exercise, but little or no ankle pressure drop after cessation of exercise. This finding suggests that, although arterial disease is present, it is not producing the symptom in question, and another cause of leg pain should be considered. The limitations imposed by cardiac, pulmonary, and musculoskeletal conditions are directly observed during exercise testing, allowing these factors to be considered in the overall management of the patient.

Follow-Up Testing

Noninvasive testing is a convenient and practical means for serial follow-up of patients after their initial evaluation. Evidence of disease progression or improvement may be observed, and the results of medical or surgical therapy can be documented objectively.

In patients who have had a successful arterial reconstruction for lower extremity occlusive disease, ankle pressures and appropriate segmental pressure gradients should be significantly improved compared with the preoperative values.[51] If a single level of disease was present preoperatively, successful bypass grafting or endarterectomy should result in normal or near-normal ankle pressures. Failure of ankle pressures to improve immediately following surgery suggests either a problem related to surgical technique or the selection of an inappropriate reconstructive procedure.[52] Deterioration of noninvasive measurements later in the postoperative period may reflect either structural changes occurring in the reconstructed segment or progression of occlusive disease at other sites.[53,54] Serial postoperative follow-up is desirable, because early identification and repair of a failing arterial reconstruction results in the greatest chance of maintaining patency. This subject is discussed further in Chapter 18.

Patients whose condition is improved after surgery but who still have not returned to normal may have their status documented by noninvasive testing. For example, a patient may show a significant improvement in treadmill walking time after arterial reconstruction despite a persistent drop in ankle pressure. This observation is common in patients with arterial occlusive disease at multiple levels who have only one level corrected; the abnormal hemodynamic response then reflects the remaining untreated disease. Figure 16–11 shows the ankle pressure changes recorded before and after an aortofemoral bypass graft in a patient who also has stenoses in both superficial femoral arteries. Although the treadmill walking time improved, an abnormal ankle pressure response is still present.

Specific Clinical Problems

Claudication

The term *intermittent claudication* refers to a muscular ache or cramp that occurs during exercise and is relieved by rest. It results from inadequate blood flow to muscle during exercise and is a definite, reproducible symptom. Claudication usually involves the calf, but the thigh or buttock may also be affected when arterial occlusions reduce blood flow to those areas. Arteriosclerosis obliterans is the most common cause of claudication; popliteal artery entrapment must be considered when claudication occurs in young adults or children.[55, 56]

When the characteristic symptoms are produced by treadmill exercise in association with a drop in ankle pressure to less than about 60 mm Hg, the clinical impression of intermittent claudication is confirmed. The walking time documents the extent of disability and serves as a baseline for subsequent follow-up. Segmental pressure gradients or plethysmography can be used to determine the approximate location of arterial occlusive lesions.

Rest Pain

Ischemic rest pain develops in the toes or forefoot when blood flow is insufficient to maintain normal cellular function at rest.

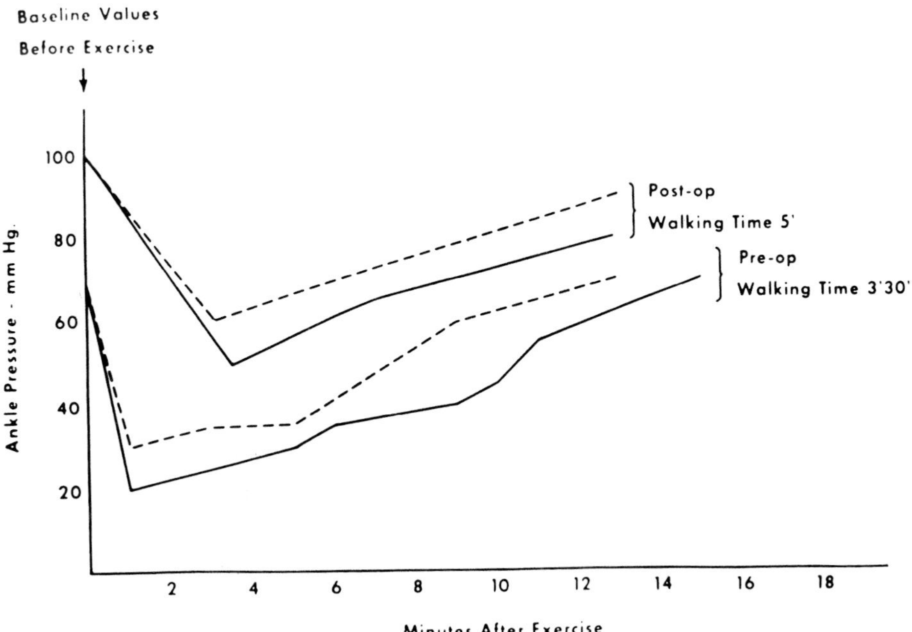

FIGURE 16–11 Ankle pressure response to treadmill exercise before and after an aortofemoral bypass graft in a patient with bilateral superficial femoral artery stenoses. The postoperative exercise test shows some improvement in walking time but remains abnormal (*dashed lines,* left ankle; *solid lines,* right ankle). (From Strandness DE: Abnormal exercise responses after successful reconstructive arterial surgery. Surgery 59:328, 1966.)

Noninvasive tests usually show multiple-level arterial occlusive disease with an ankle systolic pressure less than 40 mm Hg and an ankle pressure index less than 0.35. Treadmill exercise or reactive hyperemia testing is not necessary in patients with this degree of abnormality.

Healing of Ulcers and Amputations

Noninvasive pressure measurements can be used to assess the probability of achieving primary healing in the ischemic lower extremity. Ischemic foot ulcers are unlikely to heal if ankle systolic pressure is less than 55 mm Hg in nondiabetics or less than 80 mm Hg in diabetics.[49] The ankle pressures in diabetic patients may be falsely elevated because of medial calcification.

Ankle pressures have not been uniformly helpful in predicting healing of BK or foot amputations.[8] A BK or calf pressure greater than 70 mm Hg correlates with primary healing of BK amputations, whereas the absence of detectable Doppler flow signals at the BK level predicts failure of healing.[57] Primary healing may still be achieved with BK pressures less than 70 mm Hg, so the choice of amputation level should not be based on this pressure measurement alone.

Because lesions in the pedal or digital arteries are not detected by ankle or calf pressure measurement, toe pressure measurement may be more reliable for predicting healing of the foot. Healing of foot ulcers, toe amputations, or transmetatarsal amputations was observed in only 5% of limbs when toe pressures were less than 30 mm Hg; however, with pressures of 30 mm Hg or greater, healing occurred in approximately 90% of limbs.[38]

The transcutaneous oxygen tension ($tcPo_2$) or amount of oxygen diffusing through the skin from the dermal capillaries can be measured with an electrode applied to the skin surface. This technique has been proposed as a method for predicting wound healing and determining the most appropriate level for amputation.[58] Clinical experience has shown that $tcPo_2$ measurements are valuable for predicting healing at a particular level of the limb; however, this approach is less reliable for identifying those sites that fail to heal. In one study, successful healing of BK amputations occurred in 96% of patients with a calf $tcPo_2$ greater than 20 mm Hg but only in 50% of patients with a calf $tcPo_2$ less than 20 mm Hg.[59] Refinements of this technique, such as use of a critical Po_2 index (calf/brachial $tcPo_2$ ratio, foot/chest $tcPo_2$ ratio) or breathing supplemental oxygen, may improve the overall predictive value.[59, 60, 61] Estimation of skin blood flow by $tcPo_2$ may be more sensitive than ankle pressure measurements in the assessment of severe limb ischemia. In general, critical ischemia must be suspected whenever forefoot $tcPo_2$ is less than 40 mm Hg.[62, 63]

Predicting the Results of Arterial Surgery

Noninvasive measurements of lower extremity blood pressure have been used to predict the functional results of arterial reconstruction in terms of symptom relief and graft patency. In patients undergoing aortofemoral bypass procedures, a preoperative thigh pressure index of 0.85 or less is a reliable predictor of a good postoperative result; however, improvement may also occur in many patients with a thigh pressure index greater than 0.85.[64] The presence of occlusive disease limited to the aortoiliac arteries, as demonstrated by normal segmental pressure gradients in the leg, is also predictive of a good result after aortofemoral bypass grafting. A comparison of ankle pressure indexes before and after aortofemoral bypass showed that an increase of 0.1 or more during the first 12 hours after operation correlated highly with subsequent symptomatic improvement.[64] The preoperative ankle pressure index alone also has some predictive value.[65] When the ankle pressure index is greater than 0.8, 94% of patients obtain significant symptom relief after aortofemoral bypass, whereas only 64% of patients show the same degree of improvement if the ankle pressure index is less than 0.4. These observations indicate the aortofemoral bypass grafting is most successful in these patients with significant aortoiliac occlusive disease and normal distal arteries.

The predictive value of noninvasive pressure measurements in femoropopliteal bypass procedures has not been firmly established. An early study suggested that an ankle pressure index of greater than 0.4 predicts a high graft patency rate, whereas an ankle pressure index of less than 0.2 is associated with early graft failure.[66] Later reports have not confirmed these observations, however, and very low ankle pressures should not be regarded as a contraindication for femoropopliteal bypass.[52]

Predicting the Results of Sympathectomy

The role of sympathectomy in the management of patients with arterial disease has been controversial. Lumbar sympathectomy is sometimes considered for patients with impending limb loss caused by severe, unreconstructable occlusive disease. In this situation, ankle pressure measurements provide a means for selecting those patients most likely to benefit from the procedure.[67] An ankle pressure index greater than 0.35 predicts a favorable clinical response to sympathectomy; an index less than 0.2 correlates highly with sympathectomy failure and subsequent limb loss. The value of lumbar sympathectomy depends on the adequacy of collateral circulation in the leg, and the ankle pressure index provides an indirect assessment of the potential for increasing flow through the collateral vessels.

In addition to adequate collateral flow, the success of sympathectomy depends on the capability of the peripheral arterioles to vasodilate and on the presence of sympathetic activity in the extremity. Vasodilatation can be assessed by performing a reactive hyperemia test while monitoring a plethysmographic digit volume pulse. In normal extremities, the excursion of the volume pulse at least doubles during hyperemia, usually within the first few seconds after flow is restored. Failure of the volume pulse to increase suggests that further vasodilatation is not possible. The presence of intact sympathetic tone can be demonstrated plethysmographically by observing the response of the digit volume pulse to a deep breath. If vasodilatation or sympathetic tone is absent, sympathectomy is not beneficial.[68]

REFERENCES

1. Marinelli MR, Beach KW, Glass MJ, et al: Noninvasive testing vs. clinical evaluation of arterial disease. JAMA 241:2031–2034, 1979.
2. Beales JSM, Adcock FA, Frawley JE, et al: The radiological assessment of disease at the profunda femoris artery. Br J Radiol 44:854–857, 1971.
3. Crummy AB, Rankin RS, Turnipseed WD, et al: Biplane arteriography in ischemia of the lower extremity. Radiology 126:111–115, 1978.
4. Sethi GR, Scott SM, Takaro T: Multiple-plane angiography for more precise evaluation of aortoiliac disease. Surgery 78:154–159, 1975.
5. Thomas M, Andrews MR: Value of oblique projections in translumbar aortography. Am J Roentgenol 116:187–193, 1973.
6. Castenada-Zuniga W, Knight L, Formanek A, et al: Hemodynamic assessment of obstructive aortoiliac disease. Am J Roentgenol 127:559–561, 1976.
7. Karayannacus PE, Talukder N, Nerem RM, et al: The role of multiple noncritical arterial stenoses in the pathogenesis of ischemia. J Thorac Cardiovasc Surg 73:458–469, 1977.
8. Kempczinski RF, Rutheford RB: Current status of the vascular diagnostic laboratory. Adv Surg 12:1–52, 1978.
9. Nippa JH, Hokanson DE, Lee DR, et al: Phase rotation for separating forward and reverse blood velocity signals. IEEE Trans Sonics Ultrasonics 22:340–346, 1975.
10. Blackshear WM: Surgical indications for lower extremity arterial occlusive disease. Part I. Curr Probl Cardiol 6:22–32, 1981.
11. Baker DW: Pulsed ultrasonic Doppler blood flow sensing. IEEE Trans Sonics Ultrasonics 17:170–185, 1970.
12. Mozersky DJ, Hokanson DE, Sumner DS, et al: Ultrasonic visualization of the arterial lumen. Surgery 72:253–259, 1972.
13. Zierler RE: Carotid artery evaluation by duplex scanning. Semin Vasc Surg 1:9–16, 1988.
14. Strandness DE Jr: Ultrasound in the study of atherosclerosis. Ultrasound Med Biol 12:453–464, 1986.
15. Blackshear WM, Phillips DJ, Strandness DE: Pulsed Doppler assessment of normal human femoral artery velocity patterns. J Surg Res 27:73–83, 1979.
16. Jager KA, Phillips DJ, Martin RL, et al: Noninvasive mapping of lower limb arterial lesions. Ultrasound Med Biol 11:515–521, 1985.
17. Kohler TR, Nance DR, Cramer MM, et al: Duplex scanning for diagnosis of aortoiliac and femoropopliteal disease: A prospective study. Circulation 76:1074–1080, 1987.
18. Taylor DC, Kettler MD, Moneta GL, et al: Duplex ultrasound scanning in the diagnosis of renal artery stenosis: A prospective evaluation. J Vasc Surg 7:363–369, 1987.
19. Jager K, Bollinger A, Valli C, et al: Measurement of mesenteric blood flow by duplex scanning. J Vasc Surg 3:462–469, 1986.
20. Darling RC, Raines JK, Brener BJ, et al: Quantitative segmental pulse volume recorder: A clinical tool. Surgery 72:873–887, 1973.
21. Strandness DE Jr, Bell JW: Peripheral vascular disease: Diagnosis and objective evaluation using a mercury strain gauge. Ann Surg 161 (Suppl):1–35, 1965.
22. Hokanson DE, Sumner DS, Strandness DE Jr: An electrically calibrated plethysmograph for direct measurement of limb blood flow. IEEE Trans Biomed Eng 22:25–29, 1975.
23. Sumner DS: Volume plethysmography in vascular disease: An overview. *In* Bernstein EF (ed): Noninva-

sive Diagnostic Techniques in Vascular Disease, 3rd ed. St. Louis, CV Mosby, 1985, pp 97–118.
24. Johnston KW, Marozzo BC, Cobbold RSC: Errors and artifacts of Doppler flowmeters and their solution. Arch Surg 112:1335–1342, 1977.
25. Strandness DE, Sumner DS: Hemodynamics for Surgeons. New York, Grune & Stratton, 1975, p 29.
26. Knox RA, Strandness DE: Ultrasound techniques for evaluation of lower extremity arterial occlusion. Semin Ultrasound 2:264–275, 1981.
27. Strandness DE Jr, Zierler RE: Exercise ankle pressure measurements in arterial disease. *In* Bernstein EF (ed): Noninvasive Diagnostic Techniques in Vascular Disease, 3rd ed. St. Louis, CV Mosby, 1985, pp 575–583.
28. Strandness DE, Sumner DS: Hemodynamics for Surgeons. New York, Grune & Stratton, 1975, p 21.
29. Carter SA: Clinical measurements of systolic pressures in limbs with arterial occlusive disease. JAMA 207:1869–1874, 1969.
30. May AG, Van de Berg L, De Weese JA, et al: Clinical arterial stenosis. Surgery 54:250–259, 1963.
31. Strandness DE, Sumner DS: Hemodynamics for Surgeons. New York, Grune & Stratton, 1975, p 233.
32. Yao JST, Hobbs JT, Irvine WT: Ankle systolic pressure measurements in arterial diseases affecting the lower extremities. Br J Surg 56:676–679, 1969.
33. Sumner DS, Strandness DE: The relationship between calf blood flow and ankle blood pressure in patients with intermittent claudication. Surgery 65:763–771, 1969.
34. Yao JST: Hemodynamic studies in peripheral arterial disease. Br J Surg 57:761–766, 1970.
35. Pascarelli EF, Bertrand CA: Comparison of blood pressures in the arms and legs. N Engl J Med 270:693–698, 1964.
36. Cutajar CL, Marston A, Newcombe JF: Value of cuff occlusion pressures in assessment of peripheral vascular disease. Br J Med 2:392–395, 1973.
37. Carter SA, Lezack JD: Digital systolic pressures in the lower limbs in arterial disease. Circulation 43:905–914, 1971.
38. Ramsey DE, Manke DA, Sumner DS: Toe blood pressure—A valuable adjunct to ankle pressure measurement for assessing peripheral arterial disease. J Cardiovasc Surg 24:43–48, 1983.
39. Fronek A, Johanson K, Dilley RB, et al: Ultrasonically monitored postocclusive reactive hyperemia in the diagnosis of peripheral arterial occlusive disease. Circulation 48:149–152, 1973.
40. Hummel BW, Hummel BA, Mowbry A, et al: Reactive hyperemia vs treadmill exercise testing in arterial disease. Arch Surg 113:95–98, 1978.
41. Keagy BA, Pharr WF, Thomas D, et al: Comparison of reactive hyperemia and treadmill tests in the evaluation of peripheral vascular disease. Am J Surg 142:158–161, 1981.
42. Strandness DE, Schultz RD, Sumner DS, et al: Ultrasonic flow detection: A useful technique in the evaluation of peripheral vascular disease. Am J Surg 113:311–320, 1967.
43. Johnston KW, Taraschuk I: Validation of the role of pulsatility index in quantitation of the severity of peripheral arterial occlusive disease. Am J Surg 131:295–297, 1976.
44. Gosling RG, Dunbar G, King DH, et al: The quantitative analysis of occlusive peripheral arterial disease by a noninvasive ultrasonic technique. Angiology 22:52–55, 1971.
45. Thiele BL, Bandyk DF, Zierler RE, et al: A systematic approach to the assessment of aortoiliac disease. Arch Surg 118:477–481, 1983.
46. Baird RN, Bird DR, Clifford PC, et al: Upstream stenosis—its diagnosis by Doppler signals from the femoral artery. Arch Surg 115:1316–1322, 1980.
47. Campbell WB, Baird RN, Cole SEA, et al: Physiological interpretation of Doppler shift waveforms—the femorodistal segment in combined disease. Ultrasound Med Bio 9:265–269, 1983.
48. Baker JD, Dix D: Variability of Doppler ankle pressures with arterial occlusive disease: An evaluation of ankle index and brachial-ankle pressure gradient. Surgery 89:134–137, 1981.
49. Raines JK, Darling RC, Both K, et al: Vascular laboratory criteria for the management of peripheral vascular disease of the lower extremities. Surgery 79:21–29, 1976.
50. Winsor T: Influence of arterial disease on the systolic blood pressure gradients of the extremity. Am J Med Sci 220:117–126, 1950.
51. Strandness DE, Bell JW: Ankle pressure responses after reconstructive arterial surgery. Surgery 59:514–516, 1966.
52. Corson JD, Johnson WC, LoGerfo RS, et al: Doppler ankle systolic blood pressure: Prognostic value in vein bypass grafts of the lower extremity. Arch Surg 113:932–935, 1976.
53. Blackshear WM, Thiele BL, Strandness DE: Natural history of above- and below-knee femoropopliteal grafts. Am J Surg 140:234–241, 1980.
54. Strandness DE: Abnormal exercise responses after successful reconstructive arterial surgery. Surgery 59:325–333, 1966.
55. Insua JA, Young JR, Humphries AW: Popliteal artery entrapment syndrome. Arch Surg 101:771–775, 1970.
56. Rich NM, Collins GJ, McDonald PT, et al: Popliteal vascular entrapment: Its increasing interest. Arch Surg 114:1377–1384, 1979.
57. Barnes RW, Shanik GD, Slaymaker EE: An index of healing in below-knee amputation: Leg blood pressure by Doppler ultrasound. Surgery 79:13–20, 1976.
58. Wyss CR, Robertson C, Love SJ, et al: Relationship between transcutaneous oxygen tension, ankle blood pressure, and clinical outcome of vascular surgery in diabetic and nondiabetic patients. Surgery 101:56–62, 1987.
59. Kram HB, Appel OL, Shoemaker WC: Multisensor transcutaneous oximetric mapping to predict below-knee amputation wound healing: Use of a critical Po_2. J Vasc Surg 9:796–800, 1989.
60. Harward TRS, Volny J, Golbranson F, et al: Oxygen inhalation-induced transcutaneous Po_2 changes as a predictor of amputation level. J Vasc Surg 2:220–227, 1985.
61. Lalka SG, Malone JM, Anderson GG, et al: Transcutaneous oxygen and carbon dioxide pressure monitoring to determine severity of limb ischemia and to predict surgical outcome. J Vasc Surg 7:507–514, 1988.
62. Karanfilian RG, Lynch TG, Zirul VT, et al: The value of laser Doppler velocimetry and transcutaneous oxygen tension determination in predicting healing of ischemic forefoot ulcerations and amputations in diabetic and nondiabetic patients. J Vasc Surg 4:511–516, 1986.

63. Larsen JF, Jensen BV, Christensen KS, et al: Forefoot transcutaneous oxygen tension at different leg positions in patients with peripheral vascular disease. Eur J Vasc Surg 4:185–189, 1990.
64. Bone GE, Hayes AC, Slaymaker EE, et al: Value of segmental limb blood pressures in predicting results of aortofemoral bypass. Am J Surg 132:733–738, 1976.
65. Bernstein EF, Stuart SH, Fronek A: The predictive value of noninvasive testing in peripheral vascular disease. *In* Bernstein EF (ed): Noninvasive Diagnostic Techniques in Vascular Disease. St. Louis, CV Mosby, 1982, pp 396–403.
66. Dean RH, Yao JST, Stanton PE, et al: Prognostic indicators in femoropopliteal reconstruction. Arch Surg 110:1287–1293, 1975.
67. Yao JST, Bergan JJ: Predictability of vascular reactivity relative to sympathetic ablation. Arch Surg 107: 676–680, 1973.
68. Strandness DE Jr: Long-term value of lumbar sympathectomy. Geriatrics 21:144–155, 1966.

Chapter 17

Assessment of Upper Extremity Arteries

■ *James M. Edwards, MD* ■ *R. Eugene Zierler, MD*

Symptomatic arterial disease of the upper extremity is uncommon and accounts for approximately 5% of cases of extremity ischemia; the remaining 95% of cases occur in the lower extremity. Unlike in the lower extremity, in which atherosclerosis is by far the most common disorder, ischemia in the upper extremity may be caused by a variety of systemic diseases. Thus, the diagnosis of upper extremity arterial diseases is often complex and requires a complete medical history and physical examination, laboratory screening, and examination of the arteries of the upper extremity. With the introduction of Doppler ultrasound techniques and the development of the duplex scanner, it became possible to diagnose many upper extremity arterial abnormalities without having a patient undergo arteriography. In this chapter, we review the use of nonimaging physiologic tests and duplex scanning in the diagnosis of upper extremity arterial diseases, and we speculate on how duplex ultrasound may be used in the future.

VASCULAR ANATOMY OF THE UPPER EXTREMITY

The vascular anatomy of the upper extremity was reviewed in detail in Chapter 15, which included a discussion on anatomic variations and potential collateral routes. Readers who are unfamiliar with upper extremity arterial anatomy should review Chapter 15 before proceeding to the material contained in this chapter.

Two areas of arterial anatomy that are particularly germane to the contents of this chapter deserve special attention. These are the vascular relationships at the thoracic outlet and the arterial anatomy of the hand.

Thoracic Outlet

The subclavian artery leaves the chest via the thoracic outlet, where it passes over the first rib, behind the clavicle, and between the anterior and middle scalene muscles (Fig. 17–1). The subclavian vein passes over the first rib, behind the clavicle, and anterior to the anterior scalene muscle. The brachial plexus, which innervates the upper extremity, also exits from the thorax via the thoracic outlet between the anterior and middle scalene muscles. Because of the close confines of the thoracic outlet, the subclavian artery, the subclavian vein, and the brachial plexus are subject to impingement by the surrounding structures. Such impingement may generate upper extremity symptoms that are the subject of vascular laboratory evaluation.

Arterial Anatomy of the Hand

As illustrated in Figure 17–2, the radial and ulnar arteries cross the wrist into the hand. There the ulnar artery forms the superficial palmar arch and the radial artery forms the deep palmar arch. These arches are variable in size, origin, and anatomy. The common digital arteries usually arise from the superficial palmar arch and divide into the proper digital arteries. The proper digital arteries travel along the medial and lateral sides of each digit and join at the tip of the digit. There is abundant potential for collateral flow in the hand and across the wrist.

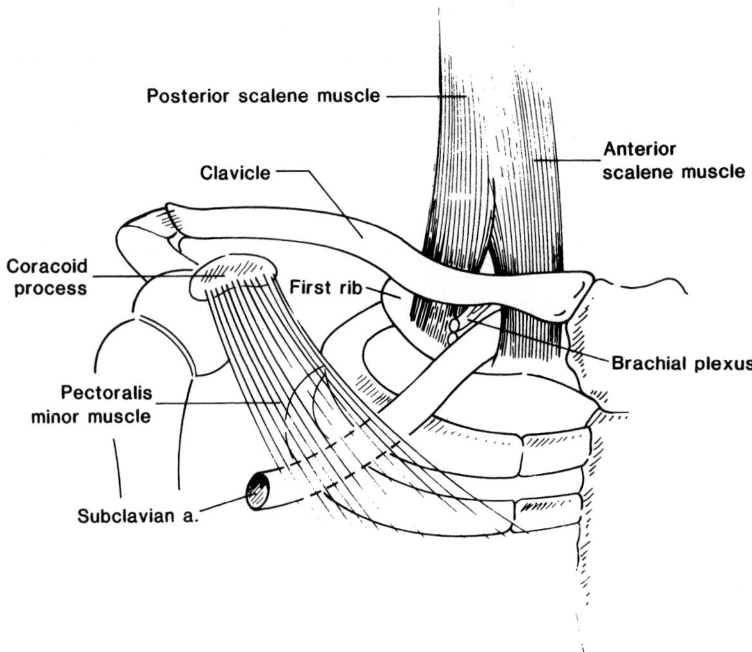

FIGURE 17–1 Thoracic outlet anatomy.

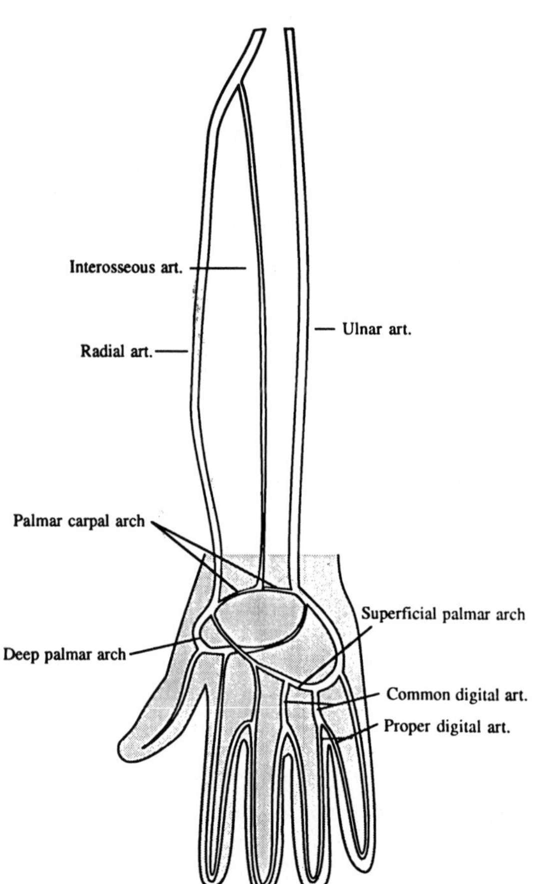

FIGURE 17–2 Forearm and hand arterial anatomy.

NONINVASIVE DIAGNOSTIC TECHNIQUES

Duplex scanning of the upper extremity arteries is generally performed in conjunction with other noninvasive vascular testing, such as digital strain-gauge plethysmography, photoplethysmography, digital and arm segmental pressures, and cold-induced vasospasm testing. These tests, in combination, usually give more information than can be obtained by arteriography alone.

Segmental Arm Pressures

Blood pressure and Doppler waveforms are measured above the elbow, below the elbow, and above the wrist while insonating the radial artery at the wrist in a similar manner to the protocol used for segmental leg pressure measurement.

Digital Pressure and Plethysmography

Digital pressure and plethysmography have proved extremely useful in the diagnosis of upper extremity arterial disease. Either photoplethysmography or strain-gauge plethysmography can be used to measure digital blood pressure and to obtain pulse waveforms. The photo cell is attached to the fingertip pulp with double-sided tape or small strain gauges are placed around the fingertip. One-inch (2.5-cm) blood pressure cuffs are placed around the proximal phalanx. Waveforms are recorded at rest, and then the cuff is inflated to measure blood pressure. It is extremely important to measure and record finger temperature before performing this test. If the finger temperature is less than 28 to 30°C, false-positive results may be obtained secondary to cold-induced vasospasm. It may be necessary to warm the hands in water or above a heating vent before testing.

Cold Challenge Testing

The simplest cold intolerance test is measuring the digital temperature recovery time after immersion of the hand in ice water for 30 seconds. A thermister probe is used to measure finger temperatures, the patient's hand is immersed in a container of ice water for 30 to 60 seconds. After the hand is dried, the fingertip pulp temperatures are measured every 5 minutes for 45 minutes or until the temperature returns to preimmersion levels. The preimmersion temperature must be above 30°C and therefore hand and body warming may be required before immersion. This test is uncomfortable and poorly tolerated by patients. A better test exists (digital hypothermic challenge test), which involves perfusing a finger cuff around the proximal phalanx on the test finger with progressively cooler fluid. The pressure in the test finger is then compared with a reference finger that is not cooled. This test requires an expensive machine and is used only in research centers.[1] Other tests for cold-induced vasospasm include thermal entrainment,[2] digital laser Doppler response to cold,[3] thermography,[4] venous occlusion plethysmography, and digital artery caliber measurement,[5] but these tests are not widely accepted or used.

Thoracic Outlet Syndrome Testing

Multiple tests for thoracic outlet syndrome have been suggested throughout the years and none have gained universal acceptance. The common denominator to all these tests is the detection of diminution of blood flow into (for suspected arterial occlusion) or out of (for suspected venous occlusion) the upper extremity with provocative positioning. Doppler waveforms, pulse volume recording, light reflection rheography,[6] laser Doppler response,[7] digital photoplethysmography, and blood pressure measurement may be used to detect arterial changes and venous outflow measurements, and clinical observation of cyanosis may be used to detect venous obstruction. Duplex scanning specifically looking for narrowing or aneurysm of the subclavian artery or vein may be used, and the technique is described in the next section.

After the selected flow detection device is positioned, the patient is placed in a seated position. One or more of the following provocative positions are then established. The elevated arm stress test (EAST) position is obtained by putting the arms in 90-degree abduction-external rotation, the hands up in the air and above the head, and the shoulders pulled back. The patient is then instructed to slowly open and close the hands for 3 minutes. The Adson maneuver is performed by having the patient turn the head toward the side being tested and then turning the head away from the side being tested, while the neck is fully extended and the chest is in full inspiratory position. The exaggerated military maneuver is performed by having the patient pull the shoulders back in an exaggerated "military attention" posture with the chest pushed out. The hyperabduction maneuver is performed by having the patient perform 180-degree abduction of the arms in 45-degree steps.

Upper Extremity Duplex Scanning

Duplex scanning of the upper extremity is carried out in similar fashion to carotid or lower extremity arterial examinations. The arteries are relatively superficial and fairly constant in location. Even digital arteries can be visualized in some patients by careful examination. Digital arterial lesions are commonly associated with more proximal disease; therefore, all arteries from the digital and palmar arteries to the subclavian arteries should be imaged, even if the suspected lesion is at one extreme of the upper extremity.

For examination of the origin of the subclavian artery, a 3- or 5-MHz probe generally gives the best images. The remaining upper extremity arteries are superficial and are best scanned with a higher frequency probe (7.5 or 10 MHz). Either a sector or a linear scan head may be used, but in either case a standoff or a mound of acoustic gel is helpful, and sometimes essential, to visualize the vessel clearly and to assess the flow pattern within it. Color-Doppler scanners facilitate identification of the vessels, and tortuosity of the upper extremity arteries may be more easily seen with color-flow imaging.

The subclavian artery (Fig. 17–3) may be visualized via a supraclavicular, infraclavicular, or sternal notch approach. The origin of the left subclavian artery from the aorta, the origin of the right subclavian artery from the innominate artery, and the origin of the innominate artery from the aorta should be visualized whenever possible. The subclavian artery should be followed distally, as it crosses under the clavicle and over the first rib, where it becomes the axillary artery. The subclavian artery is the most difficult of the upper extremity arteries to visualize. Often a single approach to the artery does not allow complete visualization of the artery, and a combination of approaches is necessary. This is particularly true if the operator is trying to visualize the subclavian artery with provoca-

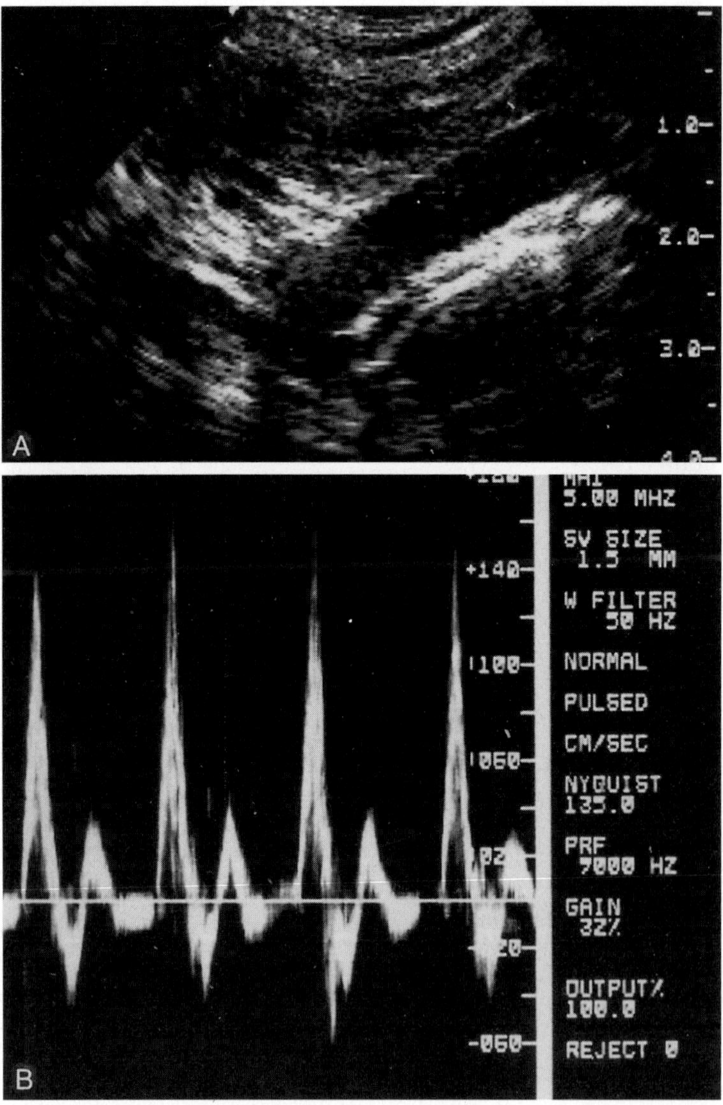

FIGURE 17–3 *A,* Normal subclavian artery. The artery is visible at the top of the display. *B,* The Doppler spectral waveform exhibits the triphasic pattern of a normal extremity artery.

tive testing, because multiple positions of the arm require constant movement of the transducer.

From an anterior transducer approach, the axillary artery (Fig. 17–4) is visible behind the pectoralis major and minor muscles. From an axillary approach, it is seen deep to the axillary fat pad. As the axillary artery travels distally, it becomes progressively more superficial. The axillary artery becomes the brachial artery at the point where it crosses the teres major muscle.

Proximally, the brachial artery (Fig. 17–5*A*) lies in a medial groove between the biceps muscle anteriorly and the triceps muscle posteriorly. The brachial artery spirals anteriorly around the humerus, as it travels distally. The profunda brachii (deep brachial) artery, which is the source of most collateral flow around the elbow, can often be visualized in the upper arm. The brachial artery is subcutaneous in the antecubital fossa and crosses the elbow joint obliquely from medial to lateral. Soon after crossing the elbow, the brachial artery is seen to bifurcate into the radial and ulnar arteries.

The forearm arteries should be followed from the antecubital fossa to the wrist. As the arteries are traced distally, they initially dive beneath the forearm flexor muscles but then become more superficial again at the wrist. The ulnar artery (see Fig. 17–5*B*) often cannot be palpated, but its location is constant at the wrist, as it emerges laterally from be-

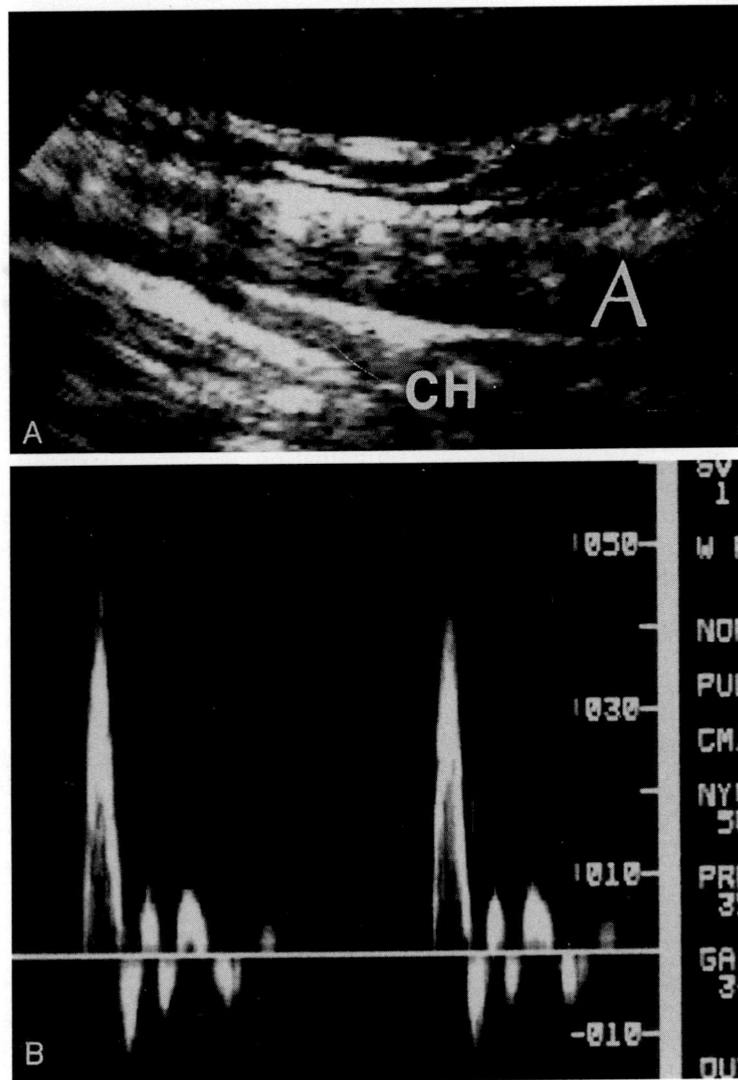

FIGURE 17–4 Normal axillary artery. *A*, The circumflex humeral branch (CH) is seen to extend posteriorly from the axillary artery (A). *B*, The Doppler spectral waveform is normal.

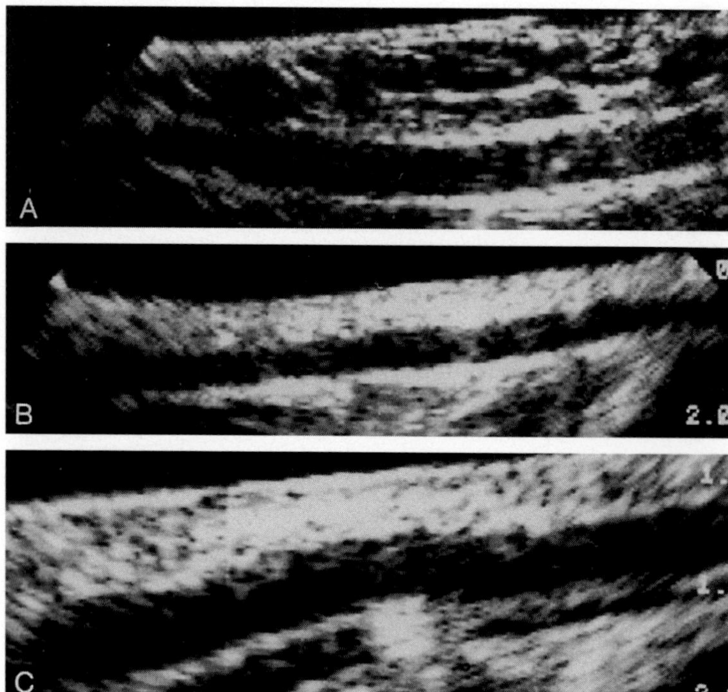

FIGURE 17–5 Duplex image of the brachial artery (*A*), ulnar artery (*B*), and radial artery (*C*), and accompanying Doppler waveforms.

hind the flexor carpi ulnaris tendon and passes over the pisiform bone. As the ulnar artery enters the palm, it travels under the hook of the hamate bone, which can make imaging difficult. This area is very important, as traumatic aneurysms of the ulnar artery are often located here. The radial artery (see Fig. 17–5*C*) is easily found by palpation at the wrist, or it can be reliably located between the flexor carpi radialis tendon and the head of the radius. The radial artery divides at the wrist into two branches. The superficial palmar branch continues into the palm and anastomoses with the superficial palmar arch. The other branch of the radial artery heads posteriorly behind the thumb before entering the palm to form the deep palmar arch.

Duplex scanning of arteriovenous dialysis fistulas and grafts is relatively simple, because these are constructed in a subcutaneous position. The use of a high-frequency probe (7.5 or 10 MHz) and a standoff or mound of acoustic gel is often necessary. The origin or arterial end of the graft or fistula should be visualized. Several centimeters of the artery proximal to the origin should also be imaged, because stenosis due to clamp injury or neointimal hyperplasia may occur just proximal to the graft origin. The body of the graft should then be imaged completely. Areas of stenosis or aneurysmal changes are common, especially in older grafts. Calcification in the walls is also common and may interfere with duplex scanning. Graft flows should be calculated in several relatively normal-appearing segments. The venous anastomosis and the native vein adjacent to the anastomosis are the most common areas for stenotic lesions. These areas must be carefully imaged because the distal veins may drain in any direction.

Table 17–1 summarizes the techniques used to visualize each upper extremity artery by duplex scanning.

TABLE 17–1 DUPLEX SCANNING TECHNIQUES FOR VISUALIZING UPPER EXTREMITY ARTERIES

Artery	Probe (MHz)	Approaches	Standoff
Subclavian	2–5	Supraclavicular Infraclavicular Sternal notch	No
Axillary	7–10	Anterior Axillary	±*
Brachial	7–10	Anterior	Yes
Radial	7–10	Anterior	Yes
Ulnar	7–10	Anterior	Yes

* ± indicates sometimes helpful.

NONINVASIVE DIAGNOSTIC TEST INTERPRETATION

Segmental Arm Pressures

Abnormal waveforms and decreased pressures at the above-elbow cuff site indicate subclavian or axillary arterial occlusive disease. Similarly, abnormalities at the below-elbow and wrist sites indicate brachial and ulnar/radial artery occlusive disease, respectively.

Digital Plethysmography

Both digital blood pressure and waveforms are part of digital plethysmography. Digital blood pressure is normally within 20 to 30 mm Hg of brachial pressure. This usually corresponds to a ratio of finger systolic pressure to brachial systolic pressure of greater than 80%. Waveforms are normal if the upstroke time is less than 0.2 second. Obstructive waveforms have a slower upstroke, and waveforms in patients with vasospasm often have an abnormal shape termed a *peaked pulse,* which is thought to represent abnormal elasticity and rebound of the digital vessels.[8] Diagrammatic representations of photoplethysmographic waveforms are shown in Figure 17–6. It is important to know that finger temperature is greater than 28 to 30°C before interpreting a test as demonstrating fixed arterial obstruction.

Cold Challenge Testing

When cold sensitivity testing is performed by immersing the patient's hands in ice water, normal individuals have a recovery time to preimmersion levels of less than 10 minutes. This test is very sensitive for detecting cold-induced vasospasm, but it is quite nonspecific in that approximately one half of patients with a positive test have no clinical symptoms of cold sensitivity.[9] The digital hypothermic challenge test is interpreted as positive for abnormal cold-induced vasospasm if the test finger pressure is reduced by more than 20% compared with the reference finger.

Thoracic Outlet Syndrome Testing

Interpretation of testing for thoracic outlet syndrome is both simple and difficult. The difficulty lies in the definition of *thoracic outlet syndrome,* as discussed in the clinical syndrome section that follows. Unfortunately, the majority of patients referred to a vascular laboratory for testing complain of neck, shoulder, arm, and hand pain. Thus, commonly, although the patient may be labeled as having thoracic outlet syndrome, arterial or venous obstruction is not suspected. Compounding this problem is the fact that many patients without complaints have a positive test for diminution in blood flow with provocative testing.

This controversy makes interpretation of the thoracic outlet tests difficult. Tests for obstruction of blood flow with provocative positioning are easily interpreted as positive or negative, but a positive test is not necessarily diagnostic for arterial or venous thoracic outlet syndrome and may have no relationship to neurogenic thoracic outlet syndrome or shoulder or neck pain.

A duplex scan demonstrating stenosis with provocative testing and a poststenotic aneurysm is diagnostic of thoracic outlet syndrome.

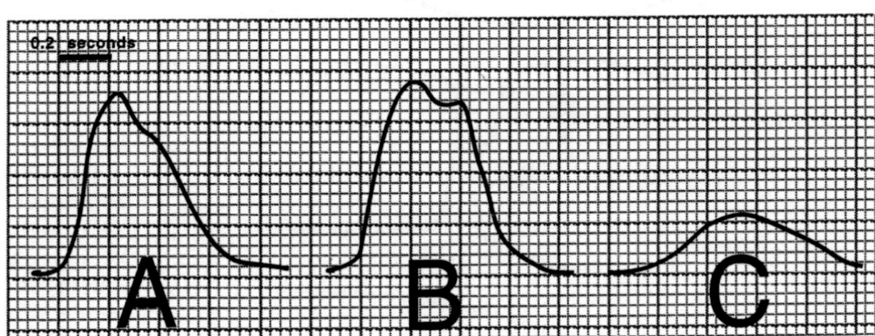

FIGURE 17–6 Diagrammatic representation of normal (*A*), obstructive (*B*), and peaked (*C*) digital photoplethysmographic waveforms.

Upper Extremity Duplex Scanning

The interpretation of duplex findings in the upper extremity is similar to the interpretation of B-mode images and Doppler signals gathered in other arterial systems. Stenoses result in high-velocity jets, poststenotic turbulence, and dampened distal waveforms (Fig. 17–7). At present no specific frequency or velocity criteria exist with which to gauge the severity of stenoses, as exist for carotid or lower extremity arteries.[10]

Normal waveforms in the upper extremity arteries are usually triphasic. In normal individuals, hemodynamic resistance in the arm may decrease markedly with arm exercise or warming of the hand, and the flow pattern may become monophasic and continue throughout diastole (Fig. 17–8). With cooling of the limb, the amplitude of the velocity waveform decreases drastically, but the triphasic pattern persists. Normal peak systolic velocity values in healthy subjects vary widely with skin temperature. As shown in Figure 17–8, radial artery velocities vary between 28 and 70 cm/sec as skin temperature goes from 18 to 35°C. Normal peak systolic velocities in the subclavian artery are in the 80 to 120 cm/sec range at room temperature, and in the radial artery they range from 40 to 60 cm/sec. Brachial artery velocities are intermediate in value.

The diagnosis of arterial occlusion is made by imaging the artery and using the Doppler instrument to show that no flow is present within the lumen. A number of structures in the arm, especially the forearm, may be mistaken for occluded arteries, including veins, tendons, and nerves. Because the upper extremity arteries are fairly constant in location, false diagnoses of occlusion can be avoided by searching carefully for the artery

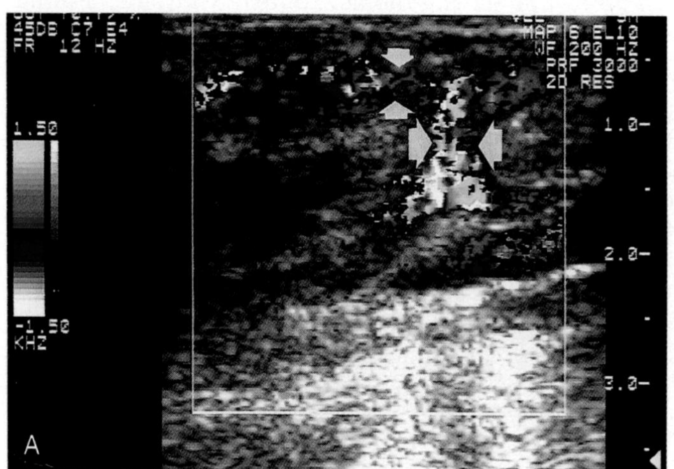

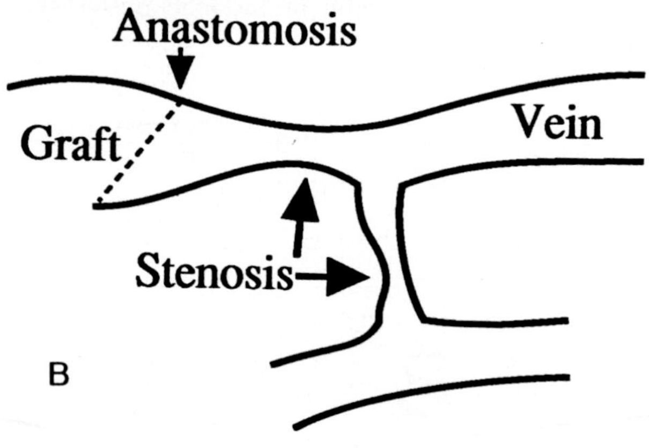

FIGURE 17–7 *A,* Color-flow duplex image of the outflow of an arteriovenous shunt demonstrating two stenoses (*small arrows,* stenosis in outflow vein; *large arrows,* stenosis in communicating vein). High velocities (yellow) and poststenotic turbulence (speckling of colors below second stenosis) are seen. *B,* A line drawing showing the anatomy seen in the color image.

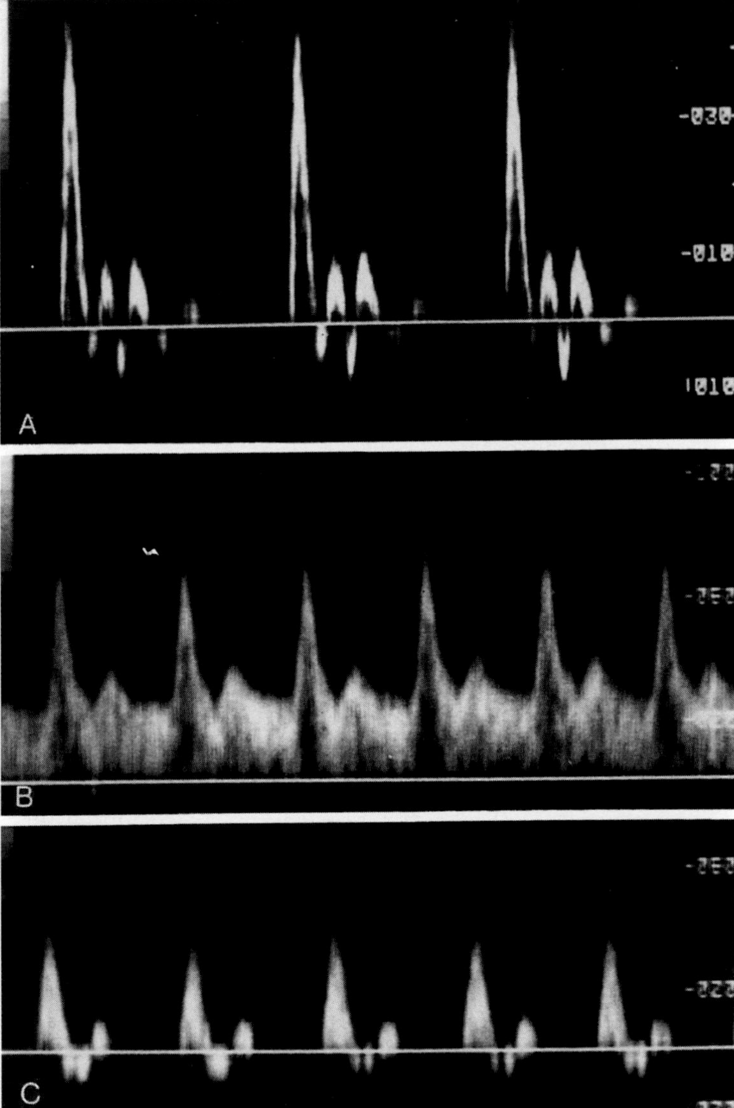

FIGURE 17–8 Doppler spectral waveforms of the radial artery showing variation with ambient temperature. Top tracing (*A*) taken at room temperature (peak systolic velocity, 45 cm/sec), middle tracing (*B*) taken after immersion in hot (40°C) water (peak systolic velocity, 70 cm/sec), bottom tracing (*C*) taken after immersion in ice (0°C) water (peak systolic velocity, 28 cm/sec).

at several levels. This can be done in a short period, especially if a color-Doppler scanner is used. Warming the extremity also decreases the possibility of a false-positive diagnosis of occlusion by increasing arterial flow to the extremity.

The introduction of color-Doppler scanners has allowed rapid identification of small arteries. Although the use of color may aid in performance of the examination, the important diagnostic information resides in the Doppler spectra. As seen in Figures 17–7, 17–9, and 17–10, the presence of various abnormalities can easily be seen using a color-Doppler scanner.

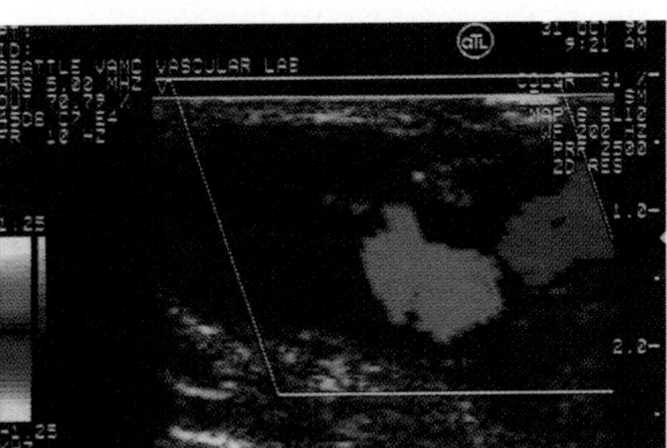

FIGURE 17–9 Color-flow duplex image of an aneurysm in an arteriovenous dialysis fistula. The maximum diameter of the vein was greater than 1.0 cm.

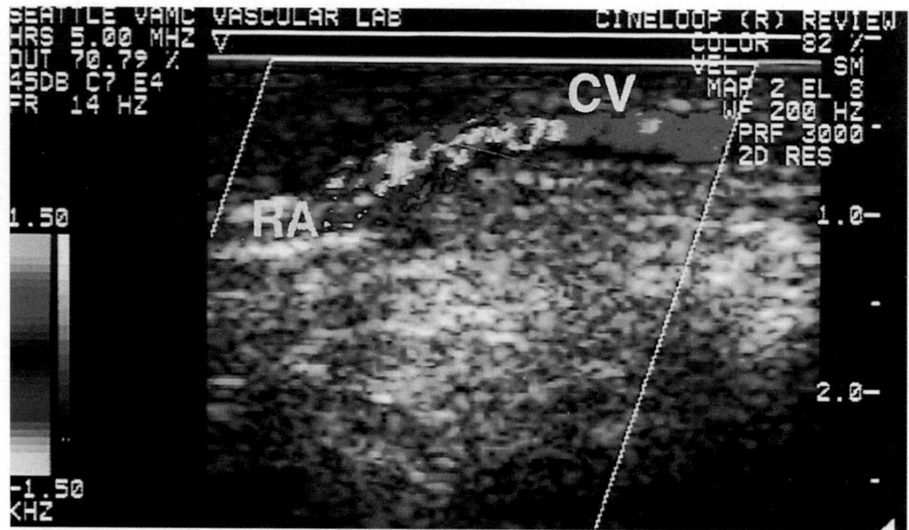

FIGURE 17–10 Black and white representation of color-flow duplex image of a normal Cimino-Brescia fistula. The radial artery (RA) is only partially in the picture, but the cephalic vein (CV) is clearly seen. Flow just distal to the anastomosis is moderately disturbed, as evidenced by the speckled pattern, but the flow pattern quickly becomes organized further downstream.

CLINICAL SYNDROMES

Raynaud's Syndrome

Most clinical syndromes involving upper extremity ischemia include Raynaud's syndrome as one of their major clinical manifestations. Raynaud's syndrome can be defined as episodic digital ischemia in response to cold or emotional stimuli. These episodes are due to spasm of the digital arteries and are clinically characterized by a series of color changes that typically consist of pallor, cyanosis, and rubor. Episodic digital ischemia is seen in association with disease involving the small vessels of the hands, embolization from an upstream lesion, occlusion of the major arteries supplying the arm or hand, and primary vasospastic disorders.

The diagnosis of Raynaud's syndrome is made on the basis of clinical presentation, but confirmatory vascular laboratory testing should include cold intolerance testing, digital plethysmography, and measurement of digital blood pressures. The important differentiation is to determine if the patient has occlusive or vasospastic Raynaud's syndrome, and if there is obstruction, determine if this is in the large or small arteries. Duplex scanning is not useful in the diagnosis of Raynaud's syndrome per se, but rather is useful in the diagnosis of a variety of conditions whose initial clinical manifestations may include Raynaud's syndrome. Thus, only selected patients being evaluated in the noninvasive vascular laboratory for Raynaud's syndrome require an upper extremity duplex examination. The most common indication is obstructive Raynaud's syndrome without evidence of an associated autoimmune disease. In this situation, the purpose of the duplex scan is to search for large arterial lesions that are obstructing blood flow directly or are a source of emboli.

Arterial Occlusive Diseases

Atherosclerosis is the most frequently encountered disease process involving the upper extremity arteries. The larger arteries are usually involved, with the lesions located proximally, particularly at the origins of the subclavian and innominate arteries. Duplex scanning can be used to diagnose stenosis and occlusion, as well as to evaluate collateral circulation patterns.[11, 12]

Takayasu's disease, an autoimmune disorder involving the arteries of the head, neck, and arms, is characterized by long segment stenoses or occlusions of the affected arteries. Although duplex scanning alone cannot be used to make this diagnosis, it is a helpful adjunct to therapy in that the progression or regression of arterial involvement can be serially assessed noninvasively to document the response to treatment.[13] Buerger's disease primarily involves the small vessels of the hand. Duplex scanning is helpful in this disease, mainly in ruling out proximal arterial lesions.

Congenital arterial abnormalities involving the upper extremity may also be detected by duplex scanning.[14] Duplex scanning has been used for diagnosing agenesis or neonatal occlusion of the subclavian artery.

Upper extremity arterial repairs may easily be followed for stenosis or occlusion with duplex scanning.[15–17] The examination techniques for postoperative surveillance are similar to those discussed in Chapter 18 for lower extremity arteries.

Aneurysms

Duplex evaluation of aneurysms is based on the B-mode image appearance, the most important feature being the size of the enlarged artery. Presence or absence of flow within the aneurysm can be determined by the Doppler component. Aneurysms in the upper extremity arteries are usually due to atherosclerosis or trauma and present with thrombosis, a pulsatile mass, or distal embolization. As a rule, an artery is considered to be aneurysmal if the diameter of the vessel at the point of interest is at least twice the diameter of the normal vessel proximally or distally. Because aneurysms may contain laminated thrombus, the measurements should be taken from outer wall to outer wall, rather than from the width of the flow stream. An example of an aneurysm is seen in Figure 17–9.

Ulnar artery aneurysms form in response to the use of the palm as a hammer (hypothenar hammer syndrome) and often present with arterial occlusion.[15] Aneurysms involving the subclavian artery often present with embolization to the digits. Aneurysms involving the axillary and brachial arteries are rare and may be caused by trauma (pseudoaneurysms), atherosclerosis, fibromuscular dysplasia, or Kawasaki's disease.[18]

Emboli

The major sources of emboli to the arm and hand are proximal aneurysms and the heart. Duplex scanning may be of use in patients with suspected embolization to identify proximal aneurysms, but the evaluation should also include echocardiography to look for mural thrombi and valvular lesions.

Trauma

The standard approach to the evaluation of arterial trauma is arteriography or surgical exploration. Unfortunately, both these methods are invasive and expensive and, in the case of surgical exploration, may fail to detect intimal injuries. Additionally, both techniques are time-consuming. For these reasons, the current trend is to observe patients with traumatic injuries that may affect major arteries if they have normal distal pressures and pulses.[19] Duplex evaluation of these patients allows for prompt identification of obstructed arteries, as well as false aneurysms and large intimal flaps. Duplex scanning can be performed rapidly, because the trauma is usually limited to a specific arterial segment. Pseudoaneurysm formation from penetrating trauma or brachial or axillary artery catheterization may also be detected with the duplex scanner.[18] As far as we are aware, only a few institutions are using duplex scanning for the initial evaluation of upper extremity arterial trauma, but as duplex scanners become more widely available in emergency departments, this application should become more common.

Thoracic Outlet Syndrome

The clinical syndrome related to compression of the neurovascular structures in the thoracic outlet has been the subject of increasing interest. The subclavian artery, subclavian vein, and brachial plexus all pass through this small anatomic space that is bordered by the first rib, the clavicle, and the scalene muscles. A cervical rib, with or without an associated fibrous band, may further narrow this anatomic space. Because multiple processes may narrow the thoracic outlet, the term *thoracic outlet syndrome* was coined in 1956.[20]

Although a variety of classifications have been suggested for the clinical manifestations of thoracic outlet syndrome, there are basically three types. The first is *true neurogenic* thoracic outlet syndrome associated with a bone abnormality, often a cervical rib, in which the diagnosis is made by electromyography. The most constant clinical features are hand weakness and wasting of the intrinsic hand muscles. Pain typically affects the hand, medial forearm, and arm, whereas any sensory deficit follows a patchy lower trunk distribution along the medial forearm and hand.[21] The second type is *vascular* thoracic outlet syndrome, which is also usually associated with a bone abnormality. An arterial or venous lesion (stenosis, occlusion, or aneurysm formation) is seen on angiography. The third type, which has been called *disputed* thoracic outlet syndrome,[21] accounts for most of the cases seen in the United States. These patients present with subjective arm and hand weakness; paresthesias; pain involving the arm, shoulder girdle, and chest wall; and headache. Although the sensory complaints are similar to those seen with neurogenic thoracic outlet syndrome, hand wasting is never found in these patients, and electromyographic testing is normal.

The proponents of disputed thoracic outlet syndrome attribute the symptoms either to only nerve compression or to combined nerve and arterial compression from bone malalignment, muscle injury, or fibrosis secondary to minor trauma. Some advocates of thoracic outlet surgery for disputed thoracic outlet syndrome believe that the syndrome is caused by a physiologic dysfunction of the scalene muscle, not a structural abnormality.[22] Although several reports have shown abnormal histologic changes in the affected muscles, this hypothesis remains to be proved.

The opponents of disputed thoracic outlet syndrome point out several problems with this diagnosis. These include the lack of an objective diagnostic test, the fact that these patients do not progress to true neurogenic or vascular thoracic outlet syndrome, the observation that this disease tends to be reported only in areas where proponents practice, and the fact that at least some of the symptoms (headache and shoulder girdle pain) cannot be anatomically related to the thoracic outlet. In other countries a similar syndrome is seen but is thought to be myofascial in nature and is called *repetitive stress injury* or *disorder*.[23] This syndrome appears to be related to fibrositis and remains poorly understood.

The role of duplex scanning in the diagnosis of thoracic outlet syndrome is not established; however, duplex scanning can detect the rare cases of vascular thoracic outlet syndrome (arterial or venous) by revealing either stenosis or aneurysmal changes. Duplex scanning of the thoracic outlet has been suggested as a sensitive test for detecting compression of the subclavian or axillary artery with provocative positioning.[24] Although there is no doubt that duplex scanning can detect narrowing or occlusion of these arteries, this finding is not diagnostic of thoracic outlet syndrome, as many normal individuals also have abnormalities produced by extreme arm positioning in the absence of any symptoms.

Arteriovenous Fistulas

Duplex scanning is a useful adjunct in the management of surgically constructed arteriovenous fistulas and grafts used for hemodialysis.[16] Several types of fistulas are currently used. A Cimino-Brescia native arteriovenous fistula is an end-to-side or a side-to-side anastomosis between the radial artery and the cephalic vein at the wrist (see Fig. 17–10). Alternatively, a prosthetic graft may be placed as a loop between the brachial artery at the elbow and an antecubital vein or as a straight graft between the radial artery at the wrist and an antecubital vein.

Both stenotic and aneurysmal lesions in the fistula, graft, or venous outflow may be detected.[25–27] As with leg bypass grafts, there appears to be a difference in the flow characteristics of venous conduits and prosthetic graft materials. Normal velocities in native arteriovenous fistulas are lower than those seen in polytetrafluoroethylene (PTFE) loop grafts. Several criteria have been described in the duplex examination of PTFE loop arteriovenous grafts that may be clinically useful. First, the mean (calculated) flow in this type of graft is normally in the range of 800 mL/min. Grafts with flows less than 450 mL/min are at high risk for thrombosis in the subsequent 2 to 6 weeks.[24] Stenoses can be detected by looking for typical areas of high velocity and poststenotic turbulence. Aneurysms are also easily visualized (see Fig. 17–9).

Tumors

Although duplex scanning is not the primary imaging modality for the detection of upper extremity tumors, evaluation of perivascular masses scanned because of their pulsating nature may lead to the diagnosis of a variety of tumors.[15]

REFERENCES

1. Nielson SL, Lassen NA: Measurement of digital blood pressure after local cooling. J Appl Physiol 43:907–910, 1977.
2. Lafferty K, de Trafford JC, Roberts VC, et al: Raynaud's phenomena and thermal entrainment: An objective test. BMJ 286:90–92, 1983.
3. Brain SD, Petty RG, Lewis JD, et al: Cutaneous blood flow responses in the forearms of Raynaud's patients induced by local cooling and intradermal injections of CGRP and histamine. Br J Clin Pharmacol 30: 853–859, 1990.
4. Chucker R, Fowler RC, Molomiza T, et al: Induced temperature gradients in Raynaud's disease measured by thermography. Angiology 22:580–593, 1971.
5. Singh S, de Trafford JC, Baskerville PA, et al: Digital artery caliber measurement—a new technique of assessing Raynaud's phenomena. Eur J Vasc Surg 5:199–203, 1991.
6. Antignani PL, Pillon S, Di Fortunato T, Bartolo M: Light reflex rheography and thoracic outlet syndrome. Angiology 41:382–386, 1990.
7. Winsor T, Winsor D, Mikail A, Sibley AE: Thoracic outlet syndromes: Application of microcirculation techniques and clinical review. Angiology 40:773–781, 1989.
8. Sumner DS, Strandness DE: An abnormal finger pulse associated with cold sensitivity. Ann Surg 175:294–298, 1972.
9. Porter JM, Snider RL, Bardana EJ, et al: The diagnosis and treatment of Raynaud's syndrome. Surgery 77:11–23, 1975.
10. Jager KA, Phillips DJ, Martin RL, et al: Noninvasive mapping of lower limb arterial lesions. Ultrasound Med Biol 11:515–521, 1985.
11. Ackerstaff RGA, Hoeneveld H, Slowikowski JM, et al: Ultrasonic duplex scanning in atherosclerotic disease of the innominate, subclavian, and vertebral arteries. A comparative study with angiography. Ultrasound Med Biol 10:409–418, 1984.
12. Grosveld WJHM, Lawson JA, Eikelboom BC, et al: Clinical and hemodynamic significance of innominate artery lesions evaluated by ultrasonography and digital angiography. Stroke 19:958–962, 1988.
13. Reed AJ, Fincher RME, Nichols FT: Takayasu arteritis in a middle-aged Caucasian woman: Clinical course correlated with duplex ultrasound and angiography. Am J Med Sci 298:324–327, 1989.
14. Merlob P, Schonfeld A, Ovadia Y, Reisner SH: Realtime echo-Doppler duplex scanner in the evaluation of patients with Poland sequence. Eur J Obstet Gynecol Reprod Bio 32:103–108, 1989.
15. Koman LA, Bond MG, Carter RE, Poehling GG: Evaluation of upper extremity vasculature with high resolution ultrasound. J Hand Surg 10A:249–255, 1985.
16. White RA, White GH, Fujitani RM, et al: Initial human evaluation of argon laser–assisted vascular anastomoses. J Vasc Surg 9:542–547, 1989.
17. Cormier JM, Amrane M, Ward A: Arterial complications of the thoracic outlet syndrome: Fifty-five operative cases. J Vasc Surg 9:778–787, 1989.
18. Thomas VC, Roder HU, Moser GH: Diagnostiche Wertigkeit der Angiodynographie bei pulsierenden Raumforderunger. ROFO Fortschr Geb Rontgenstr Nuklearmed 150:454–457, 1989.
19. Lynch K, Johansen K: Can Doppler pressure measurement replace "exclusion" arteriography in the diagnosis of occult extremity arterial trauma? Ann Surg 214:737–741, 1991.
20. Peet PM, Henriksen JD, Anderson TP, Martin GM: Thoracic outlet syndrome: Evaluation of a therapeutic exercise program. Mayo Clin Proc 31:281–287, 1956.
21. Wilbourn AJ, Porter JM: Thoracic outlet syndromes. SPINE: State of the Art Reviews, Vol 2. Philadelphia, Hanley & Belfus, 1988, pp 597–626.
22. Sanders RJ, Pearce WH: The treatment of thoracic outlet syndrome: A comparison of different operations. J Vasc Surg 10:626–634, 1989.
23. Miller MH, Topliss DJ: Chronic upper limb pain syndrome (repetitive strain injury) in the Australian workforce: A systematic cross sectional rheumatological study of 229 patients. J Rheumatol 15:1705–1712, 1988.
24. Guzzetti A, Bellotti R: Usefulness of Doppler echocardiography in the diagnosis of upper thoracic outlet syndrome. Chir Ital 40:152–155, 1988.
25. Kathrein H, Konig P, Weimann S, et al: Non-invasive morphologic and functional assessment or arteriovenous fistula in dialysis patients with duplex sonography. Ultraschall Med 10:33–40, 1989.
26. Shackleton CR, Taylor DC, Buckley AR, et al: Predicting failure in polytetrafluoroethylene vascular access grafts for hemodialysis: A pilot study. Can J Surg 30:442–444, 1987.
27. Tordoir JH, de Bruin HG, Hoeneveld H, et al: Duplex ultrasound scanning in the assessment of arteriovenous fistulas created for hemodialysis access: Comparison with digital subtraction angiography. J Vasc Surg 10:122–128, 1989.

Chapter 18

DUPLEX SONOGRAPHY OF LOWER EXTREMITY ARTERIES

■ *R. Eugene Zierler, MD* ■ *Brenda K. Zierler, PhD, RN, RVT*

The purpose of noninvasive testing for lower extremity arterial disease is to provide objective information that can be combined with the clinical history and physical examination to form the basis for decisions regarding further evaluation and treatment. One of the most critical decisions relates to whether a patient is a candidate for therapeutic intervention and should undergo arteriography. Contrast arteriography has generally been regarded as the definitive examination for lower extremity arterial disease, but this approach is invasive, expensive, and poorly suited for screening or long-term follow-up testing. In addition, arteriography provides anatomic rather than physiologic information, and it is subject to significant variability at the time of interpretation.[1,2] The most valid physiologic method for detecting hemodynamically significant lesions is direct, intra-arterial pressure measurement, but this method is also impractical in many clinical situations.

The simple and widely used indirect noninvasive tests of the lower extremity arteries, including the measurement of ankle systolic blood pressure and segmental limb pressures, provide valuable physiologic information about the arterial system, but these tests provide relatively little anatomic information.[3] Duplex scanning extends the capabilities of noninvasive testing by obtaining anatomic and physiologic information directly from sites of arterial disease. The initial application of duplex scanning concentrated on the clinically important problem of extracranial carotid artery disease. The focal nature of carotid atherosclerosis and the relatively superficial location of the carotid bifurcation contributed to the success of these early studies.[4] Continued clinical experience and advances in technology, particularly the availability of lower frequency duplex transducers, have made it possible to obtain image and flow information from deeply located vessels. Therefore, it is now feasible to perform the selective evaluation of abdominal and lower extremity arteries with ultrasound (US). The addition of color-Doppler imaging provides a visually striking method for displaying Doppler information. This article reviews the current status of lower extremity duplex scanning with color-Doppler imaging.

INSTRUMENTATION

Although the commercially available duplex scanning systems vary with respect to image quality, display capabilities, Doppler characteristics, and signal processing, they all consist of a two-dimensional B-mode imaging system, a pulsed Doppler flow detector, and a spectrum analyzer. Transducer frequencies of approximately 3 MHz are most suitable for evaluating the abdominal vessels in average-sized adults, whereas a 5-MHz transducer can be used for thin individuals. Examination of the more distal, superficially located arteries in the legs can be performed with 5-, 7.5-, or 10-MHz transducers. In general, the highest frequency scan head that provides adequate depth penetration should be used.

This chapter is adapted from Zierler RE, Zierler BK: Duplex sonography of lower extremity arteries. Semin Ultrasound CT MR 18:39–56, 1997. Reprinted with permission.

Color-Doppler instruments combine standard duplex technology with a real-time color display of blood flow. Color-Doppler imaging offers several advantages over conventional spectral waveforms for the assessment of lower extremity arteries. The color image helps identify vessels and flow abnormalities caused by arterial lesions (Figs. 18–1 and 18–2). The ability to visualize flow throughout a vessel improves the precision of Doppler sample volume placement when spectral waveforms are obtained. Thus, color-Doppler imaging has the potential for reducing examination time and improving overall accuracy. It must be emphasized, however, that color-Doppler imaging is not a replacement for conventional duplex techniques. In particular, spectral waveform analysis remains the primary source of duplex diagnostic information.[5] Furthermore, color Doppler is subject to certain artifacts and limitations with which sonographers must be familiar.

Duplex instruments (standard or color Doppler) are equipped with specific combinations of US parameters for imaging and flow detection that can be selected by the examiner for a particular application. These preset combinations can be helpful, especially during the learning process, but the parameter combinations supplied with an instrument may not be adequate for all patient examinations. A complete understanding of the US parameters that are under the technologist's control is essential for producing optimal arterial duplex scans.

DUPLEX ASSESSMENT OF NATIVE ARTERIES

Technique

In both the conventional and color-Doppler approaches to lower extremity arterial sonography, the B-mode or color image is used to identify the artery of interest and facilitate precise placement of the Doppler sample volume.[6] The image is valuable for recognizing anatomic variations and for identifying arterial disease by showing plaque or calcification. It has not been possible, however, to determine the degree of arterial narrowing from the B-mode or color image alone. Therefore, the classification of disease severity is based primarily on interpretation of the pulsed Doppler spectral waveforms.

When examining an arterial segment, it is essential to evaluate the flow pattern at closely spaced intervals. This is necessary because the flow disturbances produced by arterial lesions are only propagated along the vessel for a short distance. Experimental work has shown that the high-velocity jets and turbulence associated with arterial stenoses are damped out over a distance of only a few vessel diameters.[7] Consequently, failure to identify localized flow abnormalities could lead to underestimation of disease severity. Because local flow disturbances are usually apparent with color-Doppler imaging (see Fig. 18–1), pulsed Doppler flow samples may be obtained at more widely spaced intervals when color Doppler is used. Nonetheless, it is advisable to assess the flow characteristics with spectral waveform analysis at frequent intervals in extensively diseased vessels.

Lengths of occluded arterial segments can be measured with standard or color-Doppler scanning by imaging the point of occlusion proximally and the site where flow is reconstituted by collateral vessels distally. Because flow velocities distal to an occluded segment may be low, it is important to adjust the color-Doppler instrument properly to detect low flow rates.

For examination of the aorta and iliac arteries, patients should be fasting for 12 hours to reduce interference by bowel gas. In our experience with standard duplex instruments, satisfactory aortoiliac Doppler signals can be obtained from approximately 90% of individuals who have been prepared in this way. It is usually most convenient to examine patients early in the morning, after an overnight fast. The patient is initially positioned supine with the hips rotated externally. A left lateral decubitus position may also be advantageous for the abdominal portion of the examination. An electric blanket placed over the patient prevents vasoconstriction caused by low room temperatures.

For a complete lower extremity arterial evaluation, scanning begins with the upper portion of the abdominal aorta. An anteromidline approach to the aorta is used, with the transducer placed just below the xyphoid process. Both US images and Doppler signals are best obtained in the longitudinal plane of the aorta, but transverse views are occasionally useful to define anatomic relationships. If specifically indicated, the mesenteric and renal vessels can be examined at this time, although this does not need to be performed rou-

Text continued on page 269

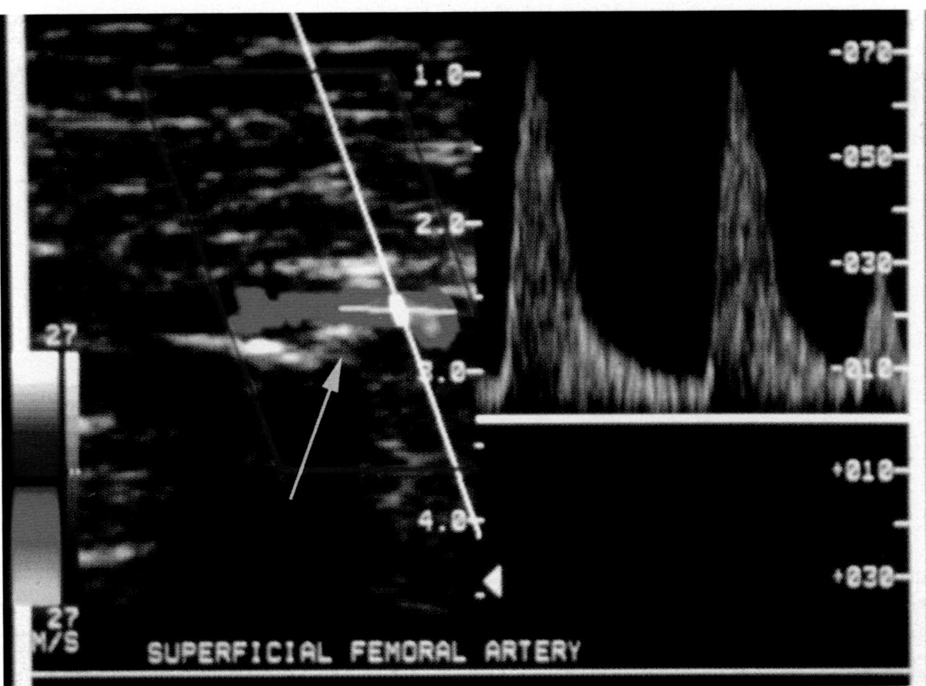

FIGURE 18–1 Moderate superficial femoral artery stenosis. Color-Doppler image shows a posterior plaque (*arrow*) and a localized, high-velocity jet. The spectral waveform from the site of stenosis indicates a 20 to 49% diameter-reducing lesion. (From Zierler RE, Zierler BK: Duplex sonography of lower extremity arteries. Semin Ultrasound CT MR 18:39–56, 1997.)

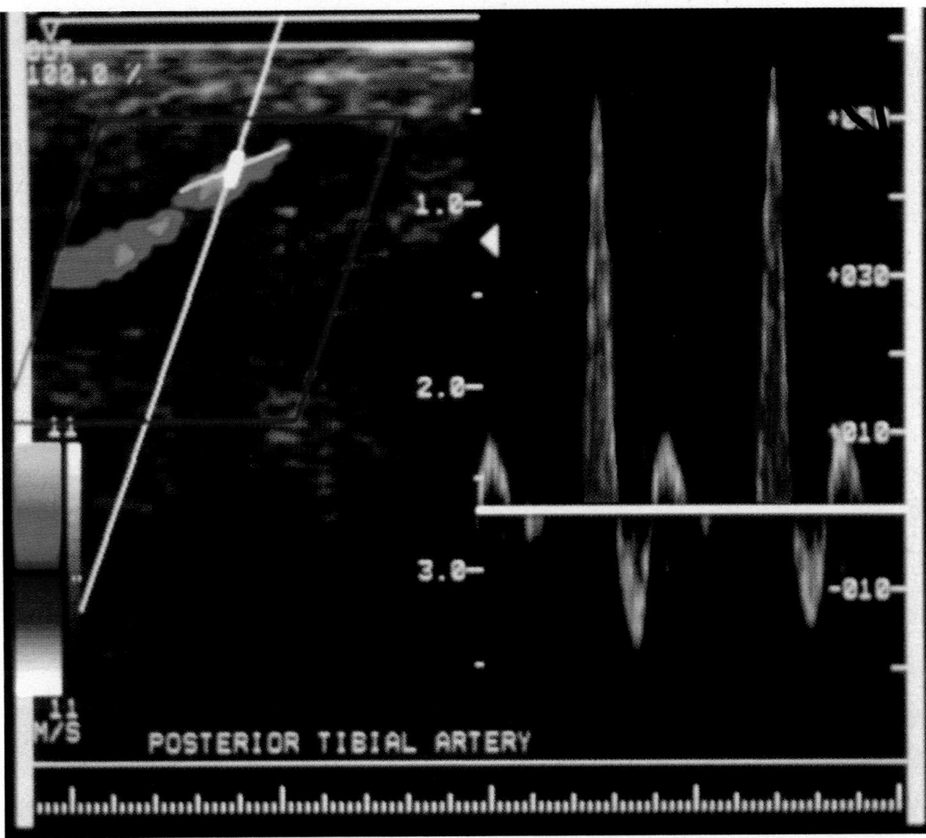

FIGURE 18–2 Color-Doppler image of a posterior tibial artery showing a small vessel with relatively low flow velocities. The corresponding normal spectral waveform is triphasic. (From Zierler RE, Zierler BK: Duplex sonography of lower extremity arteries. Semin Ultrasound CT MR 18:39–56, 1997.)

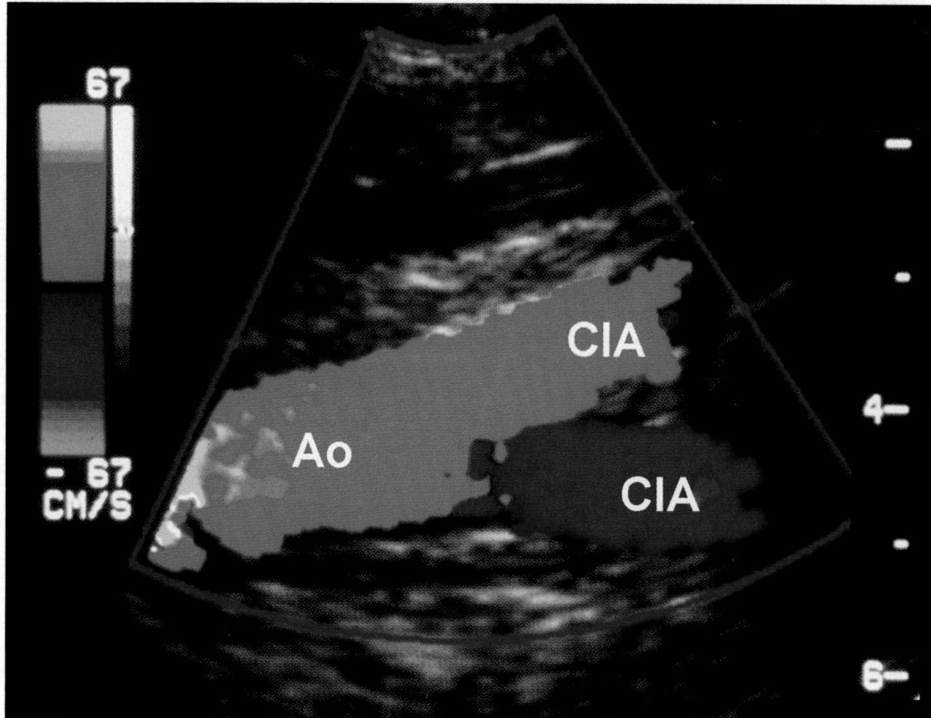

FIGURE 18–3 Color-Doppler image of the aortic bifurcation. (See p 269.) The difference in color between the common Iliac branches is the result of different flow directions with respect to the transducer. Ao = aorta; CIA = common iliac artery. (From Zierler RE, Zierler BK: Duplex sonography of lower extremity arteries. Semin Ultrasound CT MR 18:39–56, 1997.)

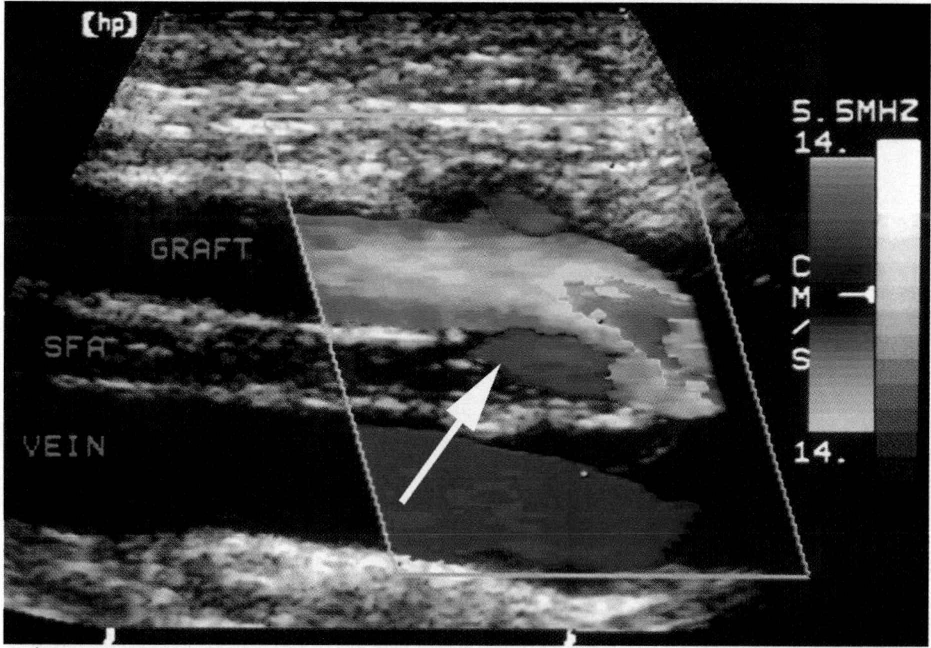

FIGURE 18–9 Color-Doppler image of the distal anastomosis of an above-knee reversed-vein femoral-popliteal bypass graft. (See p 276.) Duplex scan was performed 18 months postoperatively. Flow is visualized in the distal graft anastomosis (*arrow*), and superficial femoral artery (SFA) distal to the graft. Flow is also seen in the superficial femoral vein. (From Zierler RE, Zierler BK: Duplex sonography of lower extremity arteries. Semin Ultrasound CT MR 18:39–56, 1997.)

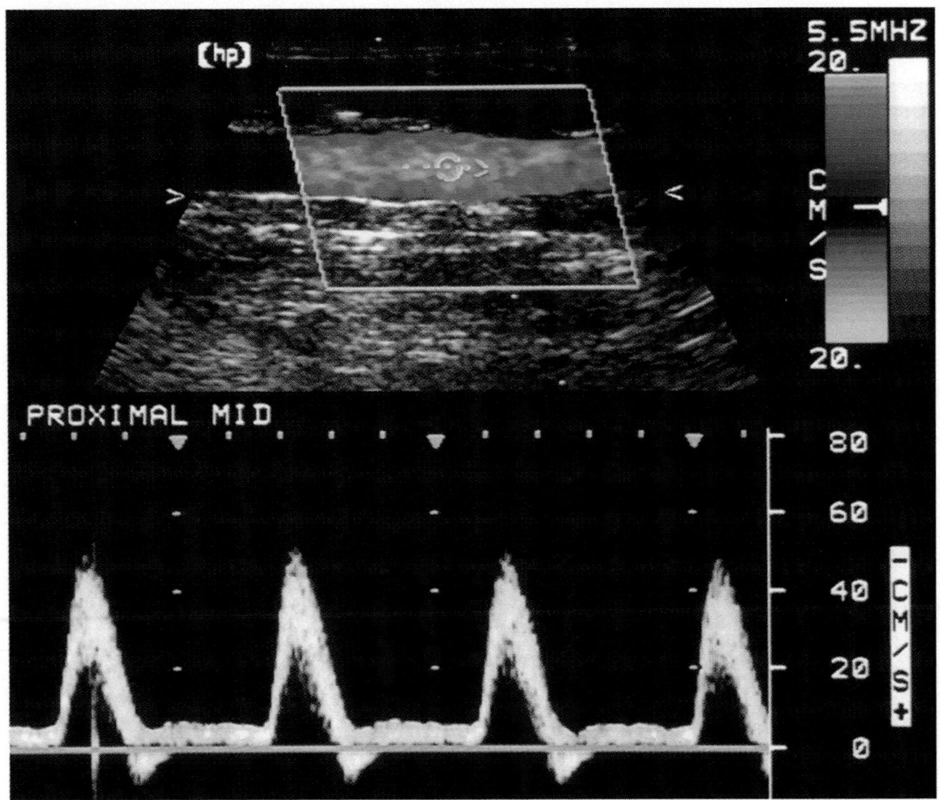

FIGURE 18–10 Normal triphasic flow pattern in a 4-year-old femoral-tibial in situ vein graft. (See p 276.) Peak systolic velocities are approximately 50 cm/sec. (From Zierler RE, Zierler BK: Duplex sonography of lower extremity arteries. Semin Ultrasound CT MR 18:39–56, 1997.)

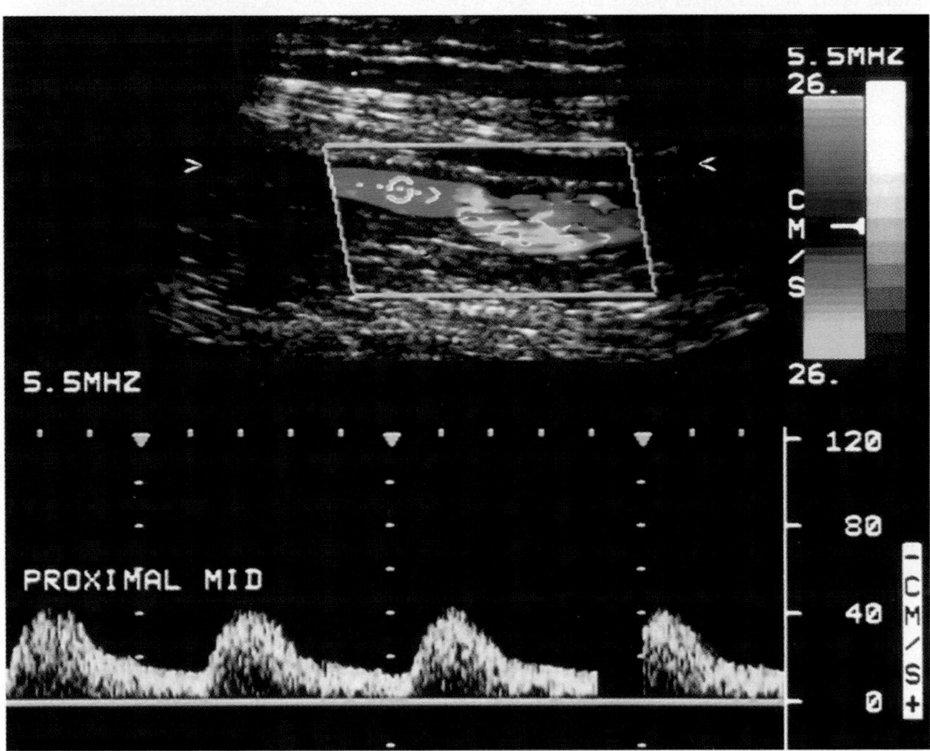

FIGURE 18–11 Damped, monophasic flow pattern proximal to a stenotic lesion in a 2-month-old femoral-popliteal bypass graft performed with reversed arm vein. (See p 276.) Peak systolic velocities are approximately 40 cm/sec. (From Zierler RE, Zierler BK: Duplex sonography of lower extremity arteries. Semin Ultrasound CT MR 18:39–56, 1997.)

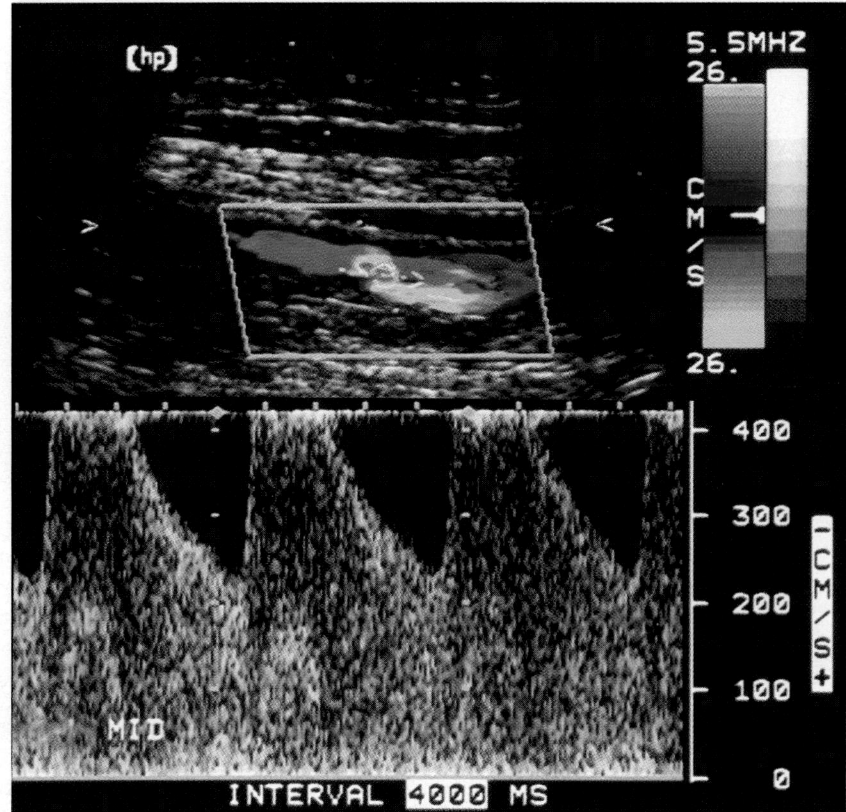

FIGURE 18–12 Color-Doppler image and velocity waveforms taken from a diameter-reducing stenosis of more than 75% in a 2-month-old femoral-popliteal bypass graft performed with reversed arm vein (same graft as Figure 18–11). (See p 277.) Peak systolic velocities are greater than 400 cm/sec, and end diastolic velocities are greater than 200 cm/sec. The velocity ratio associated with this lesion is in excess of 10. (From Zierler RE, Zierler BK: Duplex sonography of lower extremity arteries. Semin Ultrasound CT MR 18:39–56, 1997.)

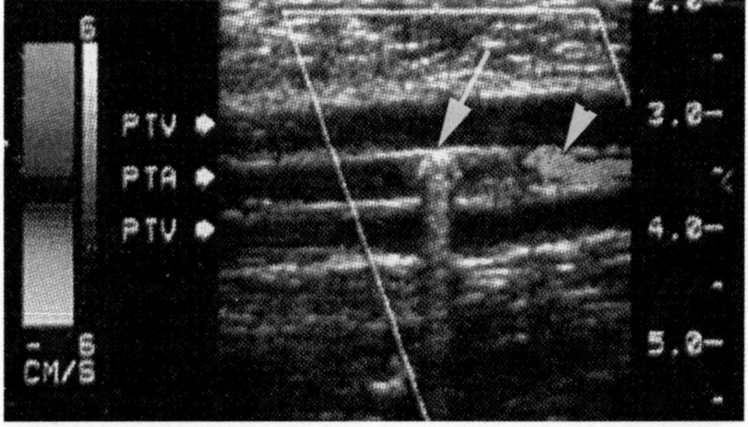

FIGURE 18–14 Color-Doppler image from a patient with a lower extremity gunshot wound showing a bullet fragment (*arrow*) in the posterior tibial artery (PTA). (See p 280.) The color-flow stream stops (*arrowhead*) at the bullet, where marked acoustic shadowing is present. Two posterior tibial veins (PTV) are also visualized. (From Zierler RE, Zierler BK: Duplex sonography of lower extremity arteries. Semin Ultrasound CT MR 18:39–56, 1997.)

tinely when evaluating the lower extremity arteries. The aorta is followed distally to its bifurcation (Fig. 18–3), and the iliac arteries are examined separately to the level of the groin.

Each lower extremity is examined in turn, beginning with the common femoral artery and working distally. After the femoral arteries are scanned throughout the thighs, it is often helpful to turn the patient to the prone position to examine the popliteal arteries. The tibial and peroneal arteries can be difficult to examine completely, but can usually be imaged with color Doppler. These vessels are best evaluated either by identifying their origins from the distal popliteal artery and scanning distally or by finding the arteries at the ankle and working proximally. Several large branches can often be seen originating from the distal superficial femoral and popliteal segments. These are readily visualized with color-Doppler imaging and represent the genicular and sural arteries.

Pulsed Doppler spectral waveforms are recorded from any areas in which increased velocities or other flow disturbances are noted with color Doppler. Recordings should also be made at the following standard locations: (1) the proximal and distal abdominal aorta; (2) the common, internal, and external iliac arteries; (3) the common and deep femoral arteries; (4) the proximal, middle, and distal superficial femoral arteries; (5) the popliteal arteries; and (6) the tibial arteries at their origin or at the level of the foot. A complete examination of the aortoiliac system and both lower extremities may require 2 hours, but a single leg can usually be evaluated in less than 1 hour.

The duplex scanning technique for arterial bypass grafts and other applications are presented elsewhere in this article.

Normal Flow Characteristics

Jager and colleagues[8] have determined standard values for arterial diameter and peak systolic flow velocity in the lower extremity arteries of 55 healthy subjects (30 males, 25 females) ranging in age from 20 to 80 years old (Table 18–1). Although women have smaller arteries than men, peak systolic velocities did not differ significantly between men and women in this study. However, the peak systolic velocities decreased steadily from the iliac to the popliteal arteries.

TABLE 18–1 MEAN ARTERIAL DIAMETERS AND PEAK SYSTOLIC FLOW VELOCITIES*

Artery	Diameter ± SD (cm)	Velocity ± SD (cm/sec)
External iliac	0.79 ± 0.13	119.3 ± 21.7
Common femoral	0.82 ± 0.14	114.1 ± 24.9
Superficial femoral (proximal)	0.60 ± 0.12	90.8 ± 13.6
Superficial femoral (distal)	0.54 ± 0.11	93.6 ± 14.1
Popliteal	0.52 ± 0.11	68.8 ± 13.5

SD = standard deviation.

* Measurements by duplex scanning in 55 healthy subjects.

Adapted from Zierler RE, Zierler BK: Duplex sonography of lower extremity arteries. Semin Ultrasound CT MR 18:42, 1997.

Duplex scans of normal lower extremity arteries show the characteristic triphasic velocity waveform that is associated with peripheral artery flow (Fig. 18–4). This flow pattern can be shown by both spectral waveforms and color-Doppler imaging.[10] The initial high-velocity, forward flow phase that results from cardiac systole is followed by a brief phase of reverse flow in early diastole and a final low-velocity, forward flow phase later in diastole. The reverse flow component is a consequence of the relatively high peripheral vascular resistance in the normal lower extremity arterial circulation. Reverse flow becomes less prominent when peripheral resistance decreases. This loss of flow reversal typically occurs in normal limbs with the vasodilatation that accompanies reactive hyperemia or limb warming. The reverse flow component is also absent distal to severe occlusive lesions.

The normal lower extremity center stream arterial flow pattern is relatively uniform, with the red blood cells all having nearly the same velocity. Therefore, the flow is laminar, and the corresponding spectral waveform contains a narrow band of frequencies with a clear area under the systolic peak (see Fig. 18–4). Arterial lesions disrupt this normal laminar flow pattern and give rise to characteristic velocity changes that produce a widening of the frequency band; this is referred to as *spectral broadening.*

Abnormal Arteries

Based on the established normal and abnormal features of spectral waveforms, a set of criteria for classifying diseased lower ex-

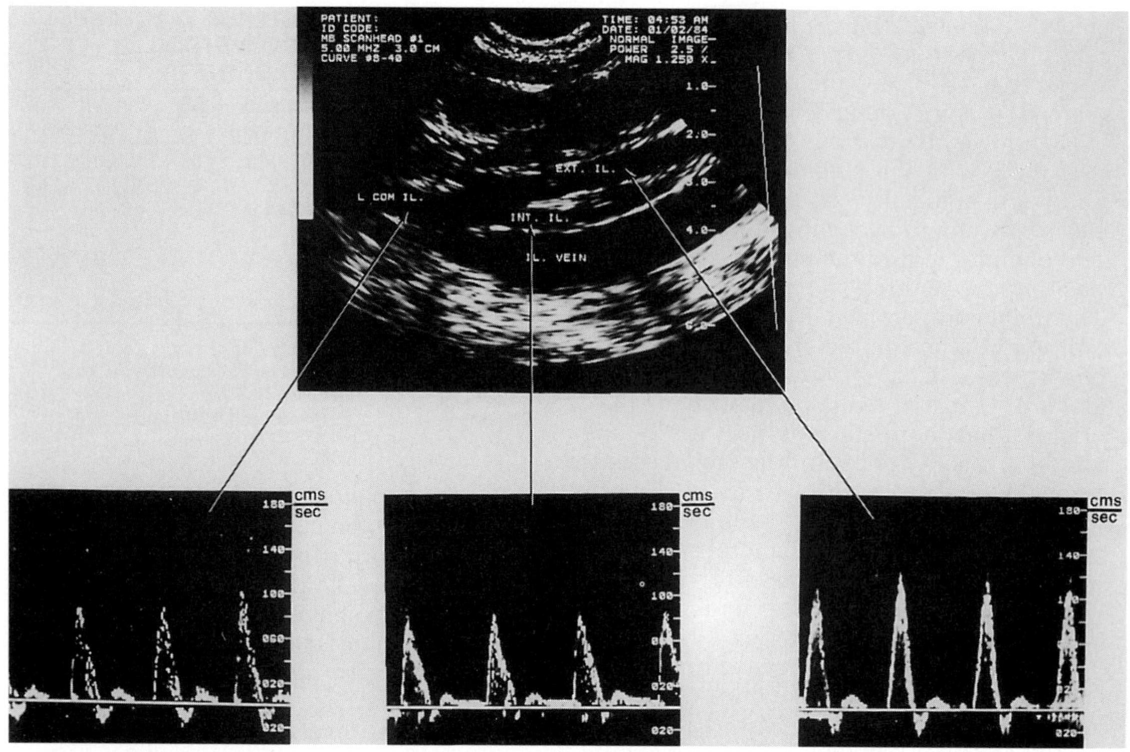

FIGURE 18–4 Spectral waveforms from a normal iliac artery segment. The waveforms are triphasic and contain a narrow band of frequencies, with a clear area under the systolic peak. Peak systolic velocities are approximately 100 cm/sec.

tremity arterial segments has been developed.[6,8] These criteria are summarized in Table 18–2 and Figure 18–5. Both the absolute velocity values and velocity ratios (stenotic jet velocities to proximal velocities) are important diagnostically. Thus, both parameters should be used for assessing extremity arterial lesions.

Minimal disease (1 to 19% diameter reduction) is indicated by a slight increase in spectral width, without a significant increase in peak systolic velocity. This minimal spectral broadening is usually found in late systole and early diastole. Moderate stenosis (20 to 49% diameter reduction) is characterized by more prominent spectral broadening and by some increase in peak systolic velocities. High-grade stenosis (50 to 99% diameter reduction) produces the most severe flow disturbance, with markedly increased peak systolic velocities, extensive spectral broadening, and loss of the reverse flow component. Occlusion of an arterial segment is documented when no Doppler flow signal can be detected in the lumen of a clearly imaged vessel. Spectral waveforms obtained distal to a high-grade stenosis or occlusion are generally monophasic, with reduced systolic velocities. The features of waveforms taken proximal to a stenotic lesion are variable and depend primarily on the status of the intervening collateral circulation. Immediately proximal to an arterial occlusion, the spectral waveforms show extremely low peak systolic velocities and little or no flow in diastole.

An important difference between spectral waveform analysis and color-Doppler imaging is that waveforms reveal the entire frequency and amplitude content of the pulsed Doppler signal at a specific site, whereas the color-Doppler image provides a single estimate of the Doppler shift frequency or flow velocity for each site within the image. Thus, spectral waveform analysis actually provides considerably more flow information from each individual site than color-Doppler imaging. The main advantage of the color display is that it presents flow information on the entire image, although the actual amount of data for each site is reduced.

Spectral waveforms contain a wide range of frequencies and amplitudes that allow determination of flow direction and parameters such as mean, mode, and peak frequency, as

TABLE 18–2 CRITERIA FOR CLASSIFYING PERIPHERAL ARTERY LESIONS*

Classification	Features
Normal	Triphasic waveform; no spectral broadening
1–19% diameter reduction	Triphasic waveform with minimal spectral broadening only; peak systolic velocities increased <30% relative to the adjacent proximal segment; proximal and distal waveforms remain normal
20–49% diameter reduction	Triphasic waveform usually maintained, although reverse flow component may be diminished; spectral broadening is prominent, with filling in of clear area under the systolic peak; peak systolic velocity is increased from 30–100% relative to the adjacent proximal segment; proximal and distal waveforms remain normal
50–99% diameter reduction	Monophasic waveform with loss of reverse flow component and forward flow throughout cardiac cycle; extensive spectral broadening; peak systolic velocity is increased >100% relative to adjacent proximal segment; distal waveform is monophasic, with reduced systolic velocity
Occlusion	No flow detected within imaged arterial segment; preocclusive "thump" may be heard just proximal to site of occlusion; distal waveforms are monophasic, with reduced systolic velocities

* Based on duplex scanning with spectral waveform analysis.
Adapted from Zierler RE, Zierler BK: Duplex sonography of lower extremity arteries. Semin Ultrasound CT MR 18:43, 1997.

well as bandwidth. In contrast, color assignments are based on flow direction and a single mean or average frequency estimate. Consequently, the peak or maximum Doppler frequency shifts found with spectral waveforms are generally higher than the frequencies indicated by the color-Doppler image. Because of this difference, the color-Doppler image may not show some high-velocity jets that are apparent on spectral waveforms.

Validation Studies

Although the criteria listed in Table 18–2 include several categories for lesions of less than 50% diameter reduction, the distinction between these categories is often subjective and is rarely of clinical importance. The most useful classification for clinical purposes recognizes those lesions of less than 50% diameter reduction, 50 to 99% diameter reduction, and occlusion. More precise classification of diameter reduction within the 50 to 99% stenosis category is not currently possible based on the commonly used spectral waveform and color-Doppler parameters.[11] Jager and associates[6] used duplex scanning to evaluate 338 arterial segments in 54 lower extremities of 30 patients and compared the severity of stenosis as classified by spectral waveform analysis to the results of independently interpreted arteriograms. For all segments, duplex scanning differentiated between normal and diseased arteries with a sensitivity of 96% and a specificity of 81%. Duplex scanning distinguished between stenoses of greater or less than 50% diameter reduction with a sensitivity of 77% and a specificity of 98%. These results compare favorably with the variability found when two different radiologists interpreted the same lower extremity arteriograms as either normal or diseased (sensitivity 98%; specificity 68%), or as greater or less than 50% diameter reduction (sensitivity 87%; specificity 94%).[2]

A second validation study was reported by Kohler and coworkers,[12] who evaluated 393 lower extremity arterial segments in 32 patients by both duplex scanning and arteriography. For correctly identifying stenoses that had a significant (measured) pressure gradient or that reduced the lumen diameter by more than 50%, duplex scanning had a sensitivity of 82%, a specificity of 92%, a positive predictive value of 80%, and a negative predictive value of 93%. The results were especially good for lesions in the iliac arteries (sensitivity 89%; specificity 90%). Lesions distal to very high-grade stenoses or complete occlusions were difficult to detect because of the low flow velocities in these segments. This limitation was also observed by Allard and colleagues,[13] who found that the presence of 50 to 99% stenoses in adjacent arterial segments decreased both the sensitivity and specificity of lower extremity duplex scanning.

Moneta and associates[14] documented the accuracy of lower extremity duplex scanning in 286 limbs of 150 patients undergoing preoperative arteriography. Ninety-nine percent of arterial segments from the common iliac to the popliteal level were successfully visualized by duplex scanning, whereas 95% of

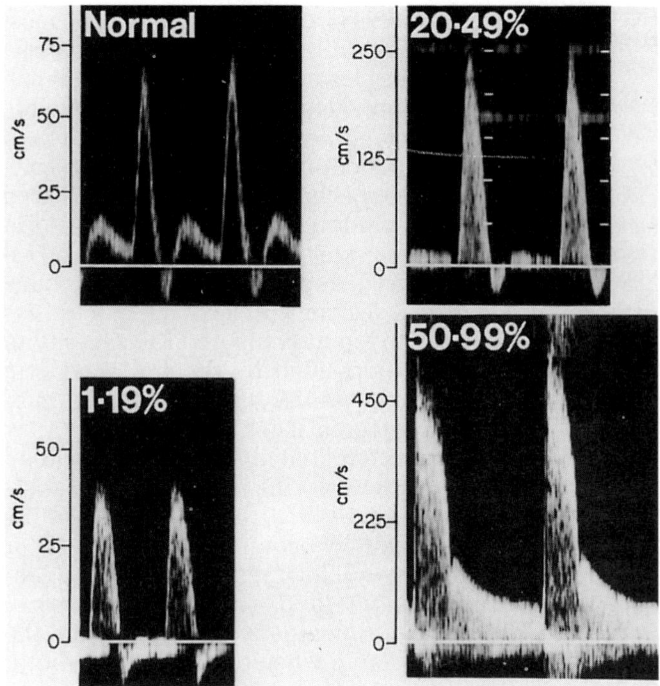

FIGURE 18–5 Lower extremity spectral waveforms. These are typical waveforms for each of the stenosis categories described in Table 18–2.

the anterior and posterior tibial arteries and 83% of the peroneal arteries were adequately imaged. For arterial segments proximal to the tibial level, duplex scanning was evaluated for its ability to identify stenoses of greater than 50% diameter reduction and for its ability to distinguish between stenosis and occlusion. In the tibial and peroneal arteries, the ability of duplex scanning to predict continuous patency from the popliteal to ankle level was assessed. In the proximal arterial segments, the overall sensitivities for detecting a greater than 50% stenosis ranged from 67% in the popliteal to 89% in the iliac arteries; corresponding specificities ranged from 97 to 99%. Stenosis was successfully distinguished from occlusion in 98% of proximal arterial lesions. For the more distal arteries, overall sensitivities for predicting continuous patency ranged from 93 to 97%. Contrary to other reported experience,[13] the accuracy of lower extremity duplex scanning was not significantly affected by the presence of multiple-level disease.

SCREENING FOR INTERVENTION

It is not essential to obtain a duplex scan on every patient who requires a lower extremity arterial evaluation. In most clinical situations, the vascular history, physical examination, and indirect measurement of ankle systolic blood pressure are sufficient to assess the presence and severity of arterial occlusive disease. Initial therapeutic plans can often be based on this information alone. If intervention is not warranted, then more sophisticated testing is usually not necessary. However, if more detailed anatomic information is needed for clinical decision making, then duplex scanning is the preferred method. Experience has shown that duplex scanning is superior to segmental pressure measurement for localization and classification of lower extremity arterial lesions.[15]

Lower extremity duplex scanning is generally most helpful for those patients who are being considered for some form of direct intervention. The goal in this setting is to determine the location and extent of arterial lesions so that decisions can be made regarding the need for arteriography and the most appropriate interventional approach. Assessment of aortoiliac disease is particularly difficult with other noninvasive methods, and duplex scanning has been especially valuable for that segment (Fig. 18–6). Whether a particular arterial segment is suitable for an endovascular procedure or direct surgical reconstruction depends on the specific features

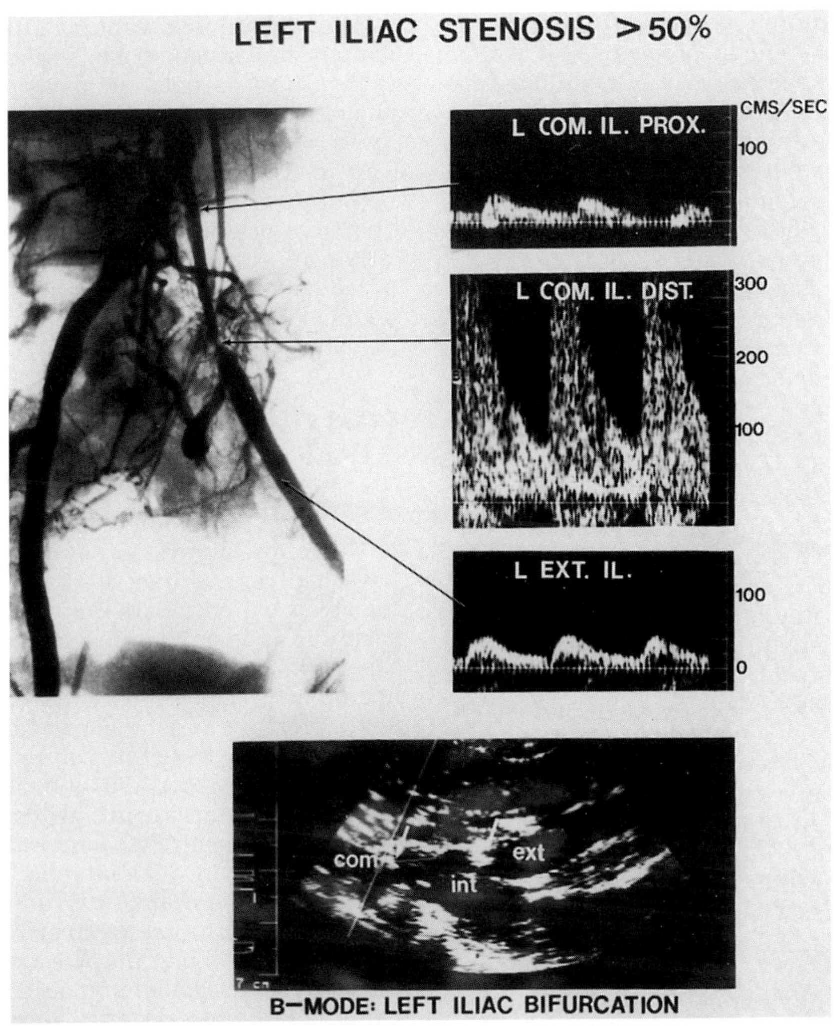

FIGURE 18–6 Left common iliac stenosis greater than 50% detected by duplex scanning. The proximal common iliac and external iliac spectral waveforms are damped and monophasic, and have markedly decreased velocities. The waveform taken in the stenotic jet (distal common iliac) shows high peak systolic velocities and extensive spectral broadening.

of the lesion. For example, focal stenoses or short occlusions in the iliac or superficial femoral arteries are usually amenable to percutaneous transluminal angioplasty, whereas arterial segments with long, irregular stenotic lesions or extensive occlusions are better treated by a surgical approach. The anatomic features that are particularly important in making this determination are the site, severity, and length of the lesion. In addition, it is essential to assess the status of the inflow and the quality of the distal run-off. Duplex scanning provides a practical means for obtaining this information without resorting to arteriography.

Edwards and coworkers[16] reported 110 patients who underwent lower extremity duplex scanning before arteriography. Based on the duplex scan findings, 50 lesions were considered suitable for balloon angioplasty. Of these, the procedure was actually performed in 47 (94%). In the remaining three cases, lesions were present as predicted by the duplex scan, but angioplasty was not performed for various technical reasons. No angioplasties were performed in patients who were found not to be candidates by duplex scanning. The characterization of lesions before arteriography and balloon angioplasty facilitates the intervention by directing attention to the appropriate arterial segment and indicating the optimal puncture site for access to the lesion.[16, 17] Thus, with a prearteriography duplex scan, it should not be necessary to perform separate diagnostic and therapeutic radiologic procedures. It is often valuable to screen elderly or debilitated patients with duplex scanning. The goal in such patients is to identify lesions that can be treated by percutaneous techniques. If such lesions are not found, and if surgery is contraindicated, further evaluation with arteriography is not necessary.

Cossman and colleagues[18] used color-Doppler scanning to examine 84 lower extremities in 61 patients undergoing evaluation for excimer laser angioplasty. There were 629 arterial sites available for comparison with contrast arteriography. The sensitivity and specificity for identifying stenoses of greater than 50% diameter reduction were 87% and 99%, respectively. Occluded arterial segments were detected with a sensitivity of 81% and a specificity of 99%. Color-Doppler imaging correctly determined the location and length of occlusion in 44 of 51 extremities (86%). In the four extremities in which color-Doppler imaging underestimated occlusion length, repeat arteriography at the time of laser angioplasty showed that the original arteriogram had not visualized a patent segment of proximal superficial femoral artery, and thus had overestimated the length of occlusion. Therefore, color-flow imaging provided accurate information on 48 of 51 arterial occlusions (94%).

The high accuracy of duplex scanning compared with arteriography, and reports of cases in which the duplex results appeared to be more reliable, have raised the issue of whether duplex scanning might replace arteriography in the evaluation of lower extremity arterial disease. Kohler and associates[19] performed a study to determine if vascular surgeons would choose different therapeutic procedures when provided with basic clinical information and the results of either lower extremity duplex scanning or arteriography. Relatively little disparity was found when decisions based on the two tests were compared for each individual surgeon. However, significant disagreement was noted among the clinical decisions made by various surgeons, even when the duplex scan and arteriogram reports agreed. These data suggest that most of the observed patient management variability was caused by diversity in the clinical approach to particular patterns of disease rather than actual differences in the results of the two diagnostic tests.

Although duplex scanning provides information similar to that obtained with arteriography, most vascular surgeons still request an arteriogram before elective operations for lower extremity arterial occlusive disease. The precise anatomic detail revealed by arteriography is considered necessary to plan operative procedures, particularly those involving the distal run-off vessels. Further experience will establish whether this type of detailed information can be obtained by noninvasive methods.

FOLLOW-UP AFTER ANGIOPLASTY

Another application of duplex scanning is in the follow-up evaluation of patients who have had various interventional procedures for lower extremity arterial disease. Duplex scanning is ideally suited for documenting the results of percutaneous transluminal angioplasty (Fig. 18–7). Although indirect ankle pressure measurements can be useful, they are unable to distinguish between recurrent disease at a previously treated site and progression of disease in a proximal or distal untreated segment. Furthermore, stenoses of moderate severity often produce only a minimal decrease in ankle systolic pressure. These limitations are overcome by duplex scanning, which permits direct examination of the treated segment and accurate classification of disease severity throughout the lower extremity.

Kinney and coworkers[20] used duplex scanning and ankle pressure measurements to monitor the results of percutaneous transluminal angioplasty in 90 lower extremities of 73 patients. Significant hemodynamic improvement was observed in 90% of the limbs. When the immediate postprocedure duplex scan detected a residual stenosis of greater than 50% diameter reduction, the rates of restenosis or clinical failure were 45% at 3 months and 88% at 1 year. However, if there was a less than 50% lesion at the angioplasty site, the subsequent failure rates were only 7% at 3 months and 20% at 18 months.

FOLLOW-UP AFTER BYPASS GRAFT SURGERY

Duplex scanning is the method of choice for monitoring the function of bypass grafts

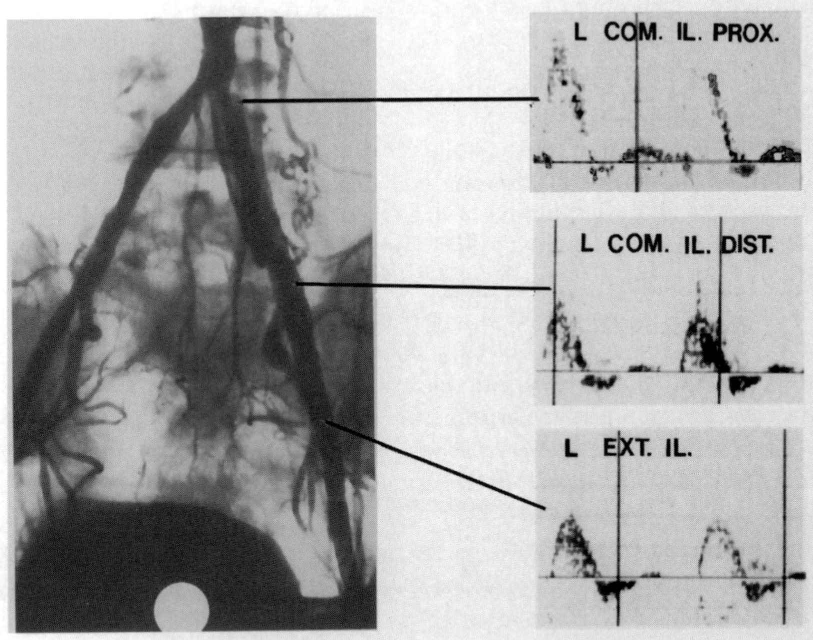

FIGURE 18–7 Left common iliac stenosis shown in Figure 18–6 after percutaneous transluminal angioplasty (PTA). Arteriogram shows the postangioplasty appearance of the artery. Spectral waveforms taken from proximal, within, and distal to the dilated lesion are now triphasic. (From Zierler RE, Zierler BK: Duplex sonography of lower extremity arteries. Semin Ultrasound CT MR 18:39–56, 1997.)

in the lower extremities. Clinical follow-up or use of ankle pressures alone is clearly inadequate for identifying those grafts that are at risk for thrombosis.[21] Experience has shown that grafts can fail without premonitory changes in ischemic symptoms or ankle pressures. The positive predictive value of the ankle-brachial systolic pressure index (when used alone) to predict graft thrombosis is in the range of 12 to 34%.[22, 23]

Because the majority of infrainguinal bypass grafts are performed with either in situ or reversed saphenous vein, most of the reported experience with graft surveillance is based on follow-up of these venous conduits. A more limited experience with duplex scanning of prosthetic bypass grafts has been reported.[24] Based on an extensive literature review, Barnes[25] found the incidence of lesions detected by postoperative graft surveillance to be 23% for in situ vein grafts and 17% for reversed vein grafts. Midgraft lesions, particularly retained valve cusps and arteriovenous fistulae, are more common with in situ conduits,[26, 27] whereas anastomotic lesions are more prevalent in reversed vein grafts.[28, 29]

The ultimate goal of graft surveillance is to identify those grafts that should undergo a revision procedure to avoid thrombosis and maintain patency. Mattos and colleagues[30] showed a 4-year patency rate of only 57% for infrainguinal vein grafts with stenoses detected by duplex scanning that were not revised. In contrast, the 4-year patency rates for normal grafts and revised grafts with stenoses were 83% and 88%, respectively. Graft intervention based on a surveillance program has resulted in 5-year patency rates in the range of 82 to 93%.[27, 31] Thus, stenotic vein grafts revised before thrombosis appear to have late patency rates equivalent to grafts without stenoses. The specific methods used for graft revision vary according to the features of the underlying lesion and include both percutaneous balloon angioplasty and direct surgical repair by patch angioplasty, interposition grafting, or extension of the graft to a more distal site. In general, routine graft surveillance by duplex scanning and appropriate intervention results in a 20 to 25% increase in long-term graft patency.[22]

Graft Scanning Technique

The scanning technique for lower extremity graft surveillance can be considered as an extension of that described previously for the native arteries. A complete duplex graft evaluation requires documenting the status of aortoiliac inflow to the graft and the distal run-off vessels, in addition to the anastomotic sites and graft conduit. The B-mode image is used to identify structural abnormalities such as aneurysmal dilatation, wall thickening, and retained valve cusps or other intraluminal defects (Fig. 18–8), whereas pulsed Doppler spectral waveforms indicate the presence of flow disturbances related to stenoses or arteriovenous fistulae. Color-Doppler imaging is valuable for showing the anatomy of bypass grafts and native arteries, as well as for rapid identification of flow disturbances (Fig. 18–9 [see p 266]). It is helpful if the examiner is familiar with the specific details of the operative procedure, including the type of conduit, the route of the graft through the leg, and the sites of anastomosis. In situ vein bypasses lie subcutaneously, just superficial to the muscular fascia; they are easily imaged throughout their length. These grafts typically have a tapered configuration with the largest diameter located proximally in the thigh. Reversed vein and prosthetic grafts may also lie in a subcutaneous position but are often placed more deeply, adjacent to the native vessels, which makes imaging more difficult.

Diagnostic Parameters

A wide range of blood flow velocities has been observed in infrainguinal vein grafts.[32] For successful bypass grafts, peak systolic velocities in the middle and distal graft segments generally exceed 40 to 45 cm/sec. In the absence of specific flow-limiting lesions, lower peak systolic velocities may be related to a conduit diameter of more than 6 mm or limited graft run-off into an isolated tibial artery segment or pedal artery. Belkin and associates[32] prospectively studied 46 infrainguinal vein grafts to identify the determinants of peak systolic velocity. Bypass grafts to the pedal arteries had significantly lower peak systolic velocities (mean, 64 ± 10 cm/sec) than grafts to the popliteal or tibial levels (mean, 90 ± 5 cm/sec). The primary factors that determined the peak systolic velocity were the measured graft outflow resistance and vein graft diameter. The investigators concluded that a single lower threshold value of peak systolic velocity could not be used to identify grafts at risk for failure and recommended reliance on the detection of focal flow disturbances within the graft.

The waveform configurations observed in infrainguinal vein grafts vary depending on the severity of ischemia in the limb and the follow-up interval. In limbs revascularized for critical ischemia, a hyperemic flow pattern is typically present in the early postoperative period, characterized by antegrade flow throughout the cardiac cycle and relatively high end diastolic velocities. These features reflect a low peripheral vascular resistance. Within a few days to several weeks after surgery, the flow pattern changes to the more typical triphasic pattern of peripheral artery flow (Fig. 18–10 [see p 267]). Subsequent transformation of the normal triphasic graft velocity waveform to a biphasic or monophasic configuration, in association with a decrease in the peak systolic velocity, is highly suggestive of an occlusive lesion proximal to, within, or distal to the graft (Fig. 18–11 [see p 267]).

The duplex criteria for classifying vein graft lesions are based on the same general principles as those described previously for native arteries. Although in situ and reversed vein grafts may have different anatomic and hemodynamic properties, the same duplex

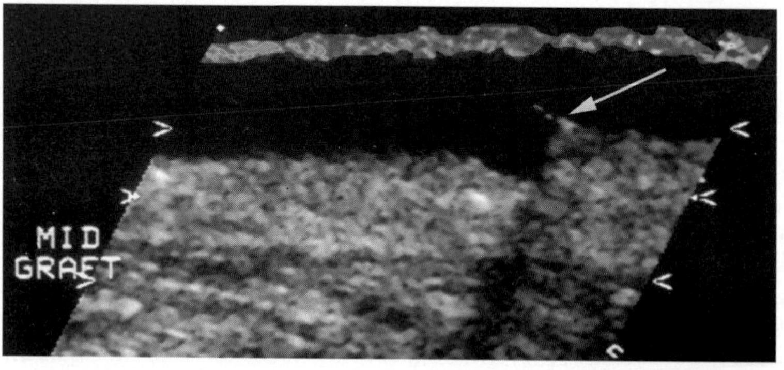

FIGURE 18–8 B-mode image of an in situ femoral-tibial vein graft. The flow direction is from left to right, and the skin line is on the top of the image. A retained valve cusp (*arrow*) is visualized on the deep wall of the graft. This was associated with a moderate flow disturbance (velocity ratio 2.5). (From Zierler RE, Zierler BK: Duplex sonography of lower extremity arteries. Semin Ultrasound CT MR 18:39–56, 1997.)

criteria are often applied to both types of grafts.[33] One widely used set of criteria is summarized in Table 18–3.[22, 33] The principal criterion for identifying a stenotic lesion is a high-velocity jet or localized increase in peak systolic velocity associated with spectral broadening. Vein graft stenoses are classified into four categories of diameter reduction based on velocity waveforms taken just proximal to, within, and distal to the lesion. The peak systolic and end diastolic velocities at these sites are recorded, and the velocity ratio (VR) is calculated as the maximum peak systolic velocity within the stenosis divided by the peak systolic velocity in the prestenotic segment. Lesions of less than 50% diameter reduction are characterized by peak systolic velocities less than 150 cm/sec and mild to moderate increases in both VR and spectral broadening. With the 50 to 75% stenoses, the peak systolic velocity is 150 cm/sec or more, VR is greater than or equal to 2.5, and marked spectral broadening is present, although the reversed flow component of the waveform is preserved. Stenoses of more than 75% diameter reduction are distinguished by a VR of 3.5 of more and an end diastolic velocity of 100 cm/sec or greater (Fig. 18–12 [see p 268]). These lesions typically have extremely high peak systolic velocities in excess of 250 cm/sec.

Clinical Implications

Caps and coworkers[33] followed 61 infrainguinal vein grafts with frequent duplex examinations and documented lesions of varying severity in 90% of these grafts, and multiple lesions in two thirds of cases. Eighty-six percent of lesions were detected within 6 months of operation. At the time of initial detection, 29% of the lesions were 0 to 19% diameter reduction, 51% were 20 to 49% diameter reduction, 17% were 50 to 75% diameter reduction, and 3% were greater than 75% diameter reduction. Disease progression, or an increase in vein graft lesion severity, was observed in 31% of the lesions by 6 months and 39% by 18 months. Regression of lesion severity was also noted and was more common for lesions of less than 50% diameter reduction. There were 32 primary revisions performed on 21 of the grafts. No significant decrease in the ankle-brachial pressure index was found before 10 of these revision procedures. The overall cumulative graft patency rate was 93% at 3 years. The investigators emphasized that the majority of vein graft lesions appear during the first 6 months after graft placement, and most of the lesions that progress do so during the first 6 months after detection. Thus, they recommended particularly frequent surveillance during the early postoperative period.

TABLE 18–3 CRITERIA FOR CLASSIFYING VEIN GRAFT LESIONS*

Classification (diameter reduction)	Features (VR, PSV, EDV)
0–19%	VR <2.0, mild spectral broadening in systole, PSV <150 cm/sec
20–49%	VR ≥2.0, spectral broadening throughout systole, no change in waveform across stenosis, PSV <150 cm/sec
50–75%	VR ≥2.5, severe spectral broadening in systole with reversed flow components, PSV ≥150 cm/sec
>75%	VR ≥3.5, EDV ≥100 cm/sec

VR = velocity ratio (PSV/prestenotic peak systolic velocity); PSV = peak systolic velocity in the stenotic jet; EDV = end-diastolic velocity in the stenotic jet.

* Based on duplex scanning with spectral waveform analysis.

Adapted from Zierler RE, Zierler BK: Duplex sonography of lower extremity arteries. Semin Ultrasound CT MR 18:49, 1997.

Based on the preceding experience and other reports,[22, 30–36] the following conclusions can be made regarding the optimal frequency of vein graft surveillance and indications for intervention. It is generally accepted that vein grafts with lesions causing greater than 75% diameter reduction are at risk for thrombosis and should be revised, even if there are no significant changes in the ipsilateral ankle-brachial pressure index. On the other extreme, it appears that vein graft lesions of less than 50% diameter reduction tend to have a relatively benign course and can be followed by serial duplex examinations. The management of lesions in the range of 50 to 75% diameter reduction is more controversial. If stenoses in this category are associated with midgraft peak systolic velocities less than 45 cm/sec or a significant decrease in the ankle-brachial pressure index, then revision should be performed; if graft velocities and ankle pressures are in the normal range, then continued duplex surveillance is warranted. Whenever possible, a baseline graft duplex examination should be obtained in the early postoperative period, preferably before hospital discharge. Follow-up examinations are then obtained routinely at 1 month after surgery and about every 3 months for the first postoperative year. The frequency of subsequent duplex graft surveillance should be adjusted according to individual graft characteristics. Stenoses of less than 50% diameter reduction that remain stable over the first 12 to 18 months can be followed at intervals of 6 to 12 months; however, if more severe lesions are present, continued surveillance at more frequent intervals may be justified.

Although duplex graft surveillance requires a substantial commitment in terms of patient time and vascular laboratory resources, it is now generally considered as "part of the service" provided by vascular surgeons after infrainguinal bypass graft procedures.[37] Because about 20% of these grafts develop significant stenotic lesions, and appropriate intervention can improve long-term patency, an improvement in limb salvage rates would be expected from an aggressive graft surveillance program. Based on the costs of graft surveillance and intervention compared with those of amputation and rehabilitation, it can be shown that duplex graft surveillance is cost-effective.[37] Other approaches to graft surveillance that may become useful in the future include three-dimensional ultrasonic imaging[38] and magnetic resonance angiography.[39]

INTRAOPERATIVE ASSESSMENT

Assessment of the technical result is an essential step in arterial reconstructive surgery. This facilitates immediate correction of any technical problems that could lead to arterial occlusion, thromboembolic complications, or graft failure.[40] Intraoperative observation and palpation of arteries or bypass grafts are not adequate for assessing technical results because these methods are subjective and may not detect significant abnormalities. For example, a strong transmitted pulse may be present in a recently occluded graft or artery. Operative arteriography has been widely used as an objective method for intraoperative assessment of arterial surgery; however, because it requires arterial puncture and injection of contrast material, it may also increase the risk of operation. Furthermore, arteriography does not provide any physiologic information on blood flow patterns in the visualized vessels. The need for a less invasive and more physiologic approach has led to the application of US methods for intraoperative assessment.

Continuous wave Doppler, pulsed Doppler, and duplex US have all been applied to the intraoperative assessment of arterial surgery. These methods have been used after carotid endarterectomy, lower extremity bypass grafting, and renal or visceral artery reconstruction.[41–47] Although the Doppler techniques alone can provide clinically valuable information, duplex scanning is now the preferred method. The combination of B-mode imaging, pulsed Doppler spectral analysis, and color-Doppler imaging is ideally suited for intraoperative assessment of lower extremity bypass grafts.

Technique and Diagnostic Parameters

The general approach to the intraoperative assessment of infrainguinal bypass grafts is analogous to that previously described for postoperative graft surveillance. A small linear array probe with a transmitting frequency of 7 to 10 MHz is typically used. The probe and cable are covered with a sterile plastic sleeve filled with acoustic gel, and a small amount of saline solution is used to couple the probe to the vessel or skin surface. Both B-mode image and velocity data are recorded from anastomotic sites, endarterectomy end points, and along vein conduits. Inflow and outflow vessels adjacent to the arterial reconstruction can also be assessed (Fig. 18–13). Immediate correction should generally be performed for lesions associated with focal flow abnormalities such as increased peak systolic velocity of greater than 180 cm/sec, extreme spectral broadening, or a VR of 2.5 or more.[45] Low midgraft velocities (less than 40 cm/sec) in vein grafts of at least 4 mm in diameter also suggest the presence of technical problems. Moderate increases in peak systolic velocity may be found in small-diameter vein grafts or distal to the anastomosis between a relatively large vein and a small tibial artery. In this situation, B-mode and color-Doppler imaging should be used to evaluate the vessel lumen for defects.

Clinical Implications

Bandyk and colleagues[45] performed intraoperative duplex scanning on 135 infraingui-

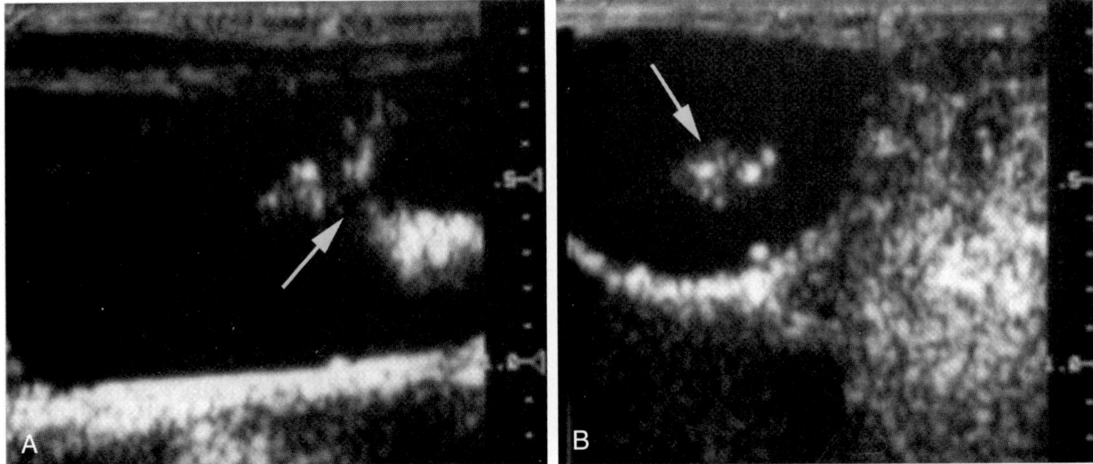

FIGURE 18–13 Longitudinal (*A*) and transverse (*B*) B-mode images of a common femoral artery taken during the intraoperative assessment of a femoral-popliteal bypass graft. A large intraluminal defect (*arrows*) is visualized, which represents residual atherosclerotic plaque from an incomplete endarterectomy. This was removed before completion of the procedure. (From Zierler RE, Zierler BK: Duplex sonography of lower extremity arteries. Semin Ultrasound CT MR 18:39–56, 1997.)

nal vein grafts and documented defects in 24 (18%), of which 19 (14%) were repaired. Of the five grafts with unrepaired lesions, one occluded in the early postoperative period, and three required revision within 30 days of the original procedure for low graft flow velocity associated with abnormalities identified by graft surveillance. None of the grafts with a normal intraoperative assessment required revision during a minimum follow-up interval of 2 months. Thus, technical defects that are noted on intraoperative assessment but are not repaired frequently result in lesions that require a secondary revision procedure.[45, 46] These grafts constitute a high-risk group that warrants close surveillance. Grafts with normal intraoperative and early duplex surveillance examinations tend to remain free of significant lesions and are at low risk for failure.

Intraoperative duplex scanning should be considered as a fundamental part of graft surveillance. By reducing the incidence of technical defects that could threaten graft patency, routine intraoperative assessment can improve the results of lower extremity bypass grafting and should decrease the need for frequent postoperative duplex surveillance.

LOWER EXTREMITY TRAUMA

Vascular injuries in the lower extremities can produce acute arterial insufficiency or exsanguinating hemorrhage that require rapid diagnosis and treatment. In this situation, the conventional history, physical examination, and diagnostic tests are usually impractical. Patients with lower extremity vascular trauma can present in two ways. Some patients have clear evidence of a vascular injury with obvious distal limb ischemia or massive hemorrhage. These patients generally undergo immediate operative exploration and repair. A second and more common presentation is when a patient has sustained blunt or penetrating trauma to an extremity but does not have specific signs or symptoms of a vascular problem. In this setting, the mechanism of trauma or location of a wound raises the clinical suspicion of an occult vascular injury.

Routine surgical exploration of vessels in proximity to traumatic wounds has been widely practiced but has a relatively low diagnostic yield. On the other extreme, the sensitivity of the physical examination alone may not be high enough to serve as a basis for treatment.[48] Consequently, arteriography has become the standard method for diagnosis of acute arterial trauma. However, in a series of 100 extremity injuries, arteriography took a mean of 2.4 hours to perform.[49] This represents an unacceptable delay in patients with major vascular injuries or multiple-system trauma who require ongoing resuscitation and immediate treatment. The use of arteriography for screening stable patients with suspected occult arterial injuries is more feasible but is associated with considerable cost and some increased risk. Furthermore, experience has shown that many post-traumatic arteriographic lesions, such as intimal flaps, pseudoaneurysms, and arteriovenous fistulae, follow a benign course and heal over time.[48]

Both indirect measurement of systolic blood pressure and duplex scanning have been used in patients with extremity trauma to avoid unnecessary arteriography and determine the need for surgical exploration. Lynch and Johansen[49] obtained Doppler pressure measurements in 100 injured limbs of 93 trauma victims who also had arteriography. An arterial pressure index (systolic pressure distal to the site of injury/brachial systolic pressure in an uninvolved arm) of greater than 0.90 was considered normal. Compared with the arteriographic findings, the arterial pressure index had a sensitivity of 87%, specificity of 97%, and overall accuracy of 95% for detecting arterial injuries. When the results of two false-positive arteriograms were excluded, the sensitivity, specificity, and accuracy increased to 95%, 98%, and 97%, respectively. The selection of trauma patients with possible occult vascular injuries for arteriography based on an arterial pressure index of less than 0.90 was prospectively evaluated in 100 limbs of 96 patients.[50] Among the 17 limbs with a decreased arterial pressure index, 16 had an abnormal arteriogram and 7 underwent arterial repair. For the 83 limbs with a normal arterial pressure index, follow-up revealed six minor lesions but no major injuries.

Although the arterial pressure index is a simple, rapid, and clinically valuable screening test, it has several important limitations. This approach cannot be used in cases where extensive wounds prevent placement of a pneumatic cuff on the injured extremity. In addition, it will not differentiate between an intrinsic arterial lesion, extrinsic compression, and vasospasm. Finally, distal limb pressure measurement will not detect non–flow-limiting lesions or injuries to non-axial arteries, such as the deep femoral artery.

Duplex scanning has been applied to the diagnosis of arterial trauma in the cervicothoracic region and the extremities.[51–54] Panetta and associates[55] reported an experimental study of duplex scanning and arteriography in a canine model of arterial injury (occlusion, laceration, intimal flap, hematoma, and arteriovenous fistula). Although duplex scanning and arteriography had equivalent overall accuracy in detecting arterial injuries, duplex scanning was significantly more sensitive (90% vs. 80%) and was more accurate than arteriography in identifying arterial lacerations. This high sensitivity makes duplex scanning particularly useful as a screening test in patients with suspected arterial injuries.

Meissner and coworkers[52] used duplex scanning as a screening test to evaluate 89 patients with suspected arterial trauma. Among 60 scans performed for wound proximity to adjacent vascular structures, only 4 (7%) were positive. Of the 19 scans done for specific clinical signs of arterial injury, 13 (68%) were positive (Fig. 18–14 [see p 268]). Clinical follow-up or arteriography confirmed that no major arterial injuries were missed. A similar experience was reported by Bynoe and colleagues[53] who prospectively evaluated 319 potential vascular injuries in 198 patients. Duplex scanning showed a sensitivity of 95%, specificity of 99%, and overall accuracy of 98%; for identifying arterial injuries.

Although most of the experience with duplex scanning for lower extremity vascular injuries has been limited to a small number of trauma centers, it is clearly effective for screening and follow-up in this clinical setting. It is particularly important to follow patients with initially negative duplex scans when there is ongoing suspicion of an arterial injury because lesions may become apparent on later examinations.[52, 56] Duplex scanning is more cost-effective than either arteriography or surgical exploration as a screening test and has replaced routine arteriography in some trauma centers.[53, 54] However, arteriography is still necessary in cases with technically difficult or equivocal duplex examinations.[57]

COMPRESSION THERAPY FOR PSEUDOANEURYSMS

The increasing use of catheter-based diagnostic and therapeutic procedures has resulted in a large number of patients undergoing common femoral artery puncture. The incidence of vascular complications after femoral artery catheterization ranges from 0.2 to 9.0%, with pseudoaneurysm formation reported in 0.05 to 5.0% of cases.[58–61] Other less frequent complications include arteriovenous fistulae and arterial thrombosis. Pseudoaneurysm formation is associated with the use of heparin after catheter removal, as well as with puncture sites located in the superficial or deep femoral arteries rather than the common femoral artery. Color-Doppler sonography is the method of choice for identifying femoral pseudoaneurysms, and this procedure avoids the need for further invasive procedures.[62, 63] Color Doppler also permits accurate determination of pseudoaneurysm size, visualization of the track between the artery and the pseudoaneurysm cavity, and assessment of the surrounding vessels. The natural history of catheter-induced femoral pseudoaneurysms appears to be variable, and spontaneous thrombosis has been observed in a significant proportion of untreated cases.[58, 64, 65] Surgical repair is recommended for pseudoaneurysms associated with rapid enlargement, rupture, compression of adjacent neurovascular structures, extreme patient discomfort, or ischemia of the overlying skin. Although direct surgical repair is effective and relatively safe, US-guided compression has emerged as an alternative to surgery for obliteration of selected catheter-induced pseudoaneurysms.[59, 60, 63, 64, 66, 67]

Compression Technique

The presence of a femoral pseudoaneurysm is confirmed when duplex scanning shows a flow-filled extraluminal cavity communicating with the common femoral artery or one of its branches. Spectral waveforms and color-Doppler imaging usually show the characteristic to-and-fro flow pattern in the neck of the pseudoaneurysm.[63] An initial trial of US-guided compression therapy is indicated for stable or slowly expanding pseudoaneurysms without skin ischemia. Oral or intravenous analgesics should be used during compression therapy to avoid excessive discomfort. Before compression is started, a baseline ankle-brachial pressure index should be recorded, and Doppler signals may be monitored in the distal arteries of the limb during the procedure.[59] The duplex US probe is positioned directly over the track connecting the artery to the pseudoaneurysm. Direct pressure is then applied with the probe until flow within the track ceases. If the track is difficult to visualize on the B-mode or color-Doppler image, sufficient probe pressure is applied to obliterate flow in the pseudoaneurysm cavity. Flow in the adjacent common, superficial, and deep femoral arteries is monitored as pressure is applied, and the amount of pressure is reduced if there is any suggestion of arterial narrowing or a decrease in the audible Doppler signal from the distal arteries. An alternative technique for patients requiring especially vigorous or prolonged compression involves application of pressure with the heel of the hand while monitoring the effect of compression with an US probe placed slightly to one side.[59]

After the first 10-minute compression period, pressure is released and the status of the pseudoaneurysm is documented by duplex scanning. Absence of flow within the track or pseudoaneurysm cavity indicates successful obliteration. If the pseudoaneurysm persists, compression is repeated for a maximum of three additional 10-minute periods (total of 40 minutes). This protocol may need to be shortened in patients with significant discomfort or if thrombus is noted in the arterial lumen. After successful obliteration of a pseudoaneurysm, patients are instructed to limit strenuous physical activity for at least 24 hours, and follow-up duplex scans are recommended at about 2 days and 1 month after the procedure to verify permanent thrombosis of the pseudoaneurysm cavity.

Results of Compression

Fellmeth and associates[64] evaluated 39 femoral artery injuries (35 pseudoaneurysms, 4 arteriovenous fistulae) detected by duplex scanning 6 hours to 14 days after catheterization. Contraindications to compression therapy were present in 10 cases, including spontaneous thrombosis in 4, unsuitable anatomy in 3, infection in 1, skin ischemia in 1, and excessive patient discomfort in 1. Of the 29 patients who underwent US-guided compression, the lesions were successfully obliterated in 27 patients (93%). No recurrences or complications were noted on follow-up evaluation extending to 15 months. In a series of 51 stable or slowly enlarging femoral pseudoaneurysms reported by Steinsapir and coworkers,[66] compression therapy was successful in 46 cases (90%). There was a single thromboembolic complication in this series, which responded to thrombolysis, and there were no late recurrences. Sorrell and colleagues[59] identified 15 femoral pseudoaneurysms that were potential candidates for US-guided compression. Four of these lesions thrombosed spontaneously before treatment, and 10 of the remaining 11 lesions (90%) underwent successful compression therapy. Compression had to be terminated in one patient because of severe discomfort. The mean total compression time required in the 10 successful cases was 30 minutes. There were no recurrences or complications attributable to compression therapy after 1 month of follow-up.

US-guided compression is a safe and effective noninvasive therapeutic approach to the initial treatment of selected catheter-induced femoral artery injuries. By avoiding direct surgical repair in a large proportion of cases, compression therapy should also be cost-effective. The technique often requires a high degree of physical effort by the physician or technologist, as well as considerable perseverance on the part of the patient.

REFERENCES

1. Slot HB, Strijbosch L, Greep JM: Interobserver variability in single-plane aortography. Surgery 90:497–503, 1981.
2. Thiele BL, Strandness DE Jr: Accuracy of angiographic quantification of peripheral atherosclerosis. Prog Cardiovasc Dis 26:223–236, 1983.
3. Zierler RE, Strandness DE Jr: Doppler techniques for lower extremity arterial diagnosis. *In* Zwiebel WJ (ed): Introduction to Vascular Ultrasonography, 2nd ed. Orlando, FL, Grune & Stratton, 1986, pp 305–331.
4. Zierler RE: Carotid artery evaluation by duplex scanning. Semin Vasc Surg 1:9–16, 1988.
5. Hatsukami TS, Primozich JF, Zierler RE, et al: Color Doppler imaging of infrainguinal arterial occlusive disease. J Vasc Surg 16:527–533, 1992.
6. Jager KA, Phillips DJ, Martin RL, et al: Noninvasive mapping of lower limb arterial lesions. Ultrasound Med Biol 11:515–521, 1985.
7. Thiele BL, Hutchinson KJ, Greene FM, et al: Pulsed Doppler waveform patterns produced by smooth stenosis in the dog thoracic aorta. *In* Taylor DEM, Stevens AL (eds): Blood Flow Theory and Practice. San Diego, CA, Academic Press, 1983, pp. 85–104.
8. Jager KA, Ricketts HJ, Strandness DE Jr: Duplex scanning for the evaluation of lower limb arterial disease *In* Bernstein EF (ed): Noninvasive Diagnostic Techniques in Vascular Disease. St Louis, Mosby, 1985, pp 619–631.
9. Blackshear WM, Phillips DJ, Strandness DE Jr: Pulsed Doppler assessment of normal human femoral artery velocity patterns. J Surg Res 27:73–83, 1979.
10. Hatsukami TS, Primozich J, Zierler RE, et al: Color Doppler characteristics in normal lower extremity arteries. Ultrasound Med Biol 18:167–171, 1992.
11. Leng GC, Whyman MR, Donnan PT, et al: Accuracy and reproducibility of duplex ultrasonography in grading femoropopliteal stenoses. J Vasc Surg 17:510–517, 1993.
12. Kohler TR, Nance DR, Cramer MM, et al: Duplex scanning for diagnosis of aortoiliac and femoropopliteal disease: A prospective study. Circulation 76:1074–1080, 1987.
13. Allard L, Cloutier G, Durand LG, et al: Limitations of ultrasonic duplex scanning for diagnosing of lower limb arterial stenoses in the presence of adjacent segment disease. J Vasc Surg 19:650–657, 1994.
14. Moneta GL, Yeager RA, Antonovic R, et al: Accuracy of lower extremity arterial duplex mapping. J Vasc Surg 15:275–284, 1992.
15. Moneta GL, Yeager RA, Lee RW, et al: Noninvasive localization of arterial occlusive disease: A comparison of segmental Doppler pressures and arterial duplex mapping. J Vasc Surg 17:578–582, 1993.
16. Edwards JM, Coldwell DM, Goldman ML, et al: The role of duplex scanning in the selection of patients for transluminal angioplasty. J Vasc Surg 13:69–74, 1991.
17. Van Der Heijden FHWM, Legemate A, van Leeuwen MS, et al: Value of duplex scanning in the selection of patients for percutaneous transluminal angioplasty. Eur J Vasc Surg 7:71–76, 1993.
18. Cossman DV, Ellison JE, Wagner WW, et al: Comparison of dye contrast arteriography to arterial mapping with color-flow duplex imaging in the lower extremities. J Vasc Surg 10:522–529, 1989.
19. Kohler T, Andros G, Porter J, et al: Can duplex scanning replace arteriography for lower extremity arterial disease? Ann Vasc Surg 4:280–287, 1990.
20. Kinney EV, Bandyk DF, Mewissen MW, et al: Monitoring functional patency of percutaneous transluminal angioplasty. Arch Surg 126:743–747, 1991.
21. Papanicolaou G, Beach KW, Zierler RE, et al: The relationship between arm-ankle pressure difference and peak systolic velocity in patients with stenotic lower extremity vein grafts. Ann Vasc Surg 9:554–560, 1995.
22. Bandyk DF: Essentials of graft surveillance. Semin Vasc Surg 6:92–102, 1993.
23. Barnes RW, Thompson BW, MacDonald CM, et al: Serial noninvasive studies do not herald postoperative failure of femoropopliteal or femorotibial bypass grafts. Ann Surg 210:486–494, 1989.
24. Sanchez LA, Suggs WD, Veith FJ, et al: Is surveillance to detect failing polytetrafluoromethylene bypasses worthwhile?: Twelve-year experience with ninety-one grafts. J Vasc Surg 18:981–989, 1993.
25. Barnes RW: How much postoperative screening is appropriate after arterial reconstruction? *In* Bernstein EF (ed): Vascular Diagnosis, 4th ed. St Louis, Mosby, 1993, pp 596–598.
26. Bandyk DF, Schmitt DD, Seabrook GR, et al: Monitoring functional patency of in situ saphenous vein bypasses: The impact of a surveillance protocol and elective revision. J Vasc Surg 9:286–294, 1989.
27. Donaldson MC, Mannick JA, Whittemore AD: Causes of primary graft failure after in situ saphenous vein bypass grafting. J Vasc Surg 15:113–120, 1992.
28. Berkowitz HD, Greenstein S, Barker CF, et al: Late failure of reversed vein bypass grafts. Ann Surg 210:782–786, 1989.
29. Mills JL, Fujitani RM, Taylor SM: The characteristics and anatomic distribution of lesions that cause re-

versed vein graft failure: A five-year prospective study. J Vasc Surg 17:195–206, 1993.
30. Mattos MA, van Bemmelen PS, Hodgson KJ, et al: Does correction of stenoses identified with color duplex scanning improve infrainguinal graft patency? J Vasc Surg 17:54–64, 1993.
31. Bergamini TM, Towne JB, Bandyk DF, et al: Experience with in situ saphenous vein bypasses during 1981 to 1989: Determinant factors of long-term patency. J Vasc Surg 13:137–149, 1993.
32. Belkin M, Raferty KB, Mackey WC, et al: A prospective study of the determinants of vein graft flow velocity: Implications for graft surveillance. J Vasc Surg 19:259–265, 1994.
33. Caps MT, Cantwell-Gab K, Bergelin RO, et al: Vein graft lesions: Time of onset and rate of progression. J Vasc Surg 22:466–475, 1995.
34. Papanicolaou G, Zierler RE, Beach KW, et al: Hemodynamic parameters of failing infrainguinal bypass grafts. Am J Surg 169:238–244, 1995.
35. Passman MA, Moneta GL, Nehler MR, et al: Do normal early color-flow duplex surveillance examination results of infrainguinal vein grafts preclude the need for late graft revision? J Vasc Surg 22:476–481, 1995.
36. Erickson CA, Towne JB, Seabrook GR, et al: Ongoing vascular laboratory surveillance is essential to maximize long-term in situ saphenous vein bypass patency. J Vasc Surg 23:18–26, 1996.
37. Bandyk DF: Cost-effectiveness of noninvasive surveillance after arterial surgery. Semin Vasc Surg 7:261–267, 1994.
38. Hodges TC, Detmer PR, Burns DH, et al: Ultrasonic three-dimensional reconstruction: In vitro and in vivo volume and area measurement. Ultrasound Med Biol 20:719–729, 1994.
39. Turnipseed WD, Sproat IA: A preliminary experience with the use of magnetic resonance angiography in assessment of failing lower extremity bypass grafts. Surgery 112:664–668, 1992.
40. Zierler RE: Intraoperative Doppler techniques for arterial evaluation. Semin Ultrasound CT MRI 6:73–84, 1985.
41. Bandyk DF, Zierler RE, Thiele BL: Detection of technical error during arterial surgery by pulsed Doppler spectral analysis. Arch Surg 119:421–428, 1984.
42. Zierler RE, Bandyk DF, Thiele BL: Intraoperative assessment of carotid endarterectomy. J Vasc Surg 1:73–81, 1984.
43. Bandyk DF, Cato RF, Towne JB: A low flow velocity predicts failure of femoropopliteal and femorotibial bypass grafts. Surgery 98:799–809, 1985.
44. Schwartz RA, Peterson GJ, Noland KA, et al: Intraoperative duplex scanning after carotid artery reconstruction: A valuable tool. J Vasc Surg 7:620–624, 1988.
45. Bandyk DF, Mills JL, Gahtan V, et al: Intraoperative duplex scanning of arterial reconstructions: Fate of repaired and unrepaired defects. J Vasc Surg 20:426–433, 1994.
46. Mills JL, Bandyk DF, Gahtan V, et al: The origin of infrainguinal vein graft stenosis: A prospective study based on duplex surveillance. J Vasc Surg 21:16–22, 1995.
47. Okuhn SP, Reilly LM, Bennett JB, et al: Intraoperative assessment of renal and visceral artery reconstruction: The role of duplex scanning and spectral analysis. J Vasc Surg 5:137–147, 1987.
48. Johansen K: Evaluation of vascular trauma. *In* Bernstein EF (ed): Vascular Diagnosis, 4th ed. St Louis, Mosby, 1993, pp 575–578.
49. Lynch K, Johansen K: Can Doppler pressure measurement replace "exclusion" arteriography in the diagnosis of occult extremity arterial trauma? Ann Surg 241:737–741, 1991.
50. Johansen K, Lynch K, Paun M, et al: Non-invasive vascular tests reliably exclude occult arterial trauma in injured extremities. J Trauma 31:515–519, 1991.
51. Fry WR, Dort JA, Smith RS, et al: Duplex scanning replaces arteriography and operative exploration in the diagnosis of potential cervical vascular injury. Am J Surg 168:693–695, 1994.
52. Meissner M, Paun M. Johansen K: Duplex scanning for arterial trauma. Am J Surg 161:552–555, 1991.
53. Bynoe RP, Miles WS, Bell RM, et al: Noninvasive diagnosis of vascular trauma by duplex ultrasonography. J Vasc Surg 14:346–352, 1991.
54. Fry WR, Smith RS, Sayers DV, et al: The success of duplex ultrasonography scanning in diagnosis of extremity vascular proximity trauma. Arch Surg 128:1368–1372, 1993.
55. Panetta TF, Hunt JP, Buechter KJ, et al: Duplex sonography versus arteriography in the diagnosis of arterial injury: An experimental study. J Trauma 33:627–635, 1992.
56. Sorrell K, Demasi R: Delayed vascular injury: The value of follow-up color flow duplex ultrasonography. J Vasc Technol 20:93–98, 1996.
57. Bergstein JM, Blair JF, Edwards J, et al: Pitfalls in the use of color-flow duplex ultrasound for screening of suspected arterial injuries in penetrated extremities. J Trauma 33:395–402, 1992.
58. Kresowik TF, Khoury MD, Miller BV, et al: A prospective study of the incidence and natural history of femoral vascular complications after percutaneous transluminal coronary angioplasty. J Vasc Surg 13:328–333, 1991.
59. Sortell KA, Feinberg RL, Wheeler JR, et al: Color-flow duplex-directed manual occlusion of femoral false aneurysms. J Vasc Surg 17:571–577, 1993.
60. Messina LM, Brothers TE, Wakefield TW, et al: Clinical characteristics and surgical management of vascular complications in patients undergoing cardiac catheterization: Interventional versus diagnostic procedures. J Vasc Surg 13:593–599, 1991.
61. Hessel SJ, Adams DF, Abrams HL: Complications of angiography. Diagn Radiol 138:273–281, 1981.
62. Coughlin BF, Paushter DM: Peripheral pseudoaneurysms: Evaluation with duplex US. Radiology 168:339–342, 1988.
63. Abu-Yosef MM, Wiese JA, Shamma AR: The "to-and-fro" sign: A new duplex Doppler sign of pseudoaneurysms complicating femoral artery catheterization. AJR Am J Roentgenol 150:632–634, 1988.
64. Fellmeth BD, Roberts AC, Bookstein JJ, et al: Postangiographic femoral artery injuries: Nonsurgical repair with US-guided compression. Radiology 178:671–675, 1991.
65. Kotval PS, Khoury A, Shah PM, et al: Doppler sonographic demonstration of the progressive spontaneous thrombosis of pseudoaneurysms. J Ultrasound Med 9:185–190, 1990.
66. Steinsapir ES, Coley BD, Fellmeth BD, et al: Selective management of iatrogenic femoral false aneurysms. J Surg Res 55:109–113, 1993.
67. Mills JL, Wiedeman JE, Robinson JG, et al: Minimizing mortality and morbidity from iatrogenic arterial injuries: The need for early recognition and prompt repair. J Vasc Surg 4:22–27, 1986.

SECTION 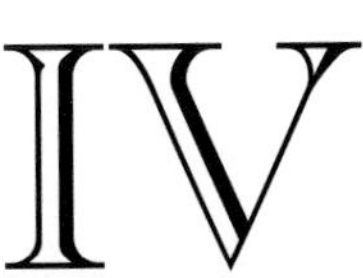

EXTREMITY VEINS

Chapter 19

Rationale for Duplex Ultrasonography Assessment of Extremity Veins

■ *Spencer W. Galt, MD* ■ *Peter F. Lawrence, MD*

To appreciate the role of duplex ultrasonography in the evaluation and treatment of venous disease, a thorough understanding of the anatomy and physiology of the venous system is necessary. This chapter principally considers the application of duplex ultrasonography in the evaluation of acute and chronic venous disease.

MAPPING FOR BYPASS SURGERY

Frequently, the astute clinician can determine whether superficial veins are suitable for use as arterial bypass conduits through careful physical examination (Fig. 19–1). Nevertheless, it is sometimes necessary to confirm the presence, location, and adequacy of the proposed bypass conduit before harvesting for coronary or peripheral vascular bypass surgery. Duplex ultrasonography can accurately accomplish these goals, and this technique should be liberally employed whenever uncertainty concerning the availability of suitable bypass conduits exists. For example, in the obese patient the course of the vein may be hidden by subcutaneous tissue. Duplex scanning can confirm the patency and location of the veins; the raising of large skin flaps is then easily avoidable. In the patient who has suffered previous saphenous vein thrombosis, duplex scanning demonstrates whether chronic occlusion or valvular insufficiency exists, conditions that obviate vein use as a bypass graft. In those patients who have undergone venous surgery or prior vein harvesting, the greater saphenous vein may be absent. A diligent search using the duplex scanner can facilitate identification of alternative bypass conduits for the planned procedure. In our experience the greater and lesser saphenous, superficial femoral, cephalic, and basilic veins are all potentially useful as bypass conduits and are easily evaluated and mapped with duplex ultrasonography.

Vein mapping may also assist in preoperative planning when a minimally invasive technique is used for vein harvest or when an in situ lower extremity saphenous vein bypass graft is anticipated. Identification of the location of valves allows lysis under angioscopic guidance; identified vein side branches may then be approached directly through small skin incisions, avoiding exposure of the entire saphenous vein and presumably reducing the frequency of wound complications.

Despite the advantages of duplex ultrasonography in determining vein patency, care must be exercised when this technique is used to exclude sections of vein from use as a bypass graft on a size criterion alone. Because veins are capacitance vessels, their size can vary greatly. Therefore, veins should be examined in the erect patient, using a tourniquet if necessary, to determine the maximal diameter. Before a vein is deemed too small for use, exploration and gentle hydrostatic dilatation are necessary, as this maneuver may be the sole means through which one may determine whether the vein is of adequate caliber to function as a bypass conduit.

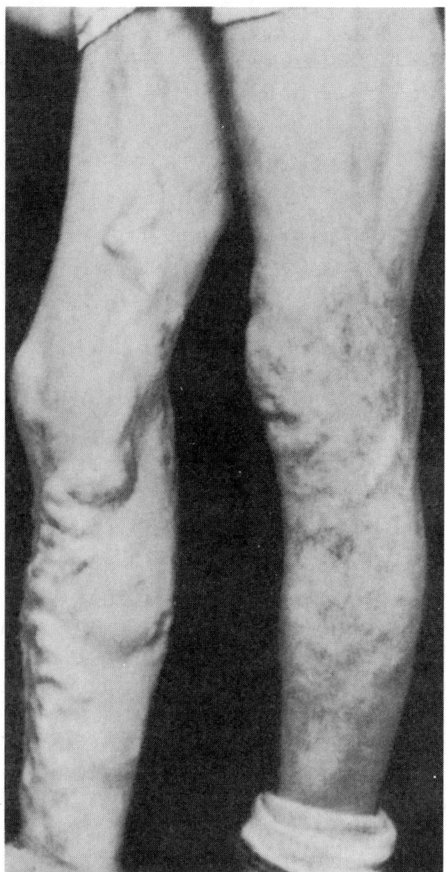

FIGURE 19–1 To distend and identify veins maximally, patients should stand for several minutes before the examination. The legs may then be elevated to collapse veins and identify the sites of incompetence.

PRIMARY VARICOSE VEINS

Primary varicose veins are abnormally dilated and tortuous veins of the superficial venous system, *in the absence of coexisting deep venous disease.* Varicose veins are classified as *secondary* when they are caused by obstruction or incompetence of the deep venous system. In most patients the medical history and physical examination provide sufficient information to distinguish between primary and secondary varicose veins. In the patient with primary varicose veins, a history of deep venous thrombosis (DVT) is rare. Physical signs of the post-thrombotic syndrome, such as brawny edema in the so-called *gaiter zone* and venous stasis ulcers, are absent. However, in the occasional patient, it can be difficult to rule out involvement of the deep venous system by the medical history and physical examination. In this instance, duplex ultrasonography can be especially helpful. Exclusion of pathology of the deep venous system confirms the diagnosis of primary varicose veins and predicts a high likelihood of cure with complete excision of the varicosities.

When surgical treatment of varicose veins is planned, sparing the normal greater saphenous vein is important, because it is the preferred bypass conduit for arterial bypass surgery. If the distal saphenous vein is uninvolved, it is appropriately spared and then available for future bypass surgery. Careful duplex interrogation identifies precisely the sites of varicosity and incompetence; it can distinguish whether the saphenous vein is involved and whether the varicosities are confined to venous tributaries or perforators (Fig. 19–2). Complete removal of diseased

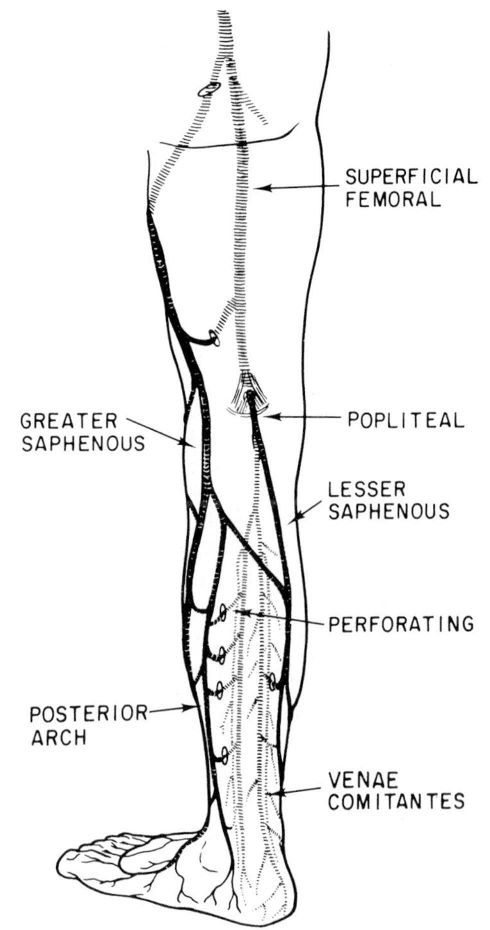

FIGURE 19–2 Superficial venous system. Shown are the sites of perforators that connect the superficial and deep venous systems. Note that most perforators arise from the superficial arch veins, rather than from the saphenous veins directly.

segments, although allowing healthy sections of the vein to be spared, is greatly facilitated.

Valvular incompetence at the saphenofemoral junction occurs in most cases of primary varicose veins. Nevertheless, the varicosities may be clinically apparent in only the calf or distal thigh (Fig. 19–3). If the saphenofemoral valve is incompetent, the saphenous vein must be ligated flush at the saphenofemoral junction, and the proximal vein must be removed. Failure to do so increases the likelihood of recurrence. Conversely, if the valve at the saphenofemoral junction is intact, the saphenous vein need not be stripped at this level. Duplex ultrasonography easily evaluates the status of the valve.

The remainder of the greater saphenous vein can be inspected similarly with duplex ultrasonography to determine the extent of varicosities. Any part of the vein found to be normal need not be stripped. If the presenting problem is calf or thigh varicosities that appear isolated from the saphenous system, the greater saphenous vein must still be examined. Even if the saphenous vein does not appear varicose, the section of saphenous vein with incompetent valves must be removed; otherwise, recurrence may be anticipated. If the saphenous vein is competent, treatment can be confined to the clinically evident varicosities.

Perforator incompetence may also cause, or accompany, varicose veins in the absence of deep venous incompetence. Occasionally, an incompetent perforator causes primary varicose veins, even though the deep venous system is intact. Ligation of the incompetent perforator is the key to successful management of the problem; perforators are easily localized with duplex ultrasonography.

RECURRENT VARICOSE VEINS

Recurrence of primary varicose veins is caused either by inadequate initial treatment or by development of new primary varicose veins. Initial treatment unwittingly directed at secondary varicose veins uniformly results in recurrence. The most easily identified and managed cause of recurrent primary varicose veins is inadequate high ligation of the greater saphenous vein at the saphenofemoral junction when an incompetent valve is present at that level (Fig. 19–4). Failure to ligate the greater saphenous vein flush with the com-

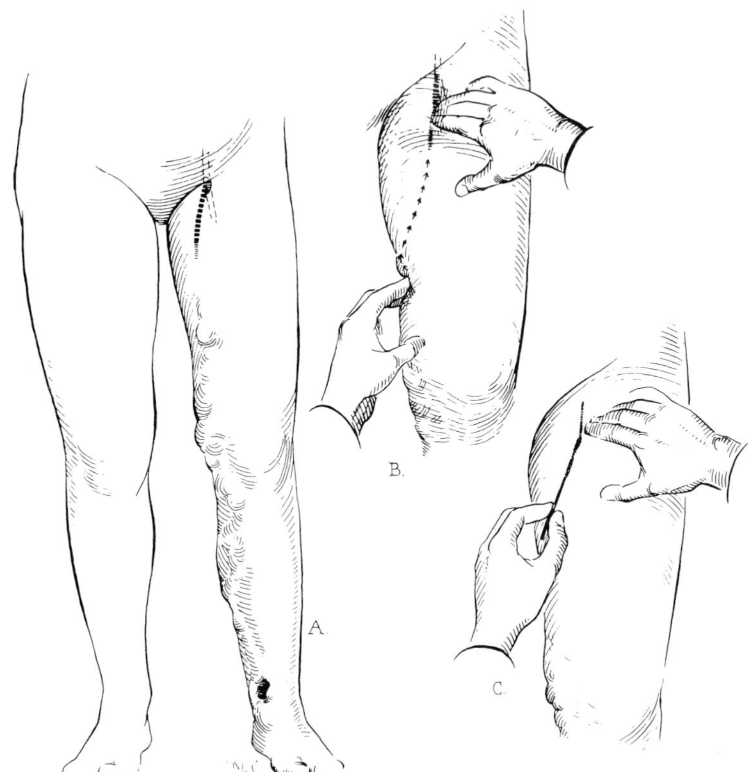

FIGURE 19–3 Varicose veins in the calf may be isolated to the superficial calf veins, or they may be associated with incompetence of the entire saphenous vein (*A*). Physical examination and duplex ultrasonography can determine the extent of superficial venous involvement (*B* and *C*).

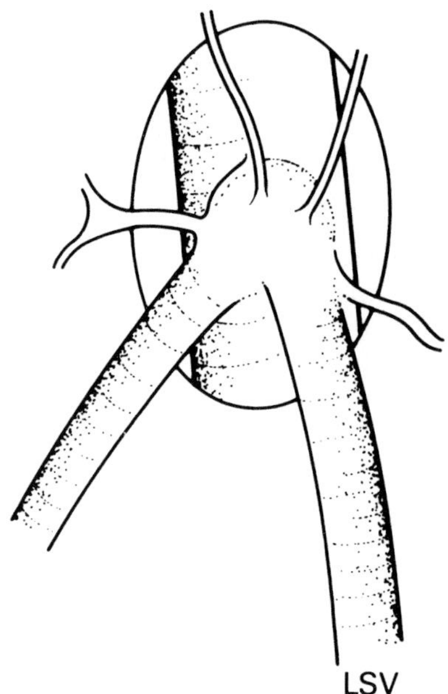

FIGURE 19–4 The greater (long) saphenous vein enters the femoral vein through the fossa ovalis. There are several large superficial branches that enter the saphenous vein at the saphenous bulb. These veins, as well as the greater saphenous vein, must be ligated to prevent recurrence of varicose veins. LSV = long saphenous vein.

mon femoral vein preserves the incompetent valve, allowing reflux into the subcutaneous branches at the saphenous bulb. This condition may be identified either by physical examination or by duplex scanning as a cluster of veins in the inguinal region. When incompetence and reflux are identified in these veins, flush ligation is curative.

A variety of other causes of recurrent primary varicosities are known, including incomplete ligation of incompetent perforators, a duplicated saphenous system, and failure to differentiate greater from lesser saphenous vein incompetence. As usual, careful physical examination complemented with duplex ultrasonography determines the cause of recurrent varicosities. The importance of evaluation of the deep venous system cannot be overstated, because secondary varicose veins, resulting from deep venous incompetence, are a common cause of recurrence.

SUPERFICIAL VENOUS THROMBOSIS

Superficial venous thrombosis has traditionally been considered a relatively benign disease. It is important, however, as a marker of coexistent DVT and hypercoagulability. The diagnosis of superficial venous thrombosis is typically made clinically. Physical findings include a painful superficial cord with surrounding erythema in the course of the vein. Treatment of patients with nonsuppurative superficial venous thrombosis is symptomatic and includes ambulation, heat application, compression, and nonsteroidal anti-inflammatory drug therapy.

Duplex evaluation of superficial venous thrombosis, especially occurring in the greater saphenous vein, is important for two reasons. First, although the clinical examination is useful in establishing the diagnosis, it is not reliable in identifying the extent of the thrombus. Particularly in the proximal thigh, the thrombus often extends beyond the apparent area of involvement.[1,2] Duplex ultrasonography documents the proximal extent and can be used to monitor progression. Although data are limited, it appears that a small proportion (approximately 10%) of patients with isolated superficial venous thrombosis of the greater saphenous vein progress to DVT if untreated; of that group, those with superficial venous thrombosis in the thigh are at highest risk, with 70% of untreated patients progressing to thrombosis of the femoral vein. Most clinicians either disconnect the saphenofemoral junction surgically or institute systemic anticoagulation if proximal saphenous thrombosis progresses to the saphenofemoral junction.

Duplex ultrasonography of extremities with superficial venous thrombosis is also useful to identify a concomitant but clinically silent DVT. Some series have demonstrated the presence of inapparent DVT in 20 to 40% of patients with superficial venous thrombosis.[3–5] Treatment is directed at DVT and superficial thrombophlebitis. Many of these patients are hypercoagulable, and the appropriate evaluation should be performed.

Occasionally, an apparent superficial phlebitis is, in fact, a soft tissue infection or hematoma. These conditions can easily be distinguished from superficial venous thrombosis with duplex scanning but may be more difficult to differentiate clinically.

DEEP VENOUS THROMBOSIS

DVT is a common and potentially fatal clinical problem in both upper and lower extremities. An accurate method of noninvasive diagnosis is important because of the variable presentation of DVT and the unreliability of the physical examination. The significant morbidity and mortality of pulmonary embolism (PE) and the potential morbidity of treatment underscore the importance of a noninvasive, accurate method of establishing the diagnosis, for which duplex ultrasound is well suited.

Pathogenesis and Risk Factors

Described in 1856 by Virchow, the triad of venous stasis, endothelial damage, and hypercoagulability remains the hallmark of risk for the development of DVT. Certain populations are at high risk for venous stasis, including patients at bedrest and surgical patients, who are often immobilized for hours on the operating table. Combined with their normal postoperative hypercoagulable state, surgical patients clearly demonstrate an increase in the likelihood of DVT. Those undergoing pelvic operations and total hip and knee arthroplasties are at highest risk for DVT because of the local trauma to the veins associated with these operations. Other predisposing factors for DVT include advanced age, limb trauma, prior DVT, varicose veins, heart failure, coagulation disorders (e.g., resistance to activated protein C), underlying malignancy, and oral contraceptive use.

Calf Vein Thrombosis

Most lower extremity DVTs become established in the deep veins of the calf,[6, 7] although acute DVT can originate anywhere in the venous system. The soleal sinuses are thought to be the most common site of origin of calf DVT,[8] which may progress into the popliteal and femoral veins. Once the popliteal or femoral vein contains thrombus, therapeutic anticoagulation or caval interruption is necessary. However, the clinical importance of isolated calf DVT remains controversial. Abundant literature has been published, but much of it is contradictory. Therefore, it is not surprising that there is no consensus over the prevalence of isolated calf DVT, the propensity for it to progress, the risk of its causing PE, and the ability of its causing postthrombotic syndrome.

The prevalence of isolated calf DVT in specific patient groups is difficult to establish because many studies include mixed patient populations and a variety of diagnostic techniques. Nevertheless, in a review of 20 studies, Philbrick and Becker[9] reported a 49% prevalence of symptomatic isolated calf DVT in medical and surgical patients. This figure has been corroborated by several other authors, albeit in mixed populations of medical and surgical patients. A recent study by Atri and colleagues[10] attempted to better separate patient populations by examining an asymptomatic postoperative high-risk group and a symptomatic ambulatory group. In the asymptomatic postoperative group, 20% of patients were found to have isolated calf DVT; in the symptomatic ambulatory group, there was a 30% prevalence. These studies indicate that although it is difficult to establish precisely, isolated calf DVT is not uncommon.

Most DVTs arise in calf veins, thus it is clear that calf DVT can propagate to the popliteal vein and more proximally. The more important issue is whether *all* calf DVTs propagate, and whether those that do can be identified, because the prognostic and therapeutic implications of isolated calf DVTs are different from DVTs in the more proximal popliteal and femoral system. The reported frequency of calf DVT propagation varies markedly in the literature. In postoperative patients, the reported rate of propagation varies from 6 to 34%.[9, 11–15] Unfortunately, it is not possible to distinguish those thrombi that are likely to propagate.

In symptomatic ambulatory patients, the chances of propagation are even less certain, because no published studies have documented the frequency of proximal propagation. Equally unclear, but probably of more importance, is the risk of PE originating from isolated calf thrombi in which no propagation into the popliteal vein has occurred. Some authors[16–18] argue that few, if any, significant pulmonary emboli arise from isolated calf DVT, and that anticoagulation is unnecessary in the absence of demonstrable propagation. Other investigators are less sanguine. They reported that patients with PE have calf-only thrombi about 5% of the time.[19, 20] Furthermore, others have reported that approximately 15% of fatal pulmonary emboli originated from isolated calf thromboses.[8, 21] These series must be interpreted with caution, because it can be difficult to be certain that PE did not originate from a more proximal source, with embolization of the entire thrombus.

In view of the variation in observed rates of proximal propagation and PE, it is not surprising that there is no general agreement on the management of isolated calf DVT. Lohr and associates[15] cited a high risk of propagation (32%) and a low incidence of PE (5%) to suggest that all patients with calf DVT should be treated with anticoagulation. Others have suggested treating only those patients with symptomatic calf vein thrombi (who appear to have a greater risk of embolism), those that demonstrate proximal propagation, or those who in follow-up are found to have developed clinically apparent PE.[22] No well-controlled, prospective randomized trial of treatment of patients with isolated calf DVT has been published; therefore, the risks and benefits of the various approaches are not established.

Currently, two approaches in the treatment of patients with isolated calf DVT seem reasonable. The patient should be maintained on therapeutic anticoagulation for 6 weeks or surveillance duplex ultrasonography should be continued for 7 to 10 days (or longer, in an immobilized patient), with institution of therapeutic anticoagulation if propagation to proximal veins is documented.

Femoropopliteal Vein Thrombosis

DVT proximal to the calf is a more serious clinical problem than isolated calf DVT. The risk of PE is greater, thus mandating therapeutic anticoagulation. For patients in whom anticoagulation is contraindicated, caval filter placement or caval interruption is necessary.

The clinical findings of DVT may change significantly as thrombus is identified more proximally. When the superficial femoral vein is involved, the calf is usually painful. Swelling and warmth are typically evident on physical examination. When thrombus extends into the common femoral or iliac vein, the patient perceives a deep leg discomfort and tightness. Swelling may be present up to the inguinal ligament, and there may be tenderness over the deep veins, particularly in the inguinal region.

Duplex ultrasonography is now accepted as the initial diagnostic test of choice in patients suspected of having femoropopliteal DVT. Duplex ultrasonography easily permits visualization of complete thrombotic occlusion, allowing accurate clot localization. Additionally, nonocclusive thrombi and free-floating thrombi that are loosely attached to the vein wall and may have a greater potential for embolization[11] can also be identified. Some clinicians also use duplex ultrasonography to follow the progression of a clot in the vein as an indicator of the effectiveness of anticoagulation therapy. Duplex ultrasonography is also a useful technique to determine both the relative age of the clot (acute vs. chronic) and the degree of spontaneous lysis, information that may provide clinical guidance in the suspected recurrence of DVT, the adequacy of anticoagulation, and the length of time anticoagulation is maintained.

Iliac Venous Thrombosis

The clinical presentation and therapeutic implications of iliac vein thrombosis resemble those of femoropopliteal vein thrombosis, and the diagnostic approach is similar. The difference between these sites of thrombosis is the inability of duplex sonography to directly image many iliac thrombi that lie deep within the pelvis. If iliac vein thrombi are visualized, the diagnosis of DVT may be made with confidence. However, despite a convincing clinical scenario, the only evidence of proximal DVT may come from the Doppler interrogation, rather than the B-mode image. Indirect Doppler evidence of proximal thrombosis includes the loss of respiratory phasicity of the signal and the inability to augment the signal with distal thigh compression, but these signs may be absent with nonocclusive thrombi. Nonocclusive thrombi, or thrombi isolated to the hypogastric vein, are likely to be missed by duplex ultrasonography. Therefore, when the clinical scenario is compelling, further evaluation of the deep venous system is indicated, usually by venography.

Because duplex ultrasound has become the diagnostic test of choice in DVT evaluation and the majority of pulmonary emboli originate in lower extremity veins, some clinicians now obtain a lower extremity duplex ultrasound as the first diagnostic study in the evaluation of possible PE. This approach is based on the noninvasive nature of the study, the portability of the machine, and the rapidity with which results may be obtained in institutions where technical support is readily available. The merit to this approach is supported when the diagnosis of DVT is confirmed, as the diagnosis of PE may be safely assumed in the appropriate clinical setting. There are potential drawbacks to this insensitive but specific approach to the diagnosis of PE.

Several investigators have addressed these issues, examining both the yield of positive results in those cases in which lower extremity duplex ultrasonography has been used as a screening test for patients with suspected PE and the frequency of detection of DVT in those patients known to have suffered PE. Beecham and colleagues[23] reviewed 225 patients who underwent both ventilation-perfusion (V/Q) scans and lower extremity duplex ultrasonography in the evaluation of suspected PE. Of 56 patients with high-probability V/Q scans, only 36% demonstrated duplex evidence of DVT. Furthermore, of 22 patients whose V/Q scans were indeterminate or low probability and who had no evidence of DVT by duplex scanning, 25% were found to have suffered PE detected by angiography. Similarly, in a study by Glover and Bendick,[24] the charts of 978 patients who were studied by duplex ultrasonography to "rule out PE" were reviewed. In a subgroup of 38 patients with acute unilateral leg swelling, acute femoropopliteal DVT was diagnosed in 68%. A second subgroup of patients included those with minimal leg symptoms who had significant risk factors for DVT. In this group, 16% of patients were found to have acute femoropopliteal or tibial DVT. In contrast, acute femoropopliteal DVT was not detected in the remaining 433 patients who had no risk factors or acute unilateral leg swelling. Three patients were found to have tibial DVT. Similar to the previous reports cited, in patients with high-probability V/Q scans but no risk factors for DVT or lower extremity symptoms, no DVT was detected in more than 60% of patients, again underscoring the inability of the lower extremity venous duplex examination to rule out PE. Killewich and coworkers[25] similarly documented the absence of duplex-diagnosed DVT in 60% of patients with PE confirmed by pulmonary angiography. Like Glover and Bendick, Eze and associates[26] demonstrated the usefulness of stratifying patients with suspected PE based on unilateral leg symptoms. In their series of 336 patients with clinically suspected PE, 7% demonstrated proximal DVT by duplex ultrasonography. However, in the 25 patients with unilateral leg swelling, 40% were found to have DVT by duplex scanning whereas DVT was evident in only 5% of patients in the absence of leg swelling. This group further confirmed that most patients with high-probability V/Q scans had no DVT visualized by duplex ultrasonography. Finally, in a study by Matteson and colleagues,[27] 664 patients who underwent venous duplex examination for the diagnosis of "rule out PE" were reviewed. For all lower extremity duplex examinations, 13% of studies were positive. Although no attempt was made to stratify patients by leg symptoms or risk factors, this study reaffirmed the overall low yield of venous duplex examination in the evaluation of PE, and the finding that the majority of patients with confirmed PE demonstrate no DVT.

In summary, it appears that the lower extremity venous duplex examination is an appropriate primary diagnostic study in the patient who is suspected of having suffered PE and has unilateral lower extremity swelling. In the absence of leg swelling, the V/Q scan is the first test of choice. Furthermore, if the venous duplex study is negative after a nondiagnostic V/Q scan, pulmonary angiography must be pursued if clinical suspicion warrants further investigation, because no DVT is demonstrated in more than one half of the patients who have suffered PE.

Axillary-Subclavian Venous Thrombosis

DVT of the upper extremities is occurring more frequently as a result of the increased use of central venous catheters.[28] Other causes of upper extremity DVT include the thoracic outlet syndrome, trauma, surgery, radiation therapy, and effort thrombosis, also known as the *Paget-Schroetter syndrome.* Presentation of upper extremity DVT can be dramatic. Marked arm swelling and prominent superficial veins leave little doubt of the diagnosis, in which the role of duplex ultrasonography is primarily confirmatory. Sometimes the presentation is more subtle. The patient may complain of vague discomfort, with minimal swelling; in these cases, duplex ultrasonography is an effective screening test to document the status of the deep venous system. Unlike the lower extremities, the proximal upper extremities are drained by a rich collateral venous network around the neck and shoulder, making the indirect evaluation of venous flow by plethysmography even less reliable than in the lower extremities, further emphasizing the value of duplex ultrasonography for upper extremity DVT. The duplex ultrasound is, however, limited by the bony structures in the neck and shoulder, impeding imaging of the proximal subclavian vein. As in the pelvis, if proximal subclavian DVT is suspected, venography should be performed.

Sequelae of DVT

The sequelae of DVT result from either proximal chronic venous obstruction or acquired incompetence of the valves of the deep venous system following recanalization, or both. In most patients who have suffered from DVT, the thrombosed vein recanalizes over a period of months, allowing adequate restoration of flow to the central circulation. Despite recanalization, the vein wall and valves are permanently damaged in at least 60% of cases,[29] leaving the valve leaflets immobile and fixed to the vein wall. Incompetence of the system results, and reflux occurs when the standing position is assumed. In some individuals the thrombosed veins do not recanalize, resulting in chronic obstruction to venous return. Regardless of whether the cause is proximal obstruction, reflux, or both, venous hypertension occurs. The venous hypertension presents clinically as chronic leg swelling, ankle pigmentation, and, ultimately, ankle ulceration in the gaiter zone. Collectively this is known as the *post-thrombotic syndrome* (Fig. 19–5).

The pathophysiology underlying the swelling and discoloration is straightforward. Increased hydrostatic pressure in the deep venous system causes extravasation of protein-rich tissue fluid, presenting clinically as interstitial edema. If venous hypertension persists, acquired incompetence of the valves of the perforating veins results in secondary varicose veins (Fig. 19–6). Red blood cells extravasate and are deposited in the subcutaneous tissue surrounding the perforators.

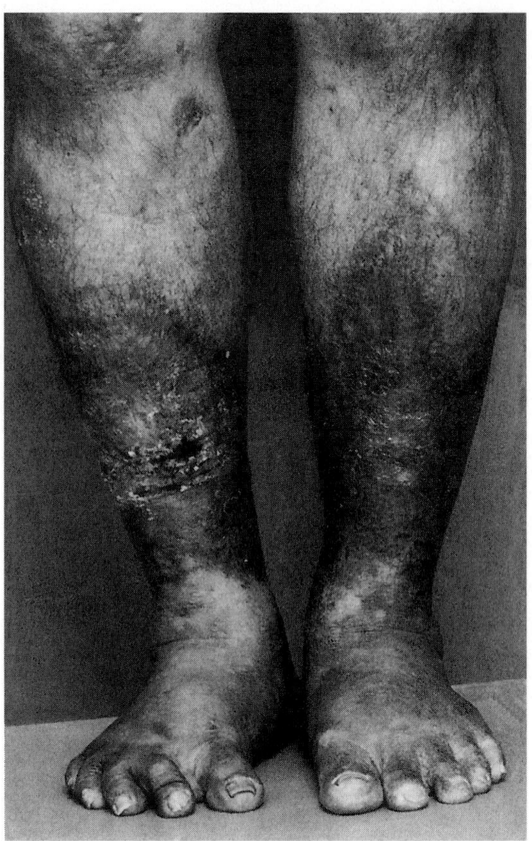

FIGURE 19–5 The *gaiter zone* is located in the lower calf and ankle. In this region the ambulatory superficial venous pressures are the highest, leading to edema, pigmentation, and ultimately ulceration. The skin, after years of edema, is difficult to examine for incompetent perforators (both clinically and with duplex ultrasonography) because of extensive fibrosis.

Metabolic breakdown of the hemoglobin is responsible for the characteristic brawny pigmentation of the postphlebitic syndrome. Eventually ulceration can develop, either spontaneously or as the result of minor trauma. Although the pathophysiology of the ulceration is not clear, it appears to be related to an inflammatory reaction in the tissue, fibrin cuffing, and eventual lipodermatosclerosis. Whatever the cause, ulceration is undoubtedly related to the persistent venous hypertension.

Duplex ultrasound of the post-thrombotic extremity is useful for both diagnosis and therapy. First, indirect confirmation of the diagnosis of venous hypertension can be made with duplex ultrasonography by direct observation of deep vein valve incompetence or documentation of chronic deep vein obstruction. The perforating veins and the su-

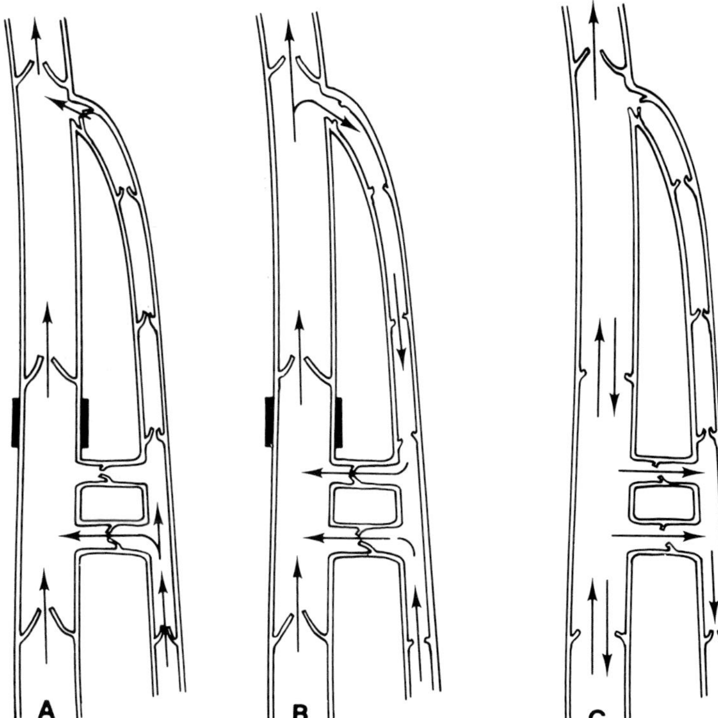

FIGURE 19–6 With incompetent deep veins and perforating veins, venous hypertension below the fascia of the leg is transmitted to the superficial system. *A,* Normal. *B,* Greater saphenous incompetence. *C,* Deep and perforator vein incompetence.

perficial venous system can be similarly assessed. This information assists in planning therapy, for example, if the deep venous system is widely incompetent, valve repair or transplantation may be required. However, if the deep venous system is competent, perforator interruption or stripping of the superficial venous system may suffice.

REFERENCES

1. Pulliam C, Barr S, Ewing A: Venous duplex scanning in the diagnosis and treatment of progressive superficial thrombophlebitis. Ann Vasc Surg 5:190–195, 1991.
2. Lohr JM, McDevitt DT, Lutter KS, et al: Operative management of greater saphenous thrombophlebitis involving the saphenofemoral junction. Am J Surg 164:269–275, 1992.
3. Lutter K, Kerr T, Roedersheimer L, et al: Superficial thrombophlebitis diagnosed by duplex scanning. Surgery 110:42–46, 1991.
4. Jorgenson J, Hanel K, Morgan A, Hunt J: The incidence of deep venous thrombosis in patients with superficial thrombophlebitis of the lower limbs. J Vasc Surg 18:70–73, 1993.
5. Ascer E, Lorensen E, Pollina R, Gennaro M: Preliminary results of nonoperative approach to saphenofemoral junction thrombophlebitis. J Vasc Surg 22:616–621, 1995.
6. Nicolaides A, Kakkar V, Renney J: The soleal sinuses: Origin of deep vein thrombosis. Br J Surg 58:307–309, 1971.
7. Rollins D, Semrow C, Friedell M, et al: Origin of deep vein thrombi in ambulatory population. Am J Surg 156:122–125, 1988.
8. Sevitt S, Gallagher N: Venous thrombosis and pulmonary embolism. A clinico-pathological study in injured and burned patients. Br J Surg 48:475–489, 1961.
9. Philbrick J, Becker D: Calf vein thrombosis: A wolf in sheep's clothing. Arch Intern Med 148:2131–2138, 1988.
10. Atri M, Herba MJ, Reinhold C, et al: Accuracy of sonography in the evaluation of calf deep vein thrombosis in both postoperative surveillance and symptomatic patients. AJR Am J Roentgenol 166:1361–1367, 1996.
11. Thomas ML, McAllister V: The radiological progression of deep venous thrombus. Radiology 99:37–40, 1971.
12. Doous T: The clinical significance of deep venous thrombosis of the calf. Br J Surg 63:377–378, 1976.
13. Kakkar V, Howe C, Flanc C, Clarke M: Natural history of postoperative deep-vein thrombosis. Lancet 230:230–232, 1969.
14. Kakkar VV, Corrigan TP: Efficacy of low-dose heparin in preventing postoperative fatal pulmonary embolism: Results of an international multicentre trial. *In* Kakker VV, Thomas DP (eds): Heparin: Chemistry and Clinical Usage. London, Academic Press, 1976, pp 229–245.
15. Lohr J, Kerr T, Lutter K, et al: Lower extremity calf thrombosis: To treat or not to treat? J Vasc Surg 14:618–623, 1991.
16. Moser KM, LeMoine JR: Is embolic risk conditioned by location of deep venous thrombosis? Ann Intern Med 94:439–444, 1981.

17. Dorfman GS, Cronan JJ, Tupper TB, et al: Occult pulmonary embolism: A common occurrence in deep venous thrombosis. AJR Am J Roentgenol 148:263–266, 1987.
18. Solis MM, Ranval TJ, Nix ML, et al: Is anticoagulation indicated for asymptomatic postoperative calf vein thrombosis? J Vasc Surg 16:414–418, 1992.
19. Haas SB, Tribus CB, Insall JN, et al: The significance of calf thrombi after total knee arthroplasty. J Bone Joint Surg Br 74:799–802, 1992.
20. Hull RD, Hirsh J, Carter CJ, et al: Pulmonary angiography, ventilation lung scanning, and venography for clinically suspected pulmonary embolism with abnormal perfusion lung scan. Ann Intern Med 98:891–899, 1983.
21. Giachino A: Relationship between deep vein thrombosis in the calf and fatal pulmonary embolism. Can J Surg 31:129–130, 1988.
22. Barnes R: Is anticoagulation indicated for postoperative or spontaneous calf vein thrombosis? *In* Veith F (ed): Current Clinical Problems in Vascular Surgery. St. Louis, Quality Medical Publishing, 1993, pp 151–155.
23. Beecham R, Dorfman G, Cronan J, et al: Is bilateral lower extremity compression sonography useful and cost-effective in the evaluation of suspected pulmonary embolism? AJR Am J Roentgenol 161:1289–1292, 1993.
24. Glover J, Bendick P: Appropriate indications for venous duplex ultrasonic examinations. Surgery 120: 725–731, 1996.
25. Killewich L, Nunless J, Auer A: Value of lower extremity venous duplex examination in the diagnosis of pulmonary embolism. J Vasc Surg 17:934–939, 1993.
26. Eze A, Comerota A, Kerr R, et al: Is venous duplex imaging an appropriate initial screening test for patients with suspected pulmonary embolism. Ann Vasc Surg 10:220–223, 1996.
27. Matteson B, Langsfeld M, Schermer C, et al: Role of venous duplex scanning in patients with suspected pulmonary embolism. J Vasc Surg 24:768–773, 1996.
28. Martin EC, Koser M, Gordon DH: Venography in axillary-subclavian vein thrombosis. Cardiovasc Radiol 2:261–266, 1979.
29. Meissner MH, Manzo RA, Bergelin RO, et al: Deep venous insufficiency: The relationship between lysis and subsequent reflux. J Vasc Surg 18:596–605, 1993.

Chapter 20

EXTREMITY VENOUS ANATOMY

■ *William J. Zwiebel, MD*

The normal anatomy of the venous system of the upper and lower extremities[1–4] is discussed in this chapter, with emphasis on those aspects of venous anatomy that are relevant to duplex imaging. In this text, the terms *proximal* and *distal* are defined in relation to the heart. Structures that are closer to the heart are described as proximal and those that are farther away are described as distal. Because most duplex examinations are conducted from proximal to distal, venous anatomy is presented in this order.

Venous valves are occasionally visualized in the course of duplex imaging. These valves are usually bicuspid, but the number of cusps varies from one to three.[1] The lumen of the vein is enlarged at the site of each valve, and the enlarged portion is called the valve sinus. The valves, which are designed to permit flow only toward the heart, increase in number from proximal to distal. In the calf, a valve is present approximately every 2 cm along the length of the tibial and peroneal veins, and the valve sinuses may produce a beaded appearance on sonographic images.

In the upper extremity, the deep veins are generally paired structures and are always accompanied by arteries. The superficial venous system is a primary route of upper extremity venous drainage; therefore, examination of the major components of the superficial system is important. In contrast, the deep system is the major route of drainage in the lower extremity, and examination of the superficial system is less important.

DEEP UPPER EXTREMITY VEINS

At its proximal end, the subclavian vein (Fig. 20–1) joins the internal jugular vein to form the brachiocephalic vein, which continues to the superior vena cava. The brachiocephalic vein usually cannot be imaged sonographically, because it is obscured by the sternum. The subclavian vein lies posterior to the medial end of the clavicle and is both posterior and inferior to the subclavian artery.

The subclavian vein becomes the axillary vein (Fig. 20–2) at the upper border of the first rib, but this point of transition cannot be identified sonographically. The axillary, brachial, radial, and ulnar veins comprise the deep venous system of the upper extremity. All of these veins are accompanied by arteries of the same name. As the axillary vein crosses the lower border of the teres major muscle, it becomes the brachial vein, but this landmark is also not readily detected sonographically. In most individuals the brachial vein is duplicated, and the two branches lie on either side of the brachial artery. The two branches generally reunite just above the elbow (see Fig. 20–2). The radial and ulnar veins are also paired and lie astride the radial and ulnar arteries, respectively. They usually join at the elbow to form a common channel that divides again to form the radial and ulnar veins. In some cases, however, they remain separate, with the radial vein joining one brachial branch and the ulnar vein joining the other brachial branch.

SUPERFICIAL UPPER EXTREMITY VEINS

The cephalic and basilic veins and their tributaries constitute the superficial venous system of the upper extremity. The cephalic vein (Fig. 20–3) joins the subclavian vein near the distal end of the clavicle. From this junction, it passes between the deltoid muscle and the clavicular portion of the pectoralis muscle. It remains deep to the deltoid muscle as it passes over the superior aspect of the shoulder. It emerges in a subcutaneous position and

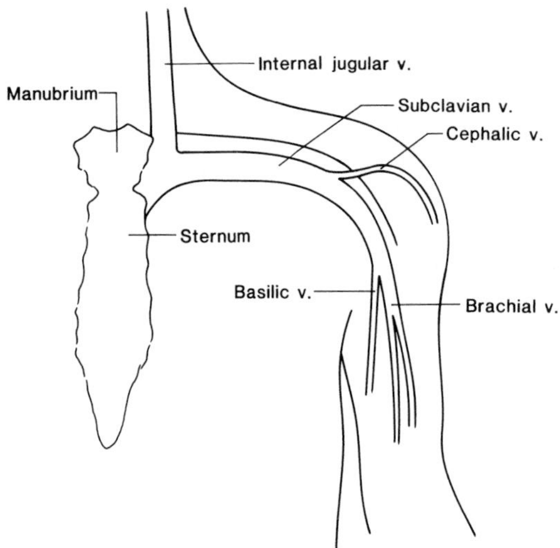

FIGURE 20–1 The subclavian vein and its tributaries.

extends the length of the arm, coursing along the biceps muscle and the lateral aspect of the cuboid fossa (at the elbow) and continuing into the forearm, to form the lateral portion of the dorsal venous arch of the hand. An important branch of the cephalic vein is the median cubital vein, which crosses the antecubital fossa obliquely (see Fig. 20–3).

The basilic vein (see Fig. 20–3) joins the axillary vein at the lower border of the teres major muscle. From this point, it courses along the medial border of the biceps muscle to the elbow. It crosses the medial aspect of the antecubital fossa, continues along the medial side of the forearm, and joins the dorsal venous arch of the hand.

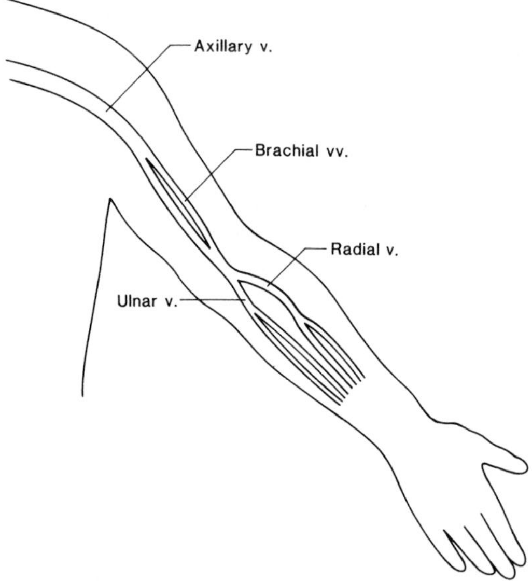

FIGURE 20–2 The deep veins of the upper extremity.

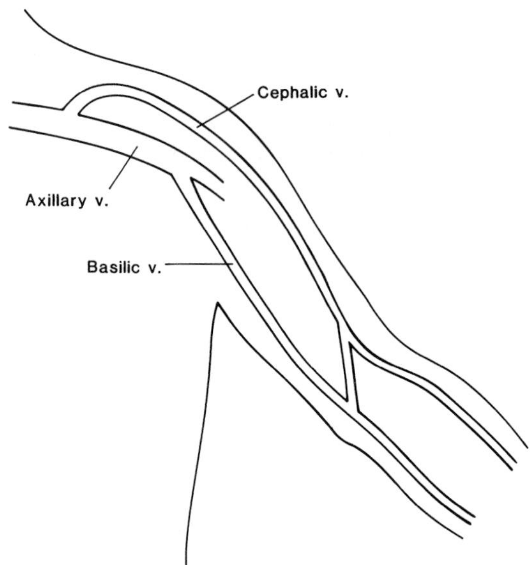

FIGURE 20–3 The superficial veins of the upper extremity.

DEEP LOWER EXTREMITY VEINS

As noted previously, most venous return from the lower extremities is channeled through the deep system. All deep veins of the lower extremity accompany correspondingly named arteries. Communications exist between the deep and superficial venous systems through perforating veins. In normally functioning perforating veins, valves maintain flow in one direction, *from superficial to deep*. Flow in the opposite direction is always abnormal.

Inferior Vena Cava and Iliac Veins

The deep veins of the lower extremity actually begin in the abdomen as the inferior vena cava and iliac veins. The inferior vena cava (Fig. 20–4) is formed by the confluence of the two common iliac veins, which unite at the L5 level. The major tributaries of the inferior vena cava are shown in Figure 20–4.

The common iliac veins are formed at the junction of the internal and external iliac veins (see Fig. 20–4), at the approximate level of the sacroiliac joints. The internal iliac

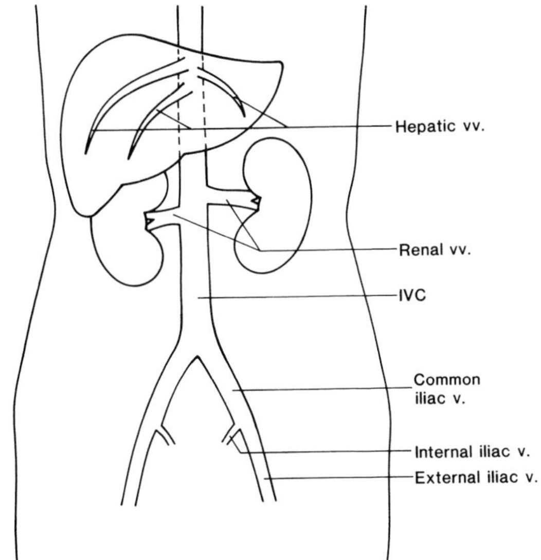

FIGURE 20–4 The inferior vena cava (IVC) and the iliac veins.

veins drain the pelvic viscera and musculature. The external iliac veins drain the lower extremities.

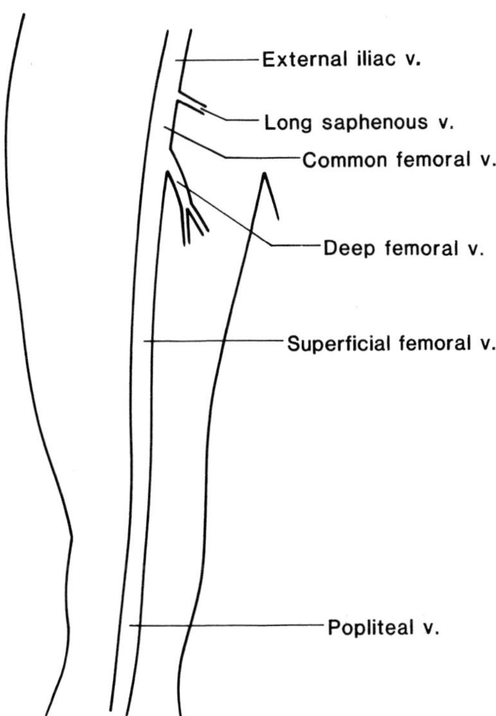

FIGURE 20–5 The femoral venous system.

Femoral Venous System

At the level of the inguinal ligament, the external iliac vein continues into the thigh as the common femoral vein (Fig. 20–5). Slightly distal to this point the common femoral vein receives two branches, the superficial femoral and deep femoral veins. The long saphenous vein also joins the anteromedial aspect of the common femoral vein. This important tributary is discussed later. The common, superficial, and deep femoral veins lie deep to the corresponding arteries, a noteworthy point with respect to duplex imaging.

The superficial femoral vein continues through the thigh as the primary route of venous drainage. This vein is bifid in approximately 25% of individuals.[2] Please note that the *superficial* femoral vein is, in fact, part of the deep venous system. This nomenclature is occasionally a point of confusion.

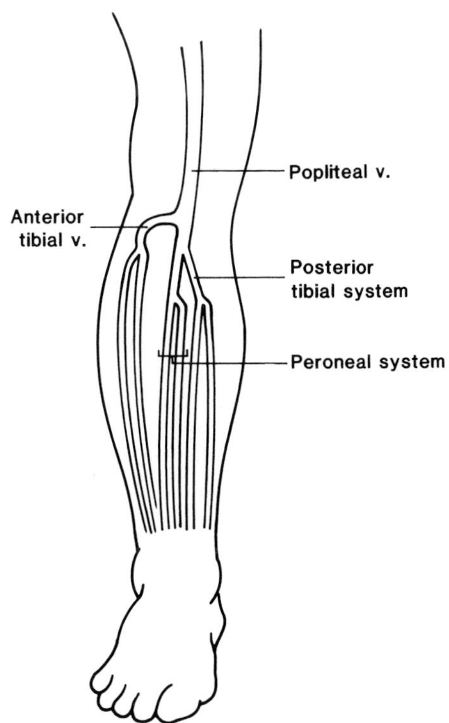

FIGURE 20–6 The popliteal vein and the calf veins.

Popliteal and Calf Veins

In the lower portion of the thigh, the superficial femoral vein dives into the adductor canal and becomes the popliteal vein. The popliteal vein (Fig. 20–6) circles around the

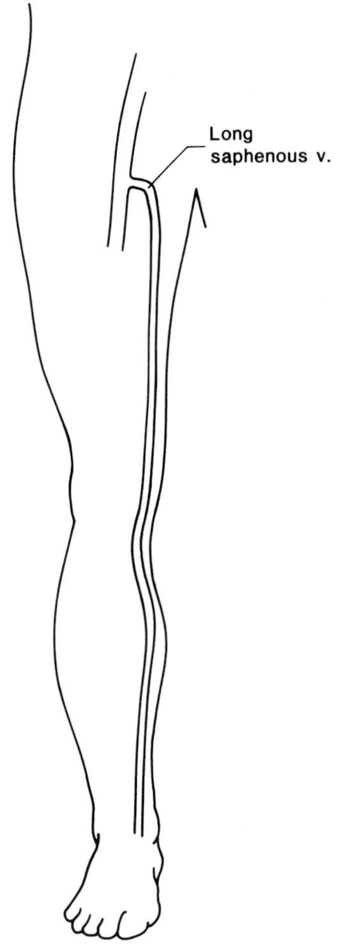

FIGURE 20–7 The long saphenous vein.

medial aspect of the thigh to the back of the knee, where it lies *superficial* to the popliteal artery. This superficial location is the inverse of that seen in the femoral area. Approximately 25% of popliteal veins are duplicated (or bifid).[2] The medial head of the gastrocnemius muscle may contain large veins called the gastrocnemius veins, which join the popliteal vein. These veins are a potential site for venous thrombosis in the calf.[5, 6]

The popliteal vein is formed at the confluence of the anterior tibial, posterior tibial, and peroneal veins (see Fig. 20–6), which drain the calf. Each of these systems consists of paired veins that accompany the artery of the same name and a trunk that is formed at the confluence of the paired veins. The posterior tibial and peroneal trunks unite in the upper portion of the calf or in the popliteal fossa to form the popliteal vein. The anterior tibial trunk has a unique anatomic configuration, in that it extends almost straight laterally from its junction with the popliteal vein. The paired anterior tibial veins often join the popliteal vein independently.

The soleal veins (or sinuses) are embedded in the soleus muscle. These important tributaries of the posterior tibial or peroneal veins may extend medially or laterally, as illustrated in Chapter 23. The soleal veins are thought to be common sites for the origin of venous thrombosis in the calf.[5, 6]

SUPERFICIAL LOWER EXTREMITY VEINS

The lower extremity is drained by an important superficial venous system, the primary components of which are the long and short saphenous veins. The long saphenous vein (Fig. 20–7), also called the greater saphenous vein, is the longest vein in the body. It joins the common femoral vein approximately 4 cm below the inguinal ligament, and from there it extends along the medial aspect of the thigh and leg to the

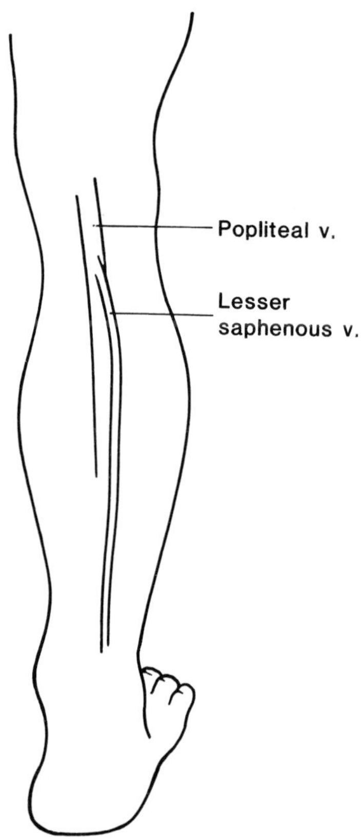

FIGURE 20–8 The lesser saphenous vein.

ankle. It then passes anterior to the medial malleolus and extends onto the foot. The long saphenous vein is a major collateral route, which functions to circumvent occlusion of the deep venous system. It also is used commonly as a conduit for arterial reconstruction and therefore is frequently the subject of duplex examination.

The lesser (small) saphenous vein (Fig. 20–8) empties into the popliteal vein posteriorly, in the popliteal space. This vein extends along the posterior aspect of the calf, between

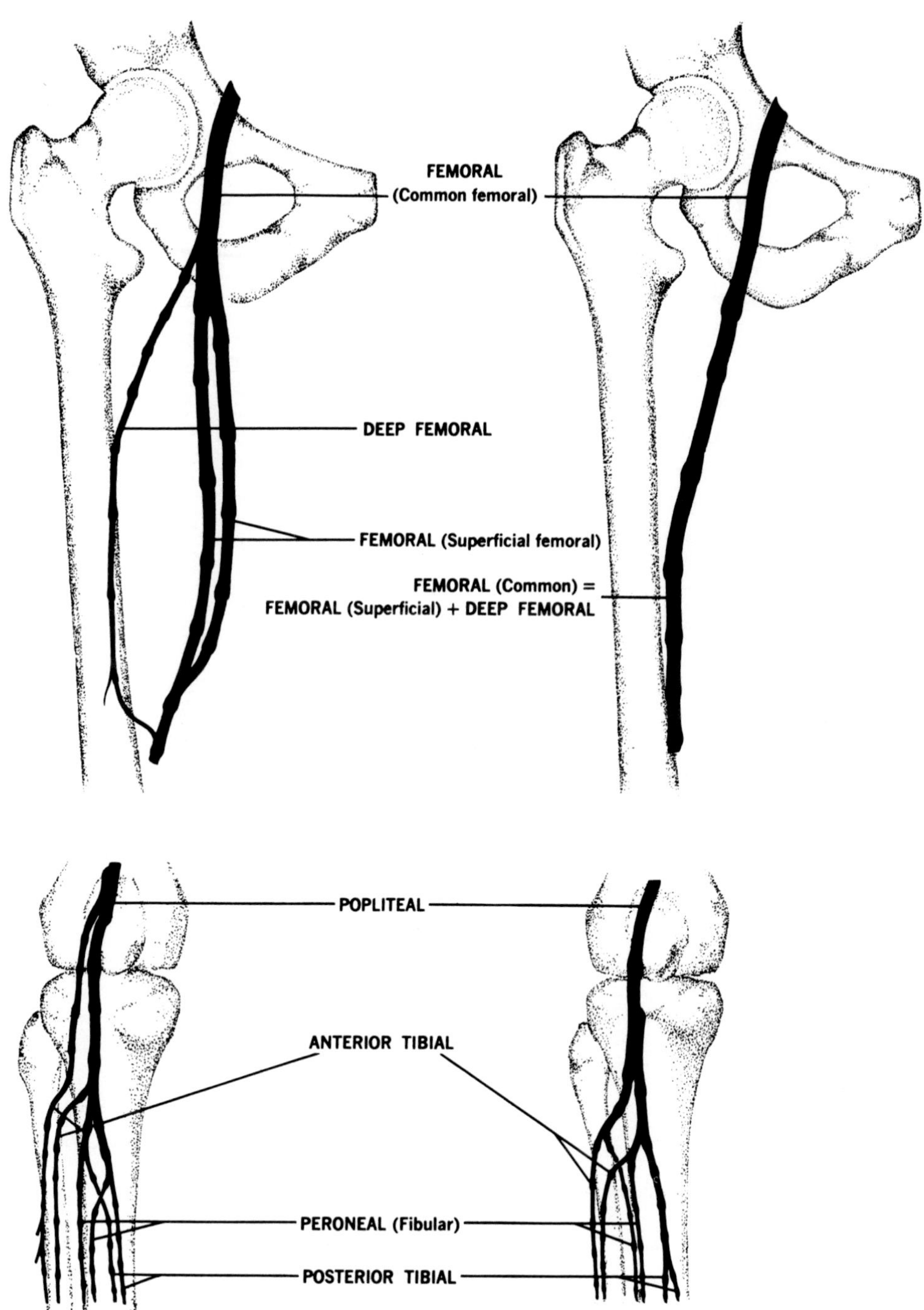

FIGURE 20–9 Common variants of lower extremity venous anatomy. (From DeWeese JA, Rogoff SM, Tobin CE: Radiographic Anatomy of Major Veins of the Lower Limb. Rochester, NY, Eastman Kodak. Reprinted courtesy of Eastman Kodak Company.)

the two heads of the gastrocnemius muscle. It lies in the same position as the seam on a stocking. A method for differentiating between the lesser saphenous and gastrocnemius veins (another popliteal vein tributary) is described in Chapter 23.

ANATOMIC VARIANTS

There are many variations of venous anatomy. For practical reasons only the more common variations are mentioned here, but the sonographer will undoubtedly encounter other variations. Common variations of lower extremity venous anatomy are illustrated in Figure 20–9. As noted previously, the superficial femoral and popliteal veins are duplicated in approximately 25% of individuals.[2] In most cases, popliteal duplication results from the union of the tibial trunks, high within the popliteal fossa. Venous duplications are important, because the unwary sonographer might overlook thrombus isolated to one of the paired veins.

Many variations can occur at the union of the tibial veins. Some of the more common are shown in Figure 20–9.[3] The frequent occurrence of variations at this location necessitates extreme care in the course of duplex examination of the calf veins.

REFERENCES

1. Hollinshead WH: Textbook of Anatomy, 3rd ed. New York, Harper & Row, 1974, p 75.
2. Kadir S: Diagnostic Angiography. Philadelphia, WB Saunders, 1986, p 541.
3. DeWeese JA, Rogoff SM, Tobin CE: Radiographic Anatomy of Major Veins of the Lower Limb. Rochester, NY, Eastman Kodak.
4. Blackburn DR: Venous anatomy. J Vasc Technol 12:78–82, 1988.
5. Cotton LT, Clark C: Anatomical localisation of venous thrombosis. Ann R Coll Surg 36:214–224, 1965.
6. Nicolaides AN, Kakkar VV, Field ES, et al: The origin of venous thrombosis: A venographic study. Br J Radiol 44:653–663, 1971.

Chapter 21

Terminology, Instrumentation, and Characteristics of Normal Veins

■ *William J. Zwiebel, MD*

Duplex examination of extremity veins has gained wide acceptance because the technique provides accurate information and is noninvasive. This chapter provides an introduction to venous imaging that includes the following: (1) a review of selected terms that apply to venous diagnosis; (2) an enumeration of the required characteristics of instruments used for venous examination; and (3) a review of the Doppler and B-mode characteristics of normal extremity veins.

TERMINOLOGY

Clot vs. Thrombus. The terms *clot* and *thrombus* are synonymous and are often used interchangeably, but clot refers to any coagulated mass of blood, and thrombus is more specific for a clot that forms in situ, within a blood vessel. Hence, thrombus is preferred with respect to the venous system.[1]

Acute and Chronic Venous Thrombosis. In terms of risk for pulmonary embolization, acute generally refers to a 2- to 3-week period,[2] after which venous thrombus is assumed to be adherent to the vein wall and not prone to embolize. In other respects, the terms *acute, subacute,* and *chronic* have not been defined as they apply to venous thrombosis, and their usage may vary from one clinician to another. From a sonographic perspective, the *appearance* of acute, subacute, and chronic thrombus has been defined only in general terms. The lack of precise clinical and sonographic definition of these terms may result in serious communication errors; therefore, they must be used with considerable caution. Generally, the use of the term "chronic venous thrombosis" is discouraged, because it is a misnomer. One may properly refer to the chronic *sequelae* of venous thrombosis but not to chronic thrombus or chronic thrombosis. Chronic thrombus is, in fact, a fibrous scar.

Thigh, Leg, and Calf. The *thigh* is the portion of the lower extremity between the hip and the knee. The *leg* is the segment between the knee and the ankle. The *calf* is the posterior, muscular portion of the leg.[1] The term "leg" is sometimes used in reference to the entire lower extremity, but this is somewhat imprecise.

Arm and Forearm. The *arm* is the portion of the upper extremity between the shoulder and the elbow, and the *forearm* is the portion from the elbow to the wrist.[1] "Arm" may properly be applied to the entire upper extremity, but this usage is imprecise.

Proximal and Distal. The terms *proximal* and *distal,*[1] as they apply to the venous system, are somewhat confusing. In the vascular system, proximal and distal are defined with respect to the heart, not with respect to flow direction. Hence, proximal means nearer to the heart and distal means farther from the heart. It is in this sense that these terms apply to the venous system.

INSTRUMENTATION

The duplex instrument chosen for extremity venous diagnosis should have the follow-

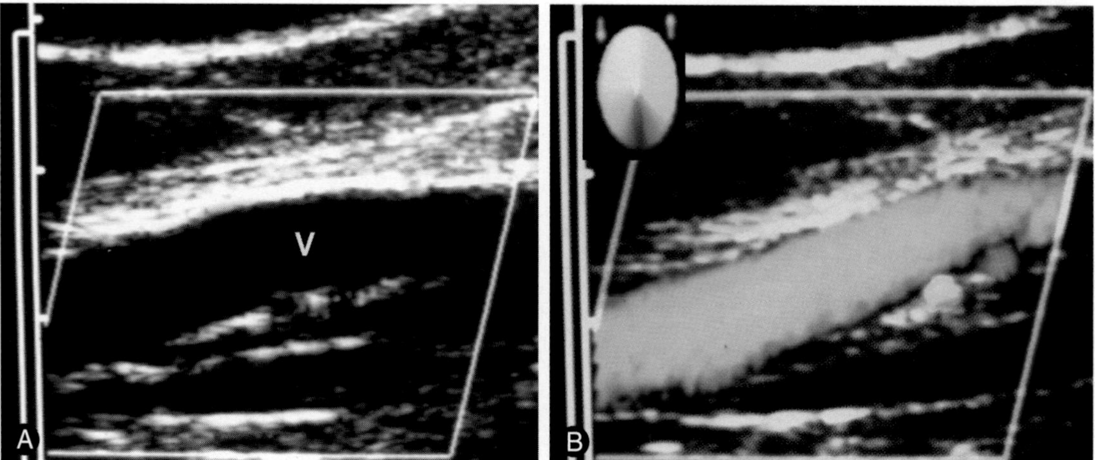

FIGURE 21–1 Color-Doppler features of a normal extremity vein. *A,* The wall of the vein (V) is clearly defined and smooth, but the wall is not visible per se. The lumen is echo free. *B,* Blood flow fills the vein lumen completely (i.e., no flow voids are present within the lumen).

ing features: (1) excellent spatial resolution, which implies incident ultrasound frequencies in the 5- to 10-MHz range; (2) excellent gray-scale resolution (dynamic range); and (3) a pulsed, range gated Doppler device that is sensitive enough to detect the low flow velocities present in smaller veins. The use of a color-Doppler instrument is desirable for venous examinations, because this facilitates both the identification of smaller veins and the confirmation of blood flow. Color Doppler is featured in this text, but accurate venous diagnosis can be accomplished without the use of color Doppler. Indeed, an accurate diagnosis may even be reached with the use of nonduplex, gray-scale instruments, but iliac vein thrombosis may be overlooked if Doppler is not available, as discussed in Chapter 22.

IMAGE CHARACTERISTICS OF NORMAL VEINS

The lumen of a normal vein[3,4] (Fig. 21–1*A*) is echo free without color Doppler, and the interior surface of the vein wall is smooth. The wall itself is so thin that it cannot be seen. Thickening of the wall suggests pathology. With many high-resolution instruments, blood flow may be visible on the B-mode image and, in such cases, the vein lumen is faintly to moderately echogenic[5] (Fig. 21–2). This normal echogenicity may be differentiated from thrombus, because movement of the blood is readily seen, whereas thrombus is stationary. Blood flow should extend all the way to the vessel margin (Fig. 21–1*B*). *The proper method for examining veins with color Doppler is to first visualize the vein wall clearly and then to demonstrate that flow is present to the wall.*

Valves, which permit only cephalad flow, are numerous within extremity veins. In general, the number of valves increases from proximal to distal. Valves may occasionally be seen with the use of duplex instruments when image quality is excellent. Valve sinuses are widened areas of the lumen that

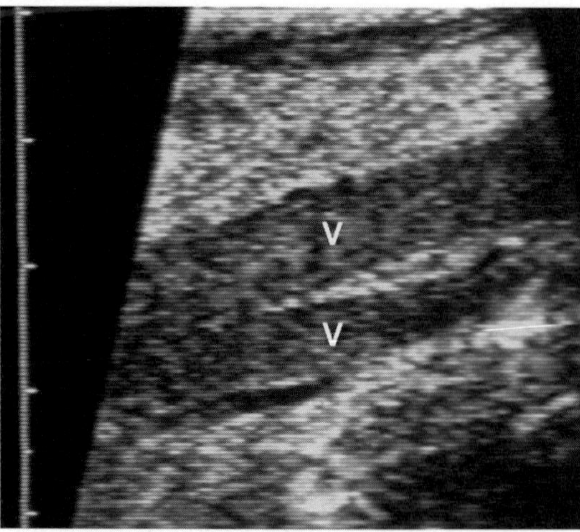

FIGURE 21–2 Echogenic blood. The blood in these veins (V) is echogenic, because flow is sluggish and red blood cells have aggregated into larger units that reflect ultrasound effectively. Movement of the blood is visible in real time, differentiating between sluggish flow and thrombus.

accommodate the valve cusps. The two cusps that constitute most valves are thin and appear delicate[5] (Fig. 21–3). The free edges of the cusps move symmetrically and freely within the flow stream. They coapt in the center of the vessel when closed, and they fold back parallel to the vein wall when open. If only the base of a cusp, near its attachment, is seen on an ultrasound image, movement of the cusp may appear restricted, even if the valve is normal. Hence, a valve that is thought to be dysfunctional should be viewed from different perspectives, if possible, to determine whether it moves freely. Dysfunctional valves generally permit reflux of blood, which is visible on the color-Doppler image or the spectrum display. Small, faintly echogenic aggregates of red blood cells may accumulate behind the valve cusps in slow flow states. These aggregates are easily displaced with vein compression, whereas thrombus in the same location is stationary.

Compressibility

Veins, as opposed to arteries, have thin walls, and the vein is held open primarily by the pressure of blood within the lumen. Thus, the vein lumen can be obliterated with a small amount of extrinsic pressure (Fig. 21–4). This simple observation is of great diagnostic importance, because the walls do not coapt when the lumen contains thrombus, even when the pressure applied is sufficient to distort the shape of an adjacent artery.[4] Vein compressibility is best tested with the image plane transverse to the vein axis. A false impression of compressibility may occur with long-axis views (parallel to the vein), because the vein may slip out of the image plane during attempted compression and disappear from view. Disappearance falsely implies compressibility.

Vein Size

The major veins of the arm and thigh are somewhat larger in diameter than corresponding arteries. If the vein is substantially larger than the artery (i.e., more than twice the arterial diameter), and if the size does not vary with respiration, thrombosis should be suspected, because thrombus distends the vein lumen. Vein size may also be increased by backpressure from congestive heart failure, proximal venous obstruction, or venous reflux. Furthermore, certain veins such as the peroneal, soleal, and gastrocnemius veins, may normally be fairly large. Enlargement, therefore, should not be the sole criterion for the diagnosis of venous thrombosis.

Small vein size may be a manifestation of a remote episode of venous thrombosis, but small vein size should not be the only criterion by which abnormality is diagnosed. If the patient is dehydrated or severely vaso-

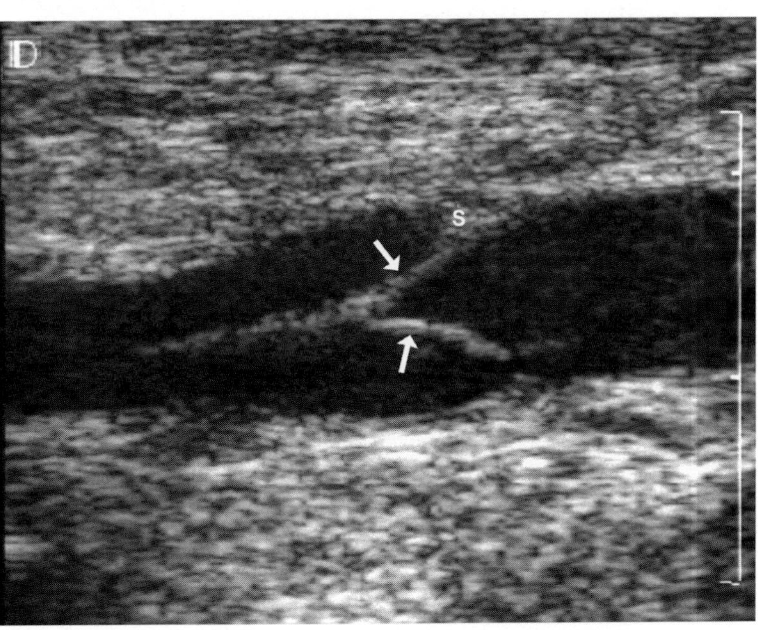

FIGURE 21–3 Venous valve. The two cusps of a valve (*arrows*) are clearly seen in this example. They are curvilinear and coapt in the center of the vessel. (It is uncommon to see venous valves with this level of clarity.) Stasis of blood (S) is evident behind one of the valve cusps. The blood is more echogenic here because of aggregation of red blood cells, as also shown in Figure 21–2.

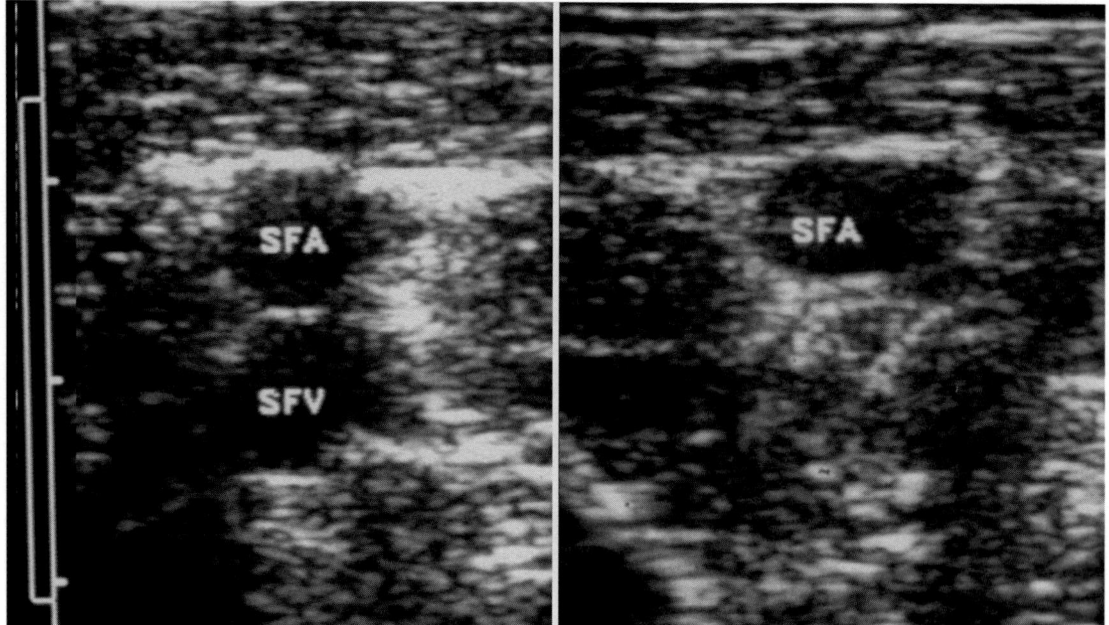

FIGURE 21–4 Vein compression. With pressure from the transducer, the superficial femoral vein (SFV) disappears from view (*right panel*), indicating that it is patent. SFA = superficial femoral artery.

constricted, the veins may be smaller than normal. Furthermore, the paired veins of the calf and forearm may be small for no apparent reason.

Respiratory Changes

The diameter of large veins (e.g., the femoral vein) increases with deep inspiration or with the Valsalva maneuver.[3] Such respiration-related changes indicate that the venous system is patent proximal to the point of examination (see discussion that follows).

DOPPLER CHARACTERISTICS OF NORMAL VEINS

Blood flow in normal veins has five important features: it is spontaneous, phasic, ceases with the Valsalva maneuver, is augmented by distal compression, and is unidirectional (toward the heart).[5–7]

Spontaneous Flow

Flow is normally present in medium-sized and large veins with the patient at rest, even if the extremity is dependent. The absence of spontaneous flow may result from thrombosis at the site of examination or from obstruction proximal or distal to that point. Flow is often *not* spontaneous in normal small veins, such as the paired tibial branches in the calf or the veins of the foot or hand.

Phasic Flow

Normal venous flow is phasic, meaning that the velocity of flow changes in response to quiet respiration and cardiac pulsation. Phasic changes in velocity are evident in the color-Doppler image, the Doppler spectrum display (Fig. 21–5), and the audible Doppler signal. The Doppler spectrum and audible signal are the best media for assessing the phasic flow pattern, because subtle abnormalities are more apparent with these media than with color-Doppler imaging. When the phasic pattern is absent, flow is described as continuous (Fig. 21–6). This flow pattern is significant, for it indicates the presence of substantial obstruction proximal, or sometimes distal, to the site of Doppler examination. With obstruction, blood trickles through diminutive collaterals or recanalization channels, and the phasic changes are

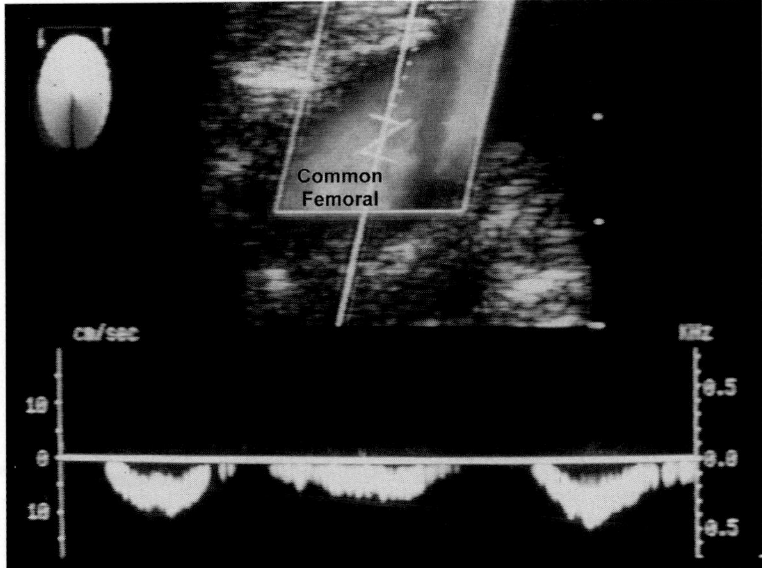

FIGURE 21–5 Spontaneous, phasic flow. The flow velocity fluctuates in response to respiration and right atrial contraction, indicating that the venous system is substantially patent between the point of Doppler examination and the chest.

lost. *The phasic pattern may persist when thrombus does not substantially obstruct the vein lumen;* therefore, the identification of a phasic flow pattern does not exclude thrombosis entirely but only excludes thrombus that occludes the vein lumen.

The Valsalva Response

Deep inspiration followed by bearing down (the Valsalva maneuver) results in the abrupt cessation of blood flow in large and medium-sized veins (Fig. 21–7). This important response documents the patency of the venous system from the point of Doppler examination to the thorax. Although cessation of flow is visible on color-Doppler images, the Valsalva response is best evaluated with the Doppler spectrum display or from the audible Doppler signal. The Valsalva maneuver is particularly useful for confirming the patency of those segments of the venous system that cannot be examined directly. It should be

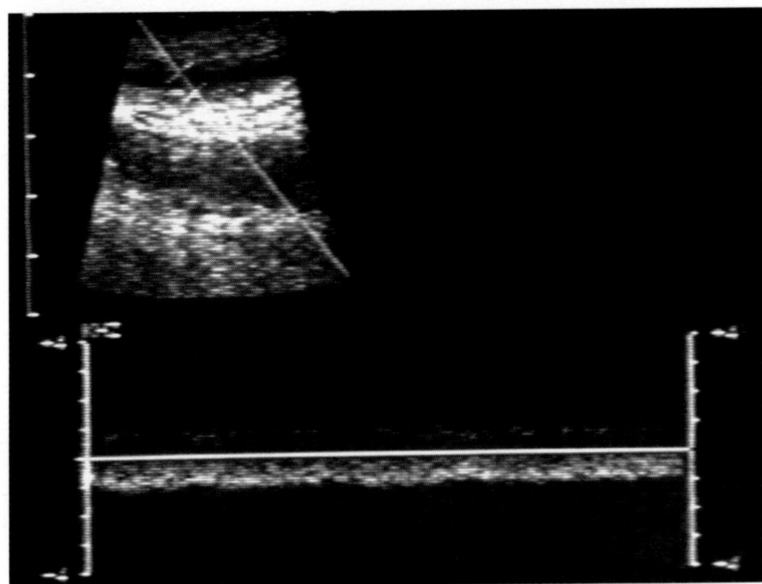

FIGURE 21–6 Continuous flow. The undulating flow pattern seen in Figure 21–5 is absent, indicating venous obstruction. The flow velocity is also low.

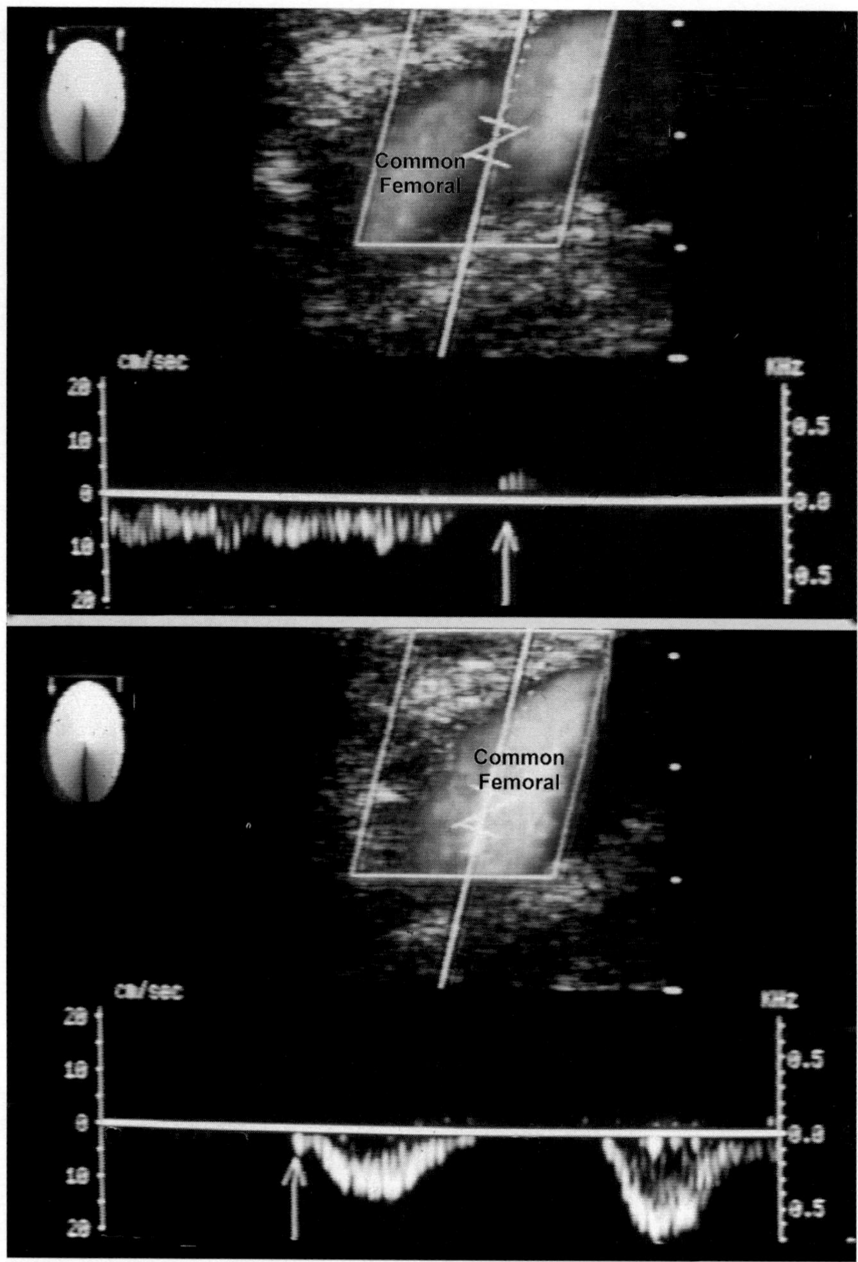

FIGURE 21–7 The Valsalva response. *Top,* As the patient bears down, elevation of intra-abdominal pressure abruptly terminates extremity venous flow (*arrow*). Reversed flow does not occur, indicating that the extremity valves are competent. *Bottom,* Flow resumes promptly with exhalation (*arrow*).

noted, however, that an abnormal response to the Valsalva maneuver occurs only with *substantial* venous obstruction. A normal response may be observed if the vein lumen is only partially blocked.

Augmentation

Manual compression of the extremity distal to the site of duplex examination increases, or augments, venous flow. The re-

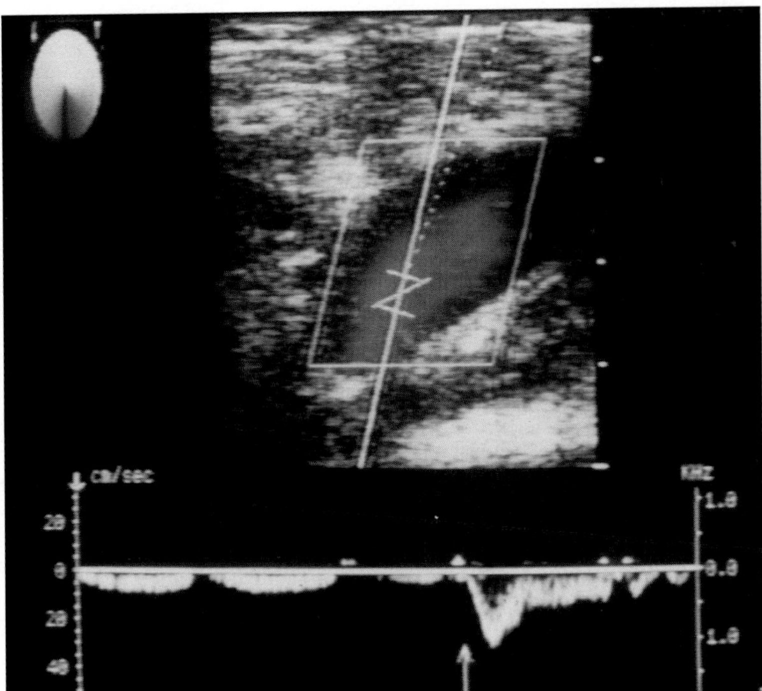

FIGURE 21–8 Flow augmentation. Calf compression results in a dramatic increase in flow velocity (*arrow*) in the common femoral vein. This finding confirms substantial patency of the veins between the calf and the common femoral area.

sulting gush of blood is recorded as an abrupt increase in the Doppler frequency shift (Fig. 21–8). This response confirms substantial patency of the veins between the site of Doppler examination and the site of venous compression. The absence of this response indicates substantial obstruction *distal to* the site of Doppler examination. Delayed or weak augmentation indicates distal obstruction that is incomplete or is circumvented by collaterals. Again, it must be noted that augmentation may be normal when a vein is only partially obstructed. The effects of augmentation are visible on color-Doppler images, but the adequacy of augmentation is best evaluated with the Doppler spectrum or audible Doppler signals.

Unidirectional Flow

In the normal venous system blood flows only toward the heart, because the valves (see Fig. 21–3) prevent flow in the opposite direction (retrograde flow). Normally functioning valves are described as competent, and valves that permit retrograde flow are described as incompetent. Valvular incompetence is diagnosed by demonstrating retrograde flow in response to the Valsalva maneuver (Fig. 21–9) or by manual compression *proximal* to the site of duplex examination. Reflux is most conveniently assessed with the color-Doppler image and may be documented with Doppler spectrum analysis.

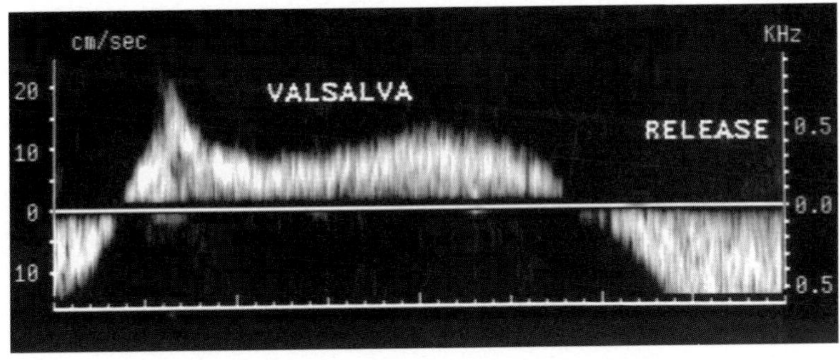

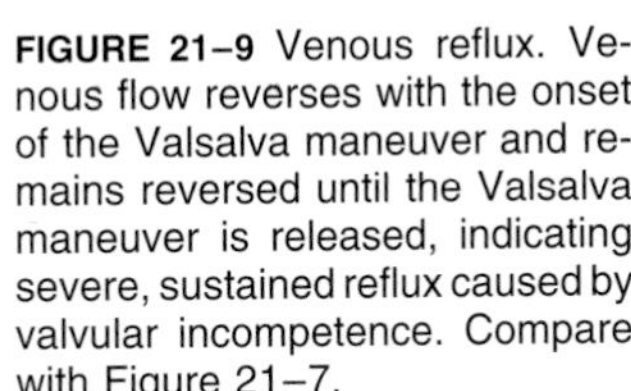
FIGURE 21–9 Venous reflux. Venous flow reverses with the onset of the Valsalva maneuver and remains reversed until the Valsalva maneuver is released, indicating severe, sustained reflux caused by valvular incompetence. Compare with Figure 21–7.

REFERENCES

1. Stedman's Medical Dictionary, 20th ed. Baltimore, Williams & Wilkins, 1961, pp 141, 249, 330, 470, 604, 837, 1233, 1527, 1533.
2. Horowitz O, Casey MP, Maslak MM: Venous thrombosis: Pulmonary embolus complex. *In* Horowitz O, McComb P, Roberts B (eds): Diseases of Blood Vessels. Philadelphia, Lea & Febiger, 1985, pp 263–289.
3. Talbot SR: B-mode evaluation of peripheral veins. Semin Ultrasound CT MR 9:295–319, 1988.
4. Effeney DJ, Friedman MB, Gooding GAW: Iliofemoral venous thrombosis: Real-time ultrasound diagnosis, normal criteria, and clinical application. Radiology 150:787–792, 1984.
5. Zwiebel WJ: Duplex examination of the carotid arteries. Semin Ultrasound CT MR 11:97–135, 1990.
6. Zwiebel WJ: Duplex sonography of the venous system. Semin Ultrasound CT MR 9:269–326, 1988.
7. Barnes RW: Doppler techniques for lower-extremity venous disease. *In* Zwiebel WJ (ed): Introduction to Vascular Ultrasonography. Orlando, FL, Grune & Stratton, 1986, pp 333–350.

Chapter 22

Extremity Venous Examination: Technical Considerations

■ *William J. Zwiebel, MD*

This chapter presents protocols for duplex ultrasound examination of both the upper and lower extremity veins.[1–15] No two ultrasound laboratories perform a given examination in exactly the same way, and it is likely that the protocols described herein will be modified to suit the needs of particular laboratories or patient populations. A consistent method of examination must be established within each laboratory, however, to ensure that examinations are comprehensive and accurate.

The orientation of the ultrasound image relative to the vein axis can be described in several ways. Images oriented along the length of the vein may be described as long axis or longitudinal. Images at right angles to the vein axis may be described as short axis or transverse. In the venous ultrasound chapters, we use the terms *long axis* and *transverse,* recognizing that transverse actually refers to the axis of the body as a whole, not to the axis of the vein.

EXAMINATION PROTOCOL FOR UPPER EXTREMITY VEINS

Extremity venous anatomy is described in detail in Chapter 20, and readers who are unfamiliar with venous anatomy should review this chapter before proceeding. A few points with respect to upper extremity venous anatomy are worthy of emphasis. First, part or all of the superior vena cava and the innominate veins generally cannot be examined with duplex scanners because these veins are obscured by the sternum and the lungs. Careful assessment of the Doppler flow characteristics is necessary, therefore, in the subclavian or axillary veins to exclude obstruction of the superior vena cava and the innominate veins. Second, anatomic variations occur frequently in the upper extremity venous system. The most common variation is duplication of the subclavian or brachial veins. Third, in the presence of venous occlusion, the neophyte may easily mistake an enlarged collateral vein for an occluded vein. Close scrutiny of venous anatomy is suggested to avoid such errors. Finally, both the superficial and deep veins are important routes of drainage in the upper extremity; therefore, both systems should be included in virtually all duplex examinations.

Patient Position

For upper extremity examinations, the patient should be recumbent on a bed or a stretcher that is sufficiently wide to comfortably support the patient's upper extremity and trunk. This is important because muscular contraction from an uncomfortable patient position can compress and occlude the veins and can limit transducer access.

Step 1. The Subclavian Vein

With the patient's upper extremity comfortably positioned along his or her side, begin by examining the subclavian vein, which may be visualized from two approaches, above and below the clavicle (Fig. 22–1). The approach from below the clavicle (through the pectoralis muscles) is generally more effective than the supraclavicular approach, as it provides

Text continued on page 318

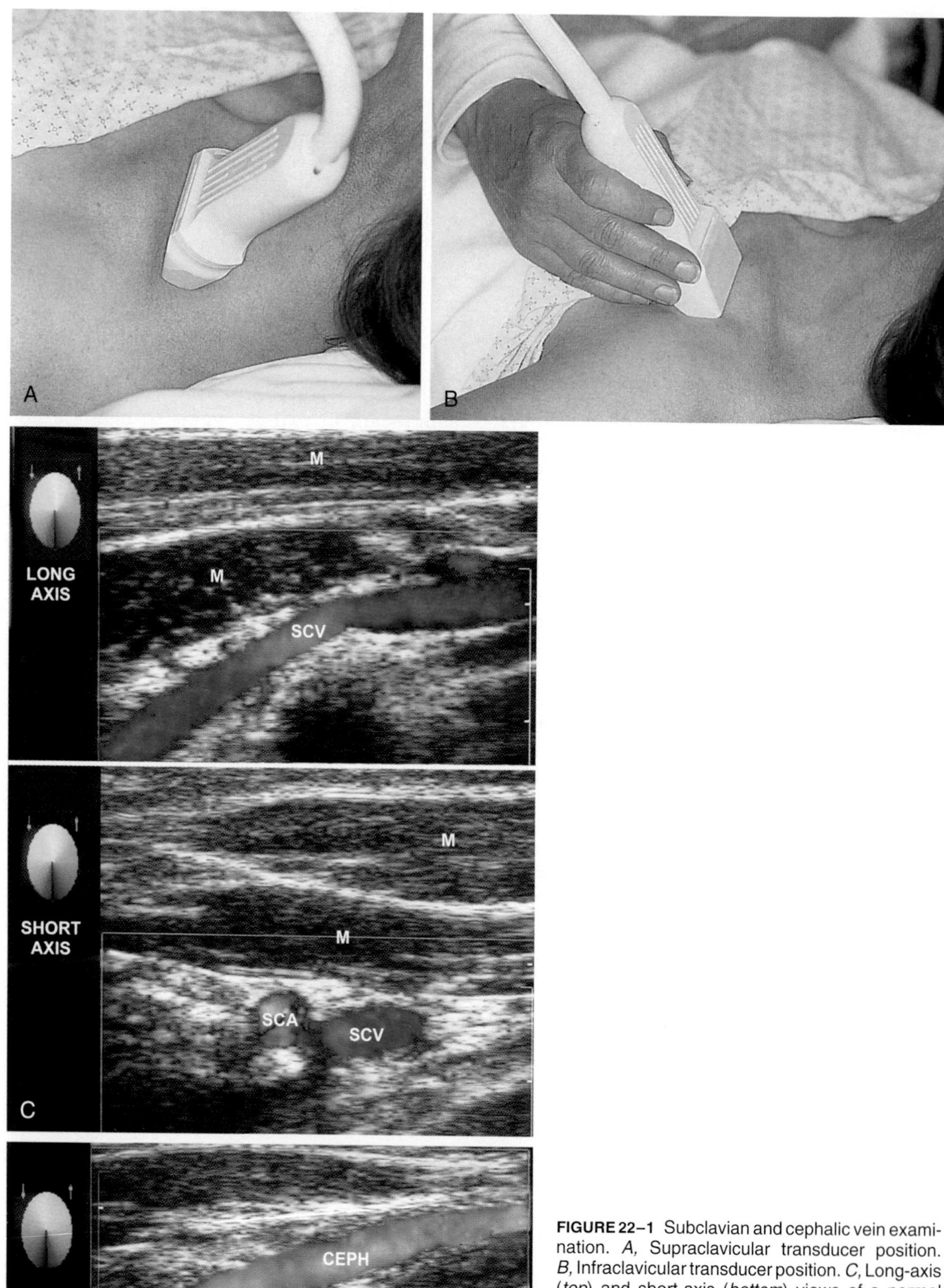

FIGURE 22–1 Subclavian and cephalic vein examination. *A,* Supraclavicular transducer position. *B,* Infraclavicular transducer position. *C,* Long-axis (*top*) and short-axis (*bottom*) views of a normal subclavian vein (SCV). Note that the vein is slightly inferior to the subclavian artery (SCA) and is deep to the pectoralis muscles (M). *D,* Supraclavicular view showing the junction of the cephalic vein (CEPH) with the subclavian vein (SCV).

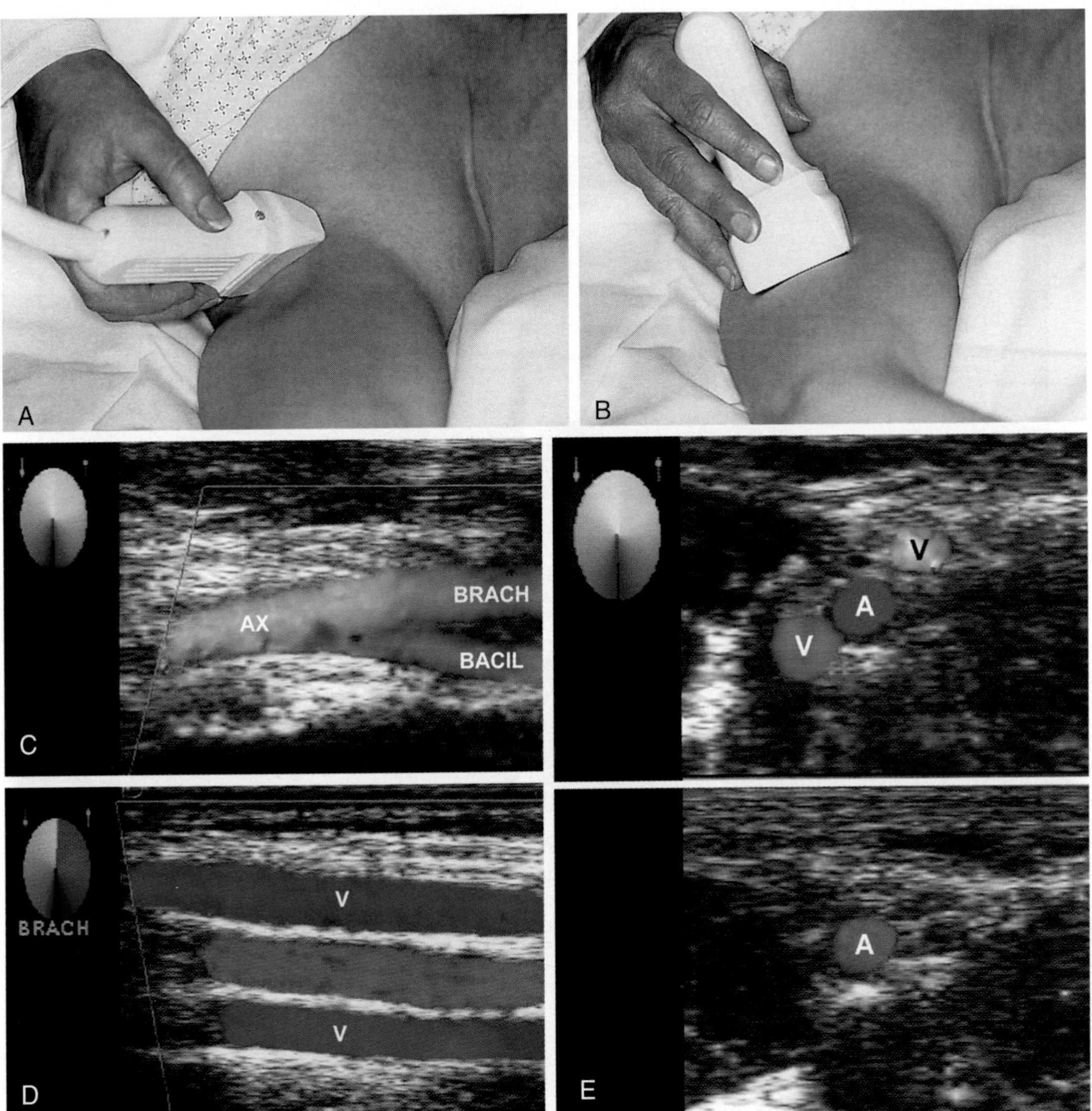

FIGURE 22–3 Axillary, basilic, and brachial vein examinations. (See p 318.) *A,* Transducer position for viewing the axillary vein. *B,* Transducer position for viewing the brachial vein. *C,* Junction of the brachial (BRACH) and the basilic (BACIL) veins, forming the axillary vein (AX). *D,* Paired brachial veins (V) lying on each side of the brachial artery. *E,* The upper image shows the brachial veins (V) adjacent to the brachial artery (A). The lower image was obtained with compression, and only the artery (A) is visible.

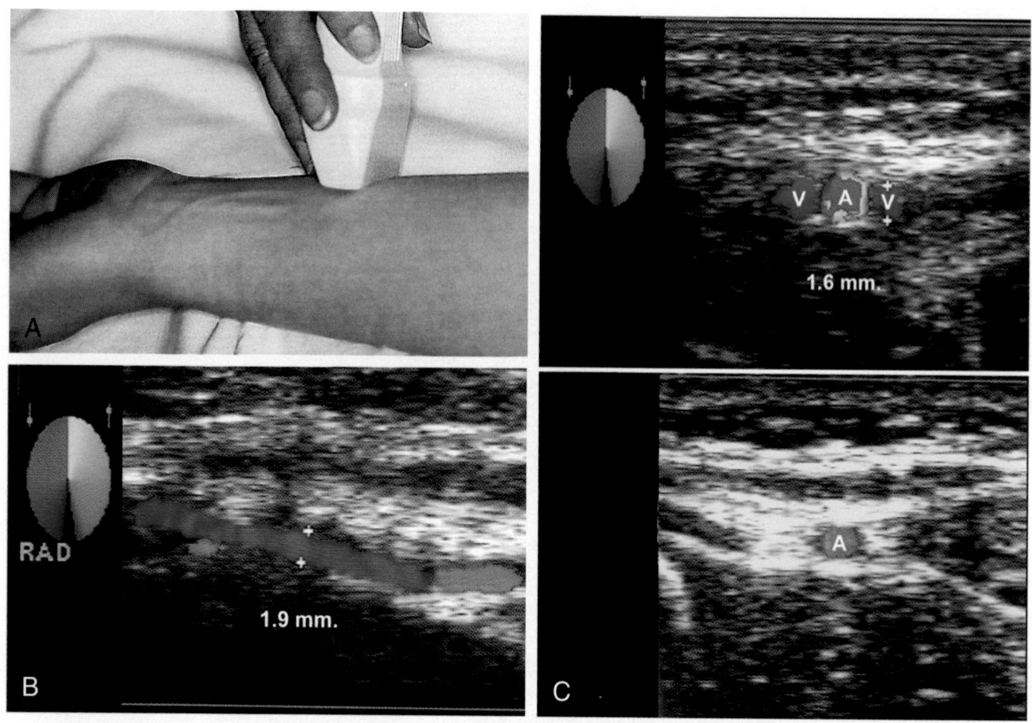

FIGURE 22–4 Forearm vein examination. (See p 319.) *A,* Transducer position for viewing the ulnar veins. *B,* Long-axis view of an ulnar vein. Note the small size (1.9 mm). *C,* The upper image is a short-axis view of the paired ulnar veins (V) adjacent to the ulnar artery (A). Note the small size of the veins (1.6 mm). In the lower image, obtained with compression, only the artery (A) is visible.

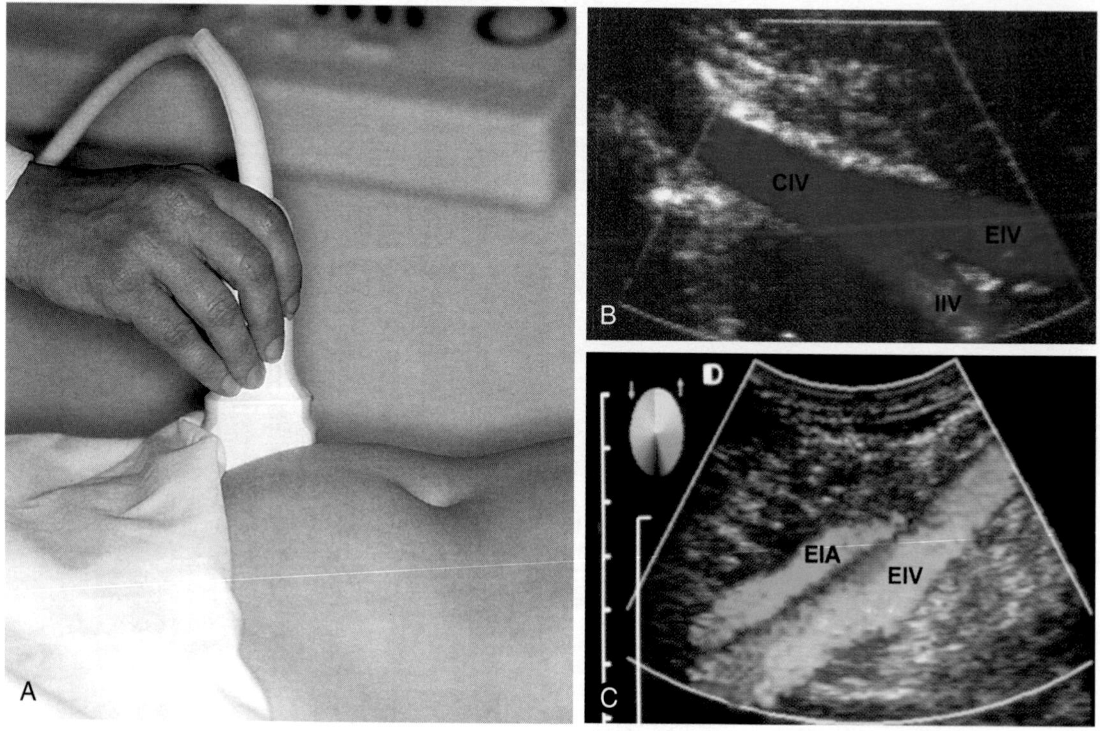

FIGURE 22–6 Iliac vein examination. (See p 321.) *A,* The transducer is positioned lateral to the rectus muscle for visualization of the iliac veins. *B,* Junction of the external (EIV) and internal (IIV) iliac veins, forming the common iliac vein (CIV). *C,* The external iliac vein (EIV), as seen just caphalad to the inguinal ligament. EIA = external iliac artery.

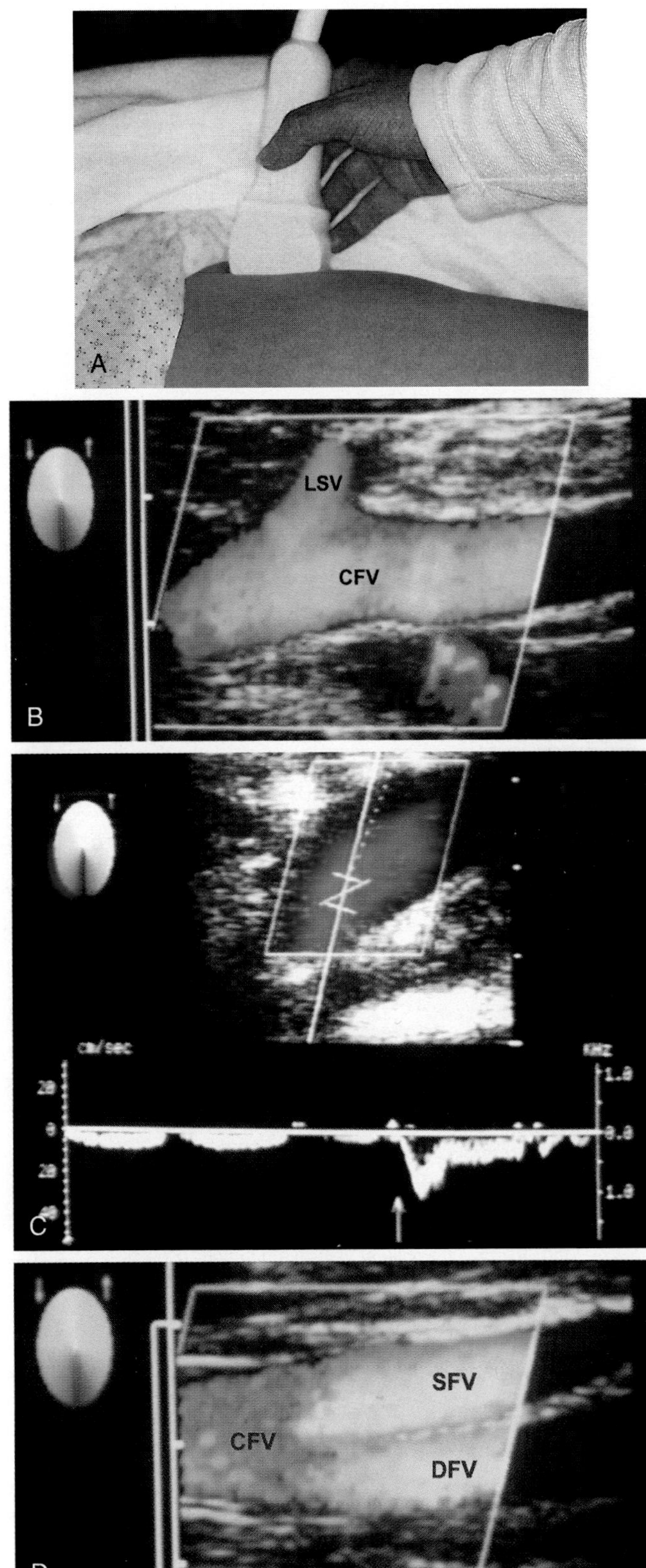

FIGURE 22–7 Long-axis femoral vein examination. (See p 321.) *A,* Transducer position, upper thigh. *B,* The junction of the long saphenous vein (LSV) with the common femoral vein (CFV) is an important landmark. *C,* Doppler signals are obtained routinely in the common femoral vein. (Phasic, spontaneous flow, with augmentation at the *arrow.*) *D,* The junction of the superficial femoral vein (SFV) and the deep femoral veins (DFV), forming the common femoral vein, is another important landmark.

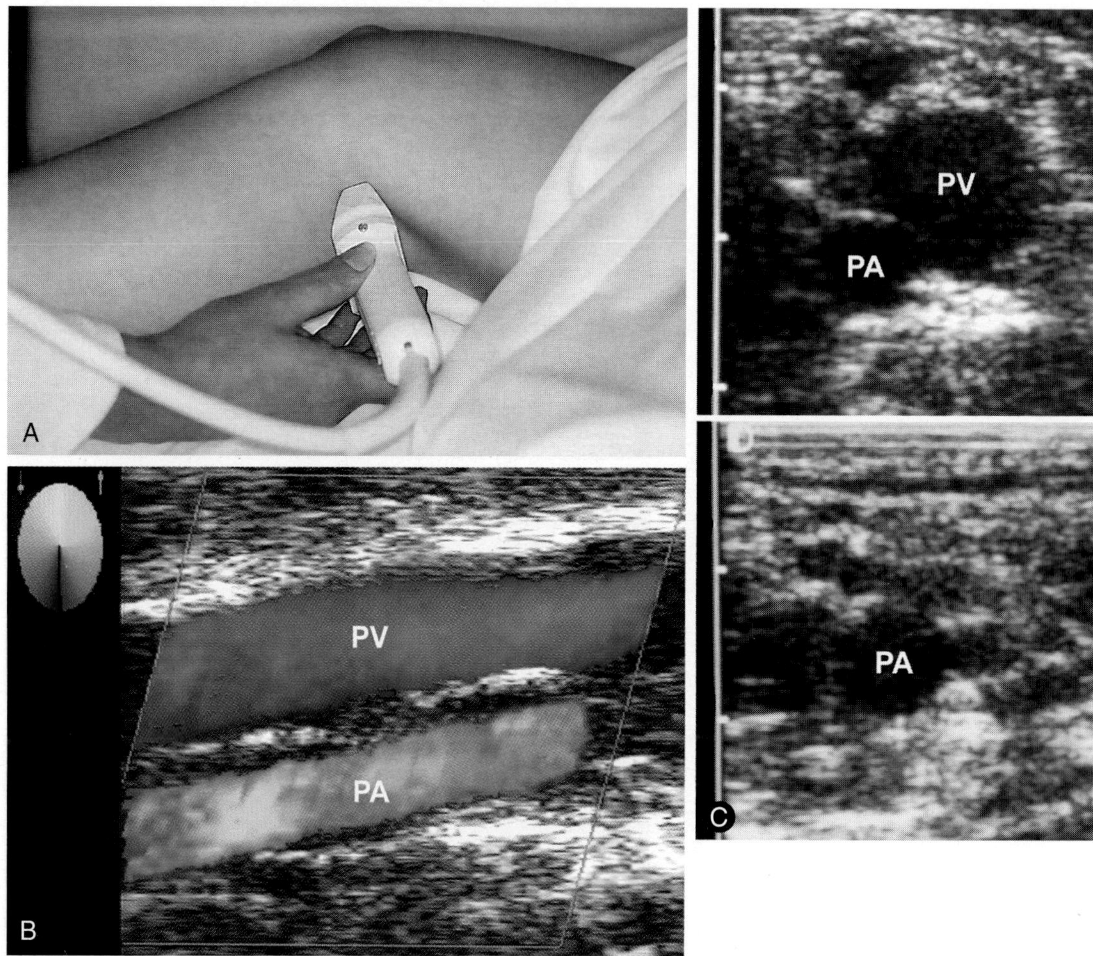

FIGURE 22–11 Popliteal vein examination. (See p 323.) *A,* Transducer positions. *B,* Long-axis view of the popliteal vein (PV). Note that the vein is *superficial* to the popliteal artery (PA). *C,* Transverse view of the popliteal vein (PV) and artery (PA), without (*top*) and with (*bottom*) compression.

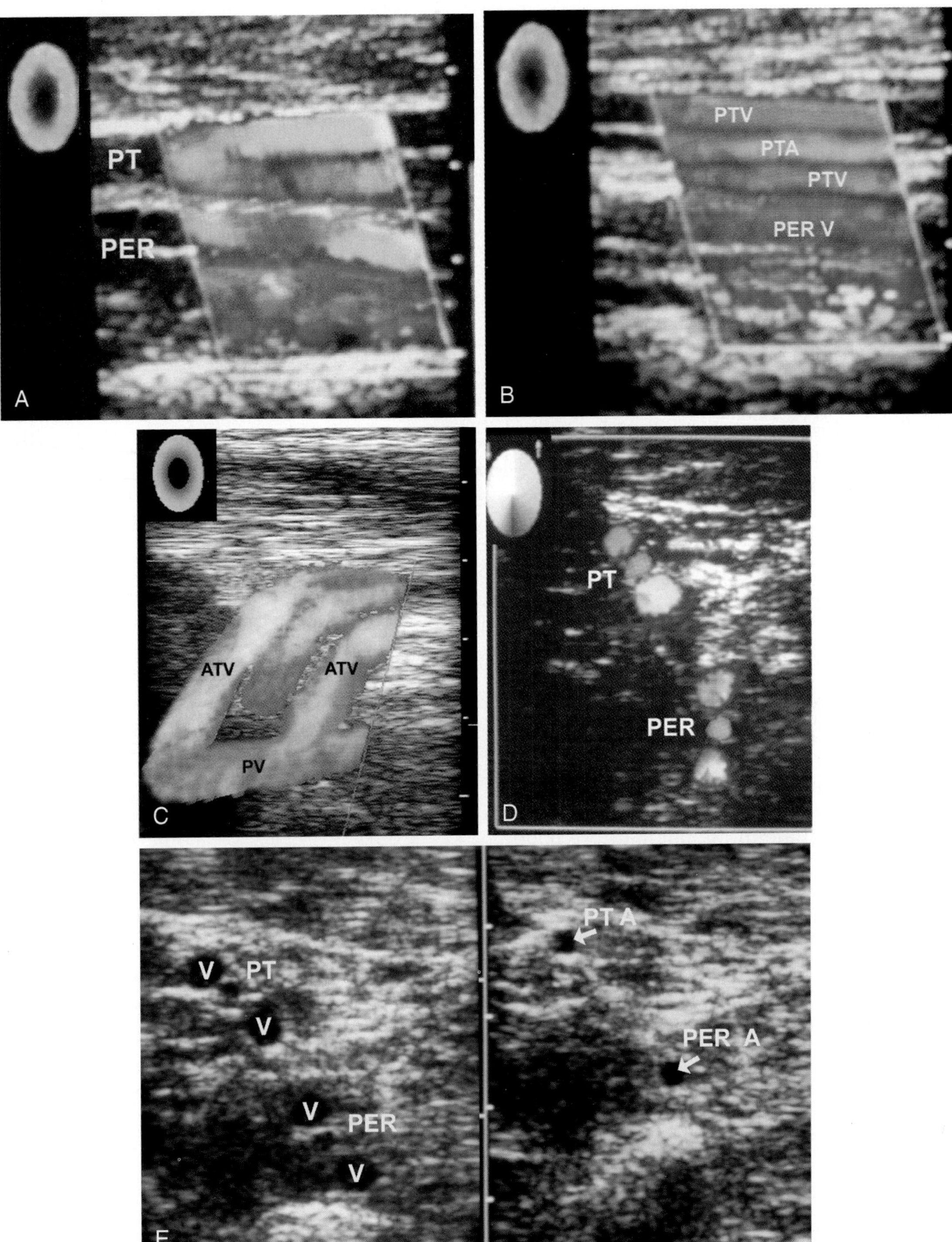

FIGURE 22–13 Representative images of normal calf veins. (See p 325.) *A,* Power Doppler view of the junction of the paired posterior tibial and peroneal veins, forming the common posterior tibial (PT) and peroneal (PER) trunks. *B,* Power Doppler view of the paired posterior tibial veins (PTV) adjacent to the posterior tibial artery (PTA). One of the peroneal veins (PER V) is also visible. *C,* Power Doppler view showing the junction of the anterior tibial veins (ATV) with the popliteal vein (PV). The anterior tibial artery lies between the anterior tibial veins. *D,* Short-axis color-Doppler view of the posterior tibial (PT) and peroneal (PER) veins. *E,* On the *left* is a short-axis view of the paired posterior tibial (PT) and peroneal (PER) veins (V) without compression. With compression (*right*), only the posterior tibial and peroneal arteries are visible (PT A and PER A, respectively).

access to a long segment of the vein. The examination is conducted almost exclusively with the image plane parallel to the vein axis. The normal vein is uniform in caliber and is larger than the adjacent artery. If doubt exists as to the identity of the vein and the artery, insert the Doppler sample volume and check the flow pattern aurally or on the Doppler spectrum display for a venous flow pattern. With vein identity confirmed, check the Doppler signal for normal flow characteristics (Fig. 22–2). Flow should be spontaneous and somewhat pulsatile (as a result of transmission of right atrial pulsations). Furthermore, flow should respond appropriately to the Valsalva maneuver. *Confirmation of normal pulsatility is particularly important,* as it confirms the patency of the innominate vein and the superior vena cava, which generally cannot be examined directly.

After the Doppler examination, look for the junction of the subclavian and internal jugular veins and confirm patency of the latter. We generally follow the internal jugular vein about half the way to the mandible. The size of the internal jugular vein changes substantially with respiration.

Next, trace the subclavian vein as far distally as possible. Watch for normal (or abnormal) flow patterns on the color-Doppler image and be careful not to slip unknowingly into an enlarged cephalic vein that is functioning as a collateral. Remember, the major deep veins of the upper extremity are accompanied by corresponding arteries. If you do not see an artery near the vein, you may be in the superficial system rather than the deep system.

Step 2. The Cephalic Vein

Locate the junction of the subclavian and cephalic veins (see Fig. 22–1*D*) and follow the cephalic vein over the deltoid muscle and down the arm to the elbow. The cephalic vein can be examined either in long-axis or in transverse view. My preference is for transverse compression examination, as this method is efficient and accurate. The vein is compressed approximately every 1 to 2 cm to confirm patency. Because the cephalic vein may be quite superficial, a light touch with the transducer is important, otherwise the vein might collapse and be lost from view.

Step 3. The Axillary and Brachial Veins

With the patient's arm abducted, place the transducer high in the axilla and identify the axillary vein in a plane parallel to the vein axis (Fig. 22–3 [see p 313]). Use the Doppler flow signals, if needed, to confirm the identity of the vein and the adjacent artery. When the Doppler examination is completed, follow the course of the axillary vein into the brachial vein. No discrete landmark indicates the junction of these segments. The brachial vein is usually duplicated, and in such cases both branches must be examined. Continue the examination of the brachial vein to the level of the elbow. Our preferred mode of examination is transverse compression, supplemented as needed with long-axis color-flow images.

Step 4. The Basilic Vein

Next, return to the axillary area and identify the junction of the basilic vein with the axillary vein, using long-axis color-flow images. Then follow the basilic vein to the elbow, using transverse compression supplemented with long-axis color-flow images as needed.

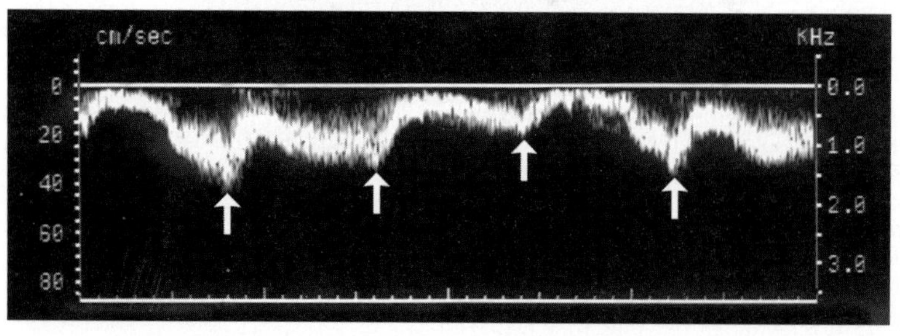

FIGURE 22–2 Normal subclavian vein Doppler signal. Note the cardiac pulsations (*arrows*) superimposed on respiratory variation.

Step 5. The Forearm Veins

In most cases, the more proximal upper extremity veins are the areas of primary clinical concern, and the venous ultrasound examination may be terminated at the elbow. If there is clinical suspicion of thrombosis in the veins of the forearm, the examination is extended beyond the elbow. For the forearm examination (Fig. 22–4 [see p 314]), trace the radial and ulnar veins from the elbow to the wrist (or vice versa), using the corresponding arteries as anatomic guides. Once again, I prefer transverse compression examination, and I use long-axis color-flow images as an ancillary method. The continuation of the cephalic and the basilic veins into the forearm may also be examined as needed.

Protocol Summary

The protocol for upper extremity venous examination is summarized in Table 22–1.

EXAMINATION PROTOCOL FOR LOWER EXTREMITY VEINS

To ensure accurate duplex diagnosis, the following features of lower extremity venous anatomy should be appreciated. Many of these features are illustrated in Chapter 20.

1. The primary venous drainage routes in the lower extremities are the deep veins, which are accompanied by arteries with corresponding names. The superficial veins are not accompanied by arteries.
2. The paired anterior tibial, posterior tibial, and peroneal veins, which are components of the deep system, are accompanied by arteries that serve as "beacons," which help to identify these veins. If an accompanying artery cannot be visualized, it may be hard to identify the deep calf veins.
3. Direct color-Doppler imaging of the common and external iliac veins is not possible in many cases, and even when these veins can be examined directly, image quality may be limited. Therefore, indirect confirmation of the patency of the iliac veins is essential, as achieved through careful examination of Doppler flow signals at the common femoral level.
4. Isolated thrombosis of the deep femoral vein is unusual, but such thrombosis poses a risk of pulmonary embolization. Therefore, routine assessment of the proximal portion of the deep femoral vein is suggested.
5. The portion of the superficial femoral vein that passes through the adductor canal is difficult to examine. This limitation should be offset with technical diligence.

TABLE 22-1 PROTOCOL FOR UPPER EXTREMITY VENOUS EXAMINATION

Step 1.	The Subclavian Vein
	Visualize with long-axis images from the manubrium as far distally as possible. Check subclavian Doppler signals. Examine the internal jugular vein.
Step 2.	The Cephalic Vein
	Identify the junction of the cephalic vein with the subclavian vein, and follow the cephalic vein over the shoulder to the elbow. Image primarily with transverse compression and supplement with long-axis views as needed.
Step 3.	The Axillary and Brachial Veins
	View the axillary vein in long axis and follow it into the brachial veins. Continue to the elbow, principally using transverse compression. Be sure to examine both branches of the brachial vein.
Step 4.	The Basilic Vein
	Identify the junction of the basilic and brachial veins, and follow the basilic vein to the elbow, principally using transverse compression.
Step 5.	The Forearm Veins
	Follow the radial and ulnar veins to the wrist if symptoms suggest abnormality in these segments. Transverse compression is recommended as the primary mode of examination.

6. Duplication of the common femoral vein in the thigh occurs in approximately 25% of normal individuals.[13] Attention to such duplication is important, as one of the branches may be patent and the other thrombosed. Duplication of the popliteal vein also occurs commonly. In most cases, popliteal duplication is caused by extension of the posterior tibial and peroneal trunks high into the popliteal space.
7. Large veins are present in the gastrocnemius muscle (particularly the medial head) and the soleus muscle. In some cases, thrombus is thought to originate in these muscular veins, and care must be taken, therefore, to identify such thrombus, which may be isolated to these branches.
8. Normal variations occur commonly in the calf veins in the form of interconnections between the posterior tibial and peroneal veins (see Chapter 20). Interconnecting channels are also common between paired calf veins. Because of these interconnections, the potential for collateralization is enormous, which is important diagnostically because blood flow may be present proximal or distal to an occluded venous segment. The identification of normal flow in one segment of a calf vein does not, therefore, exclude thrombosis elsewhere within the same system.

Patient Position

Clear visualization of the lower extremity veins requires adequate distention of the venous system. To this end, the lower extremity must be dependent, which may be accomplished by steeply elevating the head of the examination table or by examining the patient in the sitting position (Fig. 22–5). The patient should be warm to prevent vasoconstriction, which in turn results in poor venous distention. The examination room, therefore, must be reasonably warm.

Step 1. The Iliac Veins

We do not examine the iliac veins routinely in our department. Instead we rely

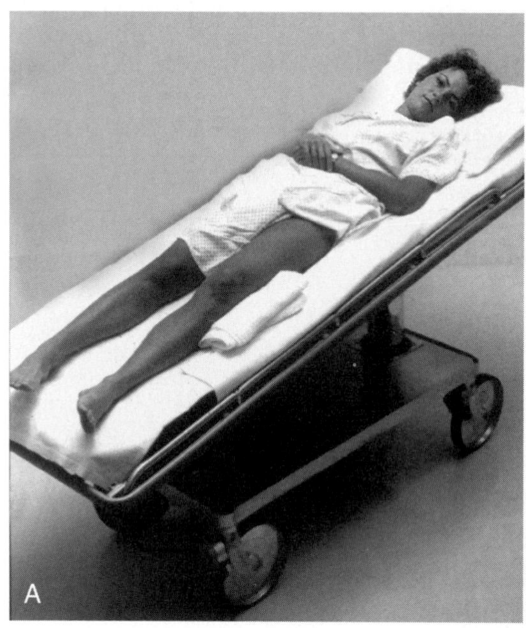

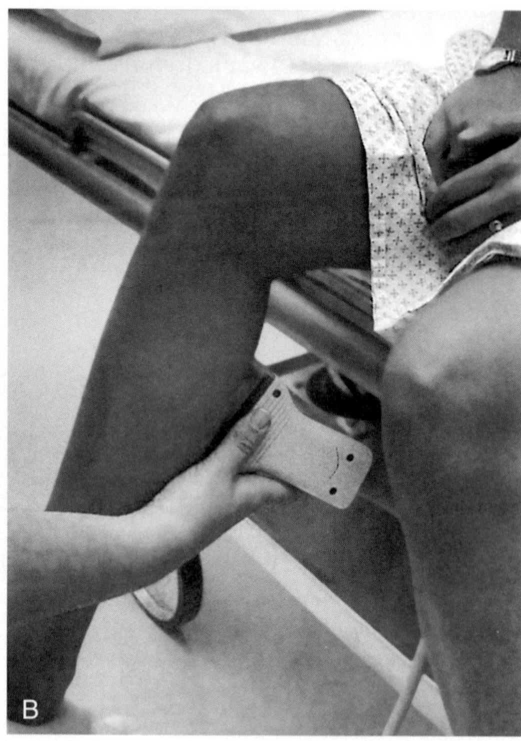

FIGURE 22–5 Patient positions for lower extremity venous examination. *A,* Supine, reverse Trendelenburg's position. *B,* Upright position. (*A, B,* Modified from Zwiebel WJ, Priest DL: Color duplex sonography of extremity veins. Semin Ultrasound CT MR 11:136–167, 1990.)

on Doppler signals obtained at the groin to exclude proximal venous occlusion. When Doppler signals are abnormal, or other reasons exist to suspect iliac vein occlusion, the iliac veins can be examined directly. A 3-MHz transducer is generally required for iliac vein examination. With the patient in a reverse Trendelenburg position, identify the external iliac vein at the groin and follow it cephalad as it dives deeply into the pelvis. From this point cephalad, the iliac system is best visualized from an anterolateral approach, with the transducer lateral to the rectus muscle (Fig. 22–6 [see p 314]). Follow the external and common iliac veins cephalad as far as possible, with a goal of tracing the iliac system all the way to the inferior vena cava. The junction of the external and common iliac veins often cannot be identified per se, but this junction is slightly inferior to the point where the iliac vessels lie most deeply within the pelvis. Examination of the iliac veins seems impossible to neophyte sonographers but becomes easier with practice; nonetheless, even experienced sonographers cannot demonstrate the iliac veins in all patients, and when the iliac veins are visualized, image quality may be suboptimal. In spite of these limitations, it is desirable to attempt the iliac examination in selected patients.

Step 2. The Femoral Segment

The examination of the venous system from the femoral level distally is usually conducted with a 5- or 7-MHz linear array transducer. With the patient in the reverse Trendelenburg position, begin the examination at the groin with long-axis views of the distal external iliac vein. Move caudad into the common femoral vein (Fig. 22–7 [see p 315]), and look for two important landmarks: the long saphenous vein and the junction of the superficial and deep femoral veins. These are the first of several landmarks that should be identified during each venous examination. Confirm the patency of the long saphenous and deep femoral veins with color-flow imaging. Next, evaluate flow in the common femoral vein with the Doppler spectrum (see Fig. 22–7*C*). Check for spontaneous and phasic flow and a normal Valsalva response. These measures are used to exclude occlusion (thrombosis) of the iliac veins or the inferior vena cava.

After the Doppler examination is complete, switch to transverse (short-axis) views and begin the transverse compression examination of the common and superficial femoral veins. *This is the primary method used in our department for lower extremity venous examination.* Beginning as high as possible in the common femoral vein and proceeding to the adductor canal, sequentially test vein compressibility at approximately 2-cm intervals (Fig. 22–8). Be sure to identify landmarks along the way that confirm anatomic location. Either the gray-scale image or the color-Doppler image may be used for the transverse compression examination, according to the technologist's preferences. Abnormal (noncompressible) areas should be assessed further with long-axis and transverse images to determine whether the material within the vein is recently formed thrombus or chronic scar, as discussed in Chapter 23.

The superficial femoral vein can be examined with transverse compression to the level of the adductor canal, at which point it dives through the adductor muscles as it courses from the medial aspect of the thigh to the popliteal space. The adductor segment of the superficial femoral vein is too deep to be compressed effectively in most patients (Fig. 22–9), and this segment must be examined only with color-Doppler imaging.

Step 3. The Long Saphenous Vein

The long saphenous vein is also called the great or greater saphenous vein.[15] We do not routinely examine the long saphenous vein in detail when searching for lower extremity venous thrombus, but we always examine the proximal 5 cm or so, at its junction with the common femoral vein. When symptoms suggest long saphenous vein thrombosis (painful, palpable subcutaneous "cord"), this vessel should be examined in detail. A superficially focused, high-frequency (7- to 10-MHz) transducer and a very light touch are required for this examination. Too much pressure obliterates the vein lumen and renders it invisible. Note that two fascial planes are visible adjacent to the long saphenous vein (Fig. 22–10) and

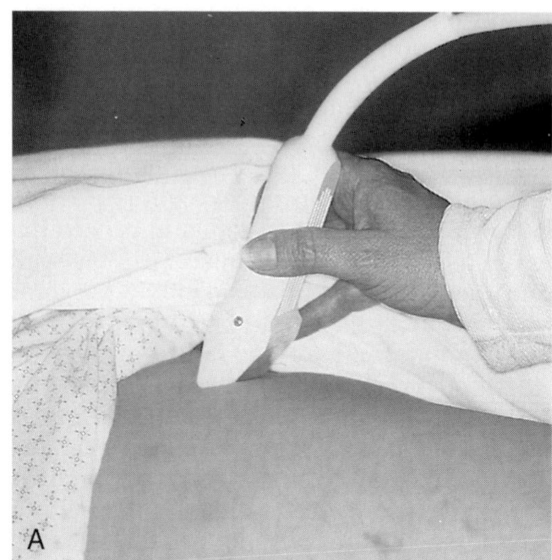

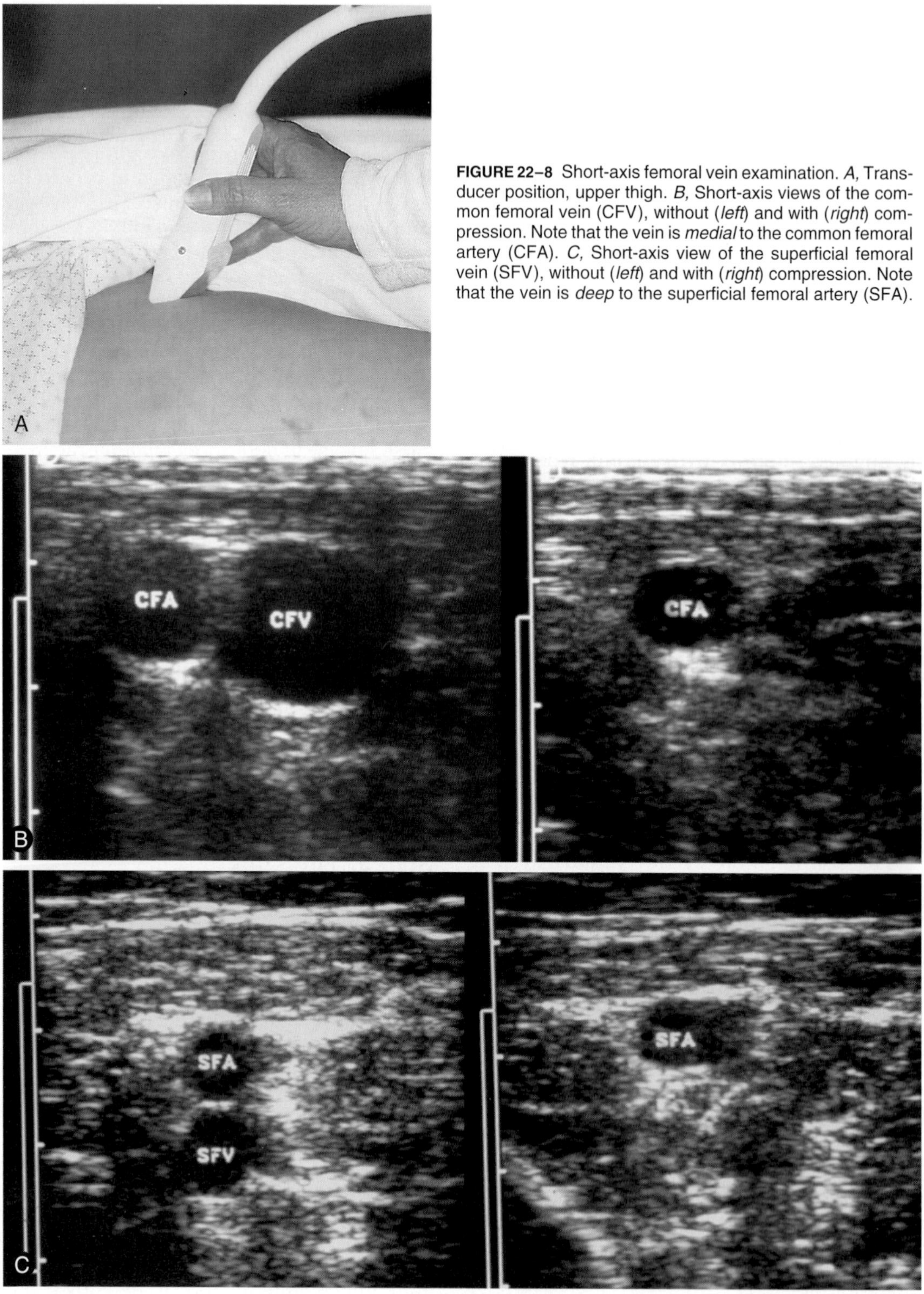

FIGURE 22–8 Short-axis femoral vein examination. *A,* Transducer position, upper thigh. *B,* Short-axis views of the common femoral vein (CFV), without (*left*) and with (*right*) compression. Note that the vein is *medial* to the common femoral artery (CFA). *C,* Short-axis view of the superficial femoral vein (SFV), without (*left*) and with (*right*) compression. Note that the vein is *deep* to the superficial femoral artery (SFA).

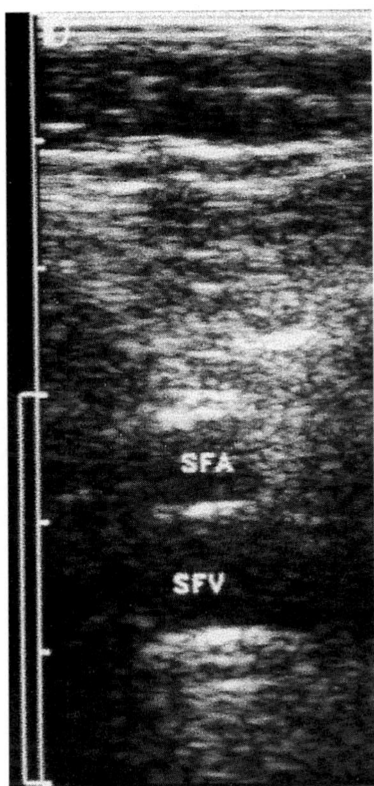

FIGURE 22–9 The adductor segment. The superficial femoral vein (SFV) is generally too deep for effective transverse compression. SFA = superficial femoral artery.

that this vein is located just outside of the muscular fascia (i.e., at the junction of the muscle and the subcutaneous fat). If the vein is just below the skin and is not invested by fascia, it probably is not the greater saphenous vein per se and probably is a subcutaneous branch or collateral. Transverse compression imaging is generally the most efficient means of saphenous vein examination.

Ultrasound is used commonly to map the course of the saphenous vein, before vein harvesting for cardiac or vascular bypass surgery. In such cases, the course of the long and sometimes short saphenous veins is traced and marked on the skin. The size of the vein is noted, as well as the presence of thrombotic scarring or other findings that might render the vein unsuitable for vascular grafting.

Step 4. The Popliteal Segment

Reposition the patient for examination of the leg, as shown in Figures 22–11 (see p 316) and 22–12. From a posteromedial transducer approach, begin the examination with long-axis views of the popliteal vein (see Fig. 22–11), and move upward into the adductor canal to examine the distal part of the superficial femoral vein. It is important to go as

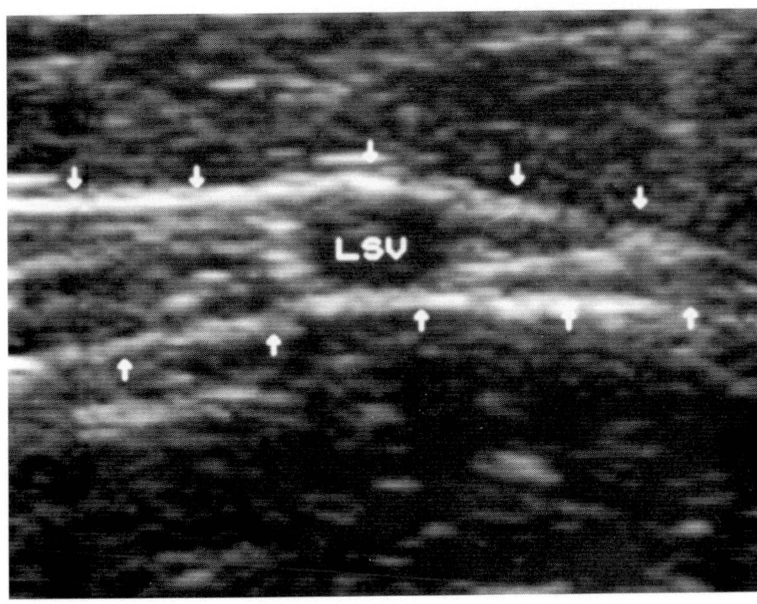

FIGURE 22–10 Short-axis view of the long saphenous vein (LSV). Note the fascial planes (*arrows*) adjacent to the vein.

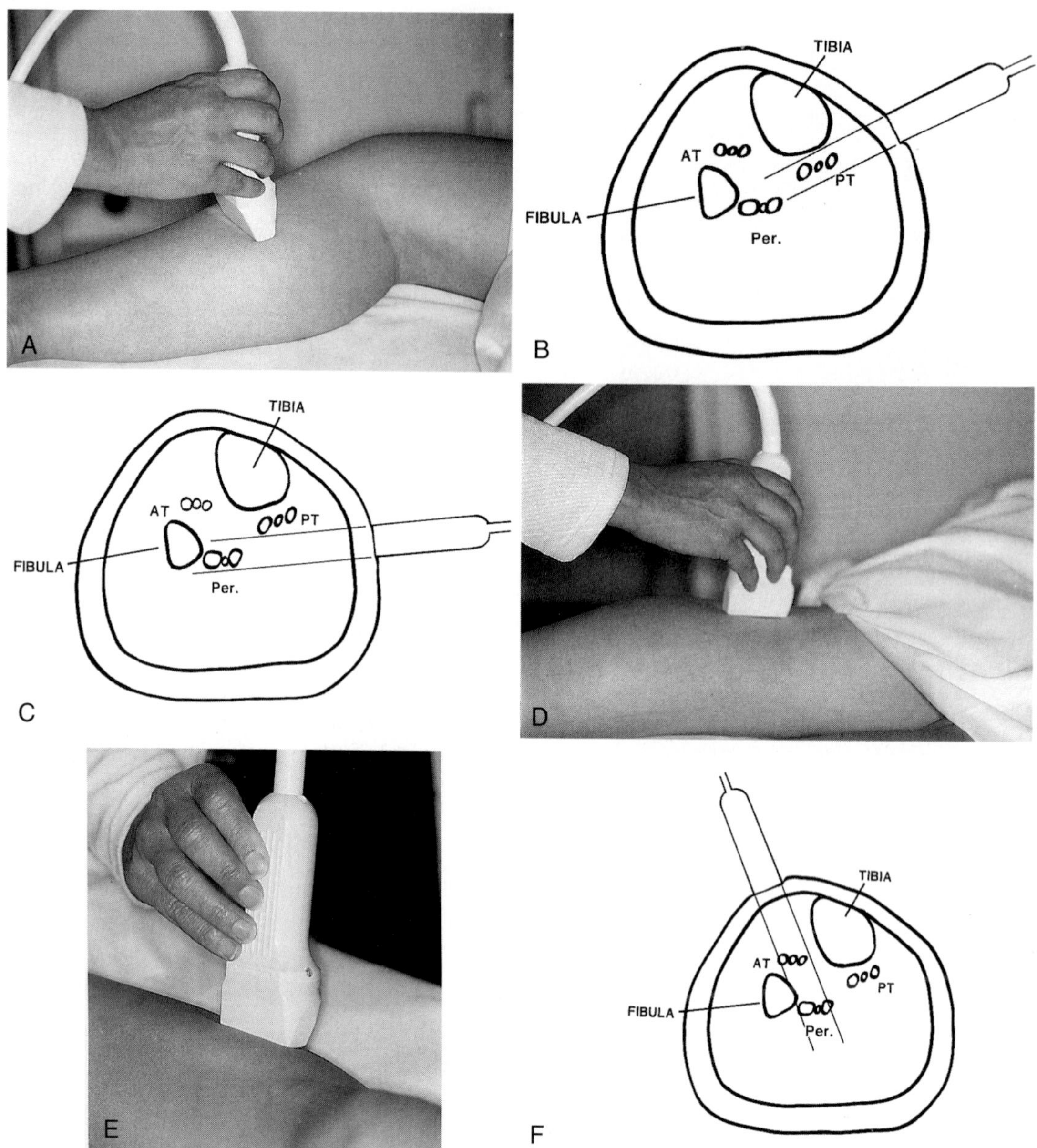

FIGURE 22–12 Calf vein transducer positions. *A,* Posteromedial position for viewing the posterior tibial and peroneal veins. *B, C,* Posterior tibial (PT) and peroneal (Per.) vein image planes. *D,* "Stocking seam" transducer approach to the peroneal veins. *E,* Anterolateral transducer position for viewing the anterior tibial veins. *F,* Anterior tibial (AT) vein image plane.

high in the adductor canal as possible to ensure that a segment of this vessel is not missed. The junction of the superficial femoral and popliteal veins is arbitrarily designated as the distal end of the adductor canal, but no sonographic landmarks identify this junction. Return to the popliteal segment, noting that the popliteal vein lies *superficial* to the popliteal artery, which is the reverse of the relationship seen in the femoral region. Continue the long-axis examination inferiorly until the popliteal vein bifurcates into the posterior tibial and peroneal trunks. This bifurcation is usually located in the inferior end of the popliteal space, but it is occasionally much higher. Next, return to the upper end of the popliteal space and test the compressibility of the popliteal vein in transverse sections (see Fig. 22–11*C*). Continue this maneuver as far distally as possible into the posterior tibial and peroneal trunks.

Step 5. The Paired Calf Veins

The transducer positions for calf vein examination are shown in Figure 22–12. There are two basic approaches to the calf veins: one may begin either at the knee or at the ankle. It is efficient to begin at the knee, as the transducer is already located here at the end of the popliteal examination. We frequently experience difficulty following the calf veins from the knee down, however, and must then go to the ankle and proceed back up to the knee.

In most instances calf vein examination is a combination of transverse compression and long-axis color-flow imaging. Because calf vein examination requires technologic creativity, it is not possible to describe a consistent examination protocol for the calf veins. The goal, however, is clear: to ensure that all three calf vein pairs (anterior tibial, posterior tibial, and peroneal) are adequately visualized.

I usually start the calf vein examination with transverse compression, which works particularly well for the paired posterior tibial and peroneal veins. The corresponding arteries are important orienting landmarks, and when the arteries are invisible (as a result of atherosclerotic occlusion), the calf vein examination is often compromised. In most cases the transverse compression examination must be supplemented with long-axis color-flow imaging, especially in the upper calf area where the paired branches unite to form common trunks. Blood flow is generally *not* spontaneous in the calf veins, and flow must be augmented by periodic manual compression of the foot or the lower portion of the calf.

The recommended approaches to the three major calf vein pairs are as follows:

POSTERIOR TIBIAL VEINS. These veins actually lie posteromedial to the tibia and are best approached from the posteromedial aspect of the leg, as shown in Figures 22–12 and 22–13) (see also p 317). As we proceed from the knee to the ankle, the posterior tibial branches gradually become more superficial. High in the calf, the paired posterior tibial veins unite to form a common trunk (which I call the posterior tibial trunk).

PERONEAL VEINS. The peroneal veins are imaged from the same transducer position as is used to visualize the posterior tibial veins (see Figs. 22–12 and 22–13). From this perspective, the peroneal veins are deep to the posterior tibial veins, but in spite of their deep location, they are well seen if the calf is not too large or edematous. The peroneal trunk must be visualized as well as the paired peroneal branches.

If the posterior tibial or peroneal veins are not well seen from a posteromedial approach, try a straight posterior approach with the patient prone, as shown in Figure 22–12*D*. In some cases, the peroneal trunk is best seen from the anterolateral approach that is used routinely to visualize the anterior tibial system (see Figs. 22–12*E* and 22–12*F*).

ANTERIOR TIBIAL VEINS. The anterior tibial veins are best visualized from an anterolateral transducer approach, with the transducer positioned between the tibia and the fibula (see Figs. 22–12 and 22–13). In many cases the paired anterior tibial veins arise directly from the popliteal vein. Alternatively, the paired veins unite and enter the popliteal vein as a common trunk. In either case, they veer off from the popliteal vein at an acute angle and then turn inferiorly after penetrating the interosseous ligament between the tibia and the fibula. The anterior tibial branches are small, and isolated thrombosis of this system is relatively uncommon[13]; nonetheless, routine examination of the anterior tibial vein is suggested. In most instances, these veins are easily visualized, and their assessment requires little examination time.

Step 6. The Gastrocnemius and Soleal Veins

In our department, we do not attempt to visualize the gastrocnemius and soleal veins routinely, but sonographers should be aware of the location of these veins to identify thrombus within these muscular branches. In some cases we have identified *isolated* muscular vein thrombus, but in most such instances the patient has been symptomatic

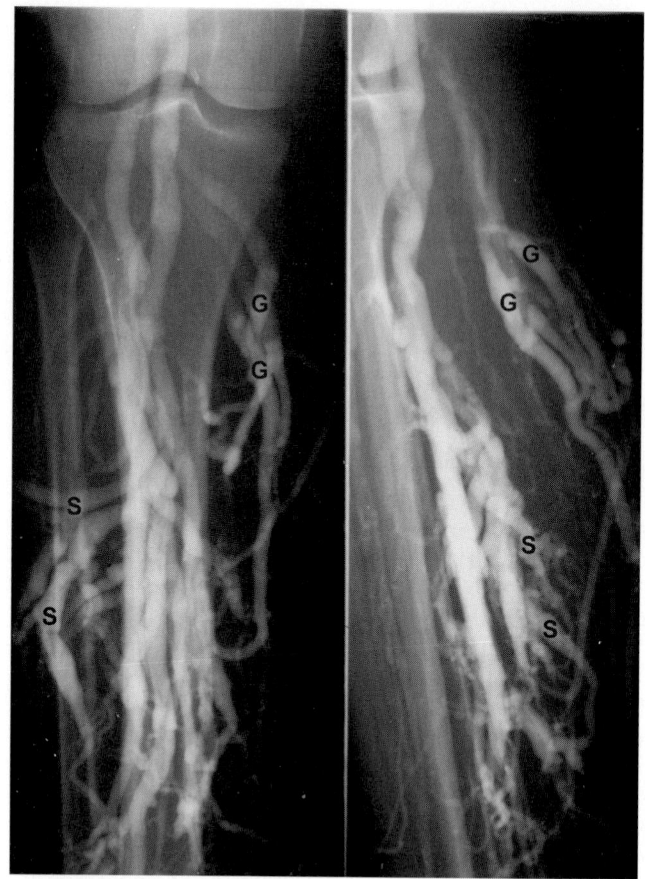

FIGURE 22–14 The gastrocnemius (G) and soleal (S) veins are shown on anteroposterior (*left*) and lateral (*right*) venograms.

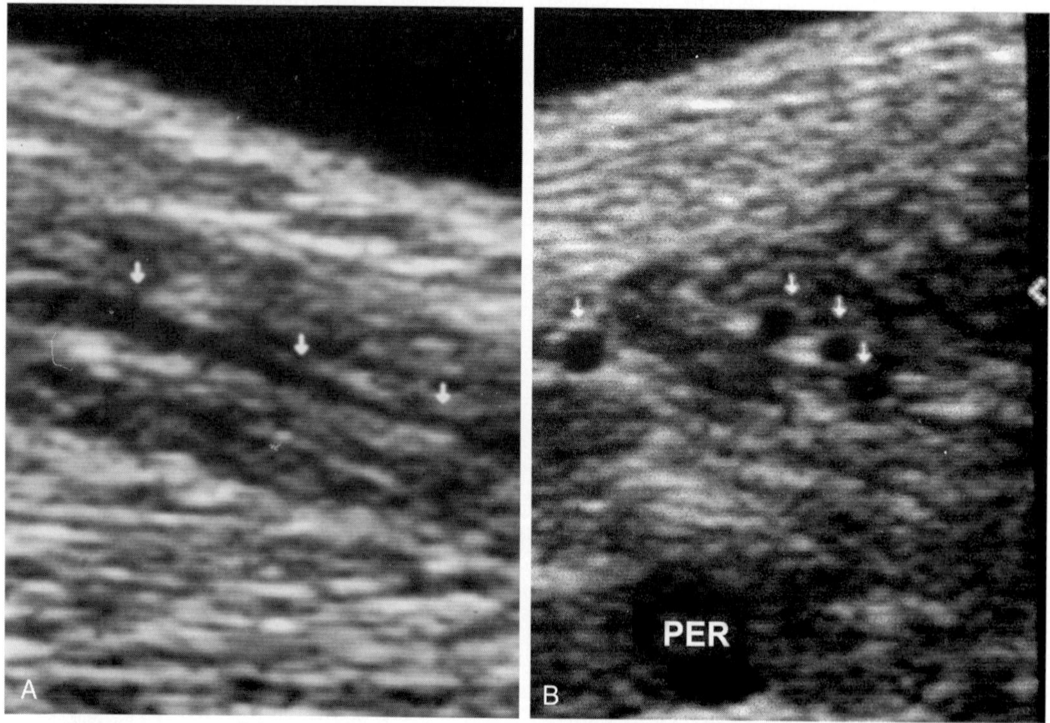

FIGURE 22–15 Soleal veins (*arrows*), as seen in long-axis (*A*) and short-axis (*B*) images. PER = peroneal vein.

and localized pain or tenderness has directed us to the thrombosed muscular vein.

The *gastrocnemius veins* are branches of the popliteal vein located in the medial head of the gastrocnemius muscle (Fig. 22–14). These veins project posteriorly and then inferiorly, beginning at the lower end of the popliteal fossa. The gastrocnemius veins are differentiated from the short (lesser or small) saphenous vein by location. The short saphenous vein is superficially located, lying between the muscular fascia and the skin. It extends down the back of the calf, in the midline, like the seam on a stocking. In contrast, the gastrocnemius veins are medially oriented and are embedded *within* the medial head of the gastrocnemius muscle. Usually, one large gastrocnemius vein is identified, but two or more veins may be present. The lateral head of the gastrocnemius muscle also contains veins, but these are usually small and are not visualized with ultrasound.

The *soleal veins* (see Fig. 22–14), which are embedded in the soleus muscle, are less easily recognizable with ultrasound than the gastrocnemius veins. Two or more soleal veins may be present (Fig. 22–15). As opposed to the gastrocnemius veins, these tend to be laterally oriented and lower in the calf. In our experience, soleal veins are only rarely

TABLE 22–2 PROTOCOL FOR LOWER EXTREMITY VENOUS EXAMINATION

Step	
Step 1.	The Iliac Segment
	Identify the external iliac vein at the groin, and follow it cephalad with long-axis images. Locate the iliac bifurcation or its approximate position. Follow the common iliac vein cephalad to the inferior vena cava. If you lose track of the vein, start at the inferior vena cava and follow the iliac vein inferiorly.
Step 2.	The Femoral Segment
	Use long-axis images to identify the external iliac vein at the groin, and follow it distally into the common femoral vein. Note the entrance of the long saphenous vein. Check Doppler characteristics at the common femoral level. Identify the deep femoral vein and confirm its patency.
	Return to the groin and check vein compressibility with transverse images from the femoral level to the adductor canal. Watch for superficial femoral vein duplication.
Step 3.	The Long Saphenous Vein
	Confirm that the proximal portion of the long saphenous vein is patent with images parallel to vein.
	Examine as much of the vein as is clinically indicated, using transverse compression.
Step 4.	The Popliteal Segment
	By imaging parallel to the vein, locate the distal portion of the superficial femoral vein as high as possible in the adductor canal. Follow the superficial femoral vein distal into the popliteal segment, to the junction of the tibial trunks.
	Confirm the compressibility of the popliteal vein and the tibial trunks in transverse section.
	Watch for popliteal vein duplication.
Step 5.	The Calf Veins
	Examine the posterior tibial veins and trunk in their entirety, starting either at the popliteal space or at the ankle. Use transverse compression as the primary mode and supplement with images parallel to veins.
	Examine the peroneal veins similarly.
	Examine the anterior tibial veins with long-axis images.
	Examine the gastrocnemius and soleal veins as clinically indicated, using images parallel or transverse to veins.

identified and are usually seen when they are painful, tender, and distended with thrombus.

Protocol Summary

The examination protocol for the lower extremity venous system is summarized in Table 22–2.

REFERENCES

1. Talbot SR: B-mode evaluation of peripheral veins. Semin Ultrasound CT MR 9:295–319, 1988.
2. Lensing AWA, Prandoni P, Brandjes D, et al: Detection of deep-vein thrombosis by real-time B-mode ultrasonography. N Engl J Med 320:341–345, 1989.
3. Effeney DJ, Friedman MB, Gooding GAW: Iliofemoral venous thrombosis: Real-time ultrasound diagnosis, normal criteria, and clinical application. Radiology 150:787–792, 1984.
4. Barnes RW: Doppler techniques for lower-extremity venous disease. *In* Zwiebel WJ (ed): Introduction to Vascular Ultrasonography. Philadelphia, Grune & Stratton, 1986, pp 333–350.
5. Sullivan ED, Peters BS, Cranley JJ: Real-time B-mode venous ultrasound. J Vasc Surg 1:465–471, 1984.
6. Oliver MA: Duplex scanning in venous disease. Bruit 9:206–209, 1985.
7. Raghavendra BN, Horii SC, Hilton S, et al: Deep venous thrombosis: Detection by probe compression of veins. J Ultrasound Med 5:89–95, 1986.
8. Dauzat MM, Laroche JP, Charras C, et al: Real-time B-mode ultrasonography for better specialty in the noninvasive diagnosis of deep venous thrombosis. J Ultrasound Med 5:625–631, 1986.
9. Cronan JJ, Dorfman GS, Scola FH, et al: Deep venous thrombosis: US assessment using vein compression. Radiology 162:191–194, 1987.
10. Vogel P, Laing FRC, Jeffrey RB, et al: Deep venous thrombosis of the lower extremity: US evaluation. Radiology 163:747–751, 1987.
11. Appelman PT, De Jong TE, Lampmann LE: Deep venous thrombosis of the leg: US findings. Radiology 163:743–746, 1987.
12. Rose SC, Zwiebel WJ, Nelson BD, et al: Symptomatic lower extremity deep venous thrombosis: Accuracy, limitations, and role of color-duplex flow imaging in diagnosis. Radiology 175:639–644, 1990.
13. Rose SC, Zwiebel WJ, Miller FJ: Distribution of acute lower extremity deep venous thrombosis in symptomatic and asymptomatic patients: Imaging implications. J Ultrasound Med 13:243–250, 1994.
14. Zwiebel WJ, Priest DL: Color Duplex sonography of extremity veins. Semin Ultrasound CT MR 11:136–167, 1990.
15. Hatch W, Hatch-Wunderle V (eds): Phlebography and Sonography of the Veins. Berlin, Springer-Verlag, 1997, pp 6–16.

Chapter 23

VENOUS THROMBOSIS

■ *William J. Zwiebel, MD*

The primary focus of this chapter is ultrasound detection and assessment of venous thrombosis, which is the principal pathology that affects the venous system. Also included is a discussion of arteriovenous fistula, which is a less common but important condition.

VENOUS THROMBOSIS

Ultrasonography is currently the principal imaging technique used for detecting venous thrombosis. Thrombus within the venous system is hypoechoic during the first few days after its formation, but with time the thrombus becomes more echogenic, and additional changes occur that permit the age of the thrombus to be approximated in most patients. The detection of thrombus and the assessment of its age require familiarity with the ultrasound findings described in the following sections on acute, subacute, and chronic thrombosis.

Acute Thrombosis

As noted in Chapter 21, the term *acute thrombosis* must be used with great caution, because the time-frame implied by the term *acute* is ambiguous. As used herein, acute refers to a thrombus that is days to perhaps 1 or 2 weeks old. Thrombus in this age range is identified by the following ultrasound findings.[1–9]

LOW ECHOGENICITY. Recently formed thrombus generates only low-level echoes and may be virtually anechoic (Fig. 23–1*A*). Because of its low echogenicity, small and nonocclusive thrombi may be difficult to visualize. The presence of such thrombi is indicated, however, by a flow void on color-Doppler images and a lack of vein compressibility (discussed later). As thrombus ages during the course of several days or weeks, echogenicity increases, but the intensity of the echoes generally remains less than that of the surrounding muscle. Blood flow persists in veins that are incompletely filled with acute thrombus, and even when the vein lumen is filled, blood flow may be demonstrated in tiny residual channels adjacent to the vein wall or within the thrombus (see Fig. 23–1*B*).

VENOUS DISTENTION. The recently thrombosed vein is generally distended to an abnormally large size (see Fig. 23–1). The exception to this rule occurs if the thrombus is small and nonocclusive. Venous distention is a significant finding, because it helps to differentiate between recently formed thrombus and older thrombus (months to years). In the latter case, either the vein size is similar to the adjacent artery or the vein is small.

LOSS OF COMPRESSIBILITY. When thrombus of any age is present, the vein lumen cannot be obliterated with compression. Lack of compressibility of the vein (Fig. 23–2 [see p 332]) is perhaps the single most reliable finding for differentiating between thrombosed and normal veins. Excellent results for diagnosing venous thrombosis have been reported on the basis of this diagnostic criterion alone.[5–7] Thrombus can only be *excluded,* however, when compression causes the vein to disappear *completely.* If the vein does not collapse completely, the lumen may be partially filled with thrombus. Resistance from surrounding musculoskeletal structures may prevent adequate compression of the vein and may result in false-positive diagnoses. To judge if compression is adequate, look at the adjacent artery. If pressure is sufficient to deform the artery substantially, the vein should collapse. When doubt remains, attempt compression from another transducer position and check for a flow void within the vein using color-Doppler imaging.

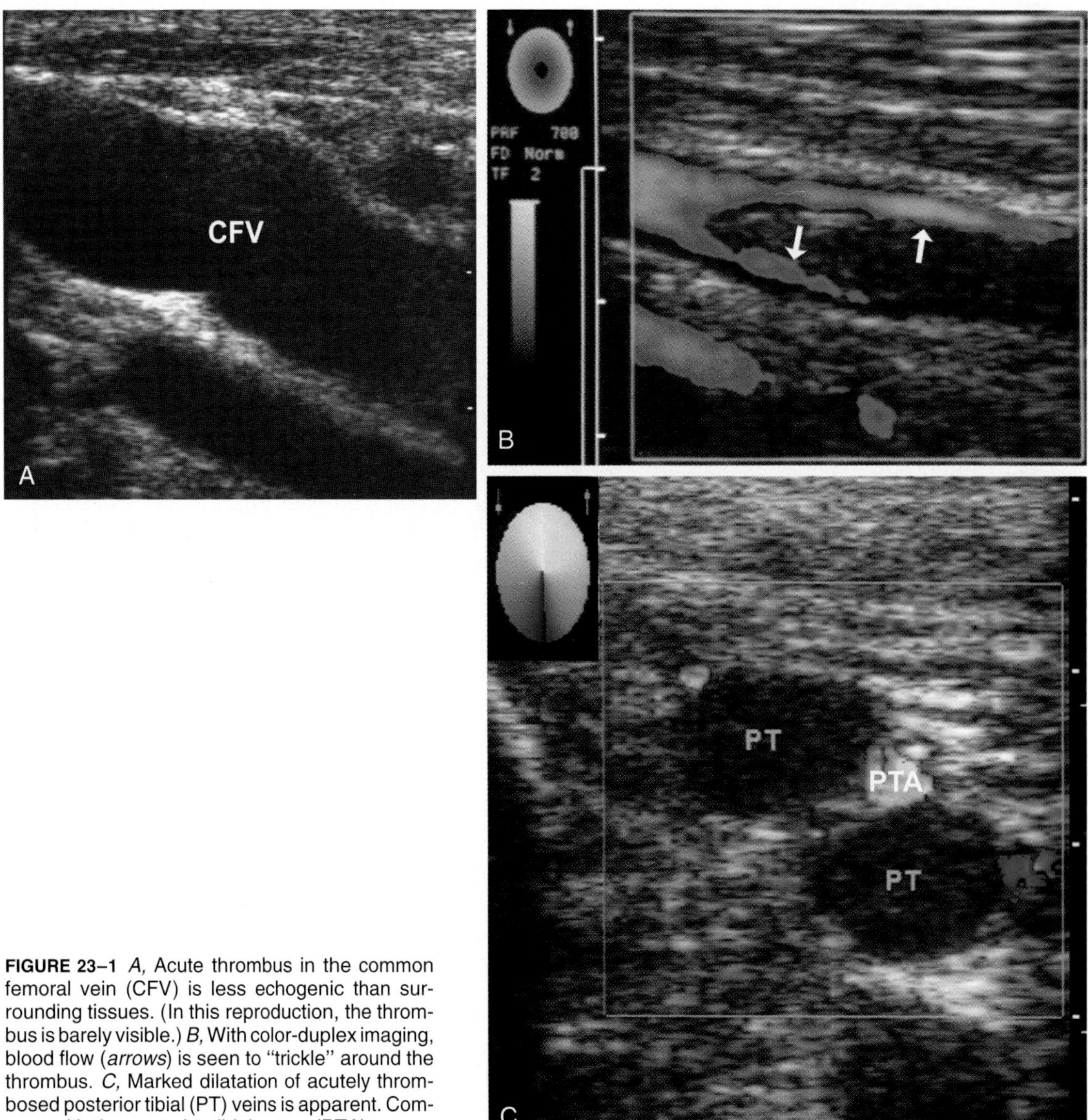

FIGURE 23–1 *A,* Acute thrombus in the common femoral vein (CFV) is less echogenic than surrounding tissues. (In this reproduction, the thrombus is barely visible.) *B,* With color-duplex imaging, blood flow (*arrows*) is seen to "trickle" around the thrombus. *C,* Marked dilatation of acutely thrombosed posterior tibial (PT) veins is apparent. Compare with the posterior tibial artery (PTA).

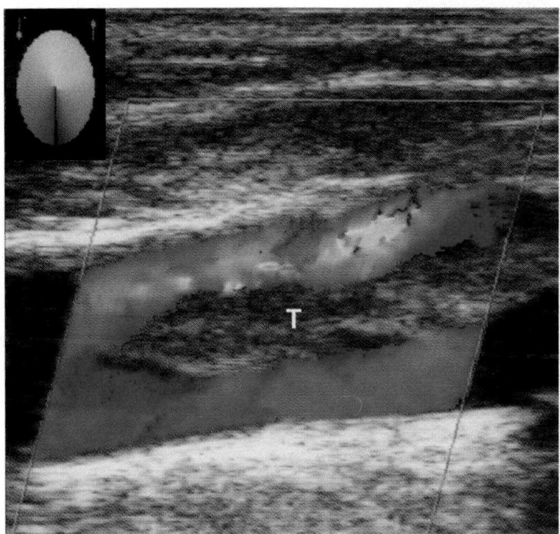

FIGURE 23–3 Free-floating thrombus. (See p 332.) Flowing blood surrounds free-floating thrombus (T) within the common femoral vein.

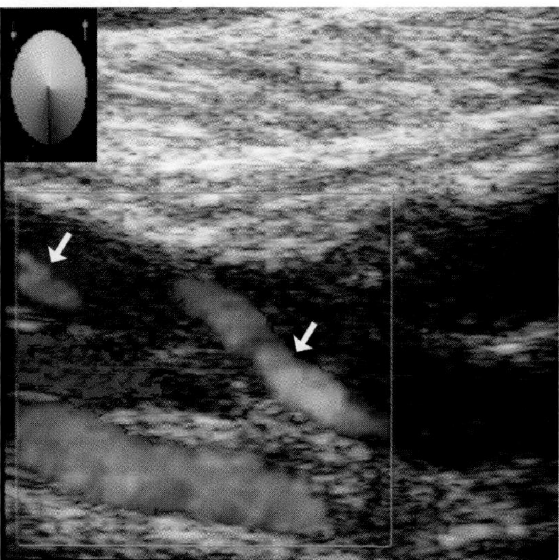

FIGURE 23–5 Recanalization. (See p 334.) Restoration of flow (*arrows*) is apparent in this 1-week-old thrombus.

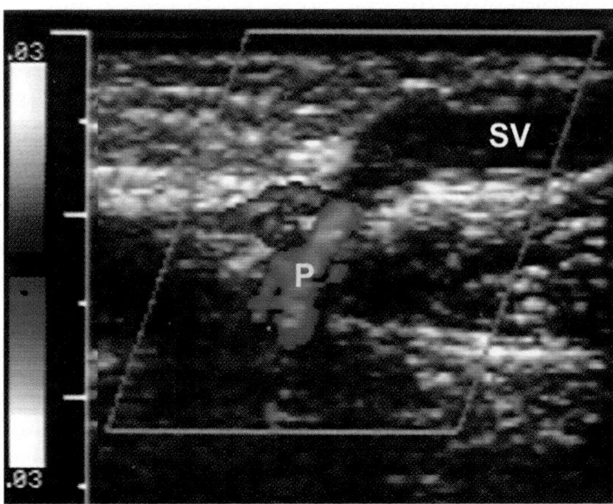

FIGURE 23–9 An acutely thrombosed superficial vein (SV) is visible just below the skin. (See p 335.) This vein communicates with a patent perforator vein (P).

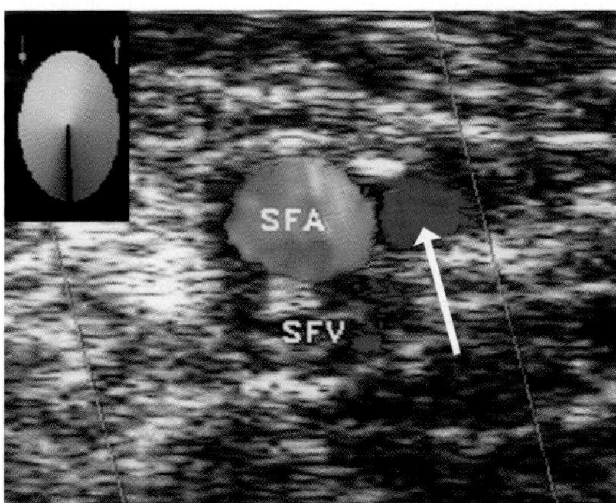

FIGURE 23–10 Duplicated superficial femoral vein. (See p 337.) The main portion of the superficial femoral vein (SFV) is occluded by 2-month-old thrombus, but the vein is duplicated and the other branch (*arrow*) is patent. SFA = superficial femoral artery.

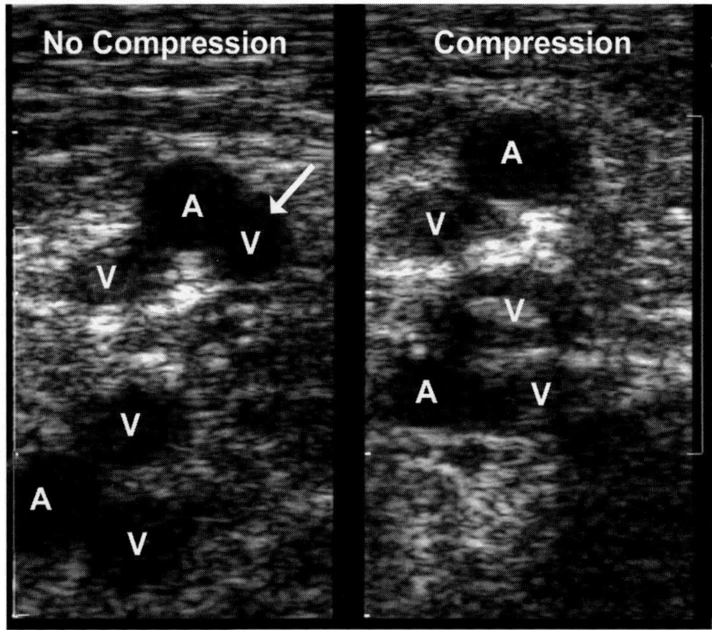

FIGURE 23–2 Lack of compressibility. (See p 329.) Four veins (V) are visible in this illustration, but only one collateral vein (*arrow*) responds to compression. The others are filled with thrombus of approximately 1 week of age. A = artery.

FREE-FLOATING THROMBUS. The proximal end of an acute thrombus may not adhere well to the vein wall, and in such cases, the thrombus is said to float freely within the lumen. The ultrasound image of free-floating thrombus (Fig. 23–3 [see p 331]) is dramatic and frightening, for it vividly depicts the potential for embolization to the pulmonary circulation. Whenever acute thrombus is identified sonographically, particularly when the thrombus is free floating, care must be taken not to dislodge the thrombus by unnecessary manipulation. The extent of thrombosis should be evaluated with as little manipulation as possible. Thereafter, the patient should remain recumbent and quiet. Dislodgement of thrombus during ultrasound examination has been reported,[10] resulting in pulmonary embolization, but this appears to occur rarely.

DOPPLER SIGNAL ABNORMALITY. When thrombus of any age substantially occludes the vein lumen, flow augmentation is diminished or absent in veins *proximal* to the thrombosed segment. Flow is continuous (see Chapter 21) rather than phasic and is *distal* to a thrombosed segment. In addition, the Valsalva response is diminished or absent.[11] These flow abnormalities only occur, however, when the vein lumen is substantially blocked by thrombus. Localized, partially occlusive thrombus may not affect flow signals. Flow signals may also be normal, or nearly so, if large collateral veins circumvent the region of obstruction.

COLLATERALIZATION. Collateral venous channels enlarge rapidly during the acute phase of venous thrombosis and these channels are often visible during ultrasound examination. The collateral may be located either adjacent to the thrombosed vein or more distant, as other veins take over for the occluded vein.

Subacute Thrombosis

By *subacute* we mean that thrombus is weeks to 1 or 2 months old. The transition from recently formed (acute) to subacute thrombus occurs gradually, and all of the so-

FIGURE 23–4 Changes in thrombus with time (long- and short-axis views). *A,* A 1-month-old thrombus within the popliteal vein (PV, *arrows*) is moderately echogenic, and the vein is substantially larger than the popliteal artery (PA). *B,* At 4 months, thrombus echogenicity is unchanged, but the size of the popliteal vein (PV, *arrows*) has decreased (about equal to the popliteal artery [PA]). *C,* At 11 months, substantial recanalization (*outlined areas*) is evident in the popliteal vein (PV, *arrows*). PA = popliteal artery. *D,* At 18 months, an echogenic area of scar (*arrows*) is all that remains at the site of popliteal vein thrombosis.

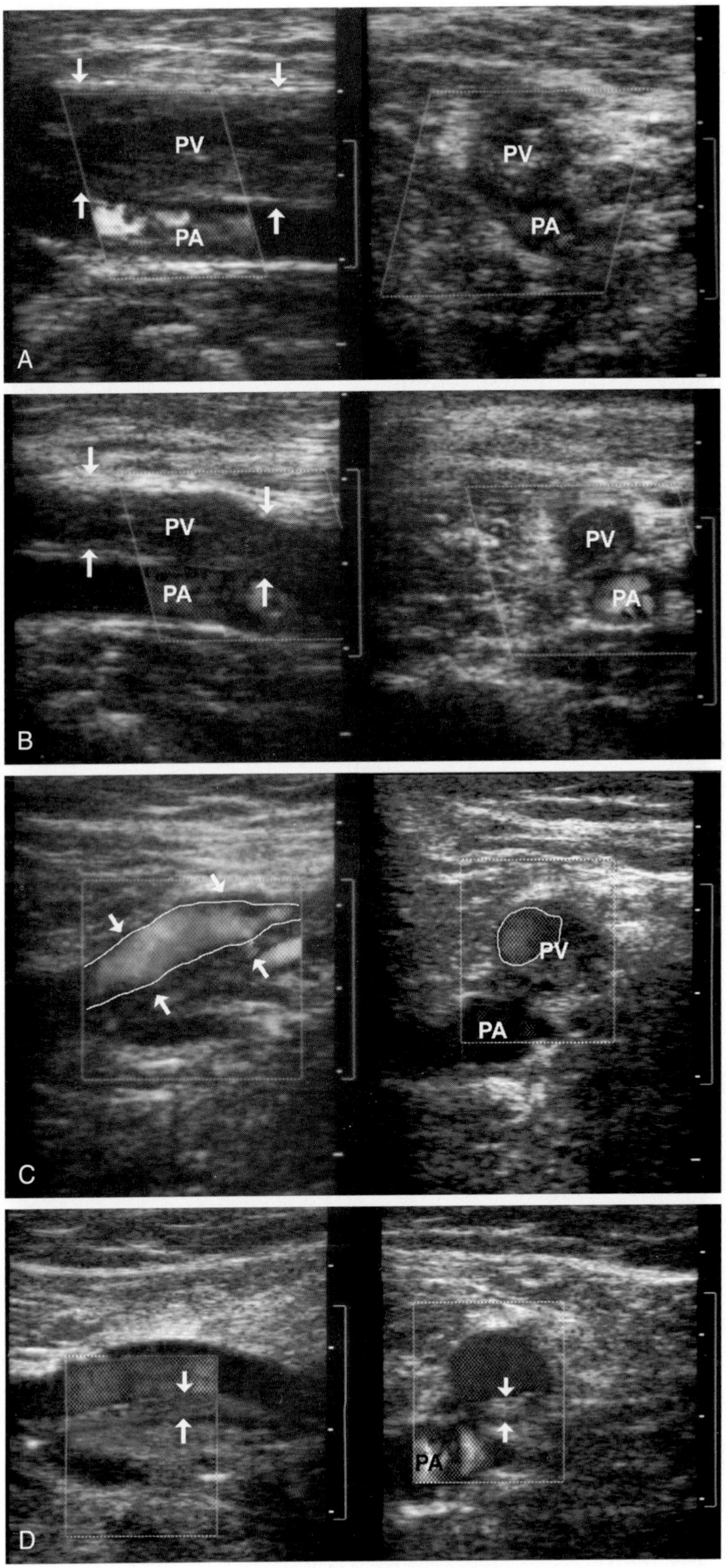

See legend on opposite page

nographic abnormalities referable to recent thrombosis persist to some extent into the subacute phase. As the thrombus ages, retracts, or lyses, however, the following changes may be seen.[1–8]

Increased Echogenicity. The thrombus gradually becomes more echogenic (Fig. 23–4). Unfortunately, it is not possible to determine the age of thrombus precisely by means of echogenicity. In my experience, thrombus that is several days old may sometimes be similar in echogenicity to thrombus that is several weeks old.

Decreased Thrombus Size. Retraction and lysis may noticeably reduce the size of thrombus, as seen on serial examinations. This may be evident on short-axis views that show a decrease in vein diameter and in long-axis views that show a decrease in the linear extent of thrombus. As venous patency is reestablished by lysis and retraction, thrombus occupies less and less of the vein lumen.

Reduced Vein Size. With retraction and lysis of thrombus, the vein becomes less distended and returns to a normal caliber. If the vein does not recanalize, it may shrink to a subnormal size as the thrombus retracts and becomes a scar.

Adherence of Thrombus. Free-floating acute thrombus becomes attached to the vein wall during the subacute period.

Resumption of Flow. With retraction and lysis of thrombus, blood flow obstruction generally diminishes, as revealed by reappearance of flow on color-Doppler examination (Fig. 23–5 [see p 331]). Not all thrombosed veins recanalize, however. Some remain permanently occluded, as discussed in the following section.

Collateralization. Collateral venous channels (Fig. 23–6) form in the acute phase of thrombosis and remain visible during the subacute phase. Such channels are commonly seen with ultrasonography.

Chronic Thrombotic Scarring

As noted in Chapter 21, the term chronic thrombosis is a misnomer and the proper term is *chronic thrombotic scarring.* I define the chronic phase of venous thrombosis as months to years after the acute episode. During this phase, thrombus that is not lysed by natural or therapeutic means is invaded by fibroblasts and becomes organized as fibrous

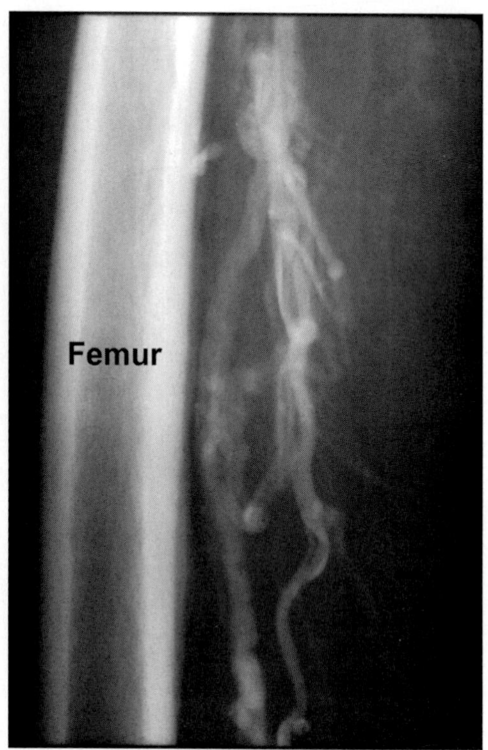

FIGURE 23–6 Collateralization. An extensive network of venous collaterals is shown on this contrast venogram. The superficial femoral vein is occluded.

tissue that persists indefinitely. Complete lysis of venous thrombus occurs in only about 20% of cases.[12] It is not surprising, therefore, that persistent abnormality is observed sonographically in many patients who have suffered venous thrombosis.[13] The following abnormalities may be seen in the chronic phase.[1, 4, 8, 13–15]

Echogenic Intraluminal Material. The organized residua of venous thrombus is moderately to markedly echogenic. The overall level of echogenicity is greater than that of adjacent muscle. This fibrous material persists as focal plaque-like thickening of the vein wall, diffuse linear thickening of the vein wall, or web-like synechiae projecting into the vein lumen (Fig. 23–7). If the vein lumen does not recanalize but instead remains occluded, the vein may be reduced to an echogenic cord with a much smaller diameter than a normal vein. In some cases, the scarred vein may disappear from sonographic view.

Valve Abnormality. Thrombus is thought to originate most commonly in the vicinity of valves. Considering this location and the fact that incomplete lysis and subsequent fi-

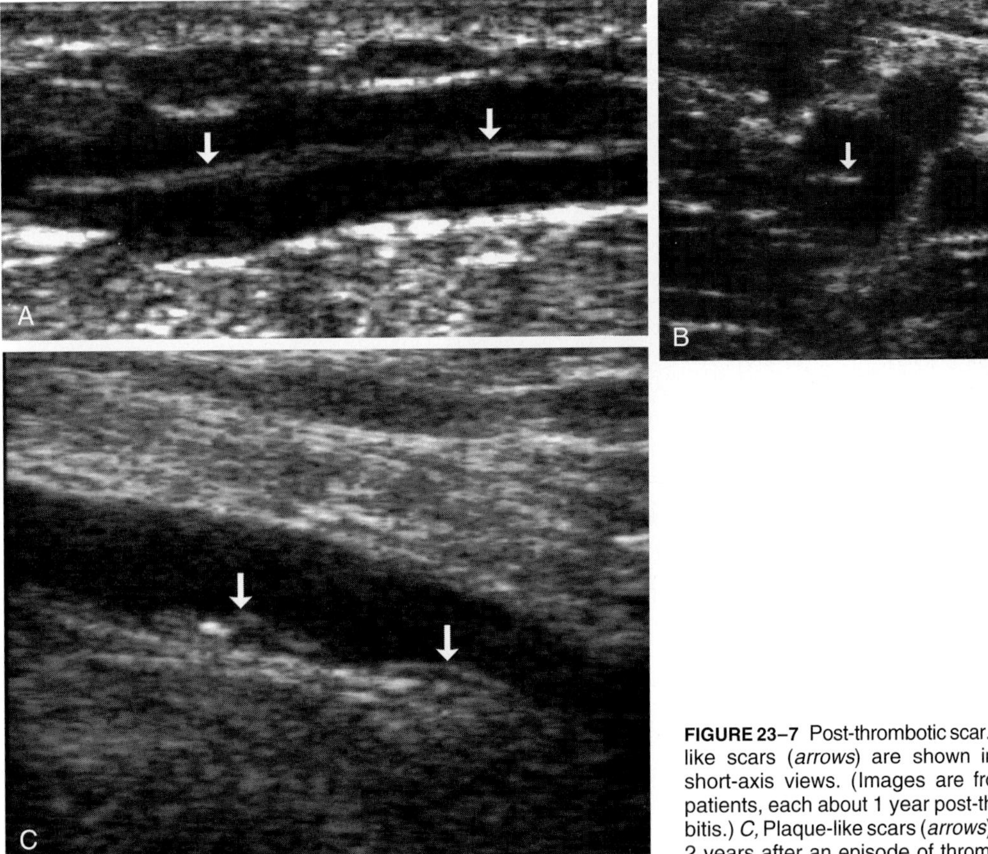

FIGURE 23–7 Post-thrombotic scar. (*A, B*) Web-like scars (*arrows*) are shown in long- and short-axis views. (Images are from different patients, each about 1 year post-thrombophlebitis.) *C,* Plaque-like scars (*arrows*) are present 2 years after an episode of thrombophlebitis.

brosis are the rule, it is not surprising that valve damage is a frequent sequela of venous thrombosis. Valve damage is manifested by thickening of the cusps, adherence of the cusps to the vein wall, restricted cusp motion (Fig. 23–8), and failure of apposition of the cusps in the center of the vessel. The physiologic consequences of valve damage are reflux and persistent venous distention that results from reflux-induced back pressure. Valvular reflux is evident on the color-Doppler image, in the audible Doppler signal, and on the Doppler spectrum display. Reflux may result in varicosities, which are abnormally large and tortuous veins, chronic edema, skin changes, and ulceration. These subjects and ultrasound assessment of venous insufficiency are covered in detail in Chapter 24.

DOPPLER FLOW ABNORMALITIES. In addition to venous reflux, other Doppler flow abnormalities may be encountered with chronic venous thrombosis because of venous obstruction. These are lack of spontaneous flow, lack of phasicity, absence of the Valsalva response, and subnormal or absent augmentation.[11]

Superficial vs. Deep Venous Thrombosis

It is important to differentiate between superficial and deep venous thrombosis (DVT). With superficial thrombosis, a palpable cord may be readily apparent in the subcutaneous tissues. On ultrasound examination, this cord reveals typical findings of venous thrombosis (Fig. 23–9 [see p 331]). In the upper extremities, both the superficial and deep venous systems have a significant role in venous drainage, and both can contribute to venous stasis problems. In the lower extremity, however, the superficial venous system is less important than the deep venous system as a conduit for venous drainage. Therefore, only supportive therapy is generally necessary when thrombus is confined to the superficial veins of the lower extremity. Venous stasis prob-

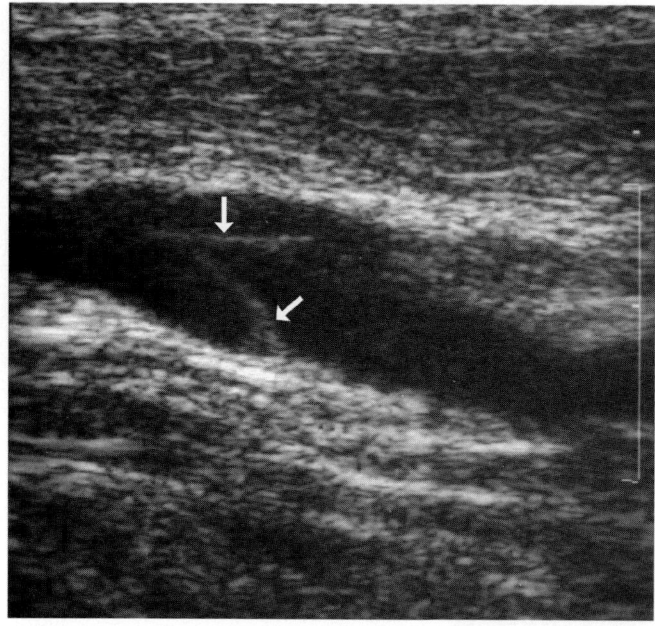

FIGURE 23–8 Immobile, or stuck, valve cusps (*arrows*) are embedded in recently formed thrombus, which is barely visible on this reproduction.

lems and varicocities can result, however, from isolated superficial vein thrombosis.

Pulmonary embolism does not generally result from superficial vein thrombosis, but thrombus located in the proximal portion of the long saphenous vein may readily extend into the common femoral vein (see Fig. 23–3), posing a risk for embolization. Careful assessment of the proximal extent of long saphenous vein thrombus is advisable, therefore.

PITFALLS IN THE DIAGNOSIS OF DEEP VENOUS THROMBOSIS

This section represents a catalog of mistakes or near-mistakes that we have made in the course of ultrasound venography. These pitfalls are grouped in several broad categories.

Suboptimal Image Quality

When the quality of the color-Doppler image is suboptimal, diagnostic error is to be expected. Many of the factors that affect image quality are beyond the sonographer's control, such as obesity and soft-tissue edema, but many factors can be controlled by the sonographer. These include the use of transducers with proper frequency and focal characteristics, the attention to gain settings and color-Doppler adjustments, and the attainment of image planes that clearly delineate the vein wall. When image quality is suboptimal, it may be possible to confirm venous patency grossly, but small and nonocclusive thrombi cannot be excluded.

Compression Difficulties

The iliac veins cannot be compressed effectively in most individuals because of resistance from overlying abdominal contents. The adductor segment of the common femoral vein and in many patients the proximal calf veins are also difficult to compress because of resistance from overlying muscle. In addition, compression may be limited in some patients by voluntary or involuntary muscle contraction. Compression difficulties can lead to a false-positive diagnosis of venous thrombosis. It is useful, therefore, to carefully assess areas in which compression is difficult with color-Doppler imaging.

Mistaken Identity

Serious errors may occur if veins are misidentified. We have seen the long saphenous vein mistaken for the superficial femoral vein, the cephalic vein mistaken for the axillary vein, the basilic vein mistaken for the brachial vein, and numerous cases of mistaken vein identity in the calf. Misidentification of veins usually occurs in the presence of venous occlusion, when a large collateral is mistaken for an occluded vein. To prevent errors of identity, *always locate* and *document major anatomic landmarks* that confirm the identity of veins. These landmarks have been described in preceding chapters.

Duplication

Unrecognized venous duplication may be a source of diagnostic error if the patent half of the duplicated system is identified and the occluded half is not. Venous duplication (Fig. 23–10 [see p 331]) should be suspected when the visualized vein is smaller than normal or the location of the vein is atypical.

Assessment of Thrombus Age

Thrombus that is extremely fresh (1 or 2 days old) is easily recognized as acute on duplex examination, because it is quite poorly echogenic. The age of a thrombotic scar that is years old is also readily recognizable because it is strongly echogenic. Between these extremes, the age of thrombus cannot be determined with certainty. A practical approach to this problem is to always ask: "Does the appearance of thrombus match the duration of the patient's symptoms?" The findings should then be reported along similar lines, for example, "Moderately echogenic thrombus is present, consistent with a 2-week history of leg swelling." Even though the age of thrombus cannot be determined precisely with ultrasonography, it is often possible to say whether its appearance is appropriate for the duration of symptoms.

Recurrent Deep Venous Thrombosis

The residua of preceding episodes of DVT poses a significant limitation for duplex examination because of the following: (1) distortion of venous anatomy; (2) development of extensive, serpiginous collaterals; and (3) residual vein wall thickening that may be difficult to differentiate from acute thrombosis. In a follow-up study of patients with DVT, Cronan and Leen[13] found persistent thrombus or wall thickening in 53% of extremities examined 6 months to 31 months after the acute thrombotic episode. Furthermore, in many of these cases it would not have been possible to differentiate between chronic abnormalities and those associated with more recent thrombosis.

In a patient with prior venous thrombosis, one of the most useful indications of new recurrence is the presence of thrombus in portions of the venous system that were previously unaffected. This finding can only be recognized if a good "road map" exists of the preceding episode of thrombosis, as illustrated in Figure 23–11. It is important for the technologist to accurately depict the location of thrombus on this road map. Of particular value is a post-treatment road map obtained at about 3 to 6 months after an episode of DVT. This post-therapy baseline shows what veins are or are not patent, and where residual thrombus is located. This information is quite valuable if the patient presents with recurrent symptoms that suggest a new episode of venous thrombosis.

We do not have a post-therapy baseline in many patients who present with recurrent DVT because they were treated previously in other institutions. Even when we have a baseline, we sometimes cannot differentiate between old and new thrombus. In such cases, we are forced to resort to contrast venography, which also may be of limited diagnostic value in patients with recurrent DVT. Magnetic resonance venography may prove to be valuable, but I believe that recurrent thrombosis is likely to remain a significant diagnostic problem.

Improper Use of the Color-Doppler Image

Color-Doppler scanning is a valuable asset to venous imaging, but it may be a source of misdiagnosis if it is used improperly. If the sensitivity or gain levels of the Doppler image are set too high, color "blooming" occurs, causing the flow information to bleed into the B-mode image. Small or even moderate-sized thrombi may be obscured by blooming. Conversely, false-positive diagnosis of thrombus may occur if spurious flow voids

Department of Veterans Affairs

Vascular Laboratory
VA Medical Center
Salt Lake City, Utah

Lower Extremity Venous Ultrasound

PATIENT IDENTIFICATION

Date: 3-23-96 Technologist: JM Tape # ______ Requested By: Bennett

Prior Exam: None Prior Treatment: ______

History: 3 Days Swelling LT Lower Extremity

EI EI
CF CF
SF SF
Gr. Saph
POP POP
AT AT
PER PT PT PER

	CIV R	CIV L	EIV R	EIV L	CFV R	CFV L	SFV R	SFV L	PFV R	PFV L	PV R	PV L	PT R	PT L	PER R	PER L	AT R	AT L	SAPH R	SAPH L
Normal		✓				✓														✓
Recent Thromb								✓		✓		✓		✓		✓				
Indeterm Thromb																				
Remote Thromb																				
Extension																				
Occluded																				
Recanalized																				
Phasic																				
Reflux																				
Non Diagnostic																				

Technologist Comments/Preliminary Report:

Hypoechoic, Veins Distended

A

4-Part – White: Radiology - Pink: Preliminary Copy - Yellow: Medical Records - Goldenrod: MD

VA Form 10-44/G (114/660)
August 1994

FIGURE 23–11 Thrombosis "road maps." Diagrams showing the extent of thrombus are made routinely in our department. In this hypothetical example, *A* shows the initial extent of thrombus, and *B* shows the extent of poststenotic scarring at the end of anticoagulant therapy.

Department of Veterans Affairs

Vascular Laboratory
VA Medical Center
Salt Lake City, Utah

Lower Extremity Venous Ultrasound

PATIENT IDENTIFICATION

Date: 6-20-96 Technologist: JM Tape # ______ Requested By: Bennett

Prior Exam: 3-23-96 Prior Treatment: ____________

History: Follow-up post therapy

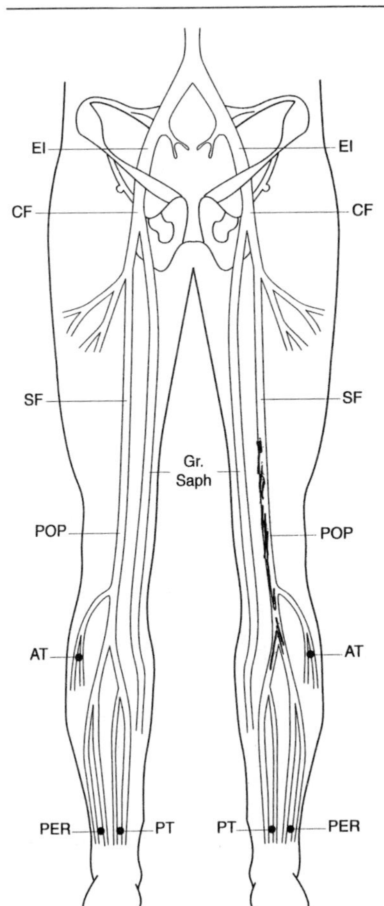

	CIV		EIV		CFV		SFV		PFV		PV		PT		PER		AT		SAPH	
	R	L	R	L	R	L	R	L	R	L	R	L	R	L	R	L	R	L	R	L
Normal		✓		✓		✓				✓						✓		✓		✓
Recent Thromb																				
Indeterm Thromb																				
Remote Thromb																				
Extension																				
Occluded																				
Recanalized								✓				✓		✓						
Phasic																				
Reflux																				
Non Diagnostic																				

Technologist Comments/Preliminary Report:
Residual thrombus
Substantial Recannalization

B

4-Part – White: Radiology - Pink: Preliminary Copy - Yellow: Medical Records - Goldenrod: MD

VA Form 10-44/G (114/660)
August 1994

FIGURE 23–11 *Continued*

are generated by an improper gain setting, an inadequate Doppler angle, or the use of the wrong velocity range.

Poor Venous Distention and Reduced Flow

The final pitfall to be considered is suboptimal venous distention. We have occasionally encountered patients without prior venous disease who were ideal candidates for duplex venography, yet visualization of the calf veins was extremely limited because of small vein caliber. This problem may be caused by vasoconstriction, which may result from an excessively cool examining room or a lack of dependency of the limb. In other instances, the lack of venous distention may be a result of hypovolemia. In still other instances, we have no explanation for the lack of venous distention.

The sonographer should do everything possible to distend the leg veins. Examination in a sitting position can be especially helpful for distending the calf veins.

REPORTED ACCURACY

Iliofemoral and Popliteal Regions

A large volume of data is available that attests to the accuracy of ultrasound for diagnosis of deep venous thrombosis in the iliofemoral and popliteal areas.[3–8, 14, 16–22] These data leave little or no doubt that duplex sonography of the femoral and popliteal veins is highly reliable in symptomatic patients. Sensitivity and specificity for acute symptomatic DVT exceeds 90% in most studies and approaches 100% in some series.

Calf Veins

Duplex sonography is also highly accurate for the diagnosis of acute calf venous thrombosis in symptomatic patients, *when the calf veins can be seen adequately.* In this circumstance, sensitivity and specificity are reported to exceed 90%.[4, 8, 21–23] The term *adequate visualization* is of great importance, however. In our patient population, all three pairs of calf veins can be seen adequately in only about 60% of patients. Success rates for calf vein assessment reported in the medical literature range from 60 to 90%,[8, 23–25] but I believe that visualization rates are population dependent. In spite of ultrasound instrument improvement, our success rate for calf vein visualization has not changed appreciably since the late 1980s.

It is well documented that the diagnostic results of calf vein sonography are poor when visualization is inadequate. However, the good news is that the *specificity* and *positive predictive value* of sonography are high, even in patients with poor visualization.[26] This means that when veins will not compress, or when you see thrombus directly, you can be confident of your diagnosis, and further studies are not needed.

Results in Asymptomatic Patients

It must be clearly understood that the excellent published results for venous sonography refer principally to symptomatic patients. Subsequent to glowing initial published reports, it was noted that sonography was generally less accurate in asymptomatic patients than in symptomatic individuals.[26–31] This seems to be largely related to selection bias, with excellent results (90% or greater sensitivity and specificity) in some series,[24] and lower levels of accuracy in others. The accuracy of sonography seems to be particularly poor in postoperative joint replacement patients, in whom sensitivity ranges from 25 to 77% overall and from 11 to 54% for calf vein thrombi.[21, 22, 26–31]*

There are three main reasons that ultrasound results are relatively poor in asymptomatic patients.[32–34] First, small, localized, nonocclusive thrombi are more prevalent in asymptomatic patients, as compared with symptomatic patients, who tend to have large segmental thrombi (e.g., the entire superficial femoral vein). Second, in some asymptomatic patient populations, the prevalence of isolated calf vein thrombosis is substantially greater than in symptomatic patients. (This has not been observed universally.[35, 36]) Because the examination success rate in the calf is relatively poor, the sensitivity for isolated

* The exception is a report of 92% sensitivity for asymptomatic calf vein thrombi.[24]

calf vein thrombus is reduced accordingly. Finally, the clarity of vein visualization may be poor in certain asymptomatic cohorts, such as the postoperative orthopedic patients who have considerable leg edema.

The bright side of ultrasound examination in asymptomatic patients is a high level of specificity. I have yet to read a published study with an ultrasound specificity of less than 90%. As noted previously, this means that when you see acute thrombus you can be confident in your diagnosis. Therefore, the use of ultrasonography as an initial examination tool for asymptomatic patients has merit. If thrombus is not seen, however, it may be advisable to proceed to other studies, such as contrast venography.

VENOUS ULTRASOUND CONTROVERSIES

Over the years that venous sonography has been used clinically, a number of controversial issues have arisen regarding the clinical applications of this diagnostic technique. These are summarized briefly as follows.

Calf Vein Examination *Is* Necessary

It is sometimes argued that there is no need to examine the calf veins because isolated calf vein thrombosis is not generally thought to pose a risk for pulmonary embolus and because some physicians feel that thrombus localized to the calf does not warrant anticoagulant therapy.[37–38] These arguments notwithstanding, the author feels that detection of calf vein thrombus is important for the following reasons:

1. *The referring physician wants to know the cause of calf symptoms* (usually pain or swelling). The practitioner must deal with a patient who wants to know *why* his or her leg hurts. Confirming or excluding DVT is key information, therefore, for both the practitioner and the patient. Furthermore, sonography may detect nonvenous causes of calf pain, such as Baker's cyst or a hematoma.

2. *Isolated calf vein thrombus may cause long-term disability.* There is increasing evidence that isolated calf vein thrombosis is not a benign condition and results in significant problems with valvular incompetence and venous stasis.[39, 40] Some practitioners treat isolated calf vein thrombosis, even in ambulatory patients, feeling that the chronic sequelae of DVT are prevented through timely and appropriate anticoagulant therapy. Treatment cannot be applied, however, without preceding ultrasound diagnosis of calf DVT.

3. *Calf vein thrombus may propagate in a cephalad direction or embolize.* Based on contrast venography series, it is estimated that only about 3% of pulmonary emboli arise from isolated calf vein thrombi.[38, 41] For this reason, the calf veins are not examined routinely in many ultrasound departments when the clinical issue is pulmonary embolus. In a recently published study, pulmonary embolization was confirmed with imaging studies in 35% of patients with isolated calf vein thrombosis *and* respiratory symptoms.[42] It may be advisable, therefore, to examine calf veins in selected patients with respiratory symptoms. Calf vein thrombus, furthermore, is known to propagate into the popliteal vein in up to 28% of cases, posing further risk of pulmonary embolization.[37, 38, 41, 43]

Origin of Pulmonary Emboli

As noted previously, thrombus is absent in lower extremity veins in about 25 to 30% of patients with arteriographically documented pulmonary emboli.[44, 45] These emboli arise in other portions of the venous system, including pelvic veins and upper extremity veins. Little information is available with respect to the incidence of embolization from these areas, but the finding of Hammers and coworkers[46] is of interest. In their study, thrombus was isolated to upper extremity veins in 30% of high-risk trauma patients with documented pulmonary embolization.

Is an Abbreviated Ultrasound Examination Adequate?

Two studies indicate that 95 to 99% of *symptomatic* acute deep venous thrombi can be detected with a limited compression ultrasound examination in which only the common femoral and popliteal veins are examined.[47–49] This technique is said to decrease examination time by slightly more than 50%. Frederick and associates[48] argue, however, that thrombus is isolated within short venous segments in a significant number of cases (22%) and that such thrombus might be overlooked, especially when it is located in the superficial femoral or deep femoral vein. They argue further that the time saved (about 5 minutes per leg) is not worth the risk of missing isolated thrombus. An additional disadvantage of the abbreviated approach is the lack of a comprehensive road map in patients with thrombus, as discussed previously. My colleagues and I have not adopted the abbreviated examination in our department.

Is Examination of Both Legs Necessary?

Before the development of ultrasound techniques for venous examination, bilateral lower extremity venous examination was the rule in noninvasive vascular laboratories, because plethysmography was the diagnostic modality employed and this method was bilateral by its very nature. When venous sonography was introduced, some vascular laboratories continued the practice of bilateral lower extremity examination, even though only one leg was symptomatic. Most radiology departments examined only the symptomatic extremity, however, because this had long been standard practice for contrast venography. There has been some controversy, therefore, concerning the need for bilateral venous studies in patients with unilateral symptoms.

I feel that the examination of both lower extremities is unnecessary in patients with unilateral extremity symptoms, and this perspective is supported by published data indicating a low incidence of thrombus in the contralateral extremity.[49, 50] Please note, however, that *the examination of both lower extremities* (at least to the popliteal level) *may be advisable in patients with signs or symptoms of pulmonary embolus,* even though only one extremity is symptomatic.

Pulmonary Embolus Screening

The noninvasive nature of venous sonography has indirectly generated considerable controversy regarding the diagnosis of pulmonary embolization. Because sonography is noninvasive there has been a tendency to use this modality wantonly. It is well recognized that pulmonary artery thromboembolism is a common and potentially life-threatening consequence of extremity venous thrombosis. This condition, which is estimated to affect 600,000 individuals in the United States annually,[51] represents a major diagnostic problem, because signs and symptoms, when present, are nonspecific.[51–53] Pulmonary arteriography offers a high level of diagnostic accuracy, but this procedure is uncomfortable, costly, and potentially hazardous. Scintigraphy (lung scan) is of some diagnostic benefit, but a high-probability ventilation/perfusion scan conveys only a 60% likelihood of pulmonary thromboembolism,[54, 55] intermediate probability lung scans are of no diagnostic value, and low probability scans have a 9% false-negative rate.[53–55] Computed tomographic angiography (CTA) and magnetic resonance angiography hold promise as direct methods for diagnosis of pulmonary embolization, and pulmonary CTA is rapidly becoming the preferred method for diagnosis of acute pulmonary embolization in the hospitals at which I practice. CTA is a simple procedure, but it requires the transportation of the patient to the radiology department, the administration of radiographic contrast, and a certain level of patient cooperation.[56, 57]

Because each method of pulmonary embolus imaging has certain disadvantages, duplex sonography is used commonly as an adjunctive diagnostic method. Pulmonary thromboembolism is implied when sonography detects thrombus in large extremity veins in a patient with appropriate signs or symptoms.[51–53] Furthermore, because therapy for extremity DVT is the same as for pulmonary thromboembolism, direct evaluation of the pulmonary circulation is unnecessary when acute DVT is diagnosed with ultrasonography. It is reasonable, therefore, to use ultrasonography as an initial study in patients suspected of pulmonary thromboembolism,[58, 59] but there are several important caveats with respect to this practice.

1. The absence of thrombus in extremity veins does not exclude pulmonary embolus. As noted previously, it is well documented that thrombus is absent in lower extremity veins in 25 to 30% of patients with documented pulmonary emboli.[43, 44]

Therefore, a negative extremity ultrasound examination must be followed with a study, such as CTA, to directly diagnose pulmonary embolus.

2. The cost-effectiveness of ultrasound screening for DVT in high-risk patient populations is subject to question. Certain patient populations, such as trauma patients in intensive care units and postoperative joint-replacement patients are known to be at risk for developing lower extremity DVT. Historically, the incidence of asymptomatic DVT was found to be greater than 80% in some of these populations,[26, 28, 34, 51, 60–63] but more recent studies in high-risk patients treated with DVT prophylaxis have shown DVT rates in the range of 6 to 10%.[36, 46, 64] Although sonography can detect DVT in these patients, potentially preventing pulmonary embolism, it is argued that a surveillance program, consisting of serial ultrasound studies, in asymptomatic high-risk patients would be far from cost-effective.[64] It is suggested, therefore, that sonography be used only in patients who develop symptoms of extremity DVT or pulmonary embolism.
3. Adequate clinical assessment is the key to cost-effective pulmonary embolus screening. Those of us working in the ultrasound business have experienced an explosion of venous ultrasound use that raises serious question about cost-effectiveness,[65, 66] and our concerns have been borne out by studies showing a low incidence of DVT in various conditions that prompt venous ultrasound referral. For example, the incidence of lower extremity venous thrombosis is only 4% in asymptomatic patients and in patients with cellulitis who are referred for venous sonography. The incidence is exceedingly low (too low to measure) in patients presenting with *bilateral* leg swelling.[49, 67] Furthermore, in 64% of patients with bilateral leg swelling (referred for sonography), a readily diagnosed cause of swelling, other than venous thrombosis, can be found if clinical assessment is adequate![67] (The usual cause is congestive heart failure.) In consideration of findings such as these, I believe ultrasound practitioners should monitor referrals for acute DVT in asymptomatic patients, in patients with bilateral leg swelling, and in patients with cellulitis. It is not the ultrasound practitioner's job to second guess a clinician's medical judgment, but he or she can help to identify practitioners who repeatedly order ultrasound studies for questionable indications.

Cancer Risk With Unexplained DVT

The final controversial issue is the rate of cancer detection in patients who present with *extensive* venous thrombosis without obvious DVT risk factors. A fairly high probability of occult malignancy has been found in such individuals. In older studies, 23 to 34% of such patients manifested a malignancy within 1 to 2 years.[68, 69] A more recent study of a large number of adults suggests that the risk of malignancy is lower than this, although it is quite significant. In this series, the cancer risk was 2.2 times greater for patients with one episode of DVT than for age-matched controls.[70] For patients with recurrent DVT, the risk was 3.2 times that of the controls. Most importantly, 40 to 60% of the patients with DVT had metastases at the time that DVT was diagnosed. In spite of these statistics, these authors felt that extensive cancer detection efforts were not warranted in adults with unexplained DVT, but that limited assessment with physical examination and laboratory studies were cost-effective.

REFERENCES

1. Talbot SR: B-mode evaluation of peripheral veins. Semin Ultrasound CT MR 9:295–319, 1988.
2. Effeney DJ, Friedman MB, Gooding GAW: Iliofemoral venous thrombosis: Real-time ultrasound diagnosis, normal criteria, and clinical application. Radiology 150:787–792, 1984.
3. Sullivan ED, Peters BS, Cranley JJ: Real-time B-mode venous ultrasound. J Vasc Surg 1:465–471, 1984.
4. Oliver MA: Duplex scanning in venous disease. Bruit IX: 206–209, 1985.
5. Raghavendra BN, Horii SC, Hilton S, et al: Deep venous thrombosis: Detection by probe compression of veins. J Ultrasound Med 5:89–95, 1986.
6. Dauzat MM, Laroche JP, Charras C, et al: Real-time B-mode ultrasonography for better specialty in the noninvasive diagnosis of deep venous thrombosis. J Ultrasound Med 5:625–631, 1986.
7. Cronan JJ, Dorfman GS, Scola FH, et al: Deep venous thrombosis: US assessment using vein compression. Radiology 162:191–194, 1987.
8. Vogel P, Laing FRC, Jeffrey RB, et al: Deep venous thrombosis of the lower extremity: US evaluation. Radiology 163:747–751, 1987.
9. Zwiebel WJ, Priest DL: Color-duplex sonography of extremity veins. Semin Ultrasound CT MR 11:136–167, 1990.

10. Schroder WB, Bealer JF: Venous duplex ultrasonography causing acute pulmonary embolism: A brief report. J Vasc Surg 15:1082–1083, 1992.
11. Barnes RW: Doppler techniques for lower-extremity venous disease. *In* Zwiebel WJ (ed): Introduction to Vascular Ultrasonography. Philadelphia, Grune & Stratton, 1986, pp 333–350.
12. Hirsh J, Genton E, Hall R: Venous thromboembolism. New York, Grune & Stratton, 1981, pp 1–4.
13. Cronan JJ, Leen V: Recurrent deep venous thrombosis: Limitations of US. Radiology 170:739–742, 1989.
14. Appelman PT, De Jong TE, Lampmann LE: Deep venous thrombosis of the leg: US findings. Radiology 163:743–746, 1987.
15. Zwiebel WJ: Sources of error in duplex venography and an algorithmic approach to the diagnosis of deep venous thrombosis. Semin Ultrasound CT MR 9:286–294, 1988.
16. O'Leary DO, Kane R, Pinel D, et al: A prospective study of the efficacy of B-scan sonography in the detection of deep venous thrombosis in the lower extremity. Presented at the American Institute of Ultrasound in Medicine Annual Convention, Las Vegas, NV, September 16–19, 1986.
17. Nix ML, Nelson CL, Harmon BH, et al: Duplex venous scanning: Image vs. Doppler accuracy. Presented at the Eleventh Annual Meeting of the Society of Vascular Technology, Chicago, IL, June 8–12, 1988.
18. Lensing AWA, Prandoni P, Brandjes D, et al: Detection of deep-vein thrombosis by real-time B-mode ultrasonography. N Engl J Med 320:341–345, 1989.
19. Foley WD, Middleton WD, Lawson TL, et al: Color Doppler ultrasound imaging of lower-extremity venous disease. AJR Am J Roentgenol 152:371–376, 1989.
20. Rose SC, Zwiebel WJ, Murdock LE, et al: Insensitivity of color Doppler flow imaging for detection of acute calf deep venous thrombosis in asymptomatic postoperative patients. J Vasc Interv Rad 4:111–117, 1993.
21. Polak JF, Culter SS, O'Leary DH: Deep vein of the calf: Assessment with color Doppler flow imaging. Radiology 171:481–485, 1989.
22. Comeroto AJ, Katz ML, Hasheim MA: Venous duplex imaging for the diagnosis of acute deep venous thrombosis. Hemostasis 23(suppl 1):61–71, 1993.
23. Semrow CM, Friedell ML, Buchbinder D, et al: The efficacy of ultrasonic venography in the detection of calf vein thrombosis. Presented at the Tenth Annual Meeting of the Society of Non-Invasive Vascular Technology, Toronto, Canada, June 4–6, 1987.
24. Atri M, Herba MK, Reinhold C, et al: Accuracy of sonography in the evaluation of calf deep vein thrombosis in both postoperative surveillance and symptomatic patients. AJR Am J Roentgenol 166:1361–1367, 1996.
25. Rose SC, Zwiebel WJ, Nelson BD, et al: Symptomatic lower extremity deep venous thrombosis: Accuracy, limitations, and role of color Doppler flow imaging in diagnosis. Radiology 175:639–644, 1990.
26. Dauzat MM, Laroche JP, Charras C, et al: Real-time B-mode ultrasonography for better specificity in the noninvasive diagnosis of deep venous thrombosis. J Ultrasound Med 5:625–631, 1986.
27. Borris LC, Christiansen JM, Lassen MR, et al: Comparison of real-time B-mode ultrasonography and bilateral ascending phlebography for detection of postoperative deep vein thrombosis following elective hip surgery. Thromb Haemost 61:363–365, 1989.
28. Manninen R, Manninen H, Soimakallio S, et al: Asymptomatic deep venous thrombosis in the calf: Accuracy and limitations of ultrasonography as a screening test after total knee arthroplasty. Br J Radiol 66:199–202, 1993.
29. Yucel EK, Fisher JS, Egglin TK, et al: Isolated calf venous thrombosis: Diagnosis with compression US. Radiology 179:443–446, 1991.
30. Midgette AS, Stuikel TA, Littenberg F: A meta-analytic method for summarizing diagnostic test performance: Receiver-operating-characteristic-summary point estimates. Medical Decis Making 13: 253–257, 1993.
31. Agnelli G, Volpato R, Radicchia S, et al: Detection of asymptomatic deep vein thrombosis by real-time B-mode ultrasonography in hip surgery patient. Thromb Haemost 68:257–260, 1992.
32. Cogo A, Lensing AW, Prandoni B, Hirsh J: Distribution of thrombosis in patients with symptomatic deep vein thrombosis. Arch Intern Med 153:2777–2780, 1993.
33. Markel A, Manzo RA, Bergelin RO, Strandness DE: Pattern and distribution of thrombi in acute venous thrombosis. Arch Surg 127:305–309, 1992.
34. Rose SC, Zwiebel WJ, Miller FJ: Distribution of acute lower extremity deep venous thrombosis in symptomatic and asymptomatic patients: Imaging implications. J Ultrasound Med 13:243–250, 1994.
35. Hill SL, Holtzman GI, Martin D, et al: The origin of lower extremity deep vein thrombi in acute venous thrombosis. Am J Surg 173:485–490, 1997.
36. Flinn WR, Sandager GP, Silva MB Jr, et al: Prospective surveillance for perioperative venous thrombosis. Experience in 2643 patients. Arch Surg 131:472–480, 1996.
37. Moreno-Cabral R, Kistner RL, Nordyke RA: Importance of calf vein thrombophlebitis. Surgery 6:735–742, 1976.
38. Hull RD, Hirsh J: Diagnostic techniques in venous thrombosis. *In* Bergan JJ, Yao JST (eds): Surgery of the Veins. New York, Grune & Stratton, 1985, pp 47–51.
39. McLafferty RB, Moneta GL, Passman MA, et al: Late clinical and hemodynamic sequelae of isolated calf vein thrombosis. J Vasc Surg 27:50–56, 1998.
40. Meissner MH, Caps MT, Bergelin RO, et al: Early outcome after isolated calf vein thrombosis. J Vasc Surg 26:749–756, 1997.
41. Horowitz O, Casey MP, Maslak MM: Venous thrombosis-pulmonary embolus complex. *In* Horowitz O, McComb P, Roberts B (eds): Diseases of Blood Vessels. Philadelphia, Lea & Febiger, 1985, pp 263–289.
42. Passman MA, Moneta GL, Taylor LM Jr, et al: Pulmonary embolism is associated with the combination of isolated calf vein thrombosis and respiratory symptoms. J Vasc Surg 25:39–45, 1997.
43. Lohr JM, James KV, Deshmukh RM, Hasselfeld KA: Allastair B. Karmody Award. Calf vein thrombi are not a benign finding. Am J Surg 170:86–90, 1995.
44. Hull RD, Hirsh J, Carter CJ, et al: Pulmonary angiography, ventilation lung scanning, and venography for clinically suspected pulmonary embolism with abnormal perfusion lung scan. Ann Intern Med 98:891–899, 1983.

45. Scigala EM, McDonnell AE, Hadcock WE, et al: Prevalence of deep venous thrombosis in patients with proven pulmonary embolism. Bruit VIII:222–224, 1984.
46. Hammers LW, Cohn SM, Brown JM, et al: Doppler color flow imaging surveillance of deep vein thrombosis in high-risk trauma patients. J Ultrasound Med 15:19–24, 1996.
47. Pezzullo JA, Perkins AB, Cronan JJ: Symptomatic deep vein thrombosis: Diagnosis with a limited compression US. Radiology 196:67–70, 1996.
48. Frederick MG, Hertzberg BS, Kliewer MA, et al: Can the US examination for lower extremity deep venous thrombosis be abbreviated? A prospective study of 755 examinations. Radiology 199:45–47, 1996.
49. Sheiman RG, Weintraub JL, McArdle CR: Bilateral lower extremity US in the patient with bilateral symptoms of deep venous thrombosis: Assessment of need. Radiology 196:379–381, 1995.
50. Strothman G, Bleba J, Fowel RJ, Rosenthal G: Contralateral duplex scanning for deep vein thrombosis is unnecessary in patients with symptoms. J Vasc Surg 22:543–547, 1995.
51. Reinmann EE, Salzman EW: Deep-vein thrombosis. N Engl J Med 331:1630–1641, 1994.
52. Hull RD, Hirsh J, Carter CJ, et al: Diagnostic value of ventilation-perfusion lung scanning in patients with suspected pulmonary embolism. Chest 88:819–828, 1985.
53. Smith LL, Iber C, Sirr S: Pulmonary embolism: Confirmation with venous duplex US as adjunct to lung scanning. Radiology 191:143–147, 1994.
54. Webber MM, Gomes AS, Roe D, et al: Comparison of Biello, McNeil, and PIOPED criteria for the diagnosis of pulmonary emboli on lung scans. AJR Am J Roentgenol 154:975–981, 1990.
55. PIOPED Data and Coordination Center: Prospective investigation of pulmonary embolism detection. Baltimore, Maryland Medical Research Institute, 7:7–8, 1986.
56. Sheedy PF, Johnson M, Welch TJ, et al: Fast CT for pulmonary embolus. Semin Ultrasound CT MRI 4:324–338, 1996.
57. Geftner WB, Hatabu H, Holland GA, Osiason AW: Pulmonary MR angiography. Semin Ultrasound CT MRI 4:316–323, 1996.
58. Hull RD, Raskob GE, Hirsh J: Cost effectiveness of noninvasive diagnosis of deep vein thrombosis in symptomatic patients. *In* Bernstein EF (ed): Vascular Diagnosis, 4th ed. St. Louis, Mosby–Year Book, 1993, pp 880–887.
59. Hull R, Hirsh J, Sackett DL, Stoddart G: Cost effectiveness of clinical diagnosis, venography, and noninvasive testing in patients with symptomatic deep-vein thrombosis. N Engl J Med 304:1561–1567, 1981.
60. Geerts WH, Code KI, Jay RM, et al: A prospective study of venous thromboembolism after major trauma. N Engl J Med 331:1601–1606, 1994.
61. Hirsch DR, Ingenito EP, Goldhaber SZ: Prevalence of deep venous thrombosis among patients in medical intensive care. JAMA 74:335–337, 1995.
62. Cronan JJ, Froehlich JA, Dorfman GS: Image-directed Doppler ultrasound: A screening technique for patients at high risk to develop deep vein thrombosis. J Clin Ultrasound 19:133–138, 1991.
63. Sevitt S, Gallagher N: Venous thrombosis and pulmonary embolism: A clinico-pathological study in injured and burned patients. Br J Surg 475–489, 1960.
64. Meyer CS, Blebea J, Davis K Jr, et al: Surveillance venous scans for deep venous thrombosis in multiple trauma patients. Ann Vasc Surg 9:109–114, 1995.
65. Zwiebel WJ: The clinical and financial impact of non-invasive vascular testing in the USA. Australas Radiol 39:309–313, 1995.
66. Matteson B, Langsfeld M, Schermer C, et al: Role of venous duplex scanning in patients with suspected pulmonary embolism. J Vasc Surg 24:768–773, 1996.
67. Cronan JJ: Venous thromboembolic disease: The role of US. Radiology 186:619–630, 1993.
68. Silverstein RK, Nachman RL: Cancer and clotting—Trousseau's warning. N Engl J Med 327:1163–1164, 1992.
69. Monreal M, Lafoz E, Casals AN, et al: Occult cancer in patients with deep venous thrombosis. Cancer 67:541–545, 1991.
70. Sorensen HT, Mellenkjaer L, Steffensen FH, et al: The risk of a diagnosis of cancer after primary deep venous thrombosis or pulmonary embolism. N Engl J Med 338:1169–1173, 1998.

Chapter 24

Definitive Diagnosis and Documentation of Chronic Venous Dysfunction

■ *Warner P. Bundens, MD, MS* ■ *John J. Bergan, MD, FACS, FRCS (Hon)*

After nearly 50 years of rapid advances in vascular surgery and after 25 years of progress in developing noninvasive vascular investigations, the venous system remains enigmatic. Its pathophysiology is a fruitful area of investigation because the component elements of venous dysfunction are incompletely understood.

As investigations into venous dysfunction proceed, research studies and individual patient examinations are being refined. Prospective, randomized studies are appearing in print, and meta-analyses are being published. Gradually, clinical examination of the dysfunctional venous system in the vascular laboratory has experienced a transition from indirect examinations, such as photoplethysmography and impedance plethysmography, to direct imaging and interrogation by means of duplex ultrasound imaging.

Fundamentally, venous conditions as studied in the clinical noninvasive laboratory can be divided into the traditional categories of *acute* and *chronic*. These in turn are investigated along anatomic lines, such as the superficial or deep venous systems and their interconnections. For the most part, acute problems consist of deep venous thrombosis (DVT) and superficial thrombophlebitis, alone or in combination. Chronic problems of venous dysfunction are due, in most cases, to reflux or backward flow through failed valves. To a lesser extent, they may be caused by obstruction. These problems may appear alone or in combination and may involve the superficial system, the deep system, or both. Outward flow through veins that perforate anatomic layers add confusing but interesting elements to the clinical examination. In summary, acute venous problems are thrombotic for the most part, and chronic difficulties are due to a failure of function called *venous stasis*.

Clinical examination, including a careful medical history and meticulous physical examination, provides a tentative but not complete diagnosis in patients with venous disorders. Further testing is often necessary. Fortunately, despite the many symptoms and findings that may be present in a single patient, the laboratory examination has to consider only two fundamental problems: obstruction and reflux. During the last several decades, numerous noninvasive methods have advanced the evaluation of venous disease. These include continuous wave Doppler imaging and various plethysmographic techniques. Color-flow sonography has rapidly become the most commonly used method of venous testing[1] (Fig. 24–1).

CLINICAL CONDITIONS

Obstruction

Venous obstruction is almost always the result of venous thrombosis. Less frequently, extrinsic compression may lead to total obstruction, such as in the subclavian vein or the left common iliac vein. Patients with one or more elements of Virchow's triad (stasis, hypercoagulability, and vein wall abnormalities) are susceptible to thrombosis.[2] The clinical presentation can be totally asymptomatic

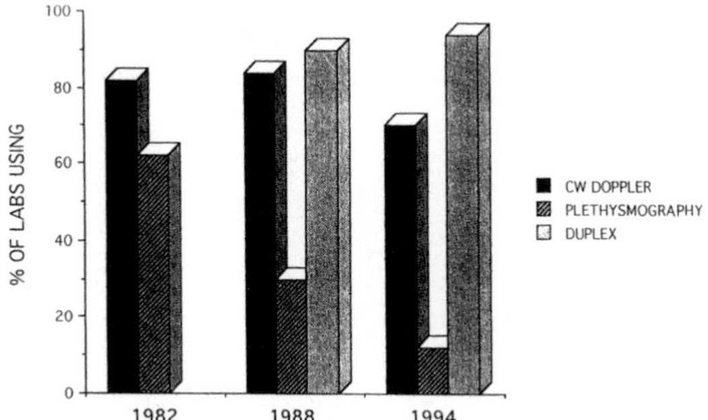

FIGURE 24–1 Modalities used by vascular laboratories for venous tests. (Data from Leers SA, Blackburn DR, Burnham SJ: Vascular technology in evolution: Results of the 1994 ARDMS task survey. J Vasc Technol 19:127, 1995.)

or may progress to flagrant phlegmasia cerulea dolens and venous gangrene. The magnitude of symptoms and findings depends to some extent on the location and number of venous segments affected by thrombus.

Superficial Thrombophlebitis

Phlebitis in a superficial vein is readily diagnosed clinically. Varicose veins in the lower extremity and intravenous therapy in the upper extremity predispose a patient to phlebitis. Although the initial diagnosis can be made clinically, approximately 20% of patients with superficial phlebitis also have associated occult DVT (Table 24–1). Furthermore, approximately one third of those who have only superficial phlebitis initially will eventually extend the thrombus to the deep system via the saphenofemoral junction or perforating veins.[8] Phlebitis of the long saphenous vein above the knee is particularly susceptible to progression to DVT.[9] Therefore, it is prudent to perform a duplex examination for DVT and, in selected cases, a follow-up examination in patients with suspected or proven ascending superficial phlebitis.

TABLE 24–2 SENSITIVITY AND SPECIFICITY OF CLINICAL FINDINGS OF DEEP VENOUS THROMBOSIS

Findings	Sensitivity (%)	Specificity (%)
Calf pain	60–85	15–20
Calf tenderness	50–75	25–50
Ankle edema	30–40	15–25
Leg or ankle swelling	35–50	10–70
Redness	5–15	80–90
Superficial vein dilatation	25–30	30–80
Homan's sign	15–40	50–80

Modified from Leclerc JR: Venous Thromboembolic Disorders. Philadelphia, Lea & Febiger, 1991.

Lower Extremity Deep Venous Thrombosis

DVT of the lower limbs is quite common. An estimated 5 million cases occur in the United States yearly.[10] In addition to the acute problem, DVT can lead to death from pulmonary embolism or significant morbidity from the postphlebitic syndrome. Assessment of this latter condition is considered in detail in this chapter. Unlike the situation of superficial phlebitis, in which the diagnosis is literally under the examining finger, the accuracy of clinical diagnosis of DVT is unreliable (Table 24–2). Clinical diagnosis of DVT has demonstrated accuracy ranging from 50 to 70% in both retrospective and prospective studies.[11] Thus, if DVT is part of a differential diagnosis, an objective test must be done to confirm or refute the diagnosis. In addition, because up to two thirds of DVTs are clinically silent,[12] screening of high-risk patients may be justified even though it may not be cost-effective.[13, 14] Duplex scanning is now used to diagnose lower extremity DVT in vir-

TABLE 24–1 INCIDENCE OF OCCULT DEEP VENOUS THROMBOSIS ASSOCIATED WITH SUPERFICIAL THROMBOPHLEBITIS

Year	Author	Method	Incidence (%)
1993	Jorgensen et al[3]	Duplex sonography	23
1991	Prountijos et al[4]	Venography	20
1991	Lutter et al[5]	Duplex sonography	28
1990	Skillman et al[6]	Impedance plethysmography and venography	12
1986	Bergqvist and Jaroszewski[7]	Venography	44*/3†

* Patients without varicose veins.
† Patients with varicose veins.

tually all vascular laboratories and ultrasound departments.

Traditional teaching, largely derived from autopsy studies, holds that most lower extremity venous thrombosis begins in soleal sinuses or calf veins. However, duplex scanning has thrown doubt on the universality of this concept. Primary iliac venous thrombosis (as considered later) is an important exception to the old dogma. Although in two thirds of cases calf DVT lyses spontaneously, the remainder may propagate into the popliteal vein or embolize directly to the lungs. Such emboli are small and often silent. There is controversy regarding how to manage patients with isolated below-knee DVT. Some disagreement comes from the fact that a single small thrombus in one paired vein is different from multiple tibial venous occlusions or total obliteration of all crural veins. Some experts recommend anticoagulation for calf DVT at the time of diagnosis, just as for above-knee DVT.[15, 16] Others advocate careful follow-up examinations until the DVT lyses or extends to the popliteal vein.[17] Some vascular laboratories completely eliminate examination of the calf veins. Despite the management controversy, such thrombi should be looked for and, if found, should not be ignored. Unfortunately, the accuracy of a duplex study for below-knee DVT is inferior to that for above-knee occlusion, as discussed elsewhere in this volume.

Iliac Venous Thrombosis

Isolated iliac venous thrombosis is said to be rare. One report using phlebography found no cases of it in 164 consecutive patients.[18] Another study using duplex scanning in 833 patients found only one case of isolated iliac (common iliac) venous thrombosis in 209 patients with DVT,[19] whereas another study of 237 patients found DVT in 56 patients and isolated iliac DVT in 3.[20] These studies included all orthopedic patients referred to a vascular laboratory with suspicion of DVT for postoperative surveillance. However, pregnancy and pelvic abnormalities, such as cancer, trauma, and recent surgery, can also predispose one to iliac thrombosis.[21] The true incidence of isolated pelvic DVT in these subgroups is not known, as duplex diagnosis of iliac venous thrombosis is often difficult, and the accuracy of this technique has not been established.

Relationship of Deep Venous Thrombosis to Chronic Venous Insufficiency

Frequently, DVT permanently damages the affected vein segment. The thrombotic obstruction may be expected to recanalize and restore flow, but recanalization produces an irregular surface that impedes flow. This leads to the opening up of venous collaterals around the obstruction, and these collaterals are usually so extensive that physiologic tests of venous function do not detect the anatomic obstruction. However, intrinsic damage to the venous valves produces shortening, thickening, and scarring, as well as splitting and perforation, which absolutely preclude normal function. Thus, the post-thrombotic venous segment can be expected to reflux. In addition to reflux through the damaged venous valve, the collateral vessels that have formed around the obstruction dilate to the point that their valves also fail, adding to reflux.

Reflux, or flow away from the heart, does not occur in every venous segment subjected to thrombosis. Nevertheless, venous reflux is so common that a physician can expect venous dysfunction after an episode of DVT.

In severe, chronic venous insufficiency (CVI), lower extremity skin changes of hyperpigmentation, induration, and ulceration occur (Fig. 24–2). The induration is commonly referred to as *lipodermatosclerosis.* In the past, such skin changes were called *post-thrombotic,* and the limb containing these changes was referred to as the *post-thrombotic* or *postphlebitic limb.* Gradually, it became known that the stigmata of the post-thrombotic limb might appear in limbs without any episode of previous DVT. As this became recognized, the terms postphlebitic and post-thrombotic became obsolete and were replaced by the term *chronic venous insufficiency.* This was important because the terms postphlebitic and post-thrombotic had a connotation of hopelessness or inevitability. Very little, after all, could be done with a partially obstructed, valveless venous segment. However, CVI carries the connotation of surgical repair. If the refluxing segments

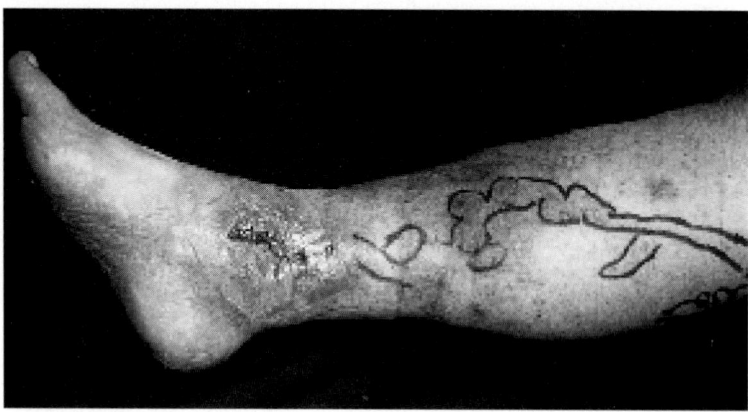

FIGURE 24–2 The limb with severe chronic venous insufficiency is characterized by edema, hyperpigmentation, and ulceration. Dilated, protuberant, saccular varicose veins are frequently present.

can be removed or repaired, the severe condition of CVI may be ameliorated. Noninvasive laboratory testing identifies the venous segments that are dysfunctional and defines the clinical procedures that may benefit the patient. Thus, the noninvasive evaluation of a limb with venous dysfunction allows the proper prescription of treatment. Examinations relevant to this are those that identify reflux, those that indicate obstruction, and those that localize perforating vein outflow.

Reflux

Although most acute venous problems are concerned with obstruction by thrombosis, most chronic venous problems are caused by reflux. *Reflux* is defined as the retrograde flow of blood in veins of the lower extremity caused by absent or incompetent valves. The result is venous hypertension, which is attributable to one of three possible mechanisms: (1) the column of blood is not interrupted by functioning valves between the right atrium and the veins of the lower extremities, which then allows full pressure of gravitational, hydrostatic forces to be exerted on the vein walls; (2) the calf muscle pump mechanism becomes ineffective, and the ejection of blood from the limb produced by muscular compression of deep veins is inadequate, increasing the residual venous volume; or (3) perforating veins, including calf perforators and the saphenofemoral or saphenopopliteal junctions, fail to function, allowing venous blood to flow distally and outward rather than proximally and inward. The failure of check valves in calf perforating veins, in particular, allows high pressures (up to 250 mm Hg) generated in the deep veins by muscular contraction to be transmitted directly to the unsupported superficial veins. The resultant venous hypertension can cause symptoms of heaviness, aching, and fatigue, as well as findings of edema and dilated veins (varicosities and telangiectasias). In some limbs, venous hypertension is associated with skin pigmentation, lipodermatosclerosis, and ulceration. In such situations, axial and perforating vein reflux is common and is directly associated with the cutaneous changes.

Uncomplicated venous reflux is common. By the age of 20 years, 20% of the population may have some reflux, although they may not have varicosities.[22] However, valves of varicose veins are always incompetent. After DVT, valve damage is common, and reflux can be detected in approximately half of the veins that were thrombosed.[23]

Although it is easy to define reflux and appreciate its importance, as yet there is no universally accepted standard of diagnosis. Of the invasive tests, ambulatory venous pressure was a historic "gold standard." However, this test is somewhat of a global measure of limb reflux. Pressures obtained in disparate categories of venous stasis may be identical, and pressures obtained do not aid in planning therapy nor do they correlate closely with stages of venous insufficiency. Descending phlebography is often used clinically to confirm and grade venous reflux, but this is occasionally inaccurate because of seepage of relatively high-density radiographic contrast media through competent valves.

EXAMINATION TECHNIQUES

Doppler Clinical Evaluation

The patient is examined in the standing position facing the examiner and supporting his or her weight on the contralateral extremity. Immobility of the lower extremity during examination is essential. Muscular contractions in the leg must be avoided. The Doppler probe is placed over the femoral triangle at an angle of 45 degrees to the horizontal. The femoral vein is identified by its location medial to the artery. Confirmation of correct probe placement is obtained by manual compression of the thigh, the calf, or the varicosities themselves. This maneuver augments blood flow in a proximal direction. After the optimum signal is obtained, the patient is asked to cough and to perform a Valsalva maneuver. Finally, the thigh, the calf, or the varicosities are manually compressed and released suddenly. Interpretation of the results of this study is obvious. After calf compression and sudden release, if there is no detectable flow, there is no reflux. Similar findings are found during the cough and the Valsalva maneuver. In contrast, flow heard on release of calf compression or during the cough or the Valsalva maneuver suggests reflux. The precise location of the reflux in the femoral or saphenous vein may be difficult to identify and, in fact, may be inaccurate. Nevertheless, this clinical evaluation aids in determining the type of intervention to be planned.

Increased accuracy of the examination can be obtained by moving the probe over the supposed location of the saphenous vein and applying a rubber tourniquet or hand pressure 10 cm below the saphenofemoral junction. If this maneuver abolishes reflux, superficial reflux is strongly suspected. Persistence of the reflux despite compression of the long saphenous vein suggests that the femoral vein itself is incompetent. Tourniquet tests are flawed by their inability to standardize pressure, failure to achieve superficial occlusion, and inadvertent deep venous occlusion.

After the femoral areas are examined bilaterally, attention is turned to each popliteal space. The saphenopopliteal junction is examined with the patient facing away from the examiner. The examination is confined to the non–weight-bearing lower extremity. The knee is slightly flexed to relax the popliteal fossa. The Doppler probe is positioned carefully with light pressure at the level of the skin crease and at a 45-degree angle to the horizontal. The popliteal vein is located lateral to the midline of the knee and is related closely to the popliteal artery. Augmentation of the venous signal by calf compression allows optimal probe positioning. The calf is once again compressed or the varicosities themselves are compressed manually. Sudden release is accomplished, and an absence of flow confirms that there is no reflux in the lesser saphenous vein or the popliteal vein. The presence of flow on release of compression suggests reflux in either the short saphenous vein or the popliteal vein. Application of a tourniquet to occlude the short saphenous vein with repetition of calf compression maneuvers may separate short saphenous from popliteal reflux, as outlined previously.

Varicose Vein Evaluation

Varicose veins are always incompetent and exhibit reflux (Fig. 24–3; see Fig. 24–2). They should be traced proximally with the Doppler transducer to determine the origin of reflux. This may lead to a saphenous vein that may be incompetent but not varicose. Alternatively, reflux may be from a named or unnamed perforating vein. The greater and lesser saphenous veins are also readily tested and should be examined segmentally throughout their length.

It is relatively easy to learn to use the hand-held Doppler transducer for venous testing, and not much experience is needed to become adept. Despite being simple to use and inexpensive, it is quite accurate. Compared with descending phlebography, the Doppler method has been found to be 92% sensitive and 73% specific.[24] The relative lack of specificity of the Doppler method is mainly a result of its inability to localize reflux at deep-to-superficial communications. For example, reflux heard with a Valsalva maneuver over the common femoral vein may be caused by deep reflux in the femoral vein or, more commonly, an incompetent saphenofemoral junction. Similar problems arise over the popliteal vein, where reflux may be in that vein or may be due to an incompetent saphenopopliteal junction. The hand-held Doppler transducer is also unreliable for locating incompetent perforating veins because they

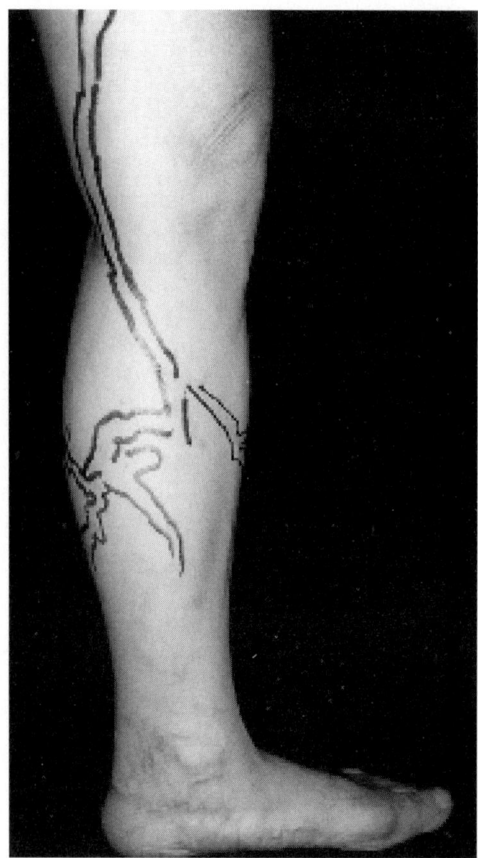

FIGURE 24–3 Illustration of tracing of varicose veins cephalad to their origin.

often connect to superficial varicosities or refluxing veins. One cannot tell if reflux is solely superficial or derives from perforating veins. Nevertheless, testing with the continuous-wave, hand-held Doppler transducer is a good clinical technique. In patients with small branch varicosities or telangiectasias, a routine examination constitutes a sufficient examination. Because of its lower specificity, a positive Doppler examination should be followed by a more definitive duplex examination.

Ambulatory Venous Pressure

In recognizing that blood pressure was important to the study of arterial disease, investigators interested in venous circulation quickly turned to venous pressure studies.[25–28] Original observations revealed a decrease in venous pressure in the foot during walking.[25] Gradual recovery to the resting basal value after walking became the basis of ambulatory venous pressure measurement. Measurement of venous pressure was done in the horizontal position, during quiet standing, and after walking, and the time for recovery to the basal level was recorded.[26, 27] It was learned that the static foot venous pressure was not related to the status of the venous valves and was equal to the pressure of a column of blood from the heart to the level of measurement. Because static pressure was not dependent on venous function, it was important to learn what was. This proved to be the magnitude of drop of the venous pressure after exercise and the time for recovery. The least pressure reduction on ambulation occurred in patients with the most severe superficial and deep valve dysfunction. It was found that if the ambulatory venous pressure decreased to less than 45 mm Hg, the risk of venous ulceration was negligible but with increasing ambulatory venous hypertension, the risk of a leg ulcer increased. A pressure of 45 to 60 mm Hg after walking indicated a 20% risk of ulceration, and a pressure greater than 60 mm Hg created a risk for ulceration of greater than 50%.[29]

A major contribution to the technique of ambulatory venous pressure measurement was the recording of venous pressure recovery time. Extrapolation of venous pressure recovery times to plethysmographic recovery times advanced the science of investigation of venous disease. After the static venous pressure was recorded, the patient was asked to perform a standard exercise. This consisted of 10 heel-raising movements at the rate of 1 per second, synchronous with a metronome. At the end of the exercise, the patient was told to remain still, and then the recovery of pressure was recorded as refilling time in seconds. That exercise was repeated after inflating a pneumatic cuff at the ankle to occlude the superficial veins. In this way it was thought that the tourniquet separated superficial reflux from deep venous reflux. Thus, limbs with primary varicose veins and competent perforating veins with a short recovery time caused by venous reflux could have recovery time prolonged, whereas limbs with pure deep venous incompetence would have a short recovery time unaffected by application of a superficial tourniquet.

Foot Volumetry

Among the various plethysmographic methods used to investigate venous insufficiency was the technique of foot volumetry. In practice, an open, water-filled bath encompassing the foot was affected by knee-bend exercise. The volume of water displaced during the knee-bend exercise related to venous function. Ejected volume was measured and was related to total foot volume. The rapid phase of refill after exercise was assessed, and that measurement related to foot volume and recovery time. This technique was capable of detecting the presence or absence of venous insufficiency, and the refilling time and refilling volume were indirect measures of venous reflux.[30] However, the method is cumbersome and, as its major flaw, is unable to determine the precise anatomic location of reflux or venous obstruction.

Photoplethysmography

Photoplethysmography uses an infrared transducer to beam light through the epidermis to the subdermal pool of skin capillaries. This pool is largely venous, and therefore, the reflected light is a measure of the venous pool. Various measurement sites have been used for the PPG examination. The most useful was found to be just proximal to the medial malleolus at the ankle. The exercise stimulus to emptying the venous pool was dorsiflexion of the foot while the patient was in the sitting position. The venous return time was found to correlate with ambulatory venous pressure recovery time, and the technique was used with tourniquet application to separate superficial from deep venous reflux.[31] As the measurement was performed on the capillary bed, the examination was highly temperature dependent. The method did not provide an estimation of venous obstruction and could not give a quantitative measure of venous function.

Light Reflection Rheography

A further refinement of the PPG is light reflection rheography. In the rheograph, the sensor head was equipped with a thermistor measuring skin temperature, so that the examination could be performed within the range of 28 to 32°C.[32] As the type of exercise and the measurement sites were comparable to those of PPG, the values obtained were similar. PPG and light reflection rheography gave a measure of combined arterial capillary inflow and capillary venous reflux. The fact that this measure may not reflect whole leg venous function has been stated as a criticism of both methods. Neither method provides a precise anatomic location of reflux and neither can reliably detect obstruction.

Mercury Strain-Gauge Plethysmography

Mercury strain-gauge plethysmography refers to the application of a mercury-filled Silastic rubber tube, which is placed around the limb. Mercury strain-gauge plethysmography has allowed the measurement of volume changes in the calf during exercise and at rest. Either heel-raising or knee-bend exercises can be used, and the method has been thoroughly investigated. Parameters of venous return time and expelled volume measured as mL/100 mL of tissue have been used.[33] As with other methods of plethysmography, mercury strain-gauge plethysmography can detect the presence or absence of venous insufficiency but can only indirectly differentiate reflux from obstruction. None of the plethysmographic methods give a precise anatomic location of reflux but tend to give a global estimate of venous function in the superficial or the deep system.

Air Plethysmography

The development of the air plethysmograph (APG) was in response to limitations of segmental measurements obtained by mercury strain-gauge plethysmography and difficulties with water-displacement plethysmography. The latter provided information on whole leg volume changes but could not be used with exercise, such as heel raising, standing, or walking. Also, gravitationally induced tissue shifts in response to postural changes interfered with segmental measurements. These were less likely to occur with the APG technique.

In practice, the APG has been standardized and consists of a 14-in.-long polyvinyl chloride air chamber. This chamber has a capacity of 5 L and surrounds the whole leg from the knee to the ankle. It is inflated to 6 mm Hg and connected to a pressure transducer, an amplifier, and a recorder. A smaller 1-L bag is placed between the air chamber and the leg and is used for calibration. With the patient supine and with the leg elevated 45 degrees, a recording is obtained. The patient is then asked to stand with the weight on the opposite extremity. The increase in leg volume between leg elevation and dependency is a result of venous filling. This is 100 to 150 mL in normal limbs and 100 to 350 mL in limbs with CVI. An index of filling is obtained by taking 90% of the venous volume and dividing it by the time taken to achieve 90% of filling. This is a measure of the average filling rate and is expressed in mL/sec. A venous filling index of 2 mL/sec or less indicates absence of significant venous reflux and confirms the fact that the veins are filling slowly from arterial inflow. A venous filling index greater than 7 mL/sec is associated with severe skin changes, chronic edema, and even ulceration. Tourniquet testing can be done, and the maneuvers repeated to separate superficial from deep venous reflux. A measure of ejection can be obtained when the patient is standing and does heel-raising movement with the weight on both legs. The volume expelled is called the *ejection fraction* and is calculated by taking the expelled volume divided by total venous volume and multiplying this by 100.

A further estimation of calf blood ejection can be obtained by asking the patient to do 10 heel-raising movements. The volume remaining in the limb is called the *residual volume,* and the residual volume fraction is calculated by dividing the residual volume by the total venous volume and multiplying this by 100. Nicolaides and colleagues[29] have shown a linear correlation between the residual volume fraction and ambulatory venous pressure.

At the present time, the APG techniques are useful in assessing therapeutic interventions, such as compression stockings and surgery. However, specific malfunctioning venous segments cannot be identified or targeted for therapeutic intervention. Investigation of the patient raises concern with one of two problems, alone or in combination. These problems are obstruction to venous flow and reflux of blood distally or outward. The APG can be used to quantify both of these abnormalities.[34] The outflow test using the APG is suitable to determine the presence or absence of outflow. An outflow fraction of less than 35% with the superficial veins occluded has been given as strong evidence for significant deep venous obstruction.[35]

Chronic venous obstruction may, however, be well compensated by the development of large collateral veins. Major venous obstructions, therefore, may produce little physiologic impairment. As has been described previously, advanced tests using the APG are possible. Some investigators have claimed that residual volume fraction, that is, the percentage of blood remaining after heel-raising movements measured by the APG, correlates directly with ambulatory venous pressure. Therefore, the noninvasive APG gives information that is comparable with the gold standard of venous pressure. However, this concept has been challenged.

The accuracy of APG indirect testing as compared with that of venous pressure measurement was challenged by Payne and colleagues[36] in 1993. That presentation compared APG with venous pressure measurements in the assessment of venous disorders and gave disappointing results. Poor correlation was found between venous filling time measured with APG and that derived from direct venous pressure. A similar discrepancy had been reported by Lees and Lambert in a 1992 presentation that was poorly circulated.[37] Those investigators, using ambulatory venous pressure as a standard, studied deep and superficial venous incompetence in 334 limbs in 176 patients. They were able to achieve a sensitivity of only 79% and a specificity of only 70% for the diagnosis of reflux in deep and superficial veins. In assessing pure deep venous incompetence, they found a sensitivity of only 48% and a specificity of 85%. This relatively poor agreement between the two investigations sharply challenged early APG reports of physiologic accuracy.

Lees and Lambert[37] further questioned whether ambulatory venous pressure should be the gold standard for venous insufficiency. They found that venous pressure was actually quite variable. An additional cause of inaccuracy was the inability to reliably occlude the superficial veins with a tourniquet without causing deep venous compression. They summarized their conclusions in a letter to the *British Journal of Surgery* saying, "we believe that the concept of being able to separate patients completely on the basis of measurements such as ambulatory venous pressure, venous refilling time, venous filling index, or residual volume fraction by correlation with the presence of skin changes is unfounded."[38]

Similar questions regarding the use of PPG and quantitative PPG have been raised by Iafrati and associates.[39] His group studied 59 legs in 45 patients with physical examination, quantitative PPG, and duplex ultrasound scanning. They demonstrated that physical examination and quantitative PPG both were 100% specific in detecting greater saphenous vein incompetence at the saphenofemoral junction. However, physical examination had a poor sensitivity of 43%, and quantitative PPG was worse with a sensitivity of 24%. van Bemmelen and colleagues[40] have also reported a poor level of sensitivity of quantitative PPG for venous insufficiency when compared with duplex scanning. They concluded that these results did not warrant the continued use of PPG for surgical decision making in patients with suspected venous insufficiency.

The Middlesex Hospital group in England also questioned the use of PPG indirect testing assessment of venous insufficiency.[41] This group attempted standardization of the PPG tracing in an effort to obtain a more accurate analysis. Even with their modification, the median trace for groups with venous disorders was different from that for normal limbs, but there was a large overlap of the interquartile values, making differentiation of normal from abnormal limbs impossible on the basis of the PPG tracing alone.

Despite advocacy of PPG as a "very simple method for recording changes in local blood volume in the ankle area,"[42] others have found that in a large experience, some 20% of the PPG investigations are not interpretable. This occurs because of inaccuracies in determining the refilling time. Furthermore, agreement between clinical evaluation combined with Doppler ultrasonography and PPG is poor.

In summary, these investigations suggest that indirect methods are not sufficient for routine evaluation of venous insufficiency.[43] It is important to recognize that testing with tourniquets is not reliable. As mentioned previously, if an abnormally short refilling time was found initially but returned to normal with tourniquet occlusion of the greater saphenous vein, it was assumed that there was no significant deep reflux. The accuracy of this assumption has been questioned,[44] and it has been learned that tourniquet application is notoriously inaccurate. Any vein under the tourniquet may be occluded or all may remain patent. Although it had also been thought that refilling time was a good screening examination for the absence or presence of reflux, it has not correlated well with the clinical severity of venous dysfunction.[45] The use of PPG as an initial screening examination has been discredited because it has been found to be only 74% sensitive and 37% specific when compared with descending phlebography.[24] Finally, plethysmography in any form does not aid in planning a definitive surgical approach to individual patient problems.

Duplex Reflux Testing

As is the case with obstructive venous disease, duplex ultrasonography has become the definitive noninvasive test for venous reflux in most medical centers. The use of duplex ultrasonography permits identification of individual veins (via gray-scale imaging) and interrogation of these veins for reflux with spectral or color Doppler imaging (Figs. 24–4 and 24–5). The valves are usually not seen per se, but incompetence is implied by backward flow in response to proximal pressure or gravity. Reverse venous flow of less than 0.5 second is taken as a sign of competency because 95% of normal valves will close in this time or less.[46] Deep, superficial, and perforating veins are readily examined with duplex sonography, permitting the location and extent of reflux to be mapped. Excellent correlation with phlebography has been shown.[47] In addition to being noninvasive, duplex sonography has the advantage of permitting skin marking for preprocedure localization of important perforating veins and the saphenopopliteal junction. The location of these structures can be quite variable.

The exact mechanism of venous valve closure has not been determined. It is not agreed on whether this is a pressure-dependent phenomenon or a venous flow velocity event. A careful study of this event using controlled limb compression revealed interesting findings.[48] When defining valve closure as an abrupt cessation of reverse flow with patients in the supine position, valve closure was achieved only after reverse venous flow velocity exceeded 30 cm/sec. This velocity was not generated by manual compression of the limb or even by a Valsalva maneuver; this

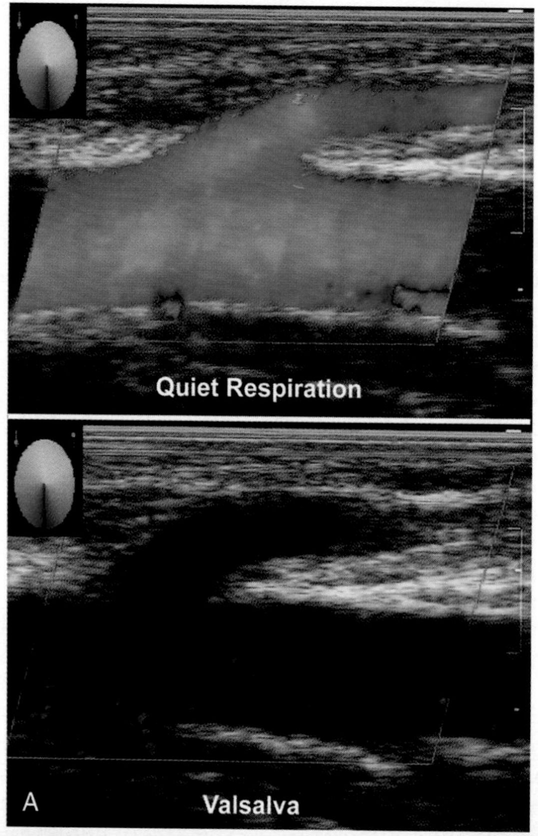

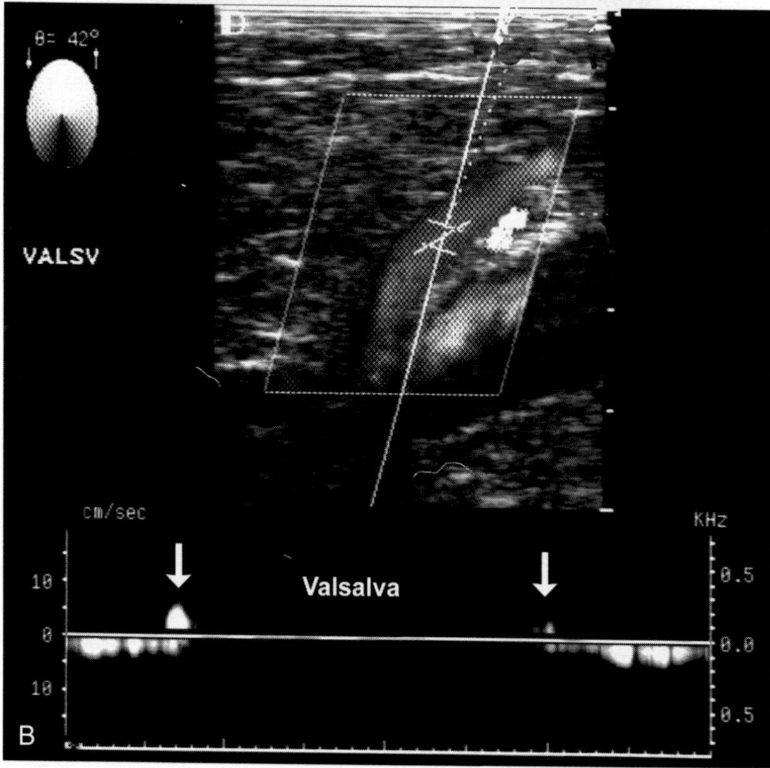

FIGURE 24–4 Normal saphenofemoral junction. *A,* During quiet respiration (*top*), cephalad blood flow is present in the greater saphenous and common femoral veins as indicated by the blue color. With the Valsalva maneuver (*bottom*), flow ceases promptly in both vessels. *B,* Spectral Doppler shows normal cessation of greater saphenous flow with the Valsalva maneuver (*arrows*) and resumption of flow after release of the maneuver.

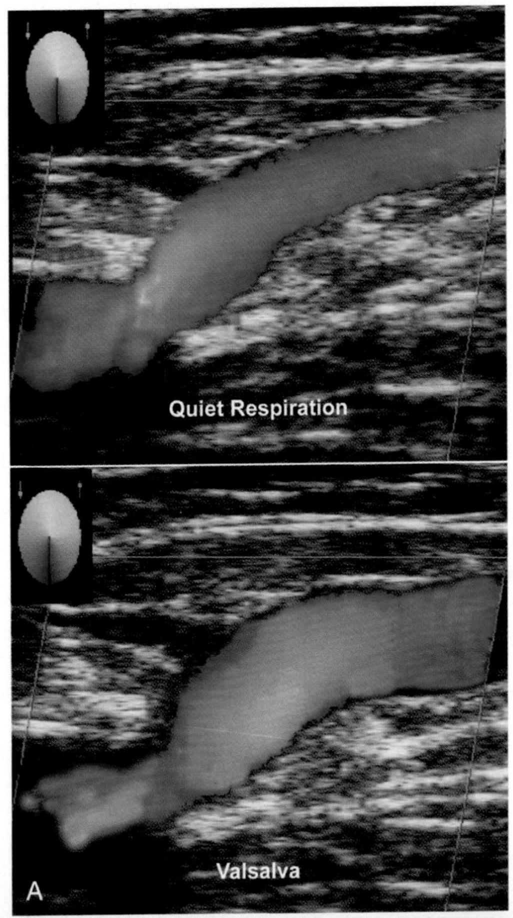

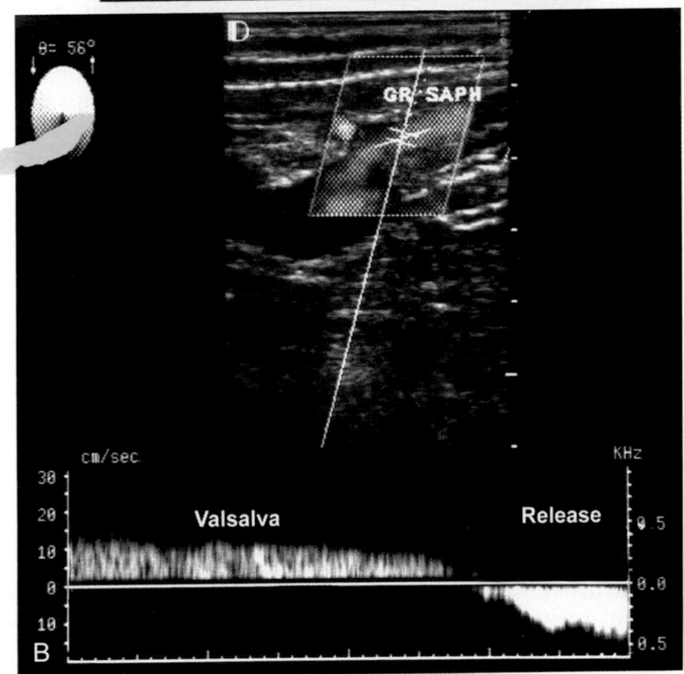

FIGURE 24–5 Greater saphenous vein reflux. *A,* In quiet respiration (*top*), blood flow is cephalad (blue) in the greater saphenous vein. During the Valsalva maneuver (*bottom*), sustained flow reversal (red) is seen in the greater saphenous vein. *B,* Doppler spectrum shows flow reversal during the Valsalva maneuver and the resumption of the normal flow direction with the Valsalva release.

velocity was achieved in the common femoral vein in only 90% of the tested individuals. The Valsalva maneuver produced progressively lower reflux velocities in distal veins, including the profunda femoris, the superficial femoral vein, and the popliteal vein. With reverse velocities lower than 30 cm/sec, the valves did not close and reflux persisted.

Quantitative Measurement of Venous Reflux

During 1989, two reports confirmed the possibility of standardizing tests of venous valve reflux with duplex scanning.[49, 50] The University of Washington group studied patients in the supine and standing positions.[50] The group from the Irvine Laboratory at St. Mary's Hospital, London, examined patients in the standing position and compared results with ambulatory venous pressure measurements.[49]

Both groups used duplex scanning and pneumatic cuffs capable of rapid inflation and deflation. The Washington group used a 24-cm thigh cuff, a 12-cm calf cuff, and a 7-cm foot cuff. The London group used a 10-cm calf cuff. The sites examined included the common femoral vein, the superficial femoral vein, the deep femoral vein, the posterior tibial vein midway between knee and ankle (the posterior tibial vein at the ankle for the Washington group), and the saphenofemoral and saphenopopliteal junctions (the medial aspect of the leg for the London group). Both groups used a standard pressure of 100 mm Hg in the calf cuff to produce cephalad flow, and records were made during deflation and 4 seconds thereafter.

Duplex scanning allows measurement of the diameter of the vessel in longitudinal and cross-sectional views. The Doppler sample volume is adjusted to insonate the whole lumen of the vessel (wall to wall). The cross-sectional area of the vessel is calculated by the system software. The average time velocity of the whole duration of reflux is calculated from the fast Fourier spectrum of the reflux when the angle of insonation and diameter of the vessel are known. Peak reflux velocity is obtained by placing the cursor at the point of peak reflux. Calculation is performed by system software.

The Washington group pointed out that the new duplex test required comparison with a standard, previously accepted test to achieve utility. However, in assessing venous reflux, the historically important tests, such as descending phlebography and recording of ambulatory venous pressures, are themselves flawed. In descending phlebography, the presence of a competent valve in the proximal system prevents evaluation of distal areas. Furthermore, examination in the upright position, as required by descending phlebography, is hampered by the higher specific gravity of the contrast media compared with that of blood. In addition, the examinations are not usually done after calf muscle pump contraction.

Ambulatory venous pressure measurements are flawed by the presence of deep venous obstruction at any level. Also, as indicated previously, the use of tourniquets during precise measurement recording fails to accurately differentiate deep, superficial, and perforator incompetence.[51]

Although the St. Mary's group described the taking of ambulatory venous pressure measurements and the performance of ascending phlebography, they failed to correlate these studies precisely with duplex quantification of venous reflux. On the other hand, they did verify the reproducibility of the duplex technique by studying seven legs 6 times on the same day. Also, in patients with severe venous stasis, separation of those with liposclerosis and ulceration from those without was demonstrated by flow at peak reflux. Reflux greater than 10 mL/sec correlated with severe skin and subcutaneous changes. Further, the St. Mary's studies showed that perforator vein reflux was important, but it was not possible to quantify perforator flow because of the irregular course of perforating veins and their location in the leg, which prevented use of a pneumatic cuff.

Scripps Memorial Hospital Method

Because of our long interest in venous pathophysiology, we quickly adopted the quantitative methods suggested by the Strandness and Nicolaides groups.[52] Patients were examined in the standing position supported by a frame with weight mainly on the opposite leg. The leg under examination was kept in a relaxed position with slight knee flexion.

TABLE 24–3 NEW CLINICAL CLASSIFICATION OF VENOUS DISEASE

Class	Symptoms and Physical Findings
0	No visible or palpable signs of venous disease
1	Telangiectasias or reticular veins
2	Varicose veins
3	Edema
4	Skin changes (pigmentation, eczema, lipodermatosclerosis)
5	Skin changes with healed ulcer
6	Skin changes with active ulceration

Modified from Phillips GWL, Paige J, Molan MP: A comparison of colour duplex ultrasound with venography and varicography in the assessment of varicose veins. Clin Radiol 50:20–25, 1995.

A duplex scanner* recorded the data. An automatic cuff inflator† was used for rapid inflation and deflation of the cuffs, which were placed at five different levels on the limb. A 10-cm thigh cuff inflated to 80 mm Hg was used proximally, and a 10-cm calf cuff inflated to 100 mm Hg was used distally. The cuffs were inflated for approximately 3 seconds and deflated within 0.3 second. A 5-MHz imaging probe attached to a 5-MHz pulsed Doppler ultrasound crystal was used to examine individual veins. Examinations were confined to the saphenofemoral and saphenopopliteal junctions. The short saphenous and popliteal veins were examined first. The probe was placed on the skin in the popliteal fossa longitudinally and the position adjusted so that the pulsating popliteal artery, the popliteal vein, and the short saphenous vein were clearly identified. Anatomic variations were recorded and the sample volume was placed on the popliteal vein 2 to 4 cm distal to the junction with the short saphenous vein. The Doppler angle was kept at approximately 45 degrees to the vessel axis, the calf cuff inflated and deflated, and the examination recording obtained. The examination was repeated by positioning the sample volume in the short saphenous vein 2 to 4 cm distal to the saphenopopliteal junction, and relevant data were obtained. If large tributary veins such as the gastrocnemius veins were found to be incompetent, they were assessed in the same manner.

Next, the saphenofemoral junction was examined with the patient facing the examiner. The femoral vein, long saphenous vein, and saphenofemoral junction were identified and the reflux was quantitated by the techniques described previously. The data obtained for each vein included the vein diameter, area, average flow (mL/min), peak reflux flow (cm/sec), and duration of reflux (seconds).

Table 24–3 shows the current clinical classification of venous disease, and Table 24–4 shows the characteristics of venous reflux in limbs in clinical classes 0 through 6.[53] As Table 24–4 demonstrates, a disappointing lack of correlation of reflux quantitation with clinical grades of venous stasis severity is evident. Possibly this can be explained by the techniques used in our early experience. At that time, only femoral and popliteal levels were interrogated. At present, other segments of the saphenous vein and the deep veins are investigated.

This early study emphasized several facts that previous studies could not show. Chief among these was the demonstration of regional venous reflux, that is, refluxing and nonrefluxing segments within the same vein. In the greater saphenous system, regional reflux was found in the upper anteromedial calf, where anterior and posterior tributaries to the saphenous vein became varicose without proximal greater saphenous incompetence. The second most important area of regional or segmental reflux was found in the distal thigh, where reflux could be demonstrated and clusters of varicosities seen without proximal saphenofemoral junction incompetence. Clearly, as shown by the early experience, axial venous incompetence was not an all-or-none phenomenon. Incompetence of the lesser saphenous vein was also found to be more often segmental than not. When found to be incompetent, it was the proximal segment of the lesser saphenous vein that was refluxing in more than 50% of patients. In at least one third of cases of lesser saphenous venous incompetence, the distal

TABLE 24–4 REFLUX IN GREATER SAPHENOUS VEIN (MEAN VALUES) ACCORDING TO CLINICAL CLASSIFICATION OF LIMB

	Clinical Class			
Measure	*0*	*1, 2*	*3*	*4, 5, 6*
Diameter (cm)	0.49	0.76	0.82	0.85
Area (cm^2)	0.2	0.56	0.69	0.58
Volume (mL/sec)	—	9.9	7.1	8.0
Peak velocity (cm/sec)	—	35.95	41.3	21.8
Time (sec*)	—	3.8	4.2	4.16

* Sensored at greater than 8 sec.

* Ultramark 9, Advanced Technology Laboratories, Bothell, WA.

† Hokanson, Bellevue, WA.

TABLE 24–5 CLINICAL CLASSIFICATION ASSIGNED TO EACH LIMB BEFORE DUPLEX STUDY

Measure	Clinical Class 0	1	2	3
Number of limbs (%)	51 (19)	139 (52)	34 (13)	42 (16)
Male	7	24	13	26
Female	44	115	21	15

half of the lesser saphenous vein was normal. Similarly, varicosities in the lesser saphenous distribution sometimes arise from veins other than the lesser saphenous vein, one of which is the ascending connection to the greater saphenous system (the vein of Giacomini). Gastrocnemius veins also contribute to lesser saphenous reflux rather than the saphenopopliteal junction.

Furthermore, the early experience made it clear that duplex scanning had its greatest value in the study of patients with recurrent varicose veins. Patients who had previous varicose vein surgery and who exhibited recurrent varicosities presented anatomic problems that were different and more difficult than those seen in patients with primary reflux. For instance, duplex scans identified retained stumps of saphenous veins, reflux through tributaries to these stumps, and origin of varicosities from major perforating veins outside of the normal anatomic locations.

QUANTIFICATION AND CLINICAL STATUS

The objective of quantification of venous pathologic function is to stratify patient limbs in such a manner that appropriate therapeutic interventions can be performed. The pneumatic cuff deflation technique allowed, for the first time, accurate quantification of various parameters of venous function. Therefore, results obtained by this method were applied through the clinical status of limbs using the then-existent clinical classification.[54]

A total of 133 patients (35 men, 98 women) were chosen for examination by duplex scanning, preliminary to decide treatment for their symptoms of venous stasis disease. Each was assigned to a clinical grade of severity of venous stasis before results of the study were known. Patients with arteriovenous malformations, known venous obstruction, or lymphedema as a cause of symptoms were excluded from the study. Patients with telangiectatic web veins; protuberant, saccular varicosities; lipodermatosclerosis; and venous ulceration were included. Patients were examined by using the technique described previously.

The data obtained for each vein in each location included vein diameter (obtained from intima to intima on the frozen image), vein area, average flow (mL/min), peak reflux flow (cm^3/sec), and duration of reflux (seconds). The normal value for the maximum duration of reflux was 0.5 second. The duration of reflux was measured for up to 8 seconds in cases of prolonged reflux. Statistical analysis was performed using the two-tailed Student *t*-test.

Table 24–5 gives the total number of limbs studied according to the clinical class assigned to each limb. Table 24–6 explains the clinical classification used in this study. Men in this study population were found to present in a higher clinical class (class 1.8, SD 1.0) than the women (class 1.0, SD 0.8; $P < .001$).

Table 24–7 gives the total population of limbs according to presence or absence of venous reflux. These are further arranged according to the sex of each patient. Vein diameter in refluxing veins was compared with veins not exhibiting reflux. Of 1013 veins studied, 266 showed venous reflux and 747 did not. Reflux was identified in 111 greater saphenous veins, 57 common femoral veins, 50 popliteal veins, and 48 lesser saphenous veins. An increased vein diameter was associated with reflux in the femoral, greater saphenous, and lesser saphenous veins. This observation did not prove to be true in the popliteal vein. A comparison of individual

TABLE 24–6 ABRIDGED EXPLANATION OF CLINICAL CLASSIFICATION

Class	Symptoms	Physical Findings
0	None	None
1	Mild swelling Heaviness Vein dilatation	Ankle edema <1 cm Dilated superficial veins Normal skin
2	Moderate swelling Heaviness Varicosities	Edema >1 cm Multiple dilated veins Mild pigmentation Mild liposclerosis
3	Severe swelling Calf pain and claudication	Edema >2 cm Multiple varicosities Marked pigmentation Severe liposclerosis

TABLE 24–7 COMPARISON OF VEIN DIAMETERS IN LIMBS WITH AND WITHOUT VENOUS REFLUX

Vein	No Reflux		Reflux		P Value
	n	*Diameter (cm)**	*n*	*Diameter (cm)**	
Total Population					
CFV	202	1.28 (0.25)	57	1.40 (0.31)	.008
GSV	116	0.58 (0.15)	111	0.76 (0.25)	<.001
POP	212	0.88 (0.19)	50	0.89 (0.24)	>.30 (NS)
LSV	215	0.45 (0.14)	48	0.57 (0.22)	≤.001
Females					
CFV	161	1.22 (0.22)	30	1.22 (0.27)	>.30 (NS)
GSV	84	0.57 (0.14)	83	0.75 (0.23)	<.001
POP	168	0.86 (0.18)	24	0.74 (0.18)	.003
LSV	173	0.43 (0.12)	20	0.53 (0.20)	.036
Males					
CFV	41	1.52 (0.21)	27	1.60 (0.20)	.14 (NS)
GSV	32	0.61 (0.17)	28	0.81 (0.31)	.005
POP	44	0.93 (0.21)	26	1.03 (0.20)	.061 (NS)
LSV	42	0.53 (0.18)	28	0.60 (0.24)	.228 (NS)

n = number of subjects; CFV = common femoral vein; GSV = greater saphenous vein; POP = popliteal vein; LSV = lesser saphenous vein; NS = not significant.

* Results expressed as mean (SD).

veins showed that men had a larger mean diameter of each vein than women. As indicated, men presented in a higher clinical class at the time of the study. Note the unexplained inverse relationship of vein diameter to reflux in the popliteal vein of women in this study.

Table 24–8 shows the percentage of veins exhibiting venous reflux in limbs grouped according to their clinical classifications. As can be seen in the table, an increased percentage of veins refluxing was seen as the clinical stage of venous reflux increased.

Table 24–9 shows that venous reflux was found in limbs that were asymptomatic and that this reflux was confined to the femoral and greater saphenous veins. As manifestations of venous stasis increased, a greater proportion of axial veins were found to be incompetent. In all clinical classes, the greater saphenous vein was most frequently incompetent.

The volume of reflux flow tended to be greater with increasing clinical classification, but no statistical correlation was found. Velocity of reflux tended to increase with clinical class in the common femoral vein, but this was not found consistently in other veins. The duration of reflux did not correlate with the clinical class.

There were certain trends in this study that may have importance. An increased vein diameter, for example, was associated with reflux. This was true particularly in the femoral, greater, and lesser saphenous veins. It is of some interest that men have a larger mean diameter of each vein than women, but this observation was flawed because the men presented with a more severe degree of venous stasis at the time of study.

Of some importance to the study of CVI was the finding that increased manifestations of chronic venous stasis were associated with a greater proportion of axial reflux through

TABLE 24–8 PERCENTAGE OF REFLUXING VEINS RANGED ACCORDING TO CLINICAL CLASSIFICATION OF AFFECTED LIMBS

Vein	Class 0		Class 1		Class 2		Class 3	
	No. Limbs	*%**	*No. Limbs*	*%**	*No. Limbs*	*%**	*No. Limbs*	*%**
CVF	51	2 (14)	136	21 (41)	34	34 (43)	40	40 (51)
GSV	46	9 (28)	125	62 (49)	28	57 (50)	31	31 (51)
POP	51	0	139	11 (31)	34	38 (49)	42	52 (51)
LSV	51	0	139	11 (31)	34	29 (46)	42	55 (50)

CFV = common femoral vein, GSV = greater saphenous vein, POP = popliteal vein, LSV = lesser saphenous vein.

* Results expressed as mean (SD); percentage = (no. refluxing veins/total no. veins) × 100.

TABLE 24-9 CORRELATION OF CLINICAL CLASSIFICATION WITH REFLUX VELOCITY—VOLUME AND DURATION (TIME)

	Class 0		Class 1		Class 2		Class 3	
Vein	*n*	*Mean (SD)*	*n*	*Mean (SD)*	*n*	*Mean (SD)*	*n*	*Mean (SD)*
CFV								
Volume (mL/sec)	1	4.0	27	13.8 (7.9)	7	26.3 (16.6)	20	20.9 (20.0)
Velocity (cm/sec)	1	10	28	17.6 (14.2)	8	23.4 (20.9)	20	28.1 (22.1)
Time (sec)	1	2.0	28	1.7 (0.85)	7	2.2 (1.2)	19	2.0 (0.78)
GSV								
Volume (mL/sec)	4	6.7 (3.3)	77	9.3 (11.1)	14	12.8 (16.8)	14	5.2 (5.7)
Velocity (cm/sec)	4	31.5 (12.7)	77	38.5 (29.2)	16	34.2 (32.3)	15	25.8 (15.0)
Time (sec)	4	3.8 (1.8)	77	3.8 (2.1)	16	3.9 (2.6)	15	3.2 (1.9)
POP								
Volume (mL/sec)	0		14	6.1 (3.3)	13	5.0 (2.5)	20	11.2 (9.5)
Velocity (cm/sec)	0		15	36.6 (29.4)	13	25.6 (16.1)	22	43.2 (31.0)
Time (sec)	0		15	0.45 (1.9)	13	3.9 (2.7)	22	3.1 (1.1)
LSV								
Volume (mL/sec)	0		15	3.2 (2.4)	6	1.3 (1.0)	22	5.2 (4.9)
Velocity (cm/sec)	0		15	33.8 (31.0)	10	29.0 (24.1)	23	42.1 (25.9)
Time (sec)	0		15	5.9 (3.1)	10	5.4 (2.7)	23	4.2 (1.9)

n = number of subjects; CFV = common femoral vein; GSV = greater saphenous vein; POP = popliteal vein; LSV = lesser saphenous vein.

the saphenous veins. In all classes of severity of venous insufficiency, the greater saphenous vein was most frequently identified as the incompetent vein.

Quantification of reflux was disappointing. The volume of reflux tended to be greater with increasing clinical classification, but this was not documented statistically. Similarly, the velocity of reflux tended to increase with the clinical classes, particularly in the common femoral vein, but this was not consistent in other veins. Quantification of reflux proved to be a cumbersome technique requiring two technicians, yet it did reveal some important physiologic changes. For the first time, it was uncovered that femoral venous reflux could be abolished by greater saphenous stripping.[55] Documentation of ablation of superficial femoral vein reflux by saphenectomy and varicectomy was an important finding that stimulated study of limbs with severe CVI. Corroboration of these observations was achieved, thus confirming this to be an important physiologic fact that might affect treatment of patients.[56]

Increased dilatation of the deep venous system accompanying superficial venous reflux had been reported by investigators on the European continent as early as 1970. This was thought to be the most important complication of superficial reflux. Because of the techniques in use in the 1970s and early 1980s, this was considered to be a purely radiologic diagnosis. An explanation for the deep venous incompetence accompanying superficial venous reflux was that the increased volume of blood flow directed distally re-entered the venous circulation through normal perforating veins. This increased venous volume was thought to elongate and kink the femoral and popliteal veins as well as the femoropopliteal junction. Measurements actually revealed the popliteal venous diameter to be one third larger in limbs with severe reflux than in limbs with lesser or no reflux. The limitations of phlebography as a method of assessment of deep vein reflux hampered development of the new knowledge that deep vein reflux could be removed by superficial vein stripping.

A further observation on the pathophysiology of venous reflux was revealed by duplex testing. Proximal femoral reflux adversely affected distal venous function.[57] When femoral venous reflux was absent in men, only 14 of 69 limbs had popliteal reflux, but when femoral vein reflux was present, 19 of 33 limbs had popliteal venous reflux (20.3% as compared with 57.5%). Similarly, when femoral vein reflux was absent in women, only 33 of 304 limbs had popliteal venous reflux; however, when femoral vein reflux was present, 12 of 48 limbs also had popliteal venous reflux (10.9% as compared with 25%).

The cumbersome nature of quantitative duplex examination using pneumatic cuff deflation discouraged many from using this technique. Instead, calf compression and the Valsalva maneuver were used. This allowed the examination to be done by a single technician much more quickly. Before turning to this much more simple method, however, it was necessary to corroborate the less cumbersome techniques with the quantitative results obtained by the pneumatic cuff deflation method. This was done by the Strandness group[58] in a study of 134 limbs in 67 patients. Both limb compression and the Valsalva maneuver were used to elicit reflux. The maneuvers, of course, were difficult to standardize. With the cuff inflation/deflation method, the normal time-to-valve closure was corroborated once again at less than 0.5 second. The specificity of the Valsalva maneuver and manual compression was very high whether used alone or in combination. Specificity exceeded 85% with the patient supine, but sensitivity was considerably reduced in the supine position. Sensitivity of the Valsalva maneuver was substantially decreased if more cephalad valves were competent, as would be expected. Manual compression achieved sensitivity in the popliteal vein of 73%, but it was surprisingly low for proximal segments, such as the common femoral vein, superficial femoral vein, and greater saphenous vein. Overall, however, it was found that the prevalence of reflux was equivalent to that obtained by the standing, cuff-deflation technique, as revealed by the Valsalva maneuver, in diseased common femoral vein segments and manual compression in diseased posterior tibial vein segments.

The grading of the degree of reflux and methods used to produce reflux are not yet standardized for duplex testing. Some laboratories merely report the presence or absence of reflux in a particular vein. Others quantitate the various parameters, including the duration of backflow, peak velocity of backflow, or the total backflow (time-average velocity × area) from all incompetent veins.[46, 48, 49] The second nonstandardized element of venous reflux testing by duplex sonography is related to the first. This is the position of the patient during examination. Some laboratories use a 15-degree reverse Trendelenburg position and a Valsalva maneuver to stimulate reflux in the proximal femoral vein. Proximal manual compression of the limb is used for the more distal vein segments. Other laboratories study the patient standing without weight bearing on the examined leg and employ the pneumatic cuff technique.

Two comparisons of these methods have been reported, as noted previously. For determining the presence or absence of reflux, both were judged to be equal.[59] However, for the quantification of reflux, the standing, cuff inflation/deflation method was superior.[60] This is logical because the standing, cuff-deflation technique produces a reproducible stimulus to reflux. The cuff is a uniform size, thus the displaced venous pool is constant. Likewise, the ultimate stimulus to reflux, gravity, is also a constant. The retrograde acceleration of blood produced by a Valsalva maneuver or by squeezing the limb is variable. The standing quantified method, however, is more time-consuming, requires more equipment, and usually requires two examiners. There is also controversy as to whether or not quantification provides more useful information on how to treat a patient and how well quantification correlates with the severity of the clinical presentation.[61] Again, this may be a fault of clinical classification.

Popliteal Fossa Anatomy

Duplex ultrasound examination of the popliteal fossa has revealed a remarkable variety of anatomic variations. These are of importance to the surgeon who approaches the lesser saphenous vein at its junction with the popliteal vein, and duplex identification of this junction should precede each surgical intervention (Figs. 24–6 and 24–7). A variety of anatomic configurations have been uncovered by duplex sonography.[62] The lesser saphenous vein was found to enter the popliteal vein alone in a majority of cases (57.8%). The vein of Giacomini was found to progress cephalad from that junction in an additional 15.7%, and both types allowed exploration of the lesser saphenous vein at the popliteal crease to proceed successfully. However, the lesser saphenous vein was seen to proceed far proximally and enter the superficial femoral vein in 10.9% of examinations, and gastrocnemius veins were found to be important in another 14%. The lesser saphenous vein was found to enter the popliteal vein below the popliteal skin crease in 1.2% of cases.

Perforating Veins

Incompetent perforating veins can also be identified by duplex sonography.[63] Color-coded duplex sonography is particularly useful (Fig. 24–8). One looks for veins coursing between the deep and superficial veins, and then during manual compression and re-

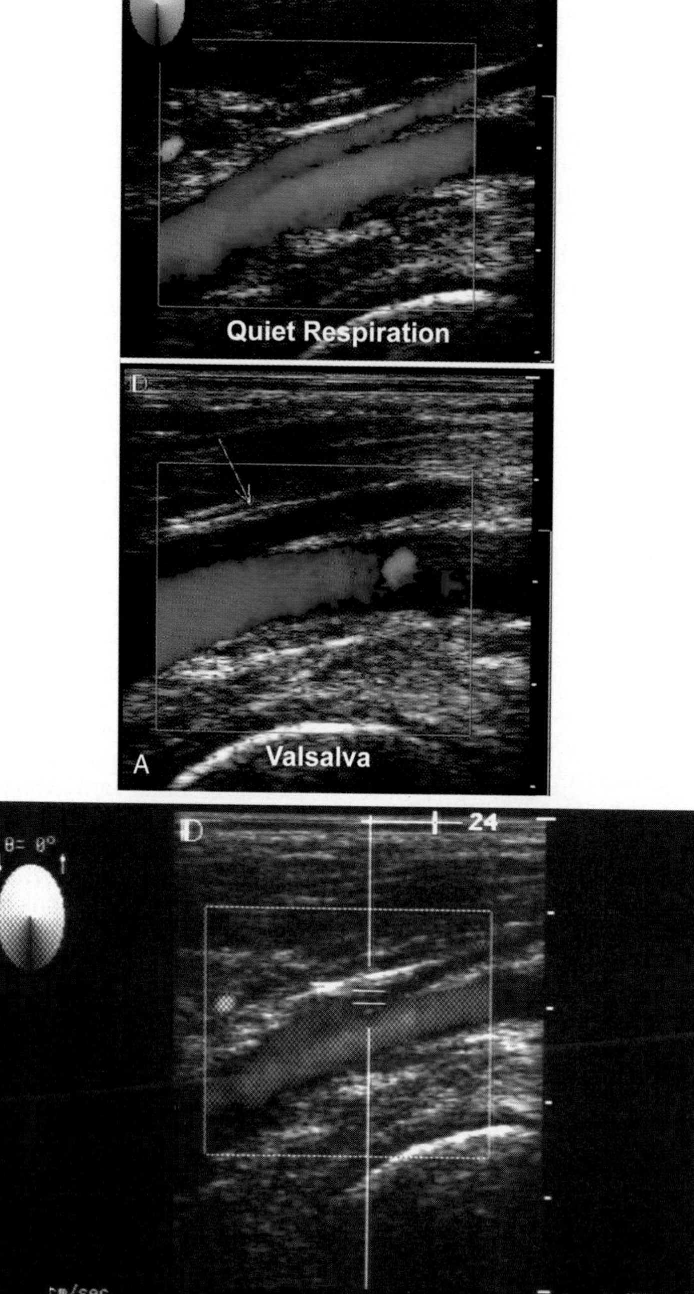

FIGURE 24–6 Competent lesser saphenous vein. *A,* With quiet respiration (*top*), blood flow is cephalad (blue) in the lesser saphenous and popliteal veins. With the Valsalva maneuver (*bottom*), flow ceases promptly in the lesser saphenous vein and a little more slowly in the popliteal vein. *B,* Doppler spectrum shows prompt cessation of blood flow in a competent lesser saphenous vein with the Valsalva maneuver.

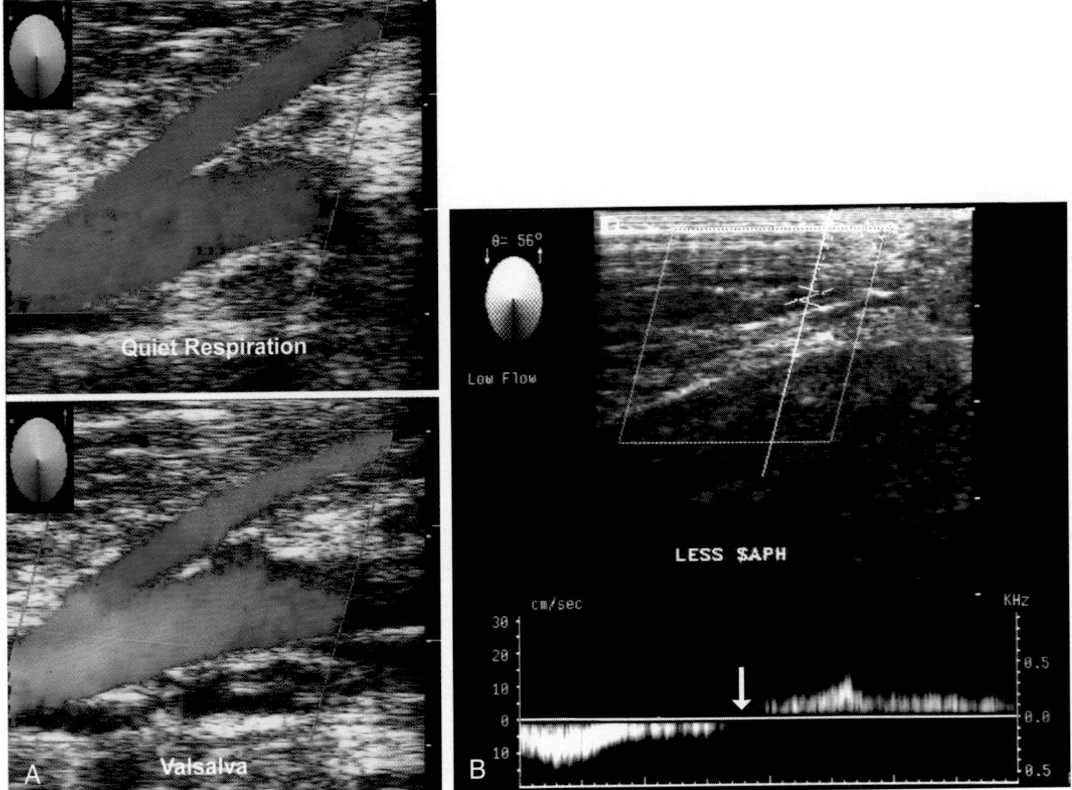

FIGURE 24–7 Lesser saphenous and popliteal vein reflux. *A,* Normal, cephalad flow (blue) is seen in the lesser saphenous and popliteal veins with quiet respiration (*top*). Flow reversal occurs in both veins with the Valsalva maneuver (*bottom*). *B,* With compression proximal to the transducer (*arrow*), lesser saphenous vein flow reverses (above baseline).

lease, one looks for bidirectional flow. Compression can be applied proximal or distal to the duplex interrogation site. A tourniquet can be applied, and compression can be exerted proximally if there is deep venous insufficiency. The technique of searching for perforating veins with outward flow has not been standardized.[64] Most incompetent perforating veins are larger than competent ones. In one study, all perforating veins larger than 4 mm in diameter were incompetent, and all those less than 3 mm were competent.[65]

Testing all perforating veins in every patient is time-consuming. In clinical practice, a search for perforating veins can be limited to limbs with lipodermatosclerosis or ulceration. In these cases, corrective surgery may be planned, and the detection of incompetent veins beneath the damaged skin or just proximal encourages surgical intervention.

RECOMMENDED TECHNIQUES

Although there are many tests of venous dysfunction, in practice only a few tests need to be done.

Telangiectasias

Before any form of treatment, including sclerotherapy, the limb should be evaluated clinically, both by inspection and palpation and by objective documentation. Objective documentation for limbs with only telangiectasias and reticular varicosities can be done with continuous wave Doppler imaging. The objective of this examination is to rule out axial reflux through the greater and lesser saphenous veins. The presence of such reflux negates the value of sclerotherapy treatment. In brief, the presence of axial reflux has been

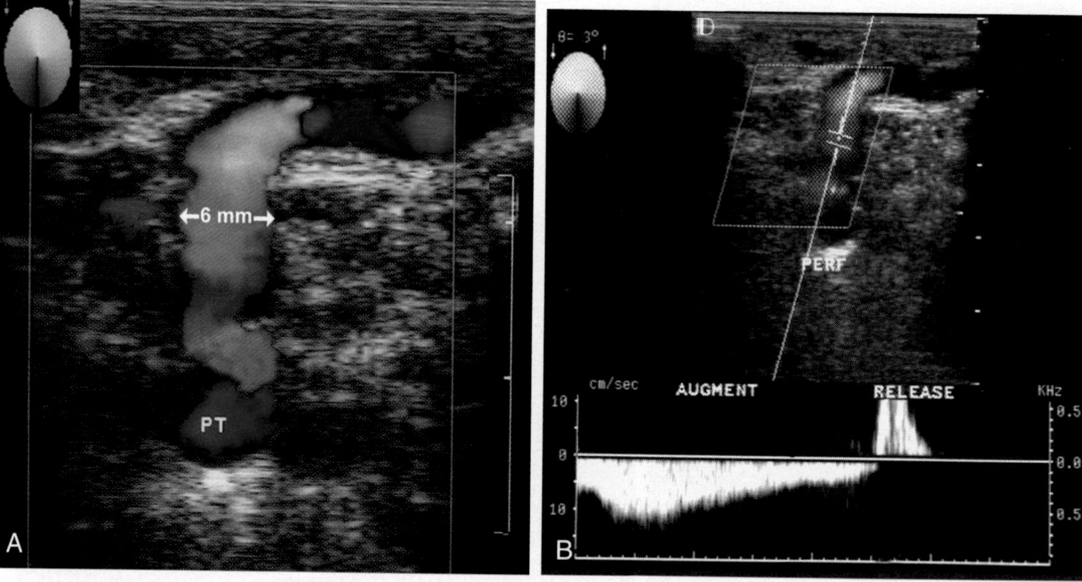

FIGURE 24–8 Incompetent perforator vein. *A,* Color-Doppler image shows a markedly dilated (6 mm) perforator vein that communicates with a superficial varix. Flow is reversed, from the posterior tibial (PT) vein toward the skin. *B,* With compression of the calf distal to the transducer (distal augmentation), sustained flow reversal (downward deflection) is seen on spectral Doppler examination.

found to correlate with recurrence of venous varicosities treated by sclerotherapy.

Varicose Veins

For the most part, varicose veins are treated by formal surgery or ambulatory phlebectomy. Formal surgery consists of ligation and division of saphenous veins at their junctions and stripping out the involved segments according to the individual practice of the surgeon. Therefore, duplex reflux examination is suggested for every limb as part of the preoperative study. The objective of this examination is to document venous reflux and provide some estimate of prognosis. For example, if a limb harboring varicose veins is found to have deep venous reflux in addition to axial saphenous venous reflux, the prognosis for cure of the symptoms may be guarded. If deep venous reflux persists after correction of the superficial reflux, certainly the chance for recurrence of varicosities and the persistence of symptoms is very good. However, if the deep venous reflux ceases after the correction of superficial reflux, then the prognosis may be quite good. Thus, a preoperative and postoperative study in patients with both superficial and deep reflux is recommended.

Chronic Venous Insufficiency

Duplex reflux study is recommended for limbs with severe CVI. A search for perforating veins on the medial and lateral aspects of the limb should be added to this examination. Limbs with severe CVI have been found to have a large component of superficial reflux as a cause of the cutaneous stigmata. Furthermore, perforating veins associated with the areas of lipodermatosclerosis or ulceration may be the target of surgical intervention. Therefore, the perforating veins should be located and measured from the sole of the heel cephalad, as an aid to their detection at the time of operation. Most operations for severe CVI consist of the correction of all areas of superficial venous reflux as well as the interruption of the perforating veins.

REFERENCES

1. Leers SA, Blackburn DR, Burnham SJ, et al: Vascular technology in evolution: Results of the 1994 ARDMS task survey. J Vasc Technol 19:127–145, 1995.
2. Virchow R: Die Cellularpathologic. *In* Hirschewald A (ed): Ihrer Begrundung auf physiologische und pathologische Gewebelehere. Berlin, A. Hirschewald, 1858.
3. Jorgensen JO, Hanel KC, Morgan AM, Hunt JM: The incidence of deep venous thrombosis in patients

with superficial thrombophlebitis of the lower limbs. J Vasc Surg 18:70–73, 1993.
4. Prountijos P, Bastounis E, Hadjinikolaou L, et al: Superficial venous thrombosis of the lower extremities coexisting with deep venous thrombosis. Int Angiol 10:63–65, 1991.
5. Lutter KS, Kerr TM, Roedersheimer LR, et al: Superficial thrombophlebitis diagnosed by duplex scanning. Surgery 110:42–46, 1991.
6. Skillman JJ, Kent KC, Porter DH, Kim D: Simultaneous occurrence of superficial and deep thrombophlebitis in the lower extremity. J Vasc Surg 11:818–824, 1990.
7. Bergqvist D, Jaroszewski H: Deep vein thrombosis in patients with superficial thrombophlebitis of the leg. Br Med J 292:658–659, 1986.
8. Bendick PJ, Ryan R, Alpers M, et al: Clinical signs of superficial thrombophlebitis. J Vasc Technol 19:57–61, 1995.
9. Moser KK: Pulmonary embolism. *In* Murray J, Nadel J (eds): Respiratory Medicine, 2nd ed. Philadelphia, WB Saunders, 1994, p 653.
10. Haeger K: Problems of acute deep venous thrombosis. The interpretation of signs and symptoms. Angiology 20:219–223, 1969.
11. Browse NL, Burnand KG, Lea Thomas M: Diseases of the Veins: Pathology, Diagnosis, and Treatment. London, Edward Arnold, 1988, p 478.
12. Salzman EW: Venous thrombosis made easy. N Engl J Med 314:847–848, 1986.
13. Mattos MA, Londrey GL, Leutz DW, et al: Color-flow duplex scanning for the surveillance and diagnosis of acute deep venous thrombosis. J Vasc Surg 15:366–376, 1992.
14. Hillner BE, Philbrick JT, Becker DM: Optimal management of suspected lower extremity deep vein thrombosis. Arch Intern Med 152:165–175, 1992.
15. Moreno-Cabral R, Kistner RL, Nordyke RA: Importance of calf vein thrombophlebitis. Surgery 80:735–742, 1976.
16. Lohr JM, James KV, Deshmukh RM, Hasselfeld KA: Calf vein thrombi are not a benign finding. Am J Surg 170:86–90, 1995.
17. Solis MM, Ranval TJ, Nix ML, et al: Is anticoagulation indicated for asymptomatic postoperative calf vein thrombosis? J Vasc Surg 16:414–419, 1992.
18. Rose SC, Zwiebel WJ, Miller FJ: Distribution of acute lower extremity deep venous thrombosis in symptomatic and asymptomatic patients: Imaging implications. J Ultrasound Med 13:243–250, 1994.
19. Markel A, Manzo RA, Bergelin RO, Strandness DE Jr: Pattern and distribution of thrombi in acute venous thrombosis. Arch Surg 127:305–309, 1992.
20. Sarpa MS, Messina LM, Smith M, et al: Reliability of venous duplex scanning to image the iliac veins and to diagnose iliac vein thrombosis in patients suspected of having acute deep venous thrombosis. J Vasc Technol 15:299–302, 1991.
21. Duddy MJ, McHugo JM. Duplex ultrasound of the common femoral vein in pregnancy and puerperium. Br J Radiol 64:785–791, 1991.
22. Schultz-Ehrenburg U, Weindorf N, Matthew U, Hirche H: New epidemiological findings with regard to initial stages of varicose veins (Bochum study I-III). *In* Raymond-Martimbeau P, Prescott R, Zummo M (eds): Phlébology 92. Paris, John Libbey Eurotext, 1992, pp 234–236.
23. van Ramshorst B, van Bemmelen PS, Hoeneveld H, Eikelboom BC: The development of valvular incompetence after deep vein thrombosis: A followup study with duplex scanning. J Vasc Surg 20:1059–1066, 1994.
24. Raju S, Fredericks R: Evaluation of methods for detecting venous reflux. Perspectives in venous insufficiency. Arch Surg 125:1463–1467, 1990.
25. Pollack AA, Wood EH: Venous pressure in the saphenous vein at the ankle in man during exercise and changes in posture. J Appl Physiol 1:649–662, 1949.
26. DeCamp PT, Schramel RJ, Ray CJ, et al: Ambulatory venous pressure determinations in postphlebitic and related syndromes. Surgery 29:44–70, 1951.
27. Decamp PT, Ward JA, Ochsner A: Ambulatory venous pressure studies in postphlebitic and other disease states. Surgery 29:365–380, 1951.
28. Hojensgard IC, Sturup H: Static and dynamic pressures in superficial and deep veins of the lower extremity in man. Acta Physiol Scand 27:49–67, 1952.
29. Nicolaides A, Christopoulos D, Vasdekis S: Progress in the investigation of chronic venous insufficiency. Ann Vasc Surg 3:278–292, 1989.
30. Thulesius O, Norgren L, Gjores JE: Foot volumetry: A new method for objective assessment of oedema and venous function. Vasa 2:325–329, 1973.
31. Abramowitz HB, Queral LA, Flinn WR, et al: The use of photoplethysmography in the assessment of venous insufficiency: A comparison to venous pressure measurements. Surgery 86:434–441, 1979.
32. O'Donnell TF, McEnroe CS, Heggerick P: Chronic venous insufficiency. Surg Clin North Am 70:159–180, 1990.
33. Struckmann JR: Ambulatory strain gauge plethysmography: Correlation to symptoms and skin changes in patients with venous insufficiency. Phlebology 2:75–80, 1987.
34. Bundens WP: Use of the air plethysmograph in the evaluation and treatment of patients with venous stasis disease. Dermatol Surg 21:67–69, 1995.
35. Christopoulos D, Nicolaides A, Szendro G: Venous reflux: Quantification and correlation with the clinical severity of chronic venous disease. Br J Surg 75:352–356, 1988.
36. Payne S, Thrush A, London N, et al: Venous assessment using air plethysmography: A comparison with clinical examination, ambulatory venous pressure measurement, and duplex scanning. Br J Surg 80:967–970, 1993.
37. Lees TA, Lambert D: A comparative study of air plethysmography and Doppler colour flow imaging with ambulatory venous pressure measurements in the diagnosis of venous reflux in the lower limb. *In* Raymond-Martimbeau P, Prescott RM, Zummo M (eds): Phlébologie 92. Paris, John Libbey Eurotext, 1992, pp 594–596.
38. Lees TA, Lambert D: Venous assessment using air plethysmography: A comparison with clinical examination, ambulatory venous pressure measurement, and duplex scanning. Br J Surg 81:314, 1994.
39. Iafrati MD, O'Donnell TF Jr, Kunkemueller A, et al: Clinical examination, duplex ultrasound, and plethysmography for varicose veins. Phlebology 9:114–118, 1994.
40. van Bemmelen PS, van Ramshorst B, Eikelbook BC: Photoplethysmography reexamined: Lack of correlation with duplex scanning. Surgery 112:544–548, 1992.
41. Sarin S, Shields DA, Scurr JH, Coleridge Smith PD: Photoplethysmography: A valuable tool in the as-

sessment of venous dysfunction? J Vasc Surg 16:154–162, 1992.
42. Fronek A: Photoplethysmography in the diagnosis of venous disease. Dermatol Surg 21:64–66, 1995.
43. Rutgers PH, Kitslaar PJEHM, Ermers EJM: Photoplethysmography in the diagnosis of superficial valvular incompetence. Br J Surg 80:351–353, 1993.
44. Bays RA, Healy DA, Atnip RG, et al: Validation of air plethysmography, photoplethysmography, and duplex ultrasonography in the evaluation of severe stasis. J Vasc Surg 20:721–727, 1994.
45. van Bemmelen PS, Mattos MA, Hodgson KJ, et al: Does air plethysmography correlate with duplex scanning in patients with chronic venous insufficiency? J Vasc Surg 18:796–807, 1993.
46. van Bemmelen PS, Bedford G, Beach K, Strandness DE Jr: Quantitative segmental evaluation of venous valvular reflux with duplex ultrasound scanning. J Vasc Surg 10:425–431, 1989.
47. Baldt MM, Böhler K, Zontsich T, et al: Preoperative imaging of lower extremity varicose veins: Color-coded duplex sonography or venography? J Ultrasound Med 15:143–154, 1996.
48. van Bemmelen P, Beach K, Bedford G, Strandness DE Jr: The mechanism of venous valve closure. Arch Surg 125:617–619, 1990.
49. Vasdekis SN, Clarke GH, Nicolaides AN: Quantification of venous reflux by means of duplex scanning. J Vasc Surg 10:670–677, 1989.
50. van Bemmelen PS, Bedford G, Beach K, Strandness DE Jr: Quantitative segmental evaluation of venous valvular reflux with duplex ultrasound scanning. J Vasc Surg 10:425–431, 1989.
51. Randhawa GK, Dhillon JS, Kistner RL, Ferris EB: Assessment of chronic venous insufficiency using dynamic venous pressure studies. Am J Surg 148: 203–209, 1984.
52. Bergan JJ, Moulton SL, Poppitti R, Beeman S: Patient selection for surgery of varicose veins using venous reflux quantification. *In* Veith FJ (ed): Current Critical Problems in Vascular Surgery. St. Louis, Quality Medical Publishing, 1992, pp 138–149.
53. Porter JM, Moneta GL, International Consensus Committee on Chronic Venous Disease: Reporting standards in venous disease. An update. J Vasc Surg 21:635–645, 1995.
54. Moulton S, Bergan JJ, Beeman S, Poppiti R: Gravitational reflux does not correlate with clinical status of venous stasis. Phlebology 8:2–6, 1993.
55. Walsh JC, Bergan JJ, Beeman S, Comer TP: Femoral venous reflux abolished by greater saphenous vein stripping. Ann Vasc Surg 8:566–570, 1994.
56. Sales SM, Bilof ML, Petrillo KA, Luka NL: Correction of lower extremity venous incompetence by ablation of superficial venous reflux. Ann Vasc Surg 10:186–190, 1996.
57. Walsh JC, Bergan JJ, Moulton SL, Beeman S: Proximal reflux adversely affects distal venous function. Vasc Surg 30:89–96, 1996.
58. Markel A, Meissner MH, Manzo RA, et al: A comparison of the cuff deflation method with Valsalva's maneuver and limb compression in detecting venous valvular reflux. Arch Surg 129:701–705, 1994.
59. Hanrahan LM, Araki CT, Rodriguez AA, et al: Distribution of valvular incompetence in patients with venous stasis ulceration. J Vasc Surg 13:805–812, 1991.
60. Masuda EM, Kister RL, Eklof B: Prospective study of duplex scanning for venous reflux: Comparison of Valsalva and pneumatic cuff techniques in the reverse Trendelenburg and standing positions. J Vasc Surg 20:711–720, 1994.
61. Weingarten MS, Branas CC, Czeredarczuk M, et al: Distribution and quantification of venous reflux in lower extremity chronic venous stasis disease with duplex scanning. J Vasc Surg 18:753–759, 1993.
62. Labropoulos N, Leon M, Nicolaides AN, et al: Superficial venous insufficiency: Correlation of anatomic extent of reflux with clinical symptoms and signs. J Vasc Surg 20:953–958, 1994.
63. Schultheiss R, Billeter M, Bollinger A, Franzeck UK: Comparison between clinical examination, cw-Doppler ultrasound, and colour-duplex sonography in the diagnosis of incompetent perforating veins. Eur J Vasc Endovasc Surg 13:122–126, 1997.
64. O'Donnell TF, Burnand KG, Clemenson G, et al: Doppler examination vs clinical and phlebographic detection of the location of incompetent perforating veins. Arch Surg 112:31–35, 1977.
65. Phillips GWL, Paige J, Molan MP: A comparison of colour duplex ultrasound with venography and varicography in the assessment of varicose veins. Clin Radiol 50:20–25, 1995.

Chapter 25

ARTERIOVENOUS FISTULA AND NONVENOUS EXTREMITY PATHOLOGY

William J. Zwiebel, MD

ARTERIOVENOUS FISTULA

A fistula is an opening that connects two epithelialized structures. In the case of an arteriovenous fistula, communication occurs between an artery and an adjacent vein. Arteriovenous fistulae almost always result from trauma, either violent or iatrogenic. The most likely site of occurrence is between the femoral artery and vein, because this is a common location for vascular catheterization. Inadvertent puncture of both the artery and the vein can result in fistulization.

The duplex ultrasound hallmarks of an arteriovenous fistula are turbulent and, in some cases, pulsatile venous flow.[1, 2] The turbulence is powerful and dramatic, and it may generate a "visible bruit," adjacent to the vein, caused by vibration of surrounding soft tissues (Fig. 25–1). In the absence of dramatic venous turbulence, the diagnosis of arteriovenous fistula should be questioned. If the injury that produced the fistula is recent, a hematoma may be present surrounding the affected vessels.

In some cases, the actual point of arteriovenous communication may be visible sonographically, but visualization of the fistula is not always possible, because the opening may be small, and turbulent effects may obscure the fistula.

CONDITIONS THAT MAY MIMIC VENOUS THROMBOSIS

Several commonly encountered conditions may mimic the signs and symptoms of venous thrombosis, and in some instances these can be identified sonographically.[3–5]

The conditions in question are congestive heart failure, abscess, hematoma, adenopathy, soft-tissue tumors, Baker's cyst, and lymphedema. Vascular technologists should be familiar with the duplex manifestations of these conditions.

Congestive Heart Failure

Bilateral lower extremity edema may result from the hydrostatic pressure induced by congestive heart failure. In such cases, the Doppler signals in large veins are pulsatile (Fig. 25–2). Pulsatility may be so striking that it is difficult, at first glance, to know whether Doppler signals are venous or arterial. However, vessel identification is easily accomplished by comparing the Doppler signals in the vein and the adjacent artery, and by noting the direction of blood flow (cephalad in the venous system). Sonography is requested frequently in patients with bilateral leg swelling and dyspnea, who are possibly suffering from pulmonary thromboembolism. In these patients, the likelihood of a positive ultrasound examination for venous thrombosis is quite low. Although it is logical, for reasons of simplicity and noninvasiveness, to begin the search for pulmonary thromboembolism with venous ultrasound, the potential for overutilization of venous ultrasound is enormous. Proper clinical screening is the only means for preventing unnecessary venous ultrasound examinations. Most importantly, a negative venous ultrasound examination does not exclude pulmonary embolus. About 25 to 30% of patients with documented pulmonary embolism do not have lower extremity venous thrombosis.[6] In such cases, the thrombus may already have embolized from

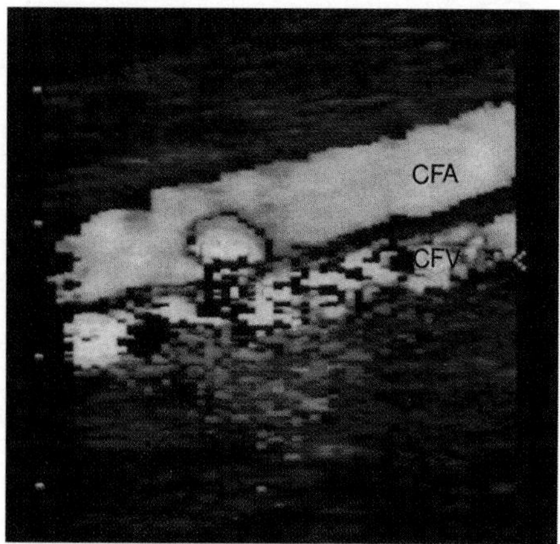

FIGURE 25–1 Arteriovenous fistula. Marked turbulence is present in the common femoral vein (CFV), as a result of an arteriovenous fistula with the common femoral artery (CFA). A visible bruit is present in the soft tissues adjacent to the vein.

the leg veins to the lungs, or the thrombus may have originated from other venous sources, including the pelvic and upper extremity veins.

Abscess and Cellulitis

Abscess and cellulitis are both manifestations of bacterial infection. The term *abscess* implies the formation of an enclosed collection of pus, whereas *cellulitis* refers to diffuse soft-tissue infection without a focal purulent collection. Abscess and cellulitis cause swelling, skin erythema, pain, and tenderness. These signs and symptoms may closely mimic the manifestations of acute venous thrombosis.

Duplex sonography plays an important diagnostic role in cases of abscess or cellulitis, by confirming that the venous system is patent and free of thrombus. If an abscess is present (Fig. 25–3), it can usually be identified with ultrasound as a circumscribed fluid collection that typically contains low-level echoes or a layer of echogenic debris. The margins of an abscess may be smooth and well defined, or shaggy and poorly defined. Extremity abscesses tend to spread out longitudinally, along the confines of the fascial planes. Therefore, they may have an elongated, fusiform shape.

The soft-tissue edema that accompanies cellulitis (Fig. 25–4) cannot be differentiated from edema generated by other conditions, such as congestive heart failure or fluid overload.

Hematoma

Extremity soft-tissue hematomas usually occur in association with one of the following: trauma (violent or iatrogenic), anticoagulation, or vigorous exercise (usually in athletes). Hematomas may cause pain and extremity swelling that are difficult to distinguish clinically from the effects of venous thrombosis.

Once again, duplex sonography plays an important diagnostic role in documenting the patency of the venous system. In addition, an acute hematoma may be directly visualized with ultrasound. Visualization, however, assumes that the blood collects locally and does not spread out within the tissues. As visualized with ultrasound, a hematoma is a hypoechoic mass (Fig. 25–5) that usually has ill-defined borders and is slightly heterogeneous. With time, the hematoma retracts, and serum is exuded. The hematoma then appears as a heterogeneous collection in which the echogenic thrombus is surrounded by anechoic fluid. With lysis of the thrombus, a hematoma may become an anechoic fluid collection.

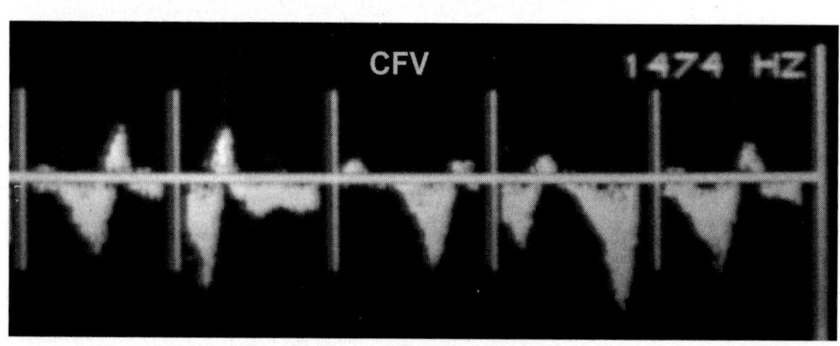

FIGURE 25–2 Pulsatile venous signal in the common femoral vein (CFV) caused by congestive heart failure. In cases such as this, it may be difficult to determine whether the flow signal is arterial or venous. Comparison with the flow signals in the adjacent artery resolves the problem, however.

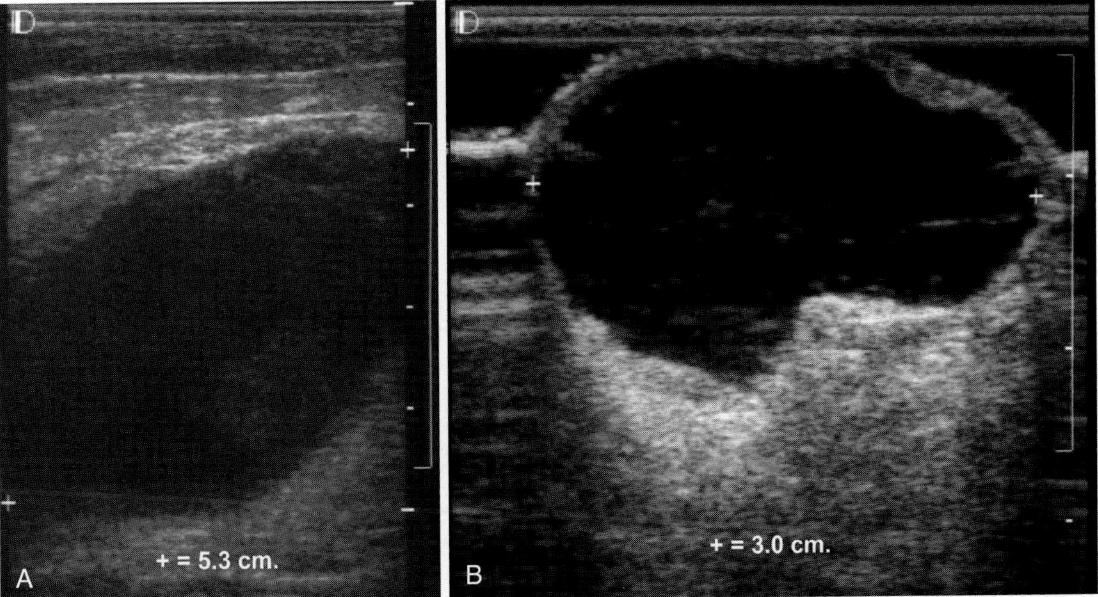

FIGURE 25–3 Soft-tissue abscess. *A,* Long-axis view of a large axillary abscess. The walls are somewhat indistinct, and some internal echoes are apparent. *B,* Incisional abscess after arterial bypass graft. The borders are defined better in this case than in *A* and enhanced through-transmission of ultrasound is more apparent.

Large hematomas may compress the venous system, causing venous distention and sluggish flow. In some cases stagnation may lead to secondary venous thrombosis.

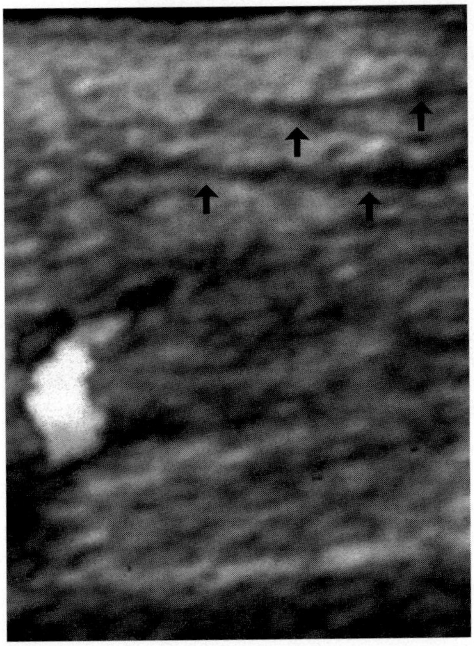

FIGURE 25–4 Soft-tissue edema. The tissue planes are poorly defined, and linear fluid collections (*arrows*) are present within the soft tissues.

Adenopathy

The term *adenopathy* refers to enlargement of lymph nodes, whether from inflammatory or neoplastic causes. Adenopathy may cause extremity swelling, either by associated obstruction of lymphatic drainage or by compression of the venous system. In some cases, the enlarged lymph nodes are tender.

Adenopathy generates hypoechoic masses that are readily identified sonographically (Fig. 25–6). These masses can generally be differentiated from abscesses or hematomas because blood flow can be demonstrated within the mass with color-Doppler ultrasound. In addition, adenopathy tends to occur at specific sites, particularly in the axilla, in the groin, along the iliac vessels, or adjacent to the inferior vena cava and the aorta. The venous system may be compressed by enlarged lymph nodes, leading to impedance of flow, as discussed previously. In patients with bilateral leg swell-

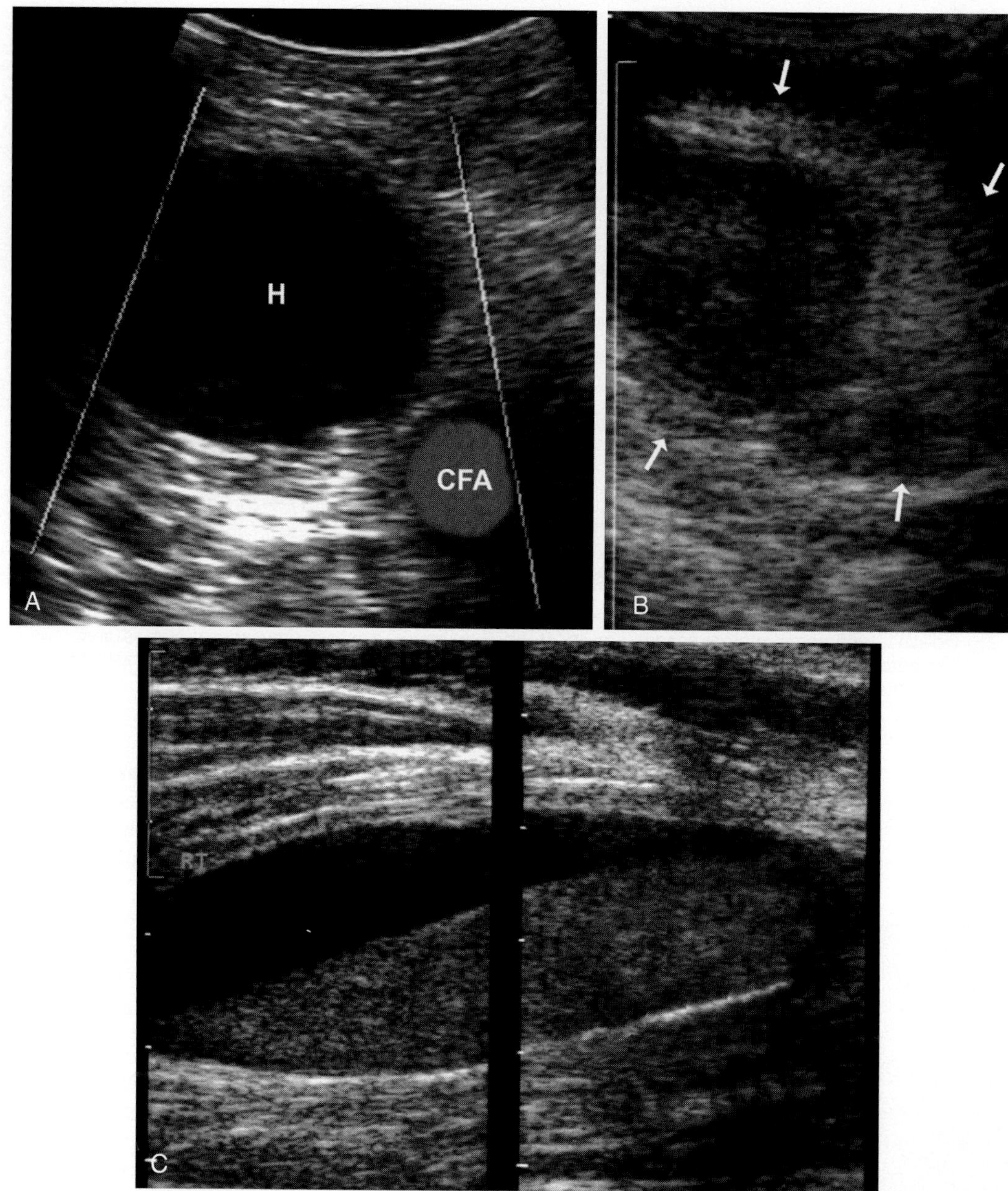

FIGURE 25–5 Soft-tissue hematoma. *A,* A rounded 1-day-old hematoma (H) is present near the common femoral artery (CFA), resulting from arterial catheterization. Note mild heterogeneity of internal signals caused by thrombus retraction. *B,* Acute (hours-old) hematoma (*arrows*) in the popliteal fossa. This hematoma is fairly echogenic, consistent with its acute state. *C,* Composite image of an acute (hours-old) arm hematoma related to poorly controlled Coumadin therapy. Note the fluid/fluid level resulting from settling of blood cells.

ing not attributable to venous thrombosis or heart failure, the sonographers should search for enlarged nodes in the pelvis or along the inferior vena cava.

Soft-Tissue Tumors

Benign or malignant soft-tissue tumors may be encountered in the course of ultra-

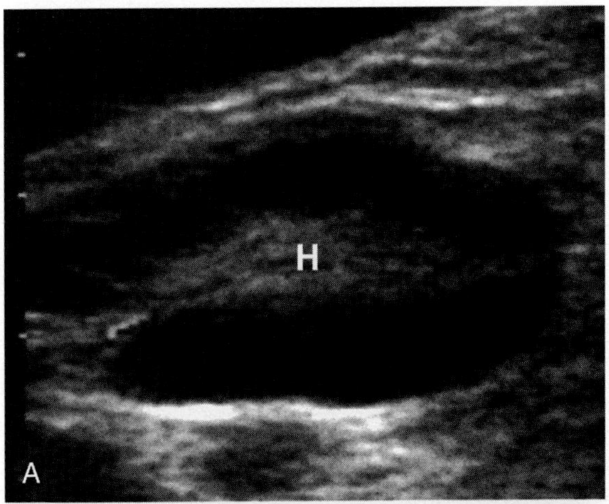

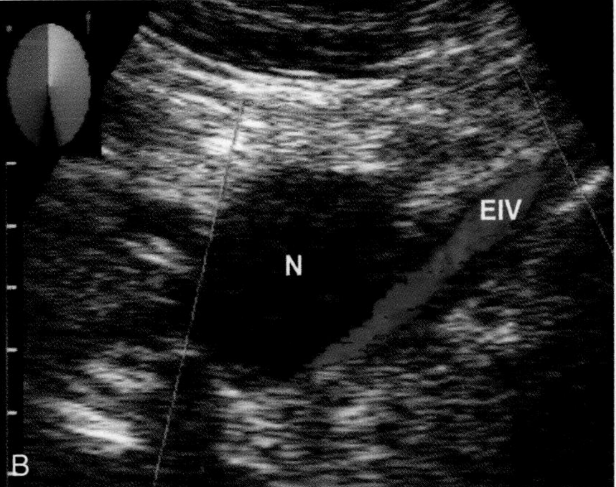

FIGURE 25–6 Adenopathy. *A,* This enlarged lymph node retains normal architecture, suggesting that it is inflamed and not neoplastic. Note the echogenic hilum (H) surrounded by markedly hypoechoic lymphoid tissue. *B,* A large nodal mass (N) is visible adjacent to the external iliac vein (EIV) in a patient who presented with leg swelling. The venous system was patent, and it was not clear whether leg swelling was due to nodal compression of the veins or lymphatic obstruction.

sound extremity examination, either as subjects of the examination or as incidental findings. The latter situation is particularly true of popliteal fossa or groin masses that are thought to be Baker's cysts or aneurysms. Primary soft-tissue tumors include leiomyomas, a variety of sarcomas, squamous cell carcinomas, and melanomas. Metastatic tumors may originate from a wide variety of sources and are usually highly malignant. The ultrasound appearance of soft-tissue tumors is variable. Some are solid, but others may contain large areas of liquefactive necrosis or hemorrhage. The latter tumors may resemble hematomas, abscesses, or cysts, but differentiation is commonly possible through the demonstration of blood flow in solid portions of the mass (Fig. 25–7).

Baker's Cysts

With chronic knee joint dysfunction, certain bursae that communicate with the knee may dilate, forming Baker's cysts. The gastrocnemiosemimembranous bursa most commonly suffers this fate. This bursa lies posterior and medial to the knee joint, between the muscles of the same names. Baker's cysts are particularly common in patients with severe degenerative joint disease and those with rheumatoid arthritis, but they are by no means exclusive to these conditions. As Baker's cysts enlarge, they dissect between the fascial planes and extend down into the calf musculature. Large cysts are prone to spontaneous rupture, which causes pain, tenderness, and swelling in the calf. These signs and symptoms are indistinguishable from the manifestations of acute deep venous thrombosis.

Duplex sonography is the primary modality for differentiation between Baker's cysts and acute deep venous thrombosis. Because most Baker's cysts arise in the gastrocnemiosemimembranous bursa, they frequently have the following characteristics (Fig

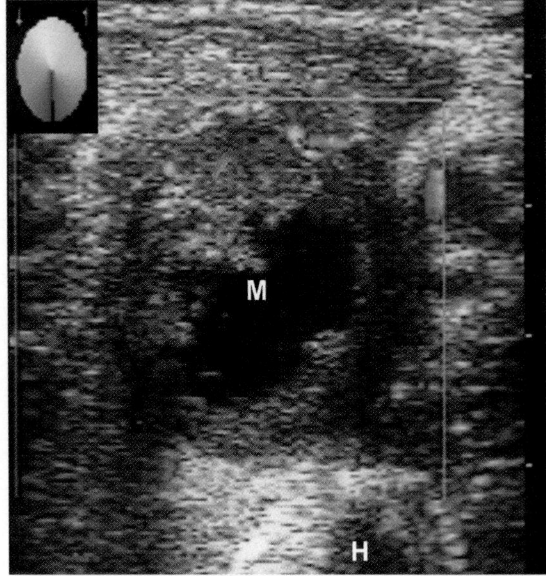

FIGURE 25–7 Soft-tissue tumor. A partially necrotic mass (M) is seen adjacent to the humerus (H). Blood flow is evident in the wall of the lesion. This is a squamous cell carcinoma metastasis from an ipsilateral digital primary.

25–8): (1) the cyst is medially located and closely associated with the medial head of the gastrocnemius muscle; (2) the cyst is crescentic, as seen in cross-section; and (3) the upper end of the cyst is at the level of the knee joint. Unfortunately, not all Baker's cysts have a typical appearance or location.

I have seen Baker's cysts that I believed were ruptured, because they trailed off inferiorly into the calf musculature without a nicely defined border, but I am not certain that cyst rupture can be confirmed sonographically. The principal role of sonography is to determine whether the venous system is the cause of calf pain. If the venous system is patent, rupture of a Baker cyst becomes one of several diagnostic possibilities. Remember, however, that the cyst may simply be an incidental finding unrelated to the patient's symptoms.

Baker's cysts are usually anechoic, but some chronic cysts may contain echogenic debris or may be diffusely echogenic (Fig. 25–9). In the latter case, soft-tissue neoplasms are a differential consideration. It is helpful in such cases to look for a cyst with

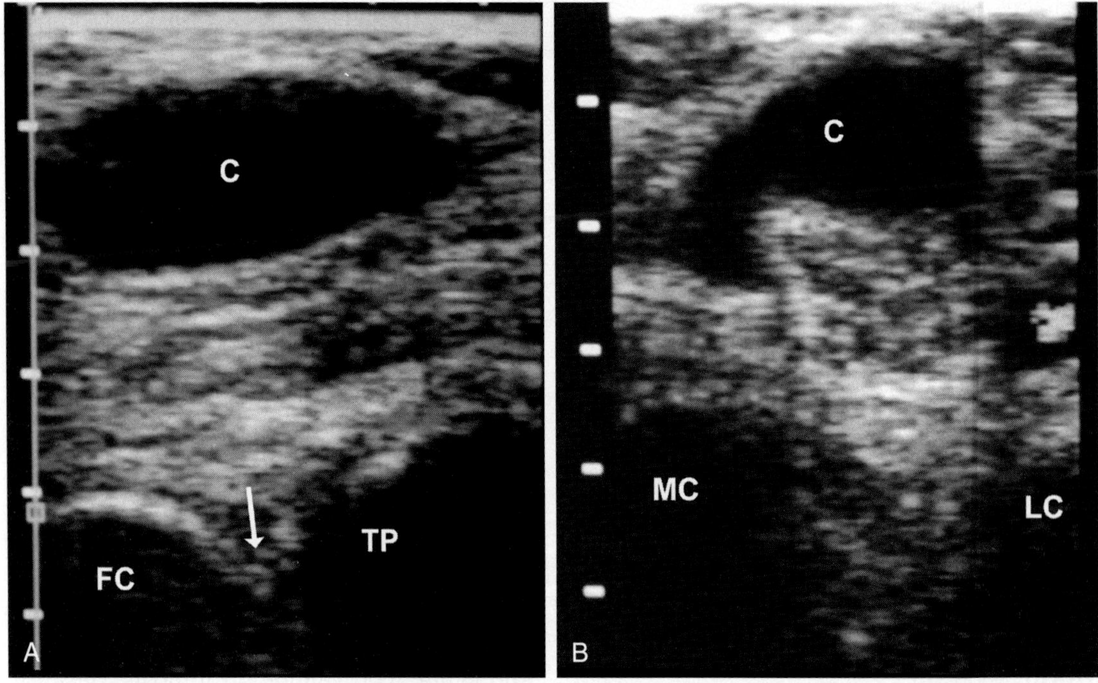

FIGURE 25–8 Baker's cyst. *A,* Longitudinal view of a Baker cyst (C). The *arrow* indicates the location of the knee joint space, between the femoral condyle (FC) and the tibial plateau (TP). *B,* A transverse scan demonstrates a medially located, crescent-shaped fluid collection (C). The location and shape are characteristic of a Baker cyst. MC = medial femoral condyle; LC = lateral femoral condyle.

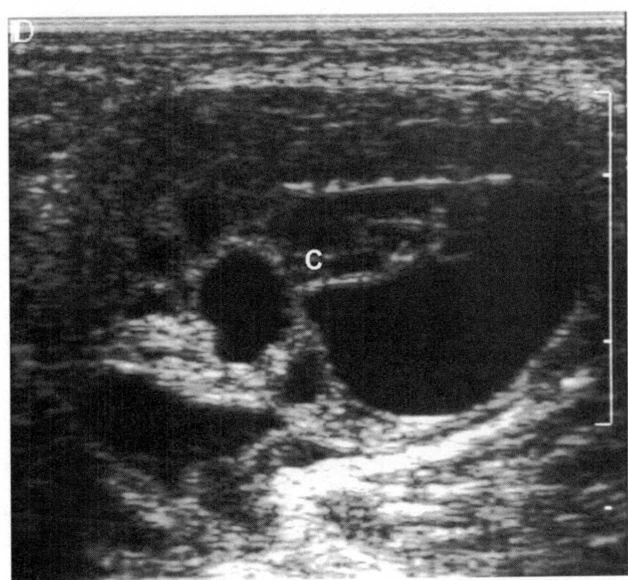

FIGURE 25–9 Multiple septa are present in Baker's cyst (C), which may contain hemorrhage or fibrinoid material.

similar echo features in the other knee. Obviously, bilateral neoplastic masses are unlikely, whereas bilateral Baker's cysts are common in patients with arthritis.

Popliteal artery aneurysms may be mistaken clinically for Baker's cysts, but differentiation is simple because blood flow is detected in the aneurysm (with the assumption that the vessel is patent).

Lymphedema

The final condition that may mimic the manifestations of venous thrombosis is lymphedema. Neoplastic or postsurgical obstruction of the lymphatic system may cause extremity swelling and pain that are difficult to differentiate from the effects of venous thrombosis. In the absence of lymph node enlargement, no specific duplex findings point to lymphatic obstruction as the cause of edema, but duplex sonography can generally confirm that the venous system is patent and is not the cause of extremity swelling.

REFERENCES

1. Needleman L, Nack TL: Vascular and nonvascular masses. J Vasc Technol 18:299–306, 1994.
2. Goldberg BB: Iatrogenic femoral arteriovenous fistula: Diagnosis with cold Doppler imaging. Radiology 170:749–752, 1989.
3. Mitchell DG, Merton DA, Liu JB, Goldberg BB: Superficial masses with color flow Doppler imaging. J Clin Ultrasound 19:555–560, 1991.
4. Borgstede JP, Clagett BS: Types, frequency and significance of alternative diagnoses found during duplex Doppler venous examination of the lower extremities. J Ultrasound Med 11:85–89, 1992.
5. Drinman KJ, Wolfson PM, Steinitz D, et al: Duplex imaging in lymphedema. J Vasc Technol 17:23–26, 1993.
6. Weinman EE, Salzman EW: Deep-vein thrombosis. N Engl J Med 331:1630–1641, 1994.

SECTION 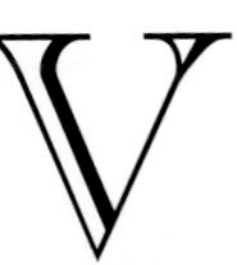

ABDOMINAL VESSELS

Chapter 26

Anatomy and Normal Doppler Signatures of Abdominal Vessels

■ *William J. Zwiebel, MD*

The correct identification of abdominal vessels and accurate assessment of blood flow in the abdomen require knowledge of vascular anatomy and of the Doppler characteristics of specific vessels. This fundamental information is presented in this chapter. The reader should be familiar with concepts of arterial pulsatility and Doppler spectrum analysis, as presented in Section 1, Basics.

CELIAC ARTERY

The celiac artery, also called the *celiac trunk* or *celiac axis,* is the most cephalad visceral branch of the abdominal aorta. It arises from the anterior aortic surface, between the diaphragmatic crura (Fig. 26–1*A*). The celiac artery bifurcates about 1 to 3 cm from its origin into the common hepatic and splenic arteries, which are readily visualized with ultrasonography. The celiac artery also gives rise to the left gastric artery, which is generally not visible sonographically. The branching pattern of the celiac artery is quite constant, occurring in approximately 93% of individuals. In the most common variations (see Fig. 26–1*B*), one or more of the celiac branches arise separately from the aorta or from the superior mesenteric artery (SMA). In less than 1% of individuals, the celiac artery and the SMA arise from the aorta as a common trunk. In such cases, the common trunk splits into the celiac artery and the SMA within 1 or 2 cm from the aorta.[1, 2]

The celiac artery (Fig. 26–2) is best visualized with ultrasonography in the transverse plane, in which the T-shaped bifurcation of the vessel is characteristic. In older individuals with tortuous vessels, the T configuration may droop to the patient's left and be less apparent. The celiac artery may also be seen readily in longitudinal images, but the T configuration is not seen in this plane. Celiac artery Doppler signals have a characteristic low-resistance flow pattern, but a slightly higher resistance pattern is seen near the origin of the vessel. The splenic and hepatic branches also exhibit a low-resistance flow pattern, with a large amount of continuous forward flow throughout diastole.[3] This pattern is induced by low-flow resistance within the microcirculation of the liver and spleen.

If the celiac artery is occluded, collateralization occurs through the pancreaticoduodenal arterial arcade, which is a network of small vessels surrounding the pancreas and duodenum. These vessels feed into the gastroduodenal artery (GDA) and then into the common hepatic artery. Because there are abundant opportunities for collateralization, hepatic or splenic artery blood flow may appear normal, even though the origin of the celiac artery is occluded, unless reversed (collateral) flow is recognized in the GDA or the proper hepatic artery.[4]

SPLENIC ARTERY

The splenic artery (the left limb of the celiac T configuration) follows a tortuous course along the posterosuperior margin of the pancreatic body and tail (Fig. 26–3*A* [see p 387]). The splenic artery gives rise to

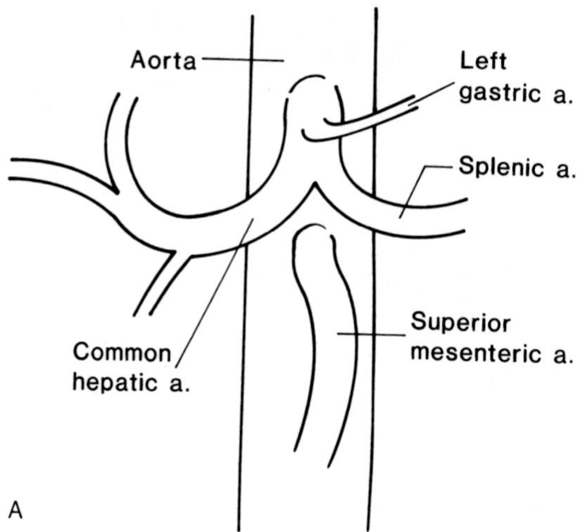

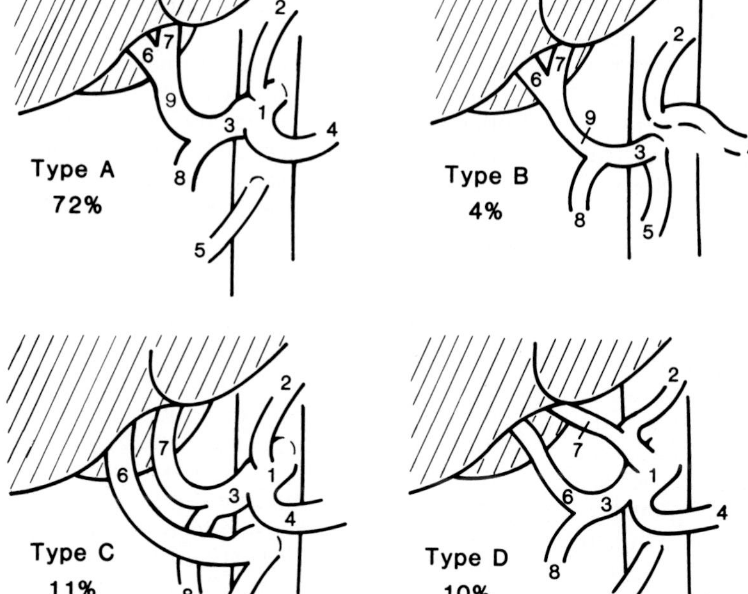

FIGURE 26–1 *A,* The celiac artery and its branches. *B,* Variations of celiac artery anatomy. 1 = celiac artery; 2 = left gastric artery; 3 = common hepatic artery; 4 = splenic artery; 5 = superior mesenteric artery; 6 = right hepatic artery; 7 = left hepatic artery; 8 = gastroduodenal artery; 9 = proper hepatic artery.

several pancreatic branches, short gastric branches, and the left gastroepiploic artery. None of these vessels can be seen with ultrasonography. The splenic artery terminates as a series of branches in the splenic hilum. Transverse scans from a midline approach usually reveal the proximal portion of the splenic artery (see Fig. 26–2*A*). The course of the distal portion of the splenic artery may be difficult to image because of tortuosity. The distal-most portion of the splenic artery may be visualized through the spleen from a left lateral approach. Because of the tortuous course of the splenic artery, flow in this vessel is typically turbulent,[5] as seen in Figure 26–3*B* (see p 387).

HEPATIC ARTERY

The common hepatic artery (Fig. 26–4 [see p 388]) is the right limb of the celiac T configuration. This vessel runs for a short distance along the superior border of the

Text continued on page 387

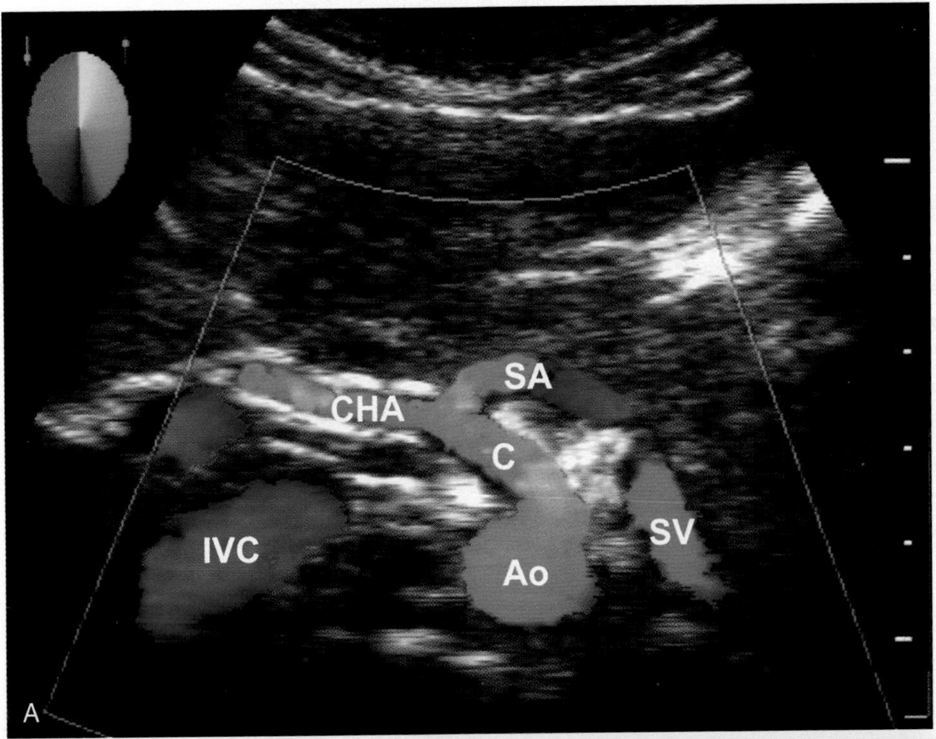

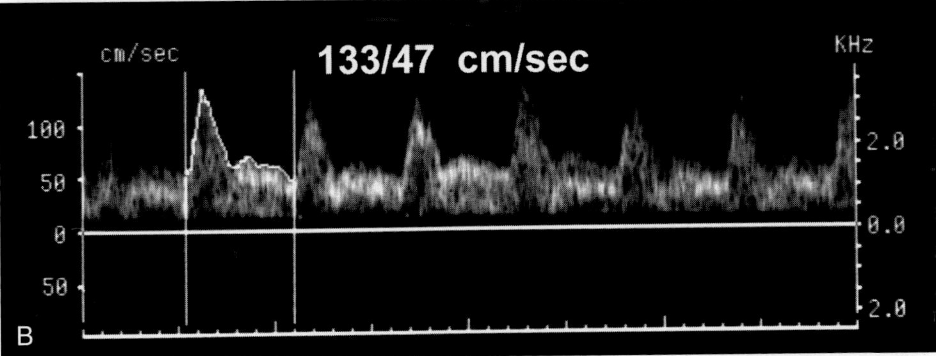

FIGURE 26–2 Celiac artery ultrasound. *A,* Transverse sonogram of the celiac axis (C) as it divides into the common hepatic artery (CHA) and splenic artery (SA). Ao = aorta; IVC = inferior vena cava; SV = a segment of the splenic vein. *B,* Normal, low-pulsatility Doppler signal in the distal portion of the celiac artery. Peak systolic velocity is 133 cm/sec, and end diastolic velocity is 47 cm/sec.

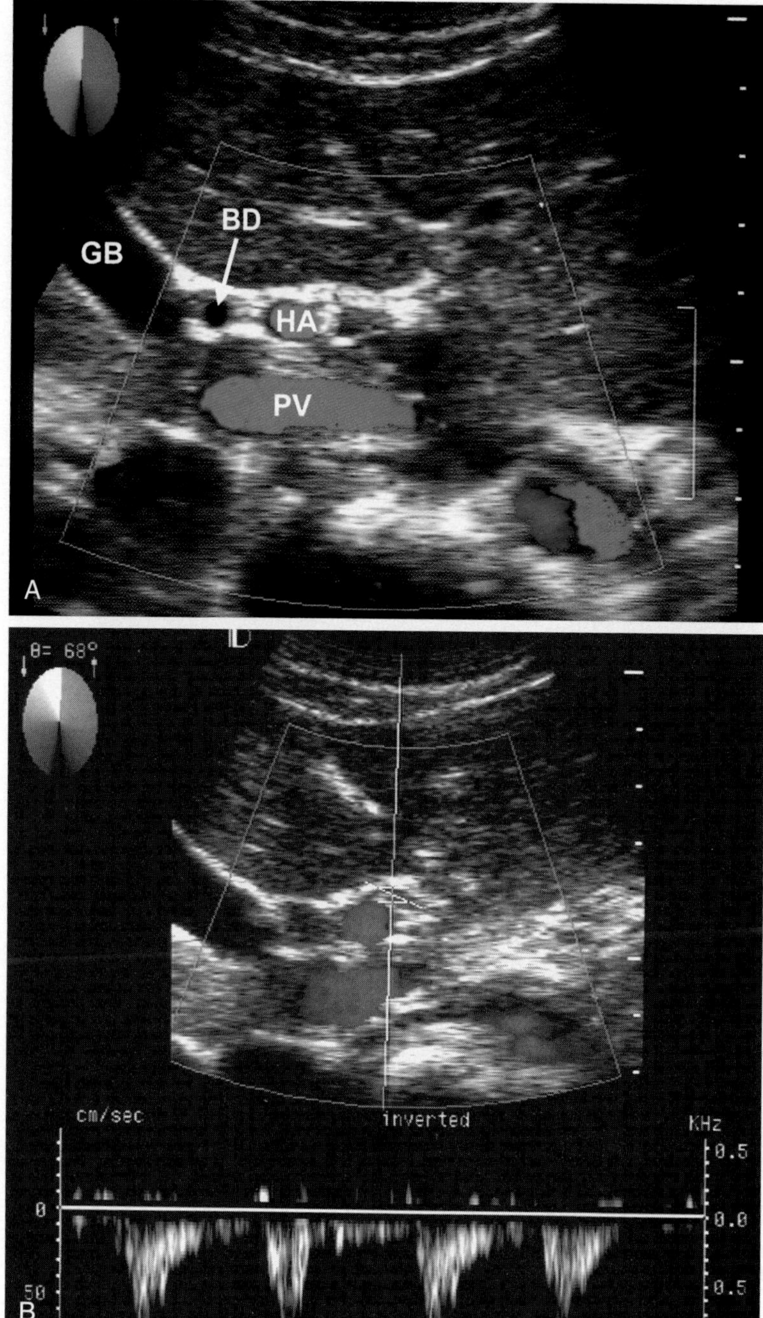

FIGURE 26–5 Ultrasonography of the hepatic artery. (See p 389.) *A,* At the porta hepatis, the hepatic artery (HA) can be differentiated from the bile duct (BD), because blood flow is present in the former and not in the latter. Blood flow is also seen in the portal vein (PV). GB =, gallbladder. *B,* Doppler examination confirms the identity of the (proper) hepatic artery, which has low-resistance arterial signals.

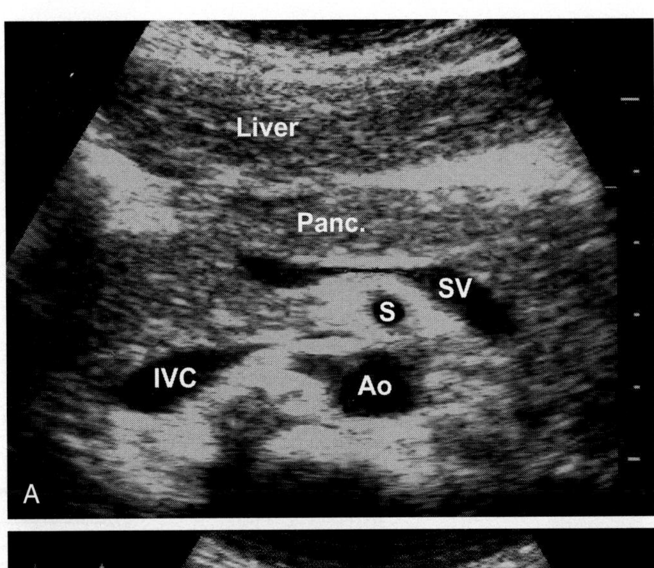

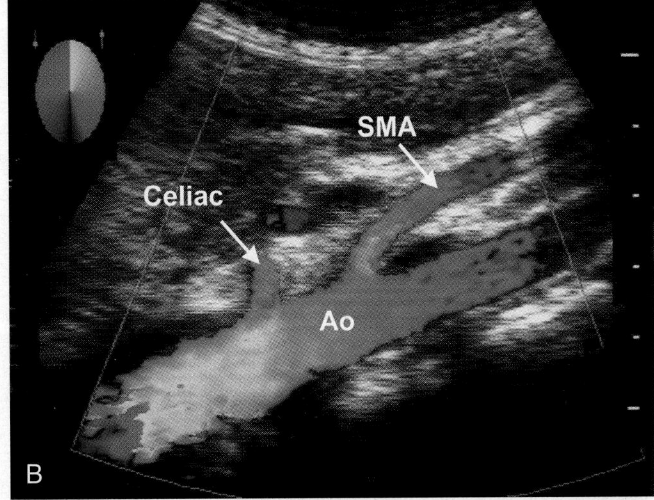

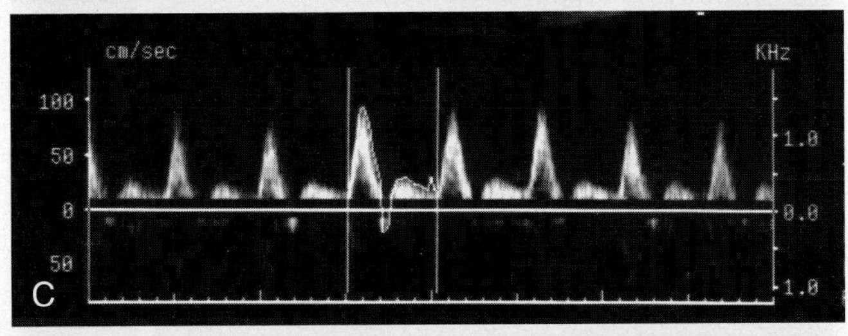

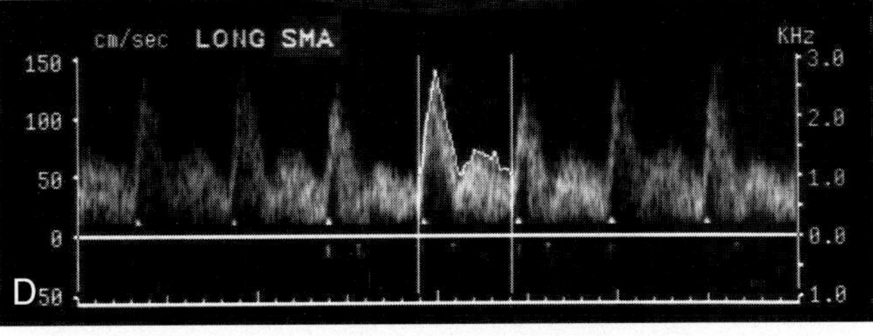

FIGURE 26–7 Ultrasound of the superior mesenteric artery. (See p 389.) *A,* Anatomic relationships of the SMA (S). Note that the SMA is surrounded by a distinctive layer of echogenic fat. The pancreas (panc.) is anterior to the SMA. The aorta (Ao) is posterior to the SMA. IVC = inferior vena cava; SV = splenic vein. *B,* A long-axis view shows the origin of the celiac artery and the SMA from the aorta (Ao). *C,* Normal, high-resistance Doppler signal in the SMA of a fasting patient. *D,* Normal low-resistance postprandial SMA Doppler signals. SMA = superior mesenteric artery.

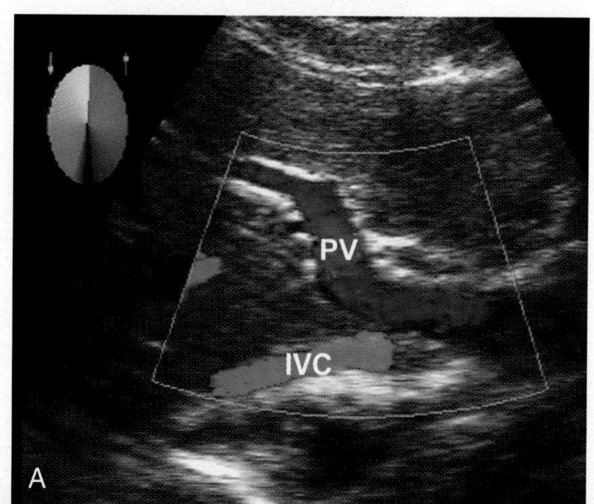

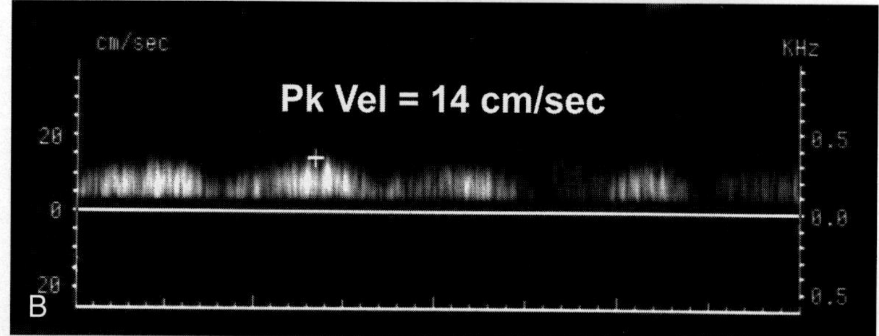

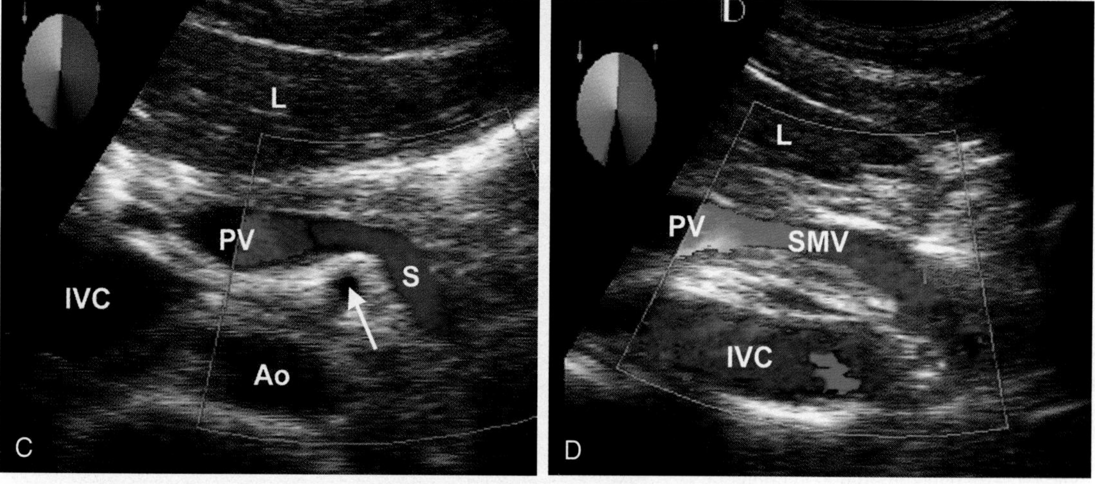

FIGURE 26–9 Ultrasound of the portal vein and its tributaries. (See p 390.) *A,* Long-axis view of the portal vein (PV). IVC = inferior vena cava. *B,* Normal phasic Doppler spectrum in the portal vein. Peak velocity (Pk Vel) is 14 cm/sec. *C,* The splenic vein (S) is seen at its junction with the portal vein (PV). *Arrow* = superior mesenteric artery; Ao = aorta; IVC = inferior vena cava; L = liver. *D,* Long-axis view of the superior mesenteric vein (SMV) as it joins the portal vein (PV). IVC = inferior vena cava; L = liver.

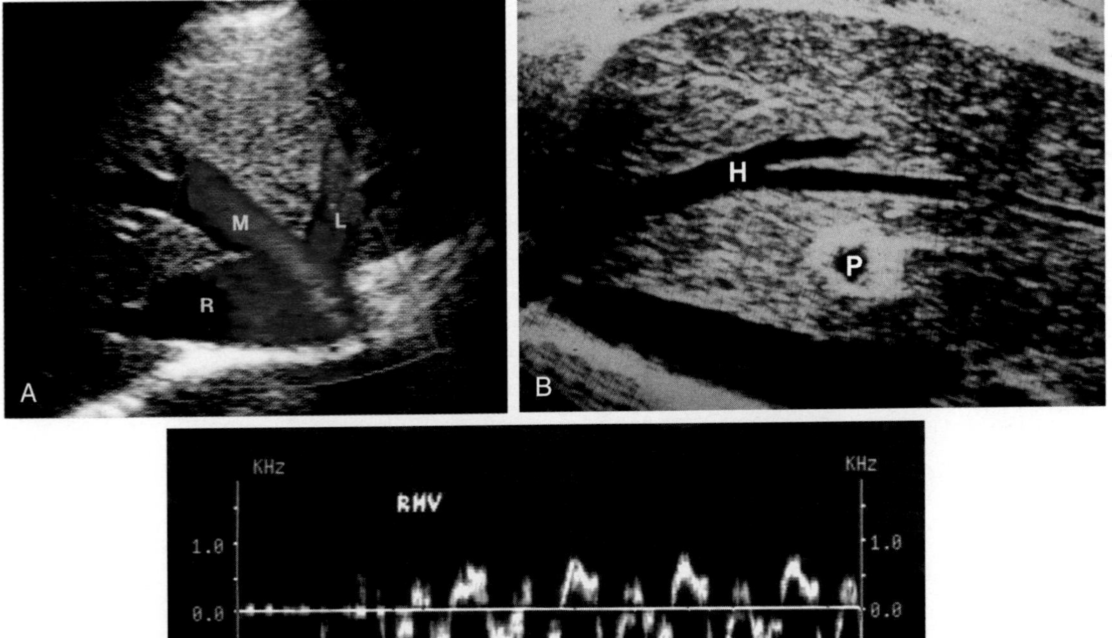

FIGURE 26–11 Hepatic vein sonography. (See p 391.) *A,* Transverse view of the three main hepatic vein trunks as they enter the inferior vena cava. R, M, and L = right, middle, and left hepatic veins. *B,* Differentiation between hepatic and portal veins. Hepatic veins (H) have naked margins, follow a longitudinal course, and become larger as they approach the diaphragm. Portal veins (P) have echogenic margins, run in transverse planes, and converge on the porta hepatis. *C,* Normal, pulsatile hepatic vein Doppler signal. RHV = right hepatic vein.

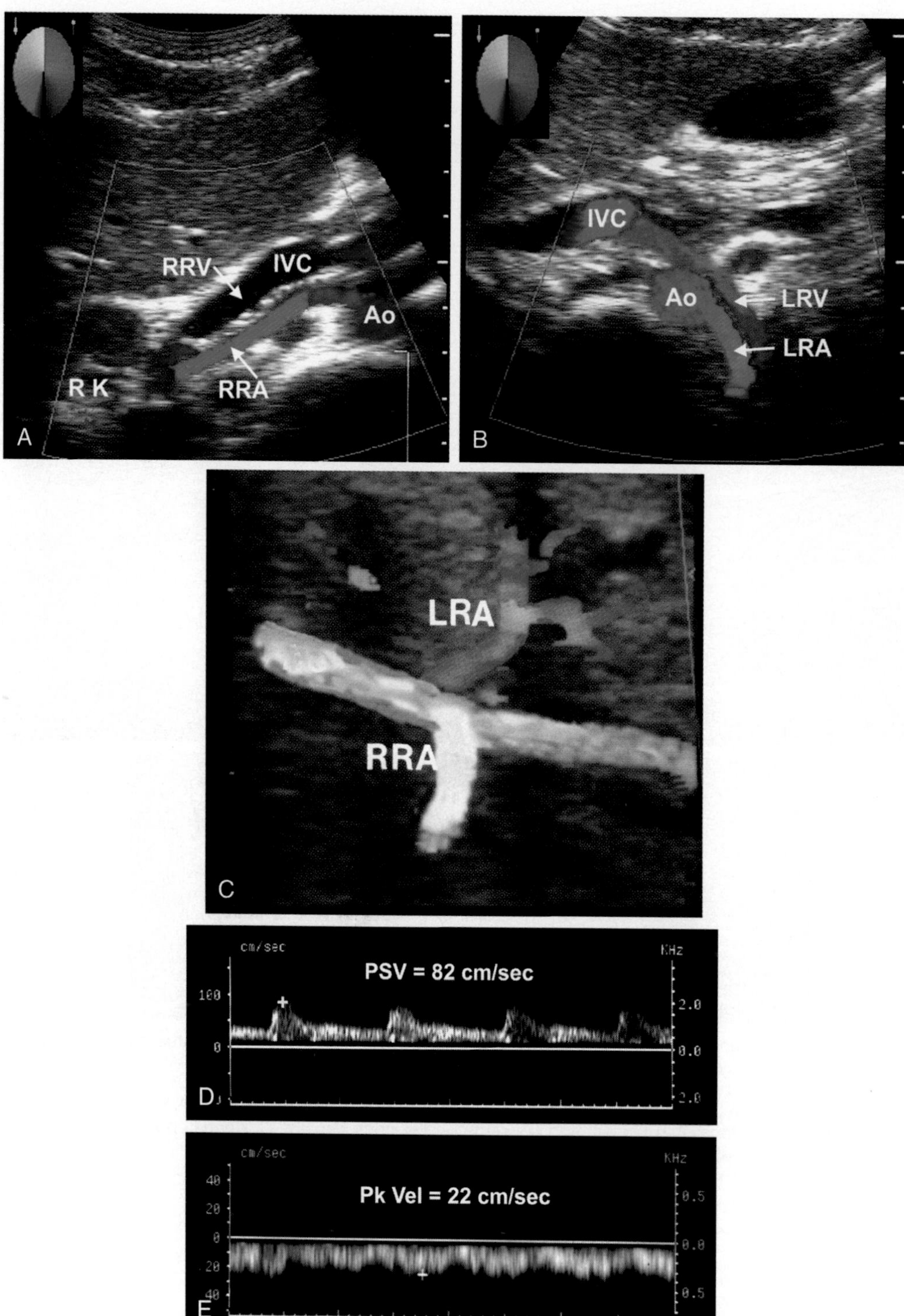

FIGURE 26–16 Sonographic appearance of the renal arteries and veins. (See p 394.) *A,* Transverse image of the right renal artery (RRA) and right renal vein (RRV). Note that the artery lies posterior to the inferior vena cava (IVC) and the renal vein. RK = right kidney; Ao = aorta. *B,* Transverse image of the left renal artery (LRA) and the left renal vein (LRV). Once again, the renal artery is posterior to the renal vein. It is important not to mistake the vein for the artery. Ao = aorta; IVC = inferior vena cava. *C,* Coronal view of the left (LRA) and right (RRA) renal arteries in a premature infant (head to left). *D,* Normal, low-pulsatility renal artery Doppler spectrum. Peak systolic velocity (PSV) is 82 cm/sec. *E,* Normal phasic renal vein Doppler spectrum. Peak velocity (Pk Vel) is 22 cm/sec.

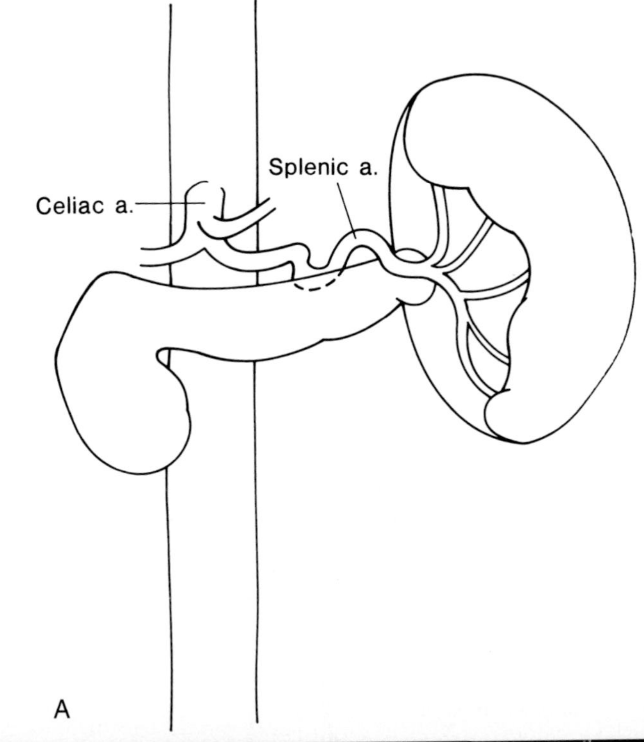

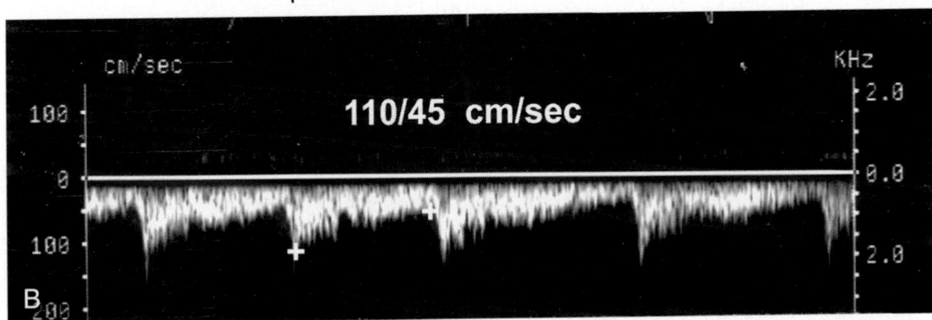

FIGURE 26–3 *A,* Splenic artery anatomy. (See p 379.) *B,* Normal, low-pulsatility Doppler signal from the splenic artery. (See p 380.) Peak systolic velocity is 110 cm/sec, and end diastolic velocity is 45 cm/sec.

pancreatic head. It then gives rise to the GDA, which can often be seen with ultrasonography at the anterosuperior border of the pancreatic head, adjacent to the duodenal bulb. After giving off the GDA, the common hepatic artery turns superiorly toward the porta hepatis and gives off the right gastric artery, which is usually not seen with ultrasonography. Beyond the GDA origin, the *common* hepatic artery becomes the *proper* hepatic artery, which follows the portal vein to the porta hepatis (entrance to the liver). At this point, it divides into the left and right hepatic arteries, which penetrate into the hepatic substance. The anatomic relationships among the hepatic artery, the portal vein, and the extrahepatic bile ducts are shown in Fig 26–4*B*.

The classic hepatic artery configuration just described is seen in 72% of individuals.[5] A number of alternative patterns may occur, including those illustrated in Figure 26–1*B*. The most noteworthy of these patterns are the following: (1) the common (4%) or right (11%) hepatic arteries may arise from the SMA, and (2) the left hepatic artery may arise from the left gastric artery (10%).[2]

The hepatic arteries are usually well visualized sonographically from an anterior abdominal approach. The common hepatic artery is most easily identified at its origin from

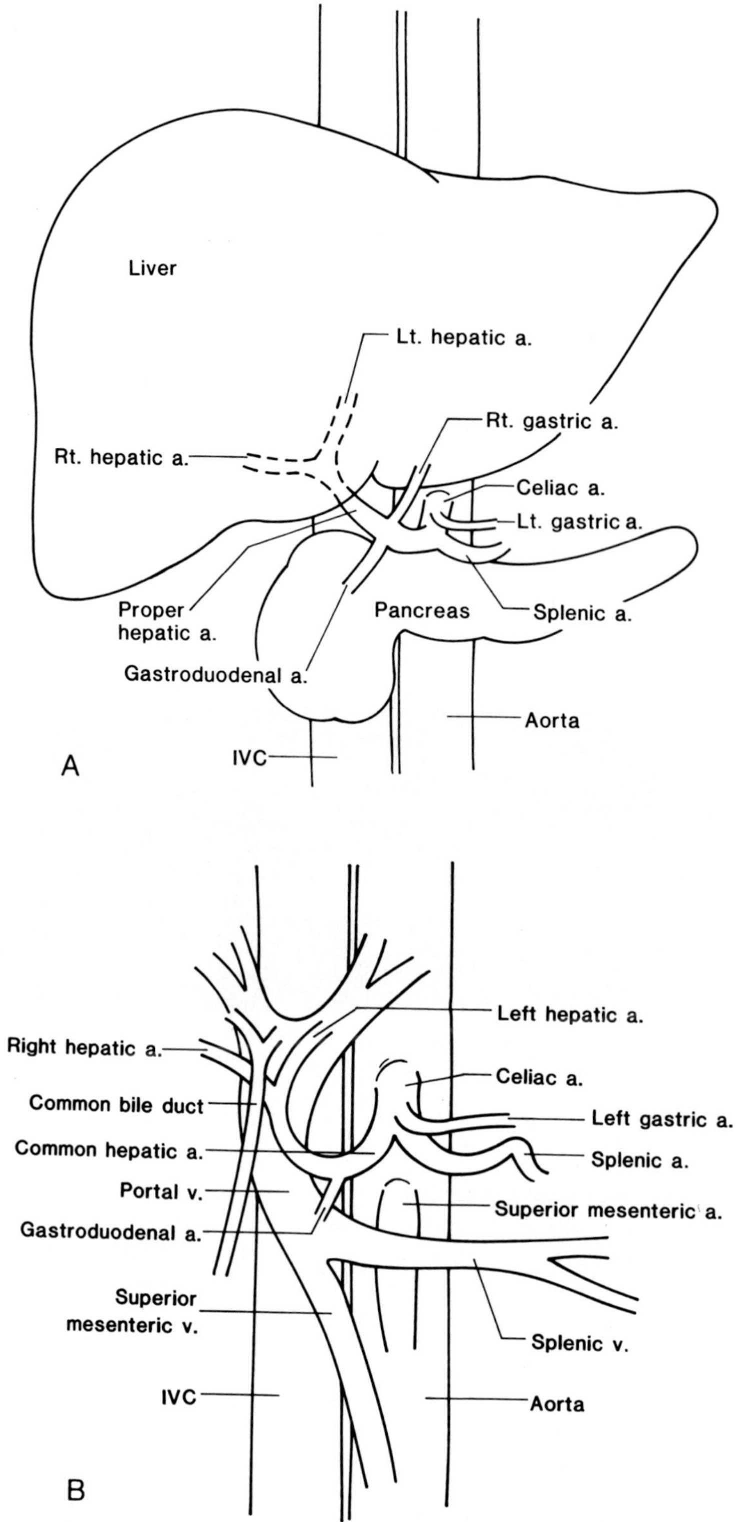

FIGURE 26–4 *A,* The hepatic artery and its branches. *B,* Anatomic relationships among the hepatic artery, the portal vein, and the extrahepatic bile ducts. IVC = inferior vena cava. (See p 380.)

the celiac artery (see Fig. 26–2*A*). The proper hepatic artery is seen on ultrasound images showing the portal vein in short or long axes, as shown in Figure 26–5*A* (see p 382). The right and left hepatic artery branches can be followed into the substance of the liver to a variable distance from the porta hepatis. As noted previously, the hepatic arterial system has low-resistance flow characteristics, with a large amount of continuous forward flow throughout diastole, as shown in Figure 26–5*B*.

SUPERIOR MESENTERIC ARTERY

The SMA arises from the anterior surface of the aorta, immediately distal to the origin of the celiac artery (Fig. 26–6). The SMA generally consists of a short, anteriorly directed segment and a much longer inferiorly directed segment that ends in the vicinity of the ileocecal valve. SMA branches supply the jejunum, ileum cecum, ascending colon, proximal two thirds of the transverse colon, and portions of the duodenum and pancreatic head. As noted previously, the SMA may also give rise to an aberrant right hepatic artery (11%) or common hepatic artery (4%).[1]

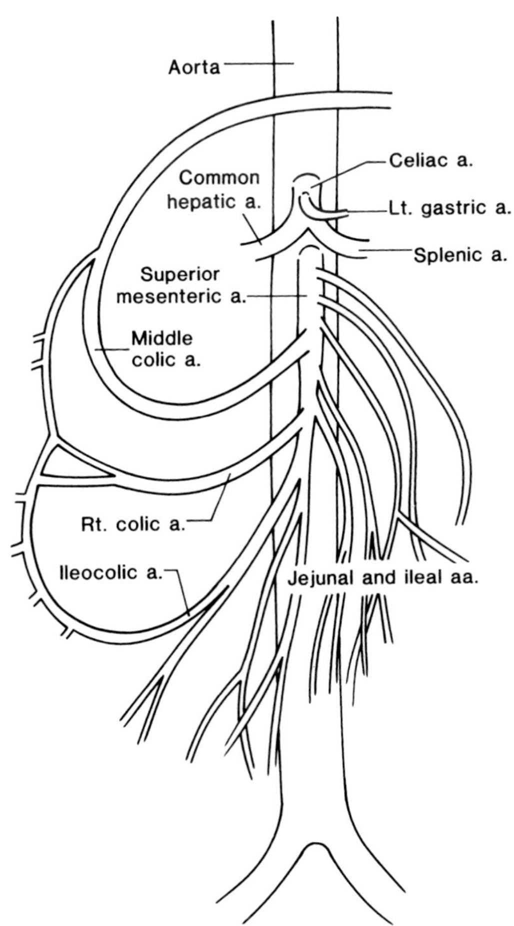

FIGURE 26–6 Superior mesenteric artery anatomy.

The SMA is most easily identified on longitudinal ultrasound images (Fig. 26–7 [see p 383]). The SMA has characteristic anatomic relationships with several epigastric structures and serves, therefore, as an important orienting landmark for scanning upper abdominal vessels. These relationships are seen on transverse ultrasound images, as illustrated in Figure 26–7*A*. First, note that the SMA is surrounded by a distinctive, triangular mantle of fat that is very useful for identifying this vessel. Second, the SMA lies to the right of the superior mesenteric vein. Third, the pancreas and the splenic vein lie anterior to the SMA. In contrast, the left renal vein (discussed later) lies posterior to the SMA (between the SMA and the aorta). These anatomic features are very distinctive, making the SMA an excellent point of orientation for abdominal scanning.

SMA blood flow is best assessed with longitudinal images, because a lengthy segment of the vessel may be evaluated from a single perspective. The SMA Doppler spectrum shows turbulent flow near the arterial origin; however, as one moves distally, flow becomes more uniform. In a fasting patient, a high-resistance flow pattern is seen in the SMA (see Fig. 26–7*C*), with sharp systolic peaks and absent late diastolic flow. Within 30 to 90 minutes after eating, SMA flow assumes a low-resistance pattern (see Fig. 26–7*D*), with broad systolic peaks and continuous diastolic flow.[3]

PORTAL VENOUS SYSTEM

The portal venous system transports blood from the bowel and spleen to the liver. The portal vein (Fig. 26–8) begins at the junction of the splenic and superior mesenteric veins, which are immediately posterior to the pancreatic neck. The portal vein courses superiorly and toward the right, passes behind the first portion of the duodenum, and terminates at the porta hepatis. At its termination, the portal vein divides into right and left portal

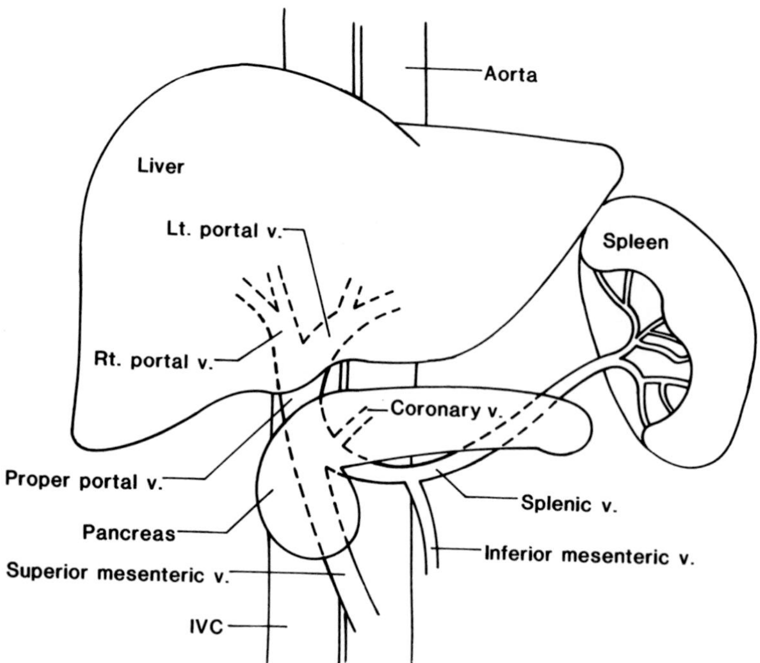

FIGURE 26–8 Portal venous system anatomy. IVC = inferior vena cava.

branches, which enter the corresponding lobes of the liver.

The splenic vein and the superior mesenteric vein are the two primary contributors to portal vein flow. The splenic vein lies posterior to the pancreas, which "follows" the splenic vein toward the hilum of the spleen. The superior mesenteric vein extends almost straight caudad from the portal vein junction and parallels the course of the SMA, which lies to its left.

Other tributaries of the portal venous system include the coronary vein and the inferior mesenteric vein (see Fig. 26–8). The latter empties into the splenic vein in 38% of individuals. Alternatively, the inferior mesenteric vein may join the splenic-superior mesenteric vein junction (32%), or the superior mesenteric vein itself (25%).[2] The coronary vein runs along the posterior aspect of the stomach toward the gastroesophageal junction. This vein usually enters the superior aspect of the portal vein near the portosplenic junction (58%), but it may also join the portal vein farther cephalad (24%), or it may join the splenic vein (16%).[2]

The portal vein is readily visualized with ultrasonography on transverse or oblique images of the porta hepatis (Fig. 26–9 [see p 384]). Flow in the portal vein and its tributaries is normally toward the liver. Portal vein Doppler waveforms exhibit subtle phasic variation, as shown in Figure 26–9*B*. This variation in flow rate is produced by a combination of respiratory and cardiac hemodynamic effects. The phasic pattern generates a "windstorm" sound in the audible Doppler signal, which is quite distinct from the pulsatile sound of the hepatic artery and other epigastric arterial branches.

The normal portal vein measures up to 13 mm in diameter (when measured in quiet respiration in a supine patient).[6] The caliber of the portal vein and its tributaries normally increases during sustained deep inspiration. This is best seen in the splenic and superior mesenteric veins, which normally increase 50 to 100% in diameter from quiet respiration to deep inspiration.[7, 8] This normal response mediates against the presence of portal hypertension.

HEPATIC VEINS

Typically, there are three major hepatic veins, as depicted in Figure 26–10, which converge on the inferior vena cava (IVC) at the diaphragm. The right hepatic vein runs in a coronal plane between the anterior and posterior segments of the right hepatic lobe. The middle hepatic vein lies between the right and left hepatic lobes and may be seen

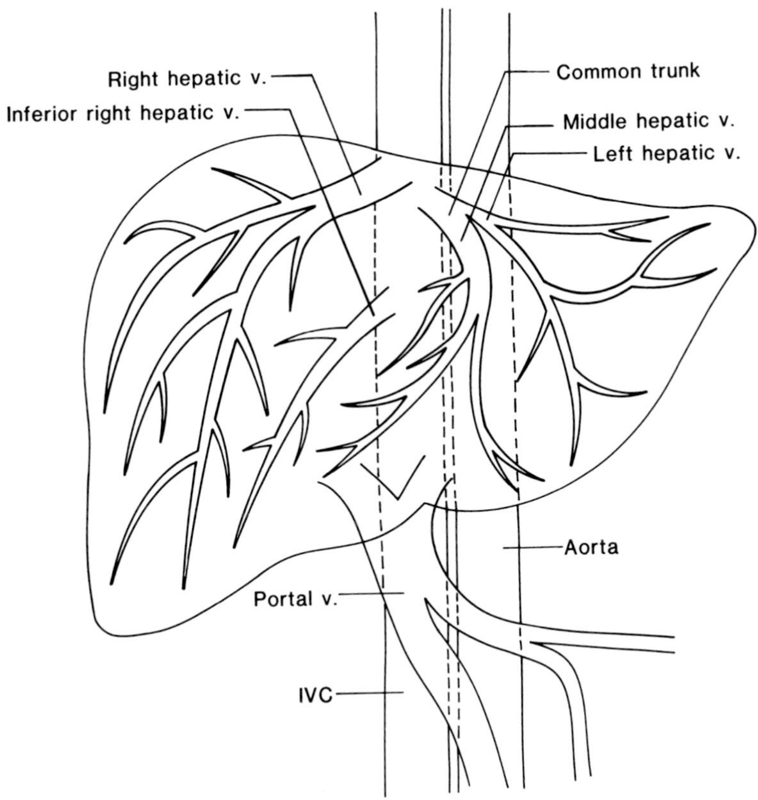

FIGURE 26–10 Hepatic vein anatomy. IVC = inferior vena cava.

prominently on sagittal or parasagittal images of the liver. The left hepatic vein runs between the medial and lateral segments of the left hepatic lobe. In 96% of individuals, the middle and left hepatic veins join to form a common trunk before entering the IVC.[9] The caudate lobe has its own venous drainage, directly into the IVC. Accessory hepatic veins are common, although they are rarely identified sonographically. An inferior right hepatic vein, as illustrated in Figure 26–10, is present in 10% of persons.[10] Occasionally, one of the three major hepatic veins is absent, and, in such cases, the right hepatic vein is usually missing (6%), or less commonly the middle or left hepatic veins. The left hepatic vein is commonly duplicated, and a number of other variations of hepatic vein anatomy may occur.[9]

The hepatic veins are frequently best visualized with ultrasonography using a transverse subxiphoid approach, which yields an image of the three main hepatic trunks converging on the IVC (Fig. 26–11 [see p 385]). From this perspective, however, flow often cannot be visualized in the right hepatic vein because the axis of this vein is perpendicular to the ultrasound beam. Flow in the right hepatic vein can be demonstrated, however, using a coronal scan plane and an intercostal transducer position. In some instances, the middle and left hepatic veins may be imaged to greater advantage in sagittal planes than on transverse scans.

The normal hepatic veins are sonolucent structures embedded within the liver parenchyma. Hepatic veins may be differentiated from portal veins by the following sonographic features:

1. Course: hepatic veins are more or less longitudinally oriented, whereas portal veins run in transverse planes.
2. Convergence: the hepatic veins converge on the IVC at the diaphragm, whereas the portal veins converge on the porta hepatis.
3. Changes in size: the hepatic veins enlarge progressively toward the diaphragm, whereas the portal veins become larger as they approach the porta hepatis.
4. Margins: hepatic veins have "naked" margins, whereas the portal veins are surrounded by a heavy sheath of echogenic fibrous tissue (see Fig. 26–11*B*).

In addition, hepatic vein Doppler signals are quite different from portal vein Doppler signals. Flow in the hepatic veins has a somewhat chaotic, pulsatile pattern that results from transmission of right atrial pulsations into the veins. The Doppler spectrum (see Fig. 26–11*C*) reflects a combination of phasic variation and transmitted pulsations.

INFERIOR VENA CAVA

The normal IVC is situated anterior to the spine and to the right of the aorta. The IVC begins at the junction of the common iliac veins and terminates in the right atrium (Fig. 26–12).

The upper abdominal portion of the IVC is easily visualized sonographically,[11–13] using the liver as an acoustic window (see Chapter 27). The inferior portion of the IVC may be difficult to visualize, depending on the body habitus of the patient and the amount of overlying bowel gas. The size of the IVC varies markedly with respiration and throughout the cardiac cycle, but the IVC seldom exceeds 2.5 cm in diameter.[13] Deep inspiration limits venous return to the chest, markedly dilating the IVC. Expiration has the opposite effect. The IVC diameter is also dependent on patient size and right atrial pressure (dilated with fluid overload or heart failure).

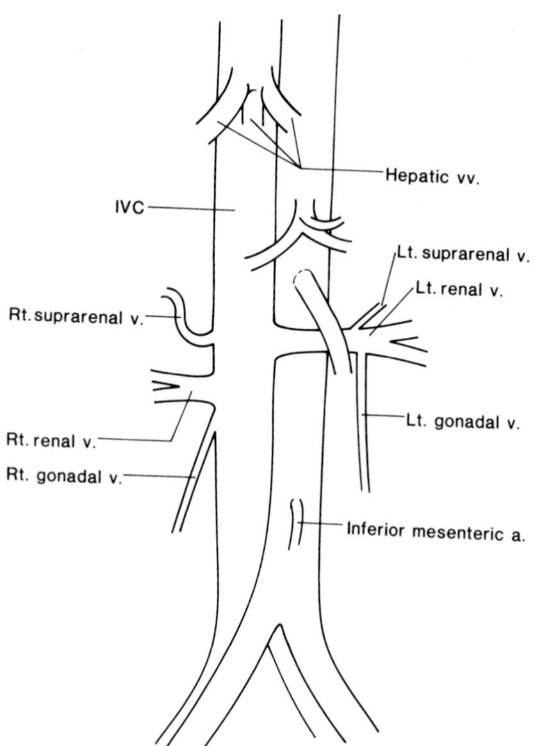

FIGURE 26–12 The inferior vena cava (IVC) and its tributaries.

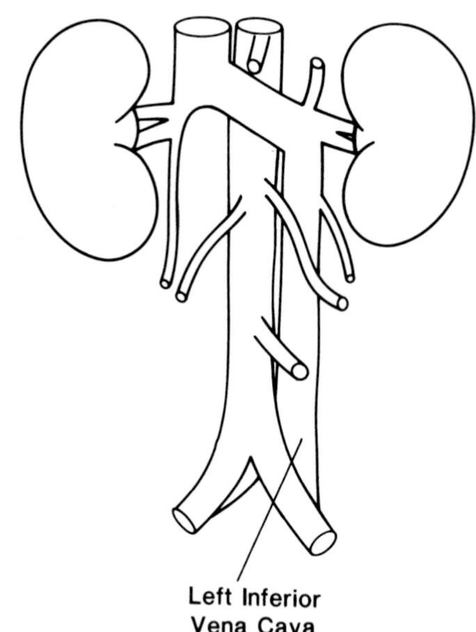

FIGURE 26–13 Anomalous, left-sided inferior vena cava.

Doppler flow signals in the IVC are somewhat pulsatile near the heart because of reflected right atrial pulsations. Farther distally, the flow pattern is phasic and is similar to the pattern seen in extremity veins.

Most anomalies of the IVC occur at and below the level of the renal veins.[10] Of these, the most common are duplication (0.2 to 3.0%) and transposition (0.2 to 0.5%). In both of these anomalies, the left-sided IVC usually crosses over to join the normal right-sided IVC at the level of the left renal vein (Fig. 26–13). Interruption of the IVC with azygos or hemiazygos continuation (0.6%) results from failure of the intrahepatic segment of the IVC to form. Flow is diverted to the heart via the azygos and hemiazygos veins, and the hepatic veins drain directly into the right atrium.

RENAL ARTERIES

The renal arteries (Fig. 26–14) arise from the aorta, slightly below the origin of the SMA. The origin of the right renal artery is usually slightly superior to the left, but this relationship is not constant. The right renal artery arises from the anterolateral aspect of

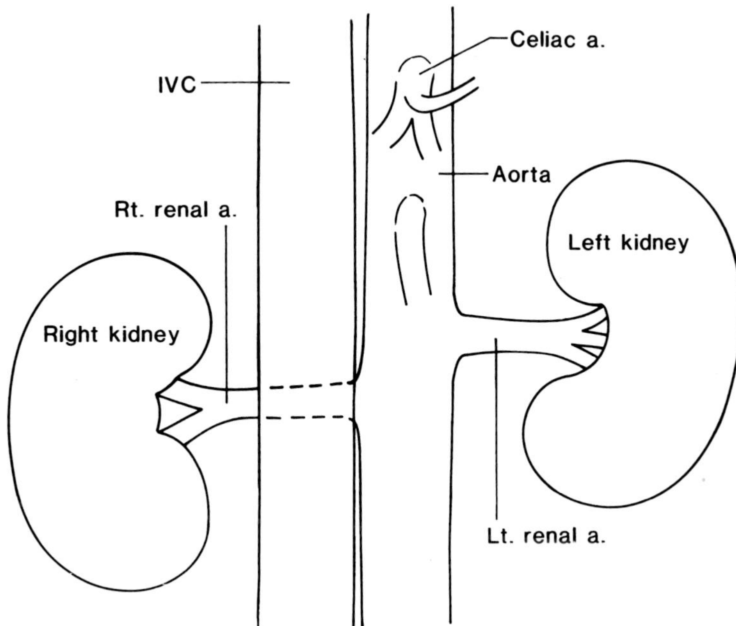

FIGURE 26–14 Renal artery anatomy. IVC = inferior vena cava.

the aorta and then passes *posterior* to the IVC as it courses toward the right renal hilum. The left renal artery arises from the lateral or posterolateral aspect of the aorta and follows a posterolateral course to the left renal hilum. Almost one third of kidneys are supplied by two or more arteries arising from the aorta.[14] In some of these cases, the main renal artery is duplicated. In other instances, accessory renal arteries are located superior or inferior to the main renal artery and may attach to the kidneys at the poles. Some polar accessory arteries arise from the common iliac arteries. Extrahilar accessory renal arteries are also fairly common. These attach to the external surface of the kidney and do not pass through the renal hilum. Extrahilar arteries may arise from the ipsilateral renal artery, the aorta, or, occasionally, from other arteries in the retroperitoneum.

The branching pattern of the renal arteries is illustrated in Figure 26–15. The renal arteries typically divide into anterior and posterior divisions that lie, respectively, anterior and posterior to the renal pelvis. The anterior division branches into four segmental arteries, whereas the posterior division supplies only a single renal segment. The segmental arteries branch farther within the renal sinus, forming interlobar arteries that penetrate the renal parenchyma. These terminate in arcuate arteries that curve around the cortico-

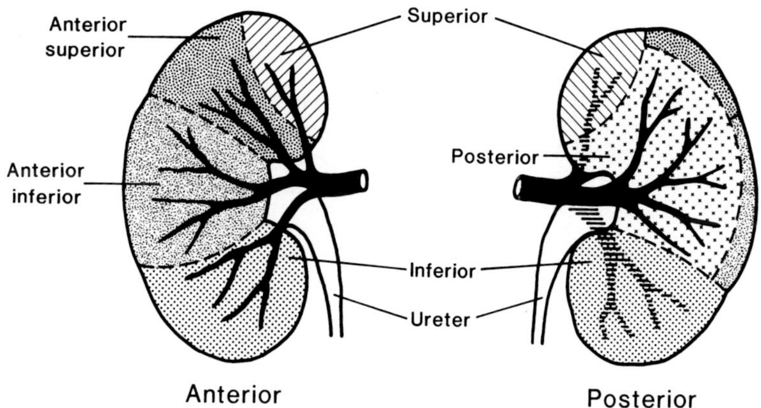

FIGURE 26–15 Distal arborization of the renal arteries.

medullary junction, giving rise to cortical branches.[14]

With ultrasonography, the renal artery origins (Fig. 26–16*A, B* [see p 386]) are usually best visualized by scanning transversely from a midline approach. In general, the right renal artery can be followed to the kidney from an anterior transducer position, but it may be difficult to trace the left renal artery to the kidney from this position. Coronal scanning from a lateral approach is a useful alternative approach in infants and small children (see Fig. 26–16*C*). This approach provides excellent Doppler angles for assessing renal artery flow.

Renal artery Doppler signals have a low-resistance flow pattern, as seen in Figure 26–16*D*. Continuous forward flow is present in diastole because of low resistance in the renal vascular bed. This flow pattern is evident at all locations in the renal arteries, including the intrarenal branches.[5]

RENAL VEINS

Each renal vein is formed from tributaries that coalesce in the renal hilum. As illustrated in Figure 26–17, the left renal vein usually receives the left suprarenal (adrenal) vein from above and the left gonadal (ovarian or testicular) vein from below. The left renal vein then passes anterior to the aorta and posterior to the SMA, to enter the left side of the IVC. The right renal vein, which is shorter than the left renal vein, extends directly to the IVC from the right renal hilum and usually receives no tributaries.

The left renal vein may be circumaortic (1.5 to 8.7%), with separate veins passing anterior and posterior to the aorta. The left renal vein may also be retroaortic in location (1.8 to 2.4%). Accessory renal veins are commonly present on the right side, draining directly into the IVC.[11, 14]

The renal veins can best be visualized with ultrasonography (see Fig. 26–16*A, B*) on transverse scans from an anterior approach. In small children, the renal veins may be seen coronally from a lateral approach. As seen on a transverse view, the left renal vein crosses the midline *between* the aorta and the SMA. This differentiates the left renal vein and the nearby splenic vein, which lies anterior to the SMA.

Doppler signals in the renal veins (see Fig. 26–16*E*) show the same phasic flow varia-

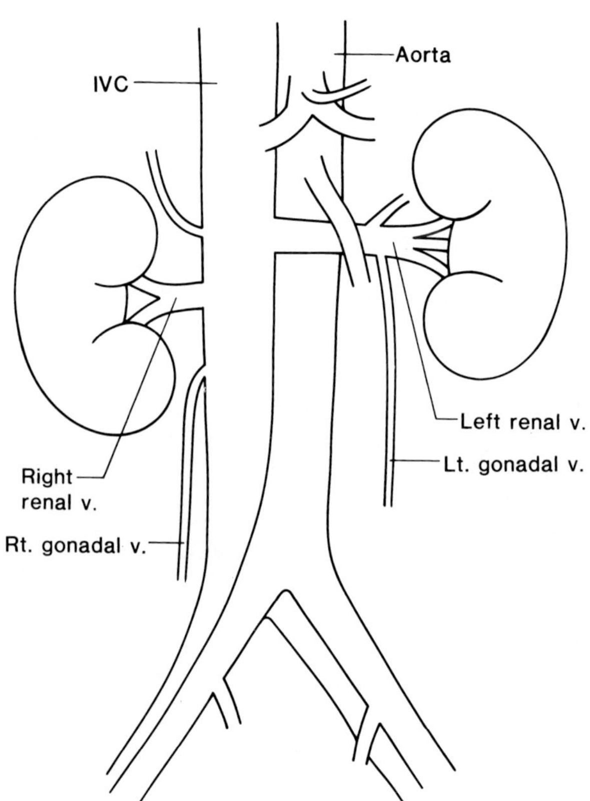

FIGURE 26–17 Renal vein anatomy. IVC = inferior vena cava.

tion as the IVC. Transmitted cardiac pulsations may be evident in the renal veins near the IVC.

REFERENCES

1. Ruzika FF Jr, Rossi P: Normal vascular anatomy of the abdominal viscera. Radiol Clin North Am 8:3–29, 1970.
2. Michels NA: Blood Supply and Anatomy of the Upper Abdominal Organs. Philadelphia, JB Lippincott, 1955.
3. Lewis BD, James EM: Current applications of duplex and color Doppler ultrasound imaging: Abdomen. Mayo Clin Proc 64:1158–1169, 1989.
4. Geelkerken RH, Delahunt TA, Schulte-Kool LJ, et al: Pitfalls in the diagnosis of origin stenosis of the coeliac and superior mesenteric arteries with transabdominal color duplex instrumentation. Ultrasound Med Biol 22:695–700, 1996.
5. Taylor KJW, Burns PN, Woodcock JP, Wells PNT: Blood flow in deep abdominal and pelvic vessels: Ultrasonic pulsed Doppler analysis. Radiology 154:487–493, 1985.
6. Weinreb J, Kumari S, Phillips G, Pochaczevsky R: Portal vein measurements by real-time sonography. AJR Am J Roentgenol 139:497–499, 1982.
7. Bolondi L, Gandolfi L, Arienti F, et al: Ultrasonography in the diagnosis of portal hypertension: Diminished response of the portal vessels to respiration. Radiology 142:167–172, 1982.
8. Bellamy EA, Bossi MC, Cosgrove DO: Ultrasound demonstration of changes in the normal portal venous system following a meal. Br J Radiol 57:147–149, 1984.
9. Cosgrove DO, Arger PH, Coleman BG: Ultrasonic anatomy of hepatic veins. J Clin Ultrasound 15:231–235, 1987.
10. Makuuchi M, Hasegawa H, Yamazaki S, et al: The inferior right hepatic vein: Ultrasonic demonstration. Radiology 148:213–217, 1983.
11. Kellman GH, Alpern MB, Sandler MA, Craig BM: Computed tomography of vena caval anomalies with embryologic correlation. Radiographics 8:533–556, 1988.
12. Needleman L, Rifkin MD: Vascular ultrasonography: Abdominal applications. Radiol Clin North Am 24: 461–484, 1986.
13. Mintz GS, Kotler MN, Parry WR, et al: Real-time inferior vena caval ultrasonography: Normal and abnormal findings and its use in assessing right-heart function. Circulation 64:1018–1024, 1981.
14. Hollinshead WH: Textbook of Anatomy, 3rd ed. Hagerstown, MD, Harper & Row, 1974, pp 521–523.

Chapter 27

AORTA, ILIAC ARTERIES, AND INFERIOR VENA CAVA

William J. Zwiebel, MD

Aneurysms of the aorta and the other abdominal vessels are potentially lethal yet are often silent clinically. Ultrasound plays an important role in the diagnosis and management of abdominal aneurysms by detecting clinically silent aneurysms, by following aneurysm enlargement over time, and by detecting complications resulting from aneurysm surgery. In this chapter, the clinical and pathologic features of abdominal arterial aneurysms are reviewed, and ultrasound techniques that ensure optimum diagnostic results are described.

AORTIC AND ILIAC ARTERIES

Normal Anatomy

Aortic and iliac artery anatomy was described and illustrated in Chapter 27. The normal abdominal aorta[1–5] (Fig. 27–1) has smooth margins and a well-defined wall, and tapers slightly below the level of the renal arteries. The maximum normal diameter of the aorta averages 2 cm in adults and varies little with respect to age, gender, race, and body size.[4, 5] The aorta is located slightly to the left of the midline and lies adjacent to the spine throughout its intra-abdominal course. In contrast, the inferior vena cava (IVC) lies to the right of the midline and gradually moves away from the spine as it passes through the liver and diaphragm. It is possible, therefore, to differentiate between the aorta and the IVC at a glance.

The normal iliac arteries (Fig. 27–2 [see p 399]) are smoothly marginated and uniform in caliber. The maximum diameter of the common iliac artery (outer to outer) is generally about 1 cm, and the external iliac artery is slightly smaller.

Terminology

The aorta is considered aneurysmal when the dilated segment is 1.5 times greater in diameter than an adjacent normal segment, or when the distal aorta exceeds 3 cm in diameter.[1–6] Aneurysmal dilatation is often localized, but some aneurysms may extend over long segments of an artery. Certain terms are used to describe the extent and shape of aneurysms, including focal aneurysm, diffuse aneurysm, saccular aneurysm, and fusiform aneurysm. The meaning of these modifiers is self-evident. Other terms describe the pathologic causes of aneurysms, including true aneurysm, false aneurysm, mycotic aneurysm, and arterial dissection. It is useful to review these terms as their meaning is not self-evident.

True Aneurysm

The composite layers of the vessel wall are intact but stretched in true aneurysms (Fig. 27–3 [see p 405]). The great majority of aortic and iliac aneurysms are true aneurysms. The precise pathogenic mechanism for aortic and iliac aneurysm formation is unknown. It frequently occurs in association with atherosclerosis, but this is a ubiquitous condition, yet aneurysms occur in relatively few individuals. Aneurysms are usually localized to the infrarenal portion of the aorta, whereas atherosclerosis is a diffuse process. Furthermore, aortoiliac aneurysms occur predomi-

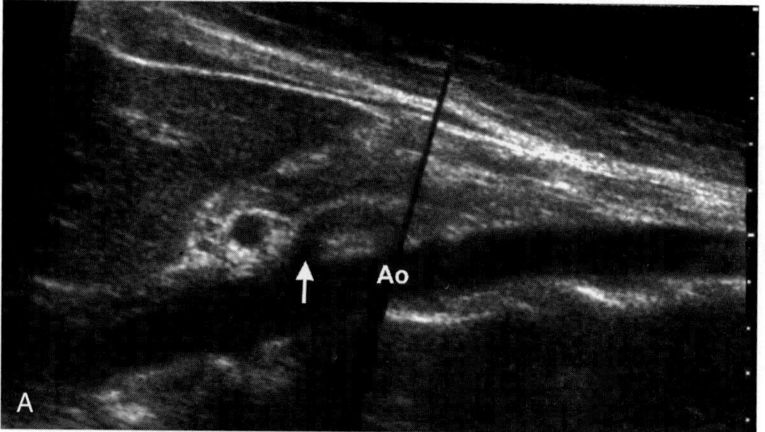

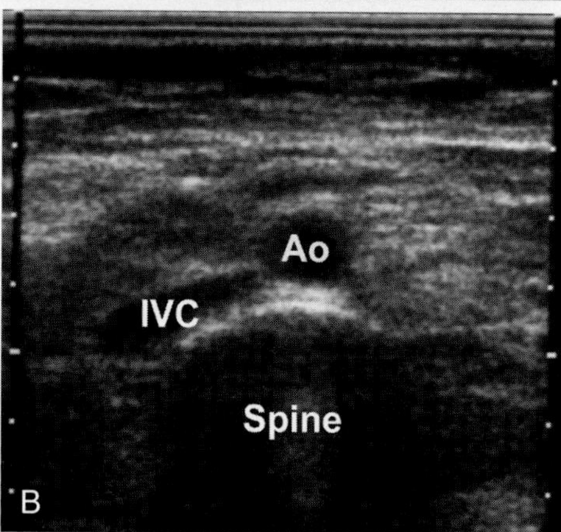

FIGURE 27–1 The normal aorta. *A,* A composite, longitudinal view demonstrates the entire aorta (Ao) from the diaphragmatic hiatus on the left, to its termination on the right. Note that the aorta tapers slightly below the level of the superior mesenteric artery (*arrow*), and that the aorta follows the course of the spine. (The IVC moves away from the spine in its cephalad portion.) *B,* Transverse view of the aorta (Ao), the inferior vena cava (IVC), and the spine. The aorta measures only about 1.5 cm in this individual.

nately (76%) in men, even though atherosclerosis occurs both in men and in women.[7]

The tendency for aortic aneurysms to occur infrarenally (below the renal arteries) is of great importance, because the surgeon may conveniently maintain perfusion of the kidneys during surgical repair by cross-clamping the aorta below the renal arteries. Surgical repair is complex for aneurysms that extend cephalad to the renal arteries and may involve reimplantation of the renal arteries or mesenteric vessels.

False Aneurysm

A false aneurysm occurs when a hole in the arterial wall permits the escape of blood, which is subsequently confined by surrounding tissues (see Fig. 27–3*C*). The extravasated blood forms a hematoma, into the center of which blood continues to circulate. The aneurysm is "false" because it is not confined by an arterial wall. Most false aneurysms result from iatrogenic arterial puncture followed by inadequate hemostasis, but false aneurysms may also result from violent trauma or localized destruction of the arterial wall by an infectious agent. The term *mycotic aneurysm* is used for infection-related lesions. False aneurysms may also occur at graft anastomoses.

Arterial Dissection

The term *dissecting aneurysm* is a misnomer, for the artery affected by dissection is not always aneurysmal (dilated). The preferred term, therefore, is *arterial dissection.*[8] This condition occurs when blood enters the media of the vessel through a rent in the intima and then dissects along the length of the artery (see Fig. 27–3*D*). The intima, and in some cases part of the media, are stripped away and a new lumen, called the *false lumen,* is formed. Blood may flow freely through both the false lumen and the original

Text continued on page 405

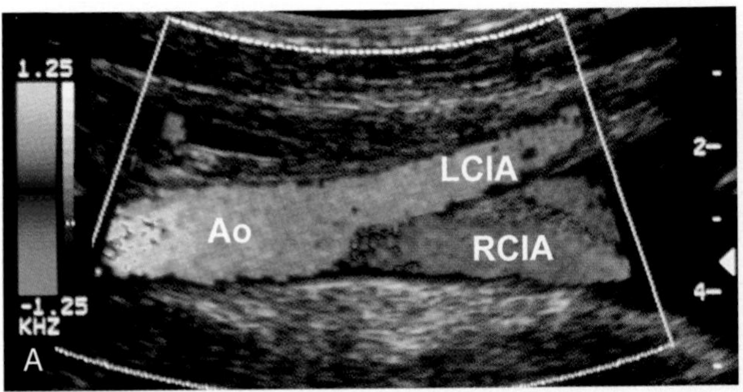

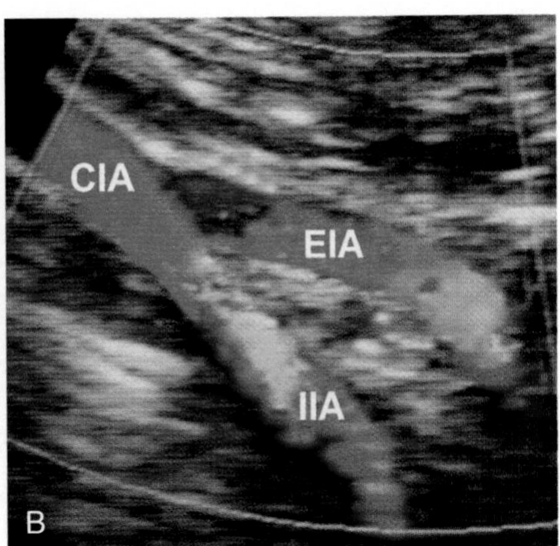

FIGURE 27–2 Normal iliac arteries. (See p 397.) *A,* A coronal view shows the bifurcation of the aorta (Ao) into the right (RCIA) and left (LCIA) common iliac arteries. *B,* The common iliac artery (CIA) is seen to divide into the external (EIA) and internal (IIA) iliac arteries.

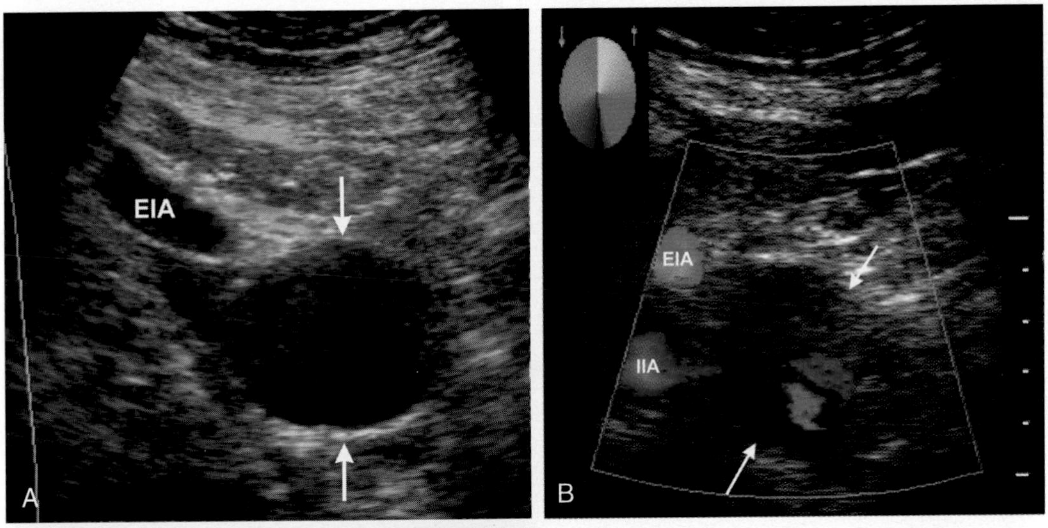

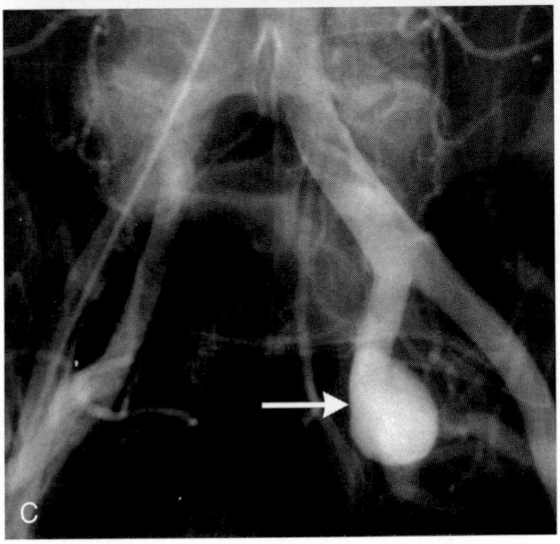

FIGURE 27–8 Isolated internal iliac artery aneurysm. (See p 410.) *A,* In this patient with lymphoma, a hypoechoic mass (*arrows*) is seen in the pelvis near the external iliac artery (EIA). This was initially thought to be a nodal mass related to lymphoma recurrence. *B,* Color-Doppler examination shows flow in the mass (*arrows*) and apparent communication with the internal iliac artery (IIA), suggesting an aneurysm. EIA = external iliac artery. *C,* Internal iliac artery aneurysm (*arrow*) is confirmed at arteriography.

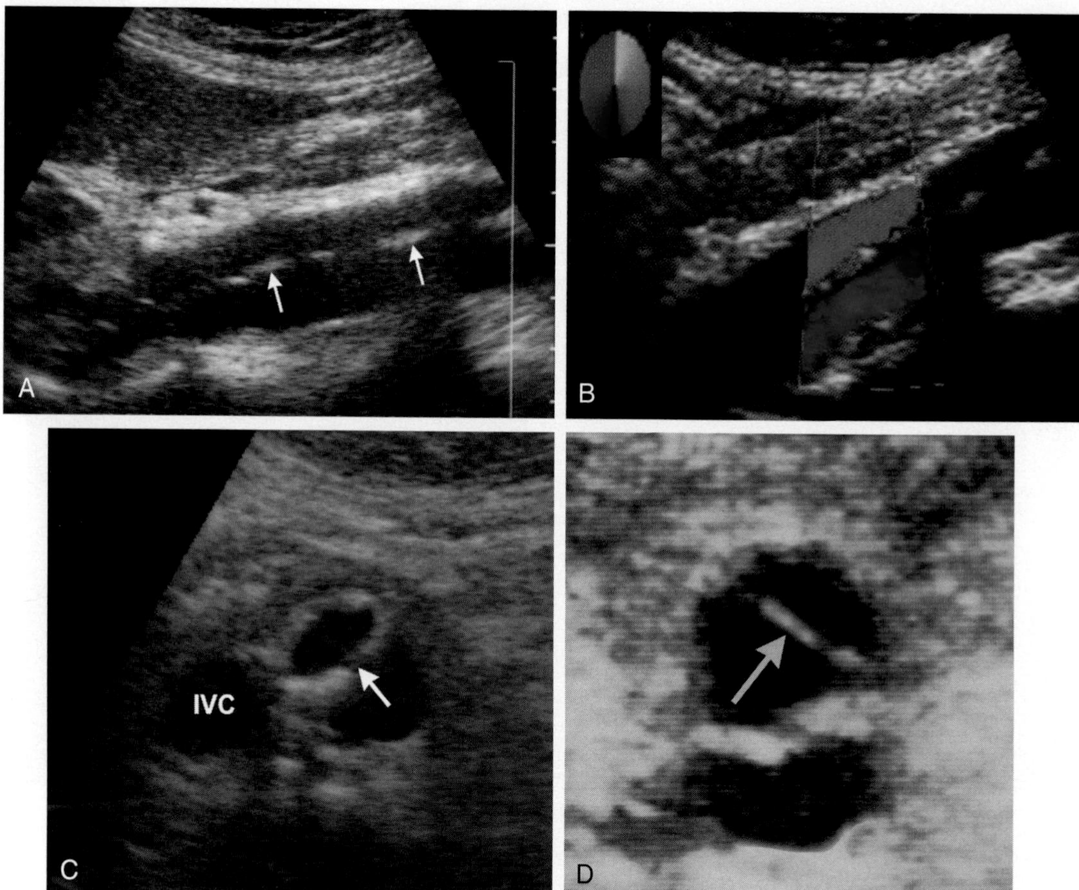

FIGURE 27–11 Aortoiliac dissection. (See p 411.) *A,* A longitudinal view of the abdominal aorta shows a dissection membrane (*arrows*). *B,* Blood flow is present in both lumina. *C,* A transverse view of the aorta shows the apparent true lumen (*arrow*) and the adjacent false lumen. IVC = inferior vena cava. *D,* in this case, dissection extended into both common iliac arteries. This short-axis image shows the dissection membrane (*arrow*) in the left common iliac artery.

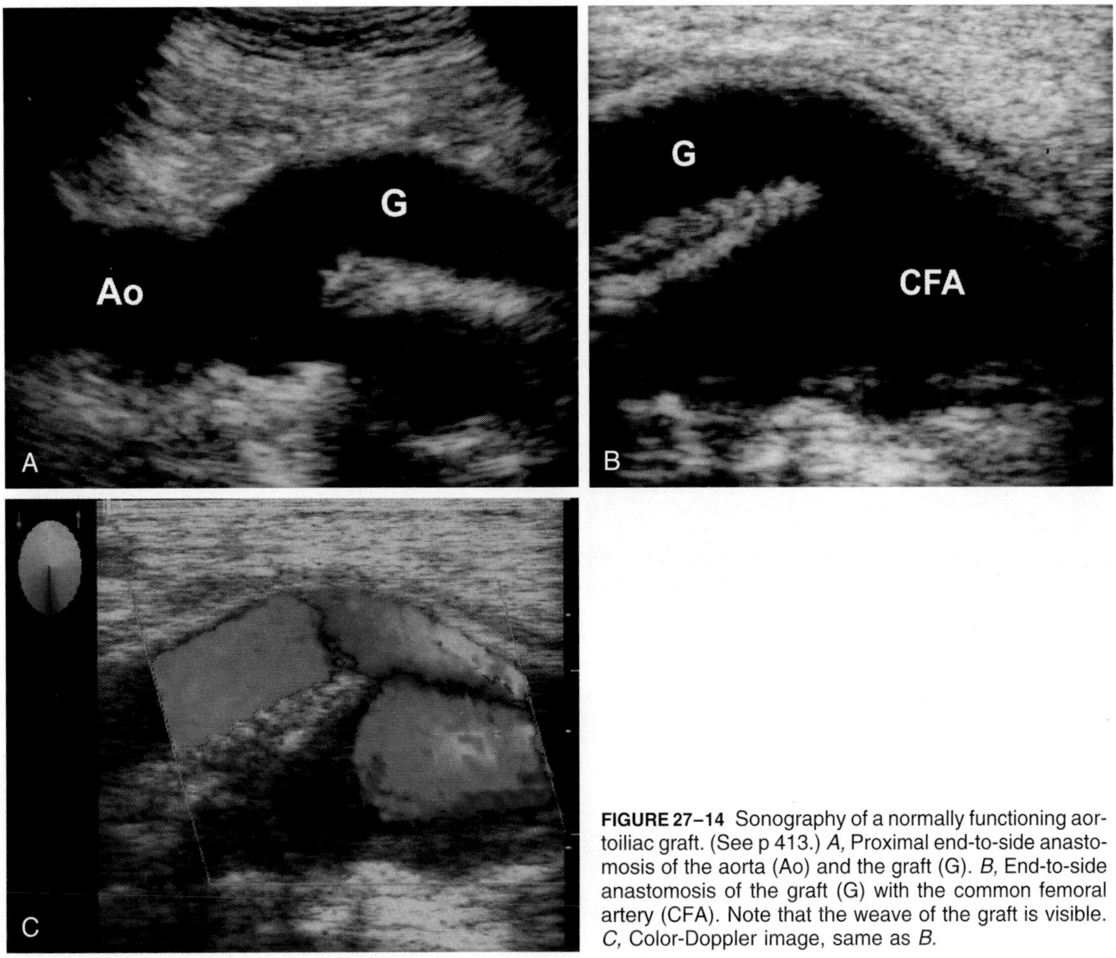

FIGURE 27–14 Sonography of a normally functioning aortoiliac graft. (See p 413.) *A,* Proximal end-to-side anastomosis of the aorta (Ao) and the graft (G). *B,* End-to-side anastomosis of the graft (G) with the common femoral artery (CFA). Note that the weave of the graft is visible. *C,* Color-Doppler image, same as *B.*

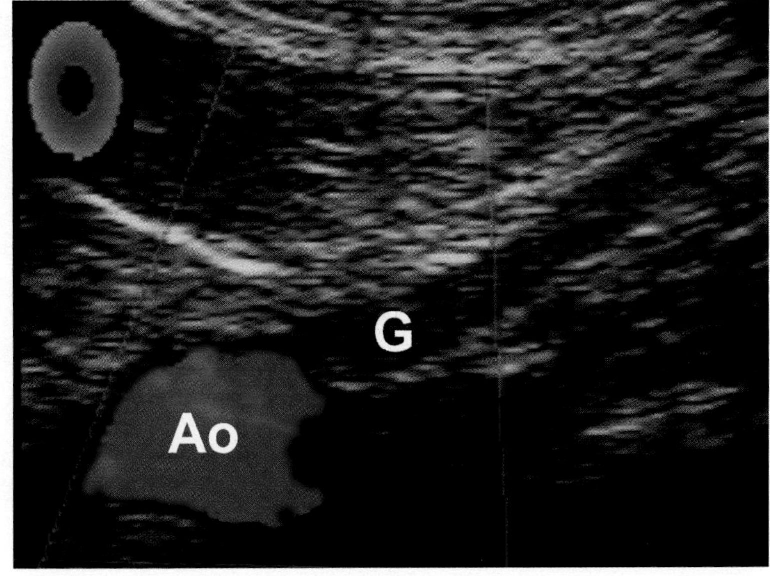

FIGURE 27–16 Graft occlusion. (See p 414.) Blood flow is present in the distal aorta (Ao) but not in the left limb (G) of this aortofemoral bypass graft.

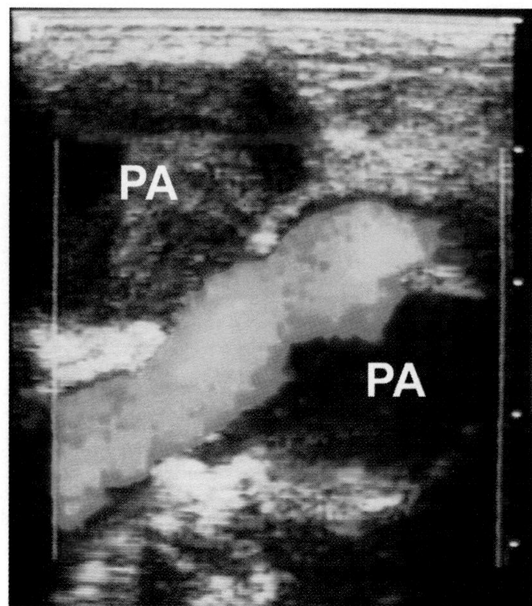

FIGURE 27–17 Graft pseudoaneurysm. (See p 414.) A large pseudoaneurysm (PA) extends both superficial and deep to the distal anastomosis of an aorto–external iliac bypass graft.

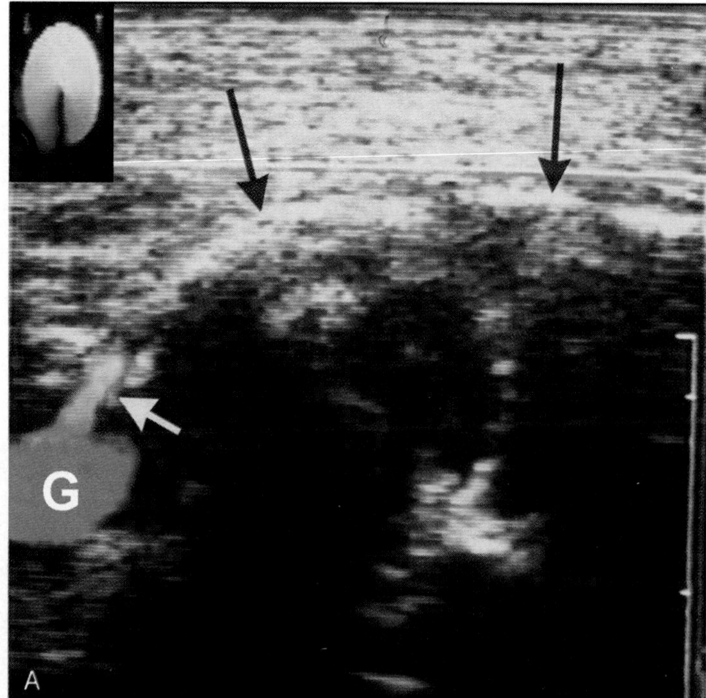

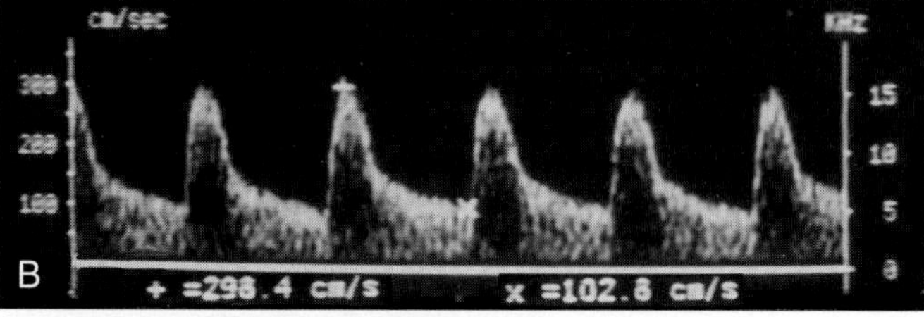

FIGURE 27–18 Graft aneurysm and stenosis (68-year-old man with claudication, 8 years after aortobifemoral graft). (See p 414.) *A,* A large aneurysm (*black arrows*) is present at the right femoral anastomosis of an aortofemoral graft (G). Only the near surface of the aneurysm is visible because extensive calcification of the aneurysm obscures deeper structures. A tiny residual lumen is present along the near surface of the aneurysm (*white arrow*). *B,* Doppler investigation of the stenotic segment shows a peak systolic velocity of 298.4 cm/sec and an end diastolic velocity of 102.8 cm/sec, consistent with severe narrowing.

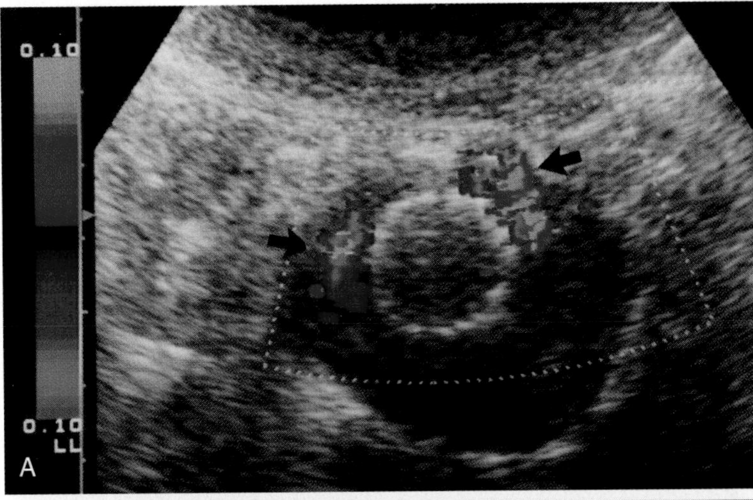

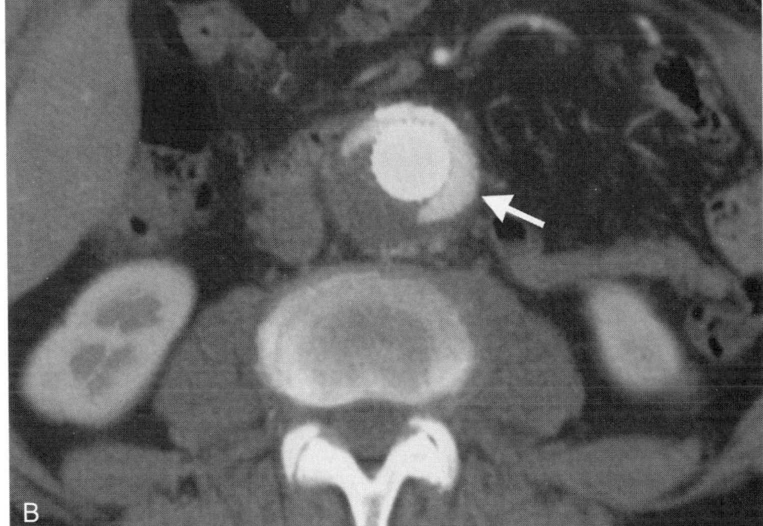

FIGURE 27–19 Leaking endoluminal prosthesis. (See p 415.) *A,* A color-Doppler image transverse to the aorta shows blood flow (*arrows*) outside of the endoluminal prosthesis. *B,* Correlative contrast–enhanced computed tomographic scan in the same patient also shows extrastent flow (*arrow*). (*A* and *B,* Courtesy of J. Golzarian, MD, Department of Radiology, Erasme Hospital, Brussels, Belgium.)

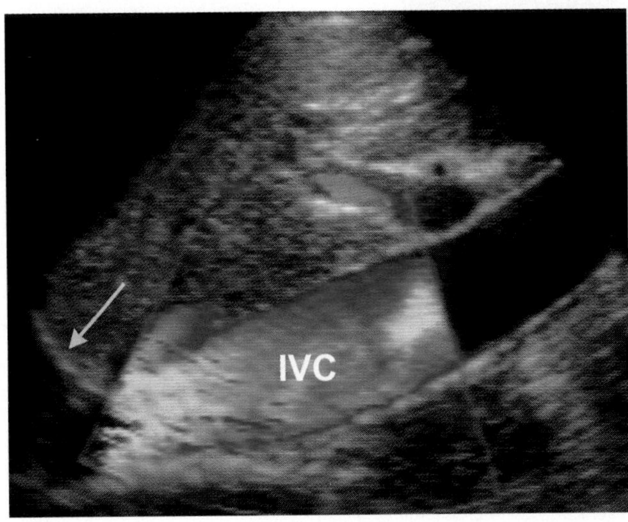

FIGURE 27–20 Normal inferior vena cava (IVC). (See p 416.) The proximal end of the IVC is seen deep to the liver in a longitudinal view. The *arrow* marks the diaphragm.

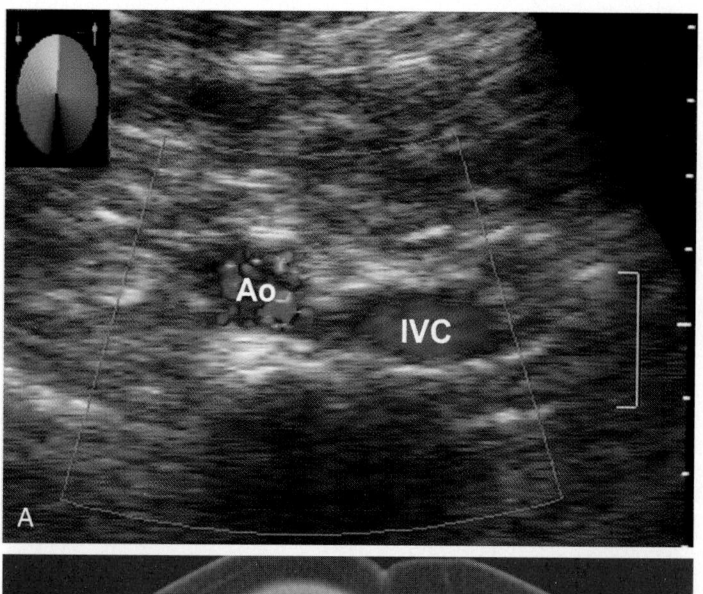

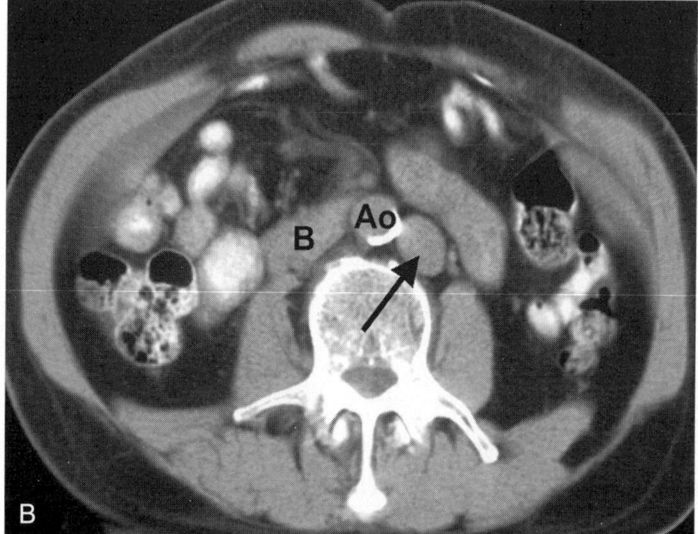

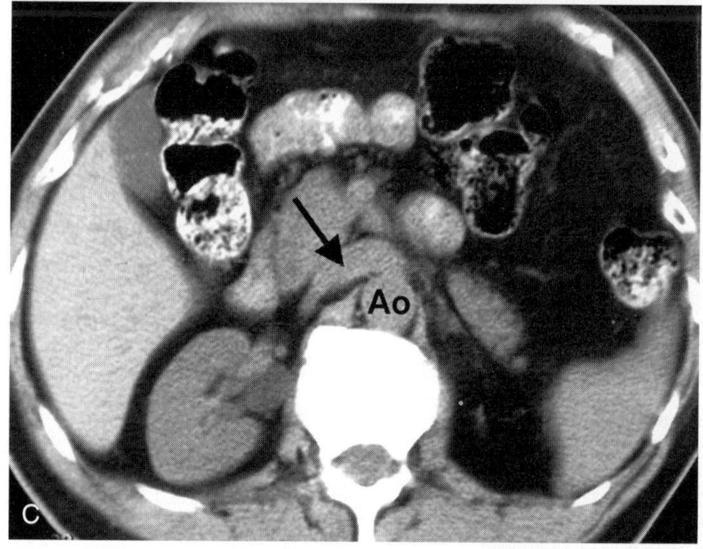

FIGURE 27–24 Left-sided inferior vena cava (IVC). (See p 417.) *A,* The IVC lies to the left of the aorta (Ao) on this transverse color-Doppler view of the lower abdomen. *B,* A computed tomogram in the same area shows the IVC (*arrow*) to the left of the aorta (Ao). B = small bowel. *C,* A computed tomogram higher in the abdomen shows the IVC (*arrow*) crossing over to the right at the level of the left renal vein.

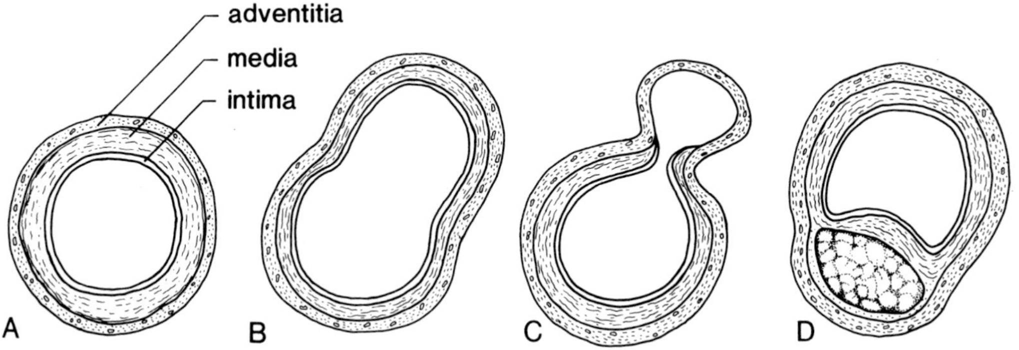

FIGURE 27–3 Types of aneurysms. *A,* Normal arterial wall components are shown. *B,* In a true aneurysm, the components of the arterial wall are "stretched." *C,* In a false aneurysm, a hole is present in the arterial wall. *D,* In arterial dissection, a hematoma forms between components of the wall.

(true) lumen to supply branch vessels. Arterial dissection requires two processes: the weakening of the media of the vessel and the development of a rent in the intima through which blood gains access to the media. Certain uncommon conditions such as Marfan's syndrome weaken the arterial media and predispose individuals to arterial dissection, but the most important predisposing condition is age and its associated weakening of the arterial media. Although arterial dissection occurs commonly in atherosclerotic vessels, it is not clear that atherosclerosis per se is a causative factor.

Aortic dissection begins almost invariably in the chest and extends into the abdomen. If the dissection begins in the ascending aorta, it may extend into the brachiocephalic vessels. The most common site at which aortic dissection begins, however, is just below the left subclavian artery. The second most common site is the ascending aorta.

Aortic Aneurysm

Presentation

Patients with aortic aneurysms may experience abdominal, back, or leg pain, but 30 to 60% of patients are asymptomatic. In asymptomatic patients, aneurysms are discovered incidentally on physical examination or imaging studies.[6, 7] It is good practice to check for silent aortic aneurysms in all elderly patients (especially men) who present for abdominal ultrasound examination.

Aortic aneurysms may also present after acute leakage or frank rupture. The signs and symptoms in such cases may include pain, prostration, or shock. Aortic aneurysm rupture is often a catastrophic event and carries a mortality rate of approximately 50%.[8–10]

Risk vs. Size

The risk that an abdominal aortic aneurysm may rupture increases with aortic aneurysm size. In a large 1998 study, the potential rupture rate was 2%/yr for aneurysms less than 4.5 cm in diameter and growth rates of less than 1 cm/yr.[11] Older studies have shown a rupture rate of only 3 to 5% over a 10-year period for aneurysms that remain less than 5 cm in diameter. In contrast, the rupture rate is increased substantially for aneurysms measuring 4.5 to 6 cm, with a rupture rate of 10%/yr reported for aneurysms of this size.[10] This figure is higher than previously reported estimates of 5%/yr for 5-cm or larger aneurysms.[6] Surgical repair is generally recommended for abdominal aortic aneurysms measuring 5 cm or greater in diameter and becomes more imperative at 6 cm in diameter because the risk of rupture increases substantially for aneurysms of this size.[12, 13]

On average the diameter of an abdominal aortic aneurysm grows 2 to 5 mm per year.[6, 14–18] Average expansion rates are not very meaningful, however, because considerable individual variation exists. When an aneurysm is discovered, therefore, serial ultrasound measurements are usually made at 6-month intervals to determine the rate of expansion. If the aneurysm is small and slow to enlarge, the follow-up interval may be increased to 1 year, but the usual interval for follow-up is 6 months.

Most iliac artery aneurysms occur in association with distal aortic aneurysms, and in

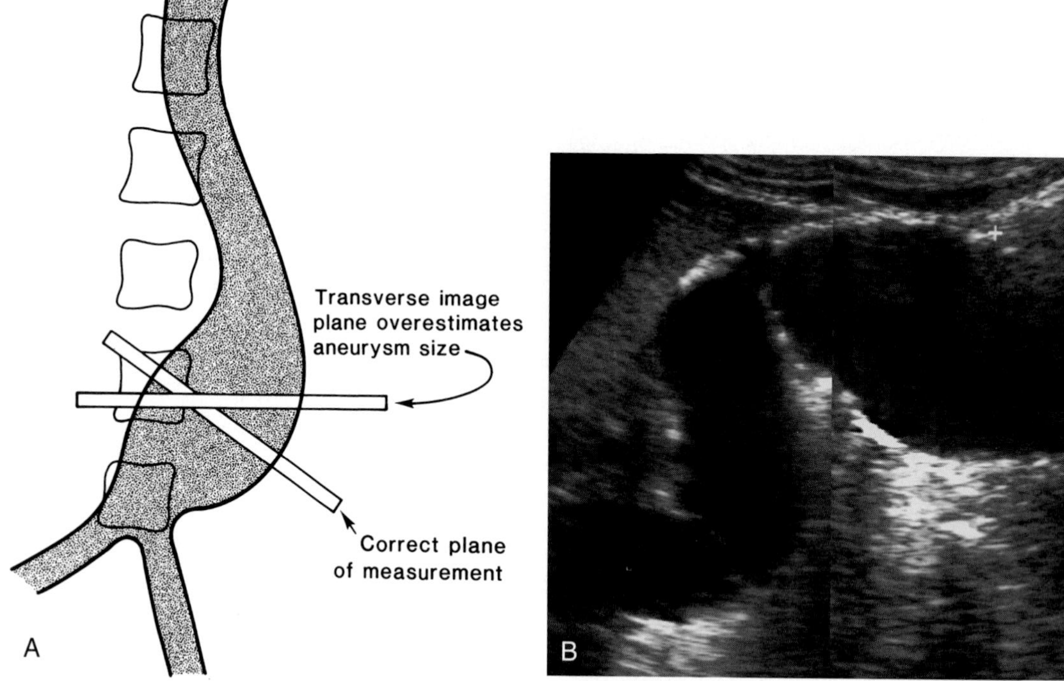

FIGURE 27–4 Measurement difficulties caused by aortic tortuosity. *A,* Note that the transverse diameter of this tortuous aorta is exaggerated with a true transverse view and is correctly measured only in an oblique view. Coronal images eliminate this problem. *B,* Composite coronal view of a markedly tortuous, aneurysmal aorta.

such cases the aortic aneurysm is generally the source of clincial concern. Isolated iliac artery aneurysms* are uncommon but may be deadly for two reasons. First, they often cannot be palpated, even when they are large, and are not detected on physical examination. Second, rupture of an iliac artery aneurysm generates nonspecific symptoms of abdominal or pelvic pain, the cause of which may not be recognized until the patient becomes hypotensive or dies. Iliac artery aneurysms 3 cm or larger are generally believed to pose significant risk of rupture, and surgical repair or percutaneous stenting is recommended for iliac aneurysms of this size. Iliac artery aneurysms are usually located in the proximal or distal portion of the common iliac arteries. *It is useful, therefore, to visualize both areas in the course of aneurysm evaluation.*

Sonographic Appearance

The primary criterion for the sonographic diagnosis of an arterial aneurysm[15, 17, 19–21] is a focal increase in the caliber of the artery, with the diameter of the dilated segment measuring at least 1.5 to 2 times greater than adjacent unaffected segments. For aortic aneurysms, an additional feature is the absence of tapering of the aorta below the mesenteric and renal vessels.

Aortic aneurysms have various gross configurations. Some are bulbous with a sharp junction, or neck, between the normal and aneurysmal portions. Others are fusiform with a gradual transition between the normal and aneurysmal portions. Many aneurysmal aortas are tortuous, for the aorta typically elongates and dilates. Tortuous aortas usually deviate to the left of the spine, as shown in Figure 27–4, but some may deviate anteriorly, creating a prominent kink at the aneurysm neck.

Concentric layers of thrombus usually line the wall of large aortic or iliac aneurysms (Fig. 27–5), and this thrombus may generate emboli that occlude distal arteries. The thrombus in an aneurysm is usually not organized, and although some evidence indicates it may reduce wall stress and risk of rupture,[15]

* Not associated with aortic aneurysm.

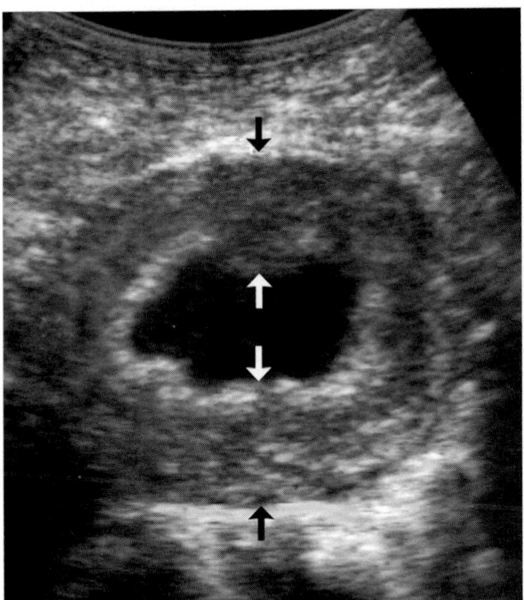

FIGURE 27–5 Thrombus within an aneurysm. Concentric layers of thrombus (*arrows*) surround the atrial lumen in this distal aortic aneurysm.

the presence or absence of thrombus does not generally affect surgical decision-making with respect to aneurysm repair.[9] Because of the presence of thrombus, the outer dimensions of an aneurysm are often much greater than the dimensions of the lumen. Therefore, arteriography usually underestimates the size of an aortic aneurysm because this technique visualizes only the arterial lumen.[19, 20]

Examination Protocol

I recommend the ultrasound examination protocol presented in Table 27–1 for assessment of aortic and iliac aneurysms. To attain the best results, the following points should be noted with respect to this protocol.

1. Always measure an aneurysm the way a surgeon does in the operating room, from the outer surfaces of the vessel (outer to outer) (Fig. 27–6).
2. Sagittal and coronal planes are recommended for aneurysm measurement, as shown in Figures 27–6*A, B.* I do not have scientific proof that this method enhances accuracy, but in my experience the use of these planes shows the point of maximum dilatation clearly, and it avoids error resulting from oblique measurement.
3. Coronal views are generally easier to obtain from the left side of the aorta than from the right side.
4. The maximum interobserver variability for aortic measurement is approximately 5 mm (95% confidence limits), and the mean variability is about 2.5 mm.[21] Therefore, an increase in size of less than 5 mm from one examination to another may not be significant.

TABLE 27–1. EXAMINATION PROTOCOL FOR AORTIC AND ILIAC ANEURYSMS

1. Longitudinal
   Examine aorta, diaphragm to bifurcation.
   Determine location and longitudinal extent of aortic aneurysm.
   Measure aortic aneurysm anteroposterior, outer to outer.
   Examine iliac arteries to iliac bifurcation.
   Measure iliac artery aneurysm(s), if present, outer to outer.
2. Transverse
   Document the maximum diameter of the aorta at the diaphragm, superior mesenteric artery, and distally near the aortic bifurcation.
   Measure aneurysm anteroposterior and transverse, outer to outer.
   Visualize the iliac arteries.
   Measure iliac artery aneurysm(s), if present, outer to outer.
3. Coronal
   Measure aortic aneurysm, *transverse* dimension, outer to outer.
   Examine iliac arteries and measure aneurysm(s), if present.
4. Color-Doppler examination
   Confirm patency of superior mesenteric, celiac, and renal arteries, and examine for flow disturbances associated with stenosis.
   Measure distance from renal arteries to aneurysm neck.
   Alternatively, measure distance from superior mesenteric artery to aneurysm neck.
5. Kidneys: longitudinal and transverse
   Document kidney length and normal features.
   Document hydronephrosis, if present.

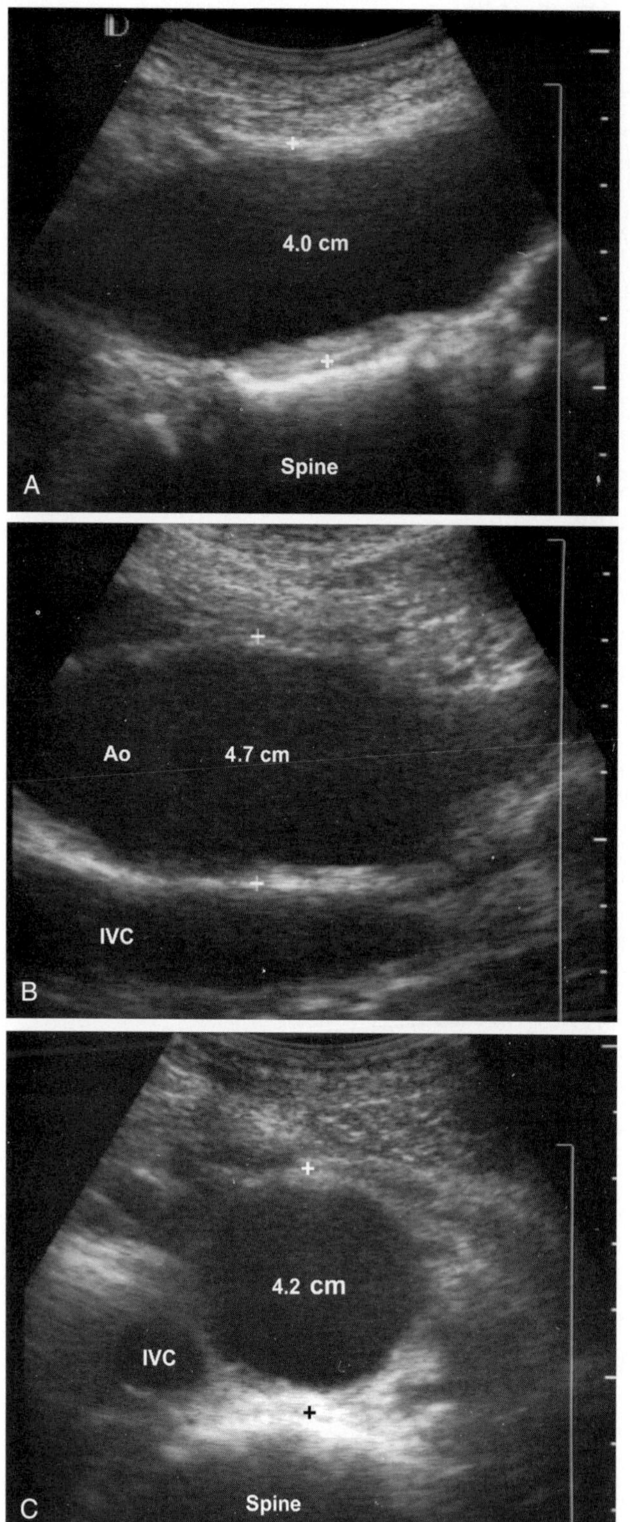

FIGURE 27–6 Aneurysm measurement technique. *A,* Longitudinal view of a distal aortic aneurysm measuring 4 cm in maximum anteroposterior dimension. The spine is visible posteriorly. *B,* As seen in the coronal scan plane, the transverse dimension is 4.7 cm. Note that both the aorta (Ao) and inferior vena cava (IVC) are visible in the coronal plane. *C,* A transverse view demonstrates the anterior and posterior surfaces of the aneurysm clearly (4.2 cm). The lateral surfaces are less clearly seen. IVC = inferior vena cava.

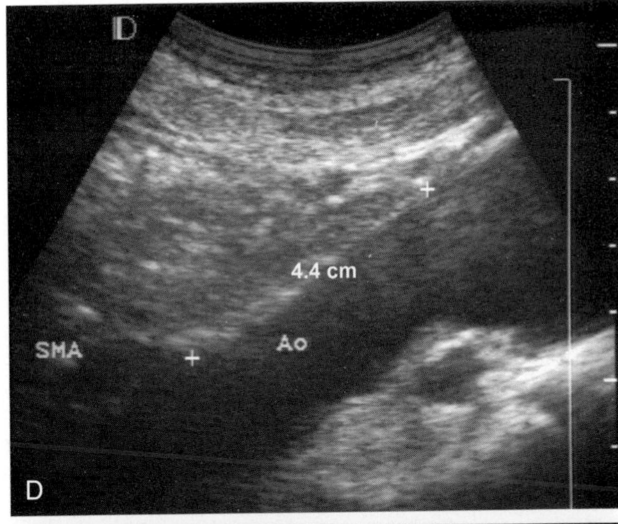

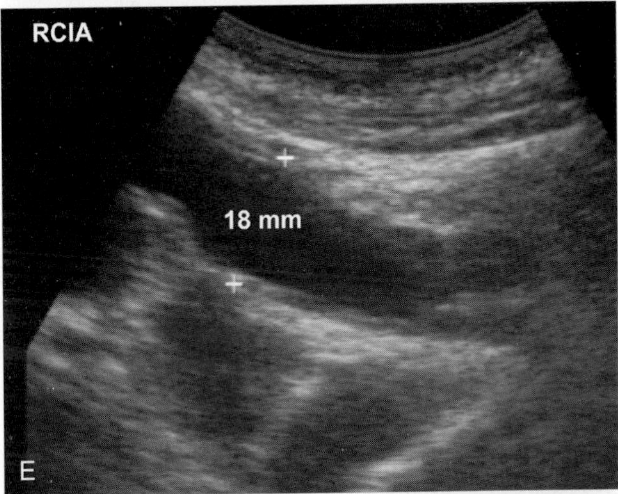

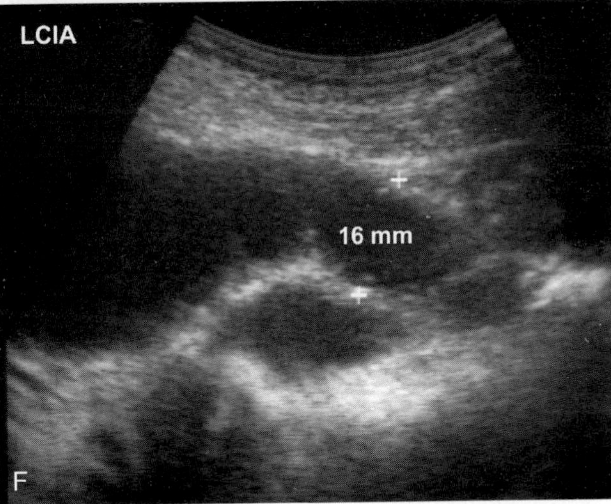

FIGURE 27–6 *Continued. D,* The distance from the superior mesenteric artery (SMA) to the neck of the aneurysm is 4.4 cm. Ao = aorta. *E,* Long-axis view of the right common iliac artery (RCIA), with focal dilatation of 18 mm diameter. *F,* Long-axis view of the left common iliac artery (LCIA), with focal dilatation of 16 mm diameter.

5. Remember, aneurysms do not decrease in size! To avoid looking foolish, be aware of the measurements reported previously before giving current measurements.
6. Always determine whether an aneurysm extends to or above the renal arteries. This is done best by directly visualizing the renal artery origins and measuring the distance from these vessels to the aneurysm. If the renal arteries cannot be visualized directly, their location may be inferred by measuring the distance from the superior mesenteric artery (SMA) to the aneurysm (see Fig. 27–6*D*). The renal arteries arise no more than 1.5 cm below the SMA; therefore, the renal arteries should be unaffected if the aneurysm begins 2 cm or more below the SMA.
7. The entire abdominal aorta must be examined to ensure that suprarenal aneurysms are not overlooked.
8. An aneurysm at the bifurcation of the iliac arteries (Figs. 27–7 and 27–8 [see p 399]) can easily be overlooked because this area is difficult to visualize. A transducer position lateral to the rectus muscles (Fig. 27–9) aids iliac artery visualization.

Aneurysm Complications

Potential complications of aortic aneurysms are atherosclerotic renal and mesenteric artery obstruction, hydronephrosis (from aneurysm compression of a ureter), retroperitoneal fibrosis, and aneurysm rupture.

Renal artery obstruction, if severe, results in shrinkage of the affected kidney. This finding, as well as hydronephrosis, is easily identified with ultrasound, and for this reason, the kidneys are always evaluated in the course of aortic examination.

Retroperitoneal fibrosis[22,23] is a rare complication of unknown etiology. Fibrosis is mani-

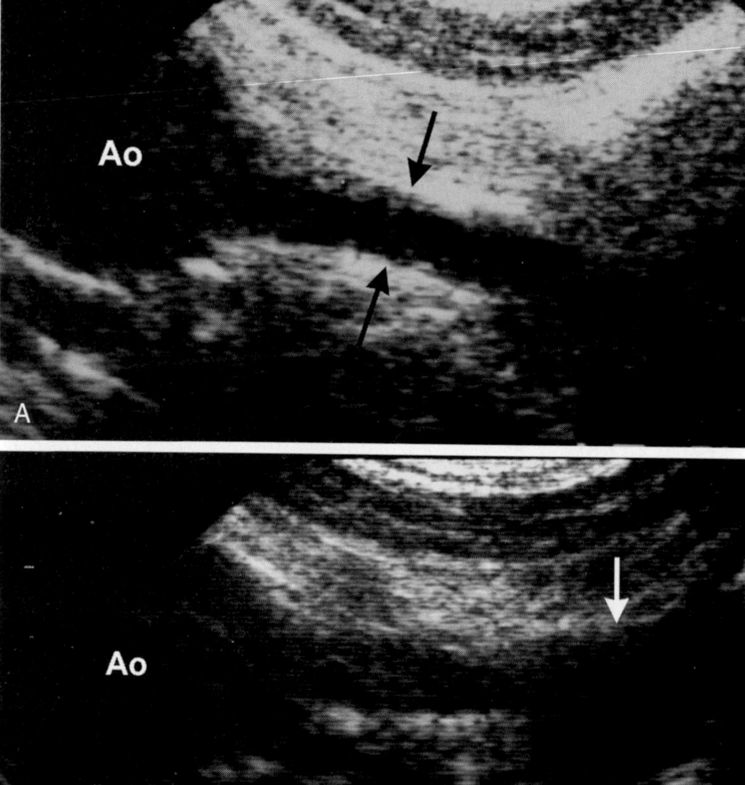

FIGURE 27–7 Aneurysms at the iliac bifurcation. *A,* An aortic aneurysm (Ao) is visible at the left. The common iliac artery (*arrows*) looks normal but the iliac bifurcation is not visualized. *B,* By tracing the iliac artery distally, an aneurysm (*arrows*) is identified in the distal common iliac artery.

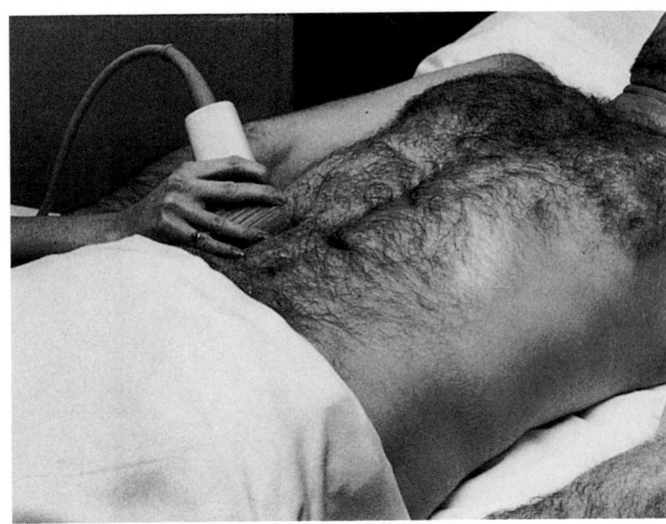

FIGURE 27–9 Transducer position lateral to the rectus muscle, for visualization of the iliac arteries.

fested as a hypoechoic soft-tissue mantle that partially or completely surrounds the aorta and may extend bilaterally into the retroperitoneum. The ureters may be entrapped in the fibrotic mass, leading to hydronephrosis.

The most disastrous complication of aortic or iliac aneurysm is rupture.[5, 6, 24, 25] Sonography is only rarely used when aneurysm rupture is suspected, because immediate surgery is often required to maintain life. In some cases, however, leakage of blood is contained by surrounding tissues, lessening the acuteness of the clinical situation. In such instances, imaging is used to confirm that aneurysm leakage is the cause of the patient's symptoms. Computed tomography (CT) is the preferred method for this task,[24] but as an expedient, sonography sometimes is used merely to confirm the presence of an aortic aneurysm, implying that rupture is the cause of symptoms. The demonstration of a retroperitoneal hematoma provides direct evidence of aortic rupture (Fig. 27–10). The hematoma is hypoechoic and is usually unilateral or asymmetric. It typically displaces the ipsilateral kidney. Peritoneal fluid may also be present if the aneurysm has leaked into the peritoneal space.

Arterial Dissection

CT and magnetic resonance imaging are the primary imaging methods used for detecting and evaluating arterial dissection in the thorax and the abdomen. Arterial dissection may be encountered incidentally, however, during ultrasound examination. Therefore, it is important for sonographers to recognize this condition. The distinguishing ultrasound finding in arterial dissection is a membrane that divides the arterial lumen into two compartments (Fig. 27–11 [see p 400]). This membrane consists of the intima and in some cases a portion of the media. The membrane moves freely with arterial pulsations if it is thin and if both the true and false lumina are patent. If the membrane is thick or if one lumen is thrombosed, however, the membrane may move little or not at all. Duplex examination may demonstrate flow in both lumina, but different flow rates may be present, and in some cases flow in the false lumen may be too slow to be detected.

The diameter of the aorta is generally increased by dissection but not as dramatically as with true aneurysms. In addition, the proximal and distal ends of the dissection may not be sharply defined, as with true aneurysms. Aortic dissection virtually always originates in the chest and extends into the abdominal aorta. Dissection may also extend into the iliac arteries or into the other aortic branches. The sonographer should try to determine the extent of dissection within the abdomen (if this is not already known) and should look for extension into major aortic branches. Stenosis or occlusion of branch vessels com-

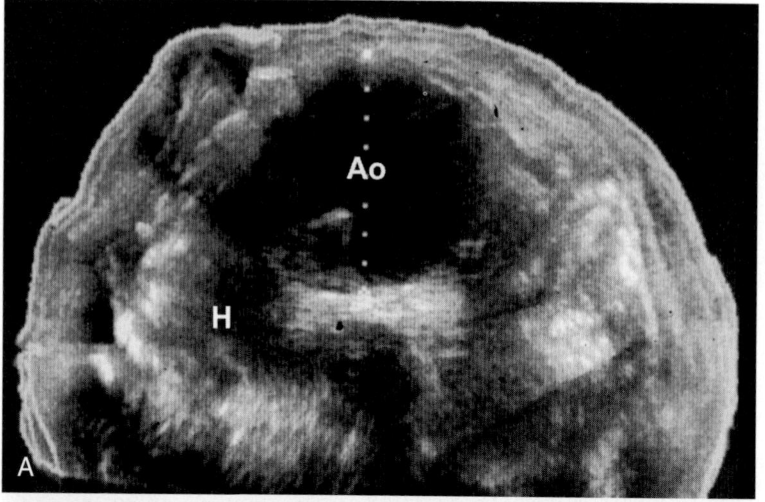

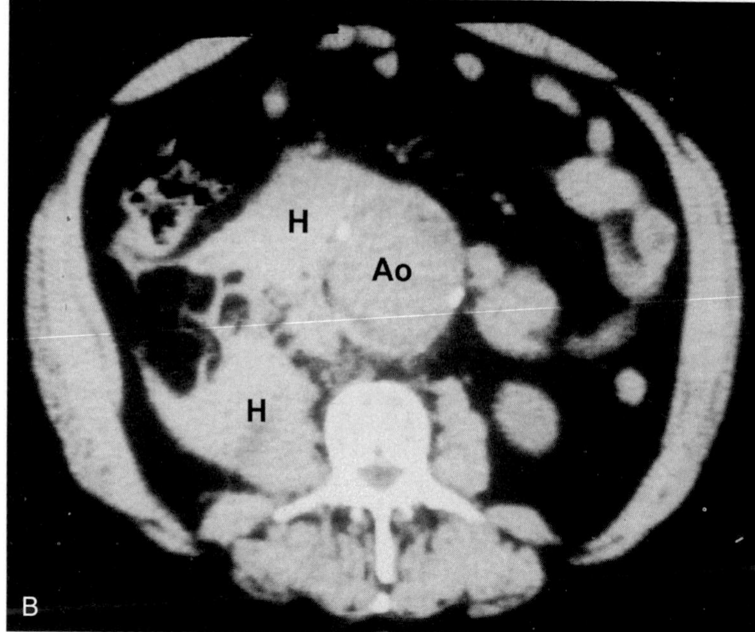

FIGURE 27–10 Aneurysm rupture. *A,* A transverse abdominal sonogram demonstrates a large hematoma (H) that has dissected posterolaterally from an 8-cm aortic aneurysm (Ao). *B,* Computed tomography demonstrates the hematoma (H) more clearly. Ao = aortic aneurysm.

monly accompanies dissection, and duplex sonography can provide valuable information about these complications.

Aneurysms of Epigastric Aortic Branches

Aneurysms form uncommonly in aortic branch arteries, including the SMA, the splenic artery, the hepatic artery, and the renal arteries.[26, 27] Although these aneurysms are uncommon, they are of considerable importance, for they may be mistaken for abdominal masses arising from the pancreas, the liver, or other epigastric structures. This error is particularly apt to occur if the aneurysm does not pulsate because of surrounding fibrosis or intraluminal thrombus. The correct diagnosis in such cases can be made only if "aneurysm" comes to the sonographer's mind and Doppler imaging is used to detect flow within the lesion, as shown in Figure 27–12.

Postoperative Assessment

Three types of surgical graft procedures are commonly used for aortic aneurysm repair

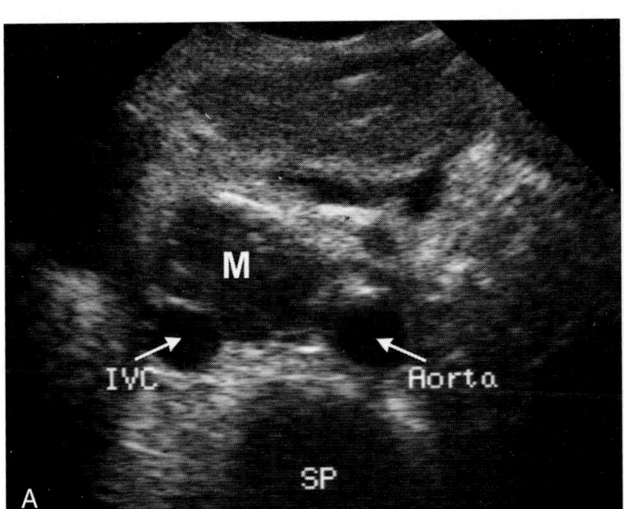

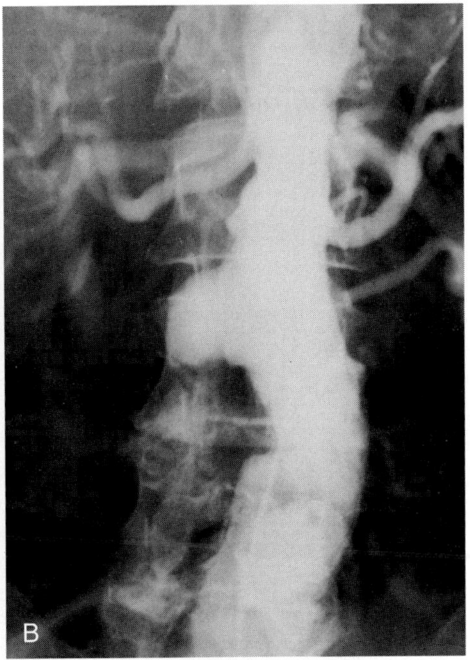

FIGURE 27–12 Mass-like epigastric aneurysm. This 75-year-old man, who presented with upper abdominal pain, had undergone aortic aneurysm repair approximately 15 years ago, but he had not received regular follow-up. *A,* Sonography demonstrated a hypoechoic mass (M) Located slightly to the right of the aorta, in the vicinity of the pancreatic head. The mass did not pulsate, and Doppler examination was not done. Initially, the mass was thought to be a pancreatic pseudocyst or a necrotic tumor in or near the pancreatic head. IVC = inferior vena cava; SP = spine. *B,* An arteriogram showed that the mass communicated with the aortic lumen, confirming the diagnosis of pseudoaneurysm.

(Fig. 27–13): (1) simple tube grafts, for aneurysms limited to the aorta; (2) aortoiliac grafts; and (3) aortobifemoral grafts. In some cases, the aneurysmal aorta is opened longitudinally, the graft is placed inside, and the native aorta is wrapped around the graft. This is done to isolate the graft and the duodenum, lessening the chance of graft infection. The wrapping procedure creates a potential space that normally contains fluid during the immediate postoperative periods.[28, 29]

As of the late 1990s, percutaneous, endoluminal repair of aortic aneurysms has come into clinical usage, and it seems likely that this method of aortoiliac aneurysm repair will be widely used in the future.[30–33] Endoluminal prostheses are specialized expandable wall stents that are placed within the dilated arterial lumen via a cutdown in a peripheral artery. CT is the preferred imaging method for surgical planning and for follow-up, but it is likely that duplex ultrasound also has a follow-up role.

Technique and Normal Appearance of Grafts

The objectives of postoperative ultrasound examination are to examine the full length of the graft to evaluate blood flow, to detect pathologic fluid collections, and to detect aneurysms. In general, the graft examination is fairly quick and easy. The sonographer begins at the proximal end and follows the graft to the distal end (or vice versa) using color-flow imaging. As long as there are no flow disturbances, we simply document the appearance of the proximal and distal anastomoses and obtain Doppler waveforms and velocities in the runoff vessels, just beyond the distal anastomoses.

The graft material used for aortic bypass has a textured appearance and is quite echogenic (Fig. 27–14 [see p 401]); therefore, the graft can usually be identified easily. Slight puckering of the graft and the native artery occurs at the suture lines, causing visible thickening of the artery wall at the anastomo-

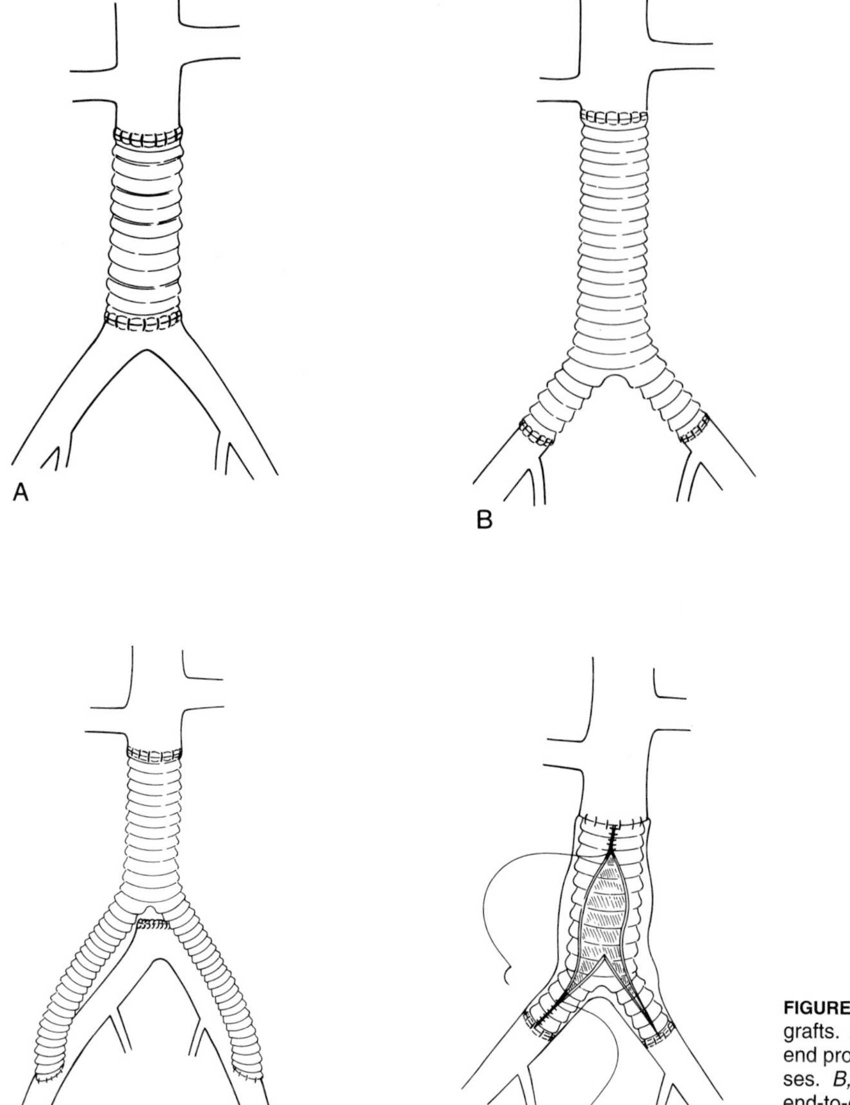

FIGURE 27–13 Types of aortic grafts. *A,* Tube graft with end-to-end proximal and distal anastomoses. *B,* Aortobifemoral graft with end-to-end distal anastomoses. *C,* Aortoiliac graft with end-to-side distal anastomoses. *D,* The native aorta is wrapped around the graft and sewn closed.

sis. A small layer of fluid is normally present around the graft during the postoperative period. This fluid may be focal or diffuse and may persist for more than a week.

Endoluminal stent grafts (Fig. 27–15) are moderately echogenic and easily visualized. The stent weave is readily apparent. Although the stents are made of metallic wire, the weave is coarse, allowing for transmission of ultrasound and the detection of flow with color-Doppler and spectral Doppler imaging.

Complications

The primary complications of aortic graft surgery are hematoma, infection, pseudoaneurysm, true aneurysm, stenosis, and occlusion. Most graft complications occur at the anastomoses; therefore, it is imperative to examine the proximal and distal anastomoses carefully. Several graft complications are illustrated in Figures 27–16 through 27–18 (see pp 401–402). Hematomas and seromas cannot be differentiated sonographically

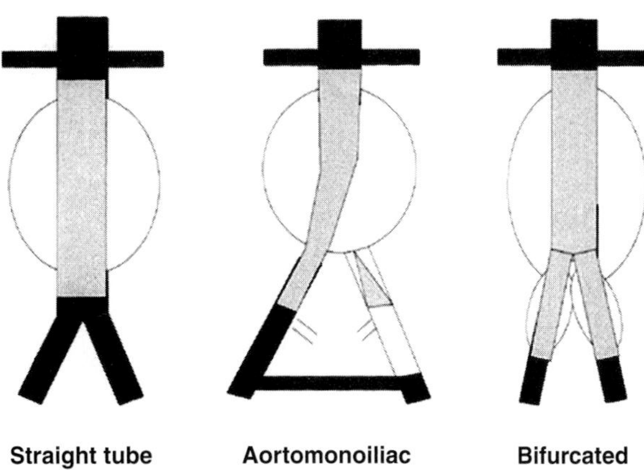

FIGURE 27–15 Types of endoluminal prostheses. The straight tube prosthesis can be used only if there is a "cuff" of normal aorta at the distal end of the aneurysm and the iliac arteries are not aneurysmal. With the aortomonoiliac prosthesis, one common iliac artery is surgically occluded and a femorofemoral bypass graft supplies blood to the occluded side. The bifurcated graft is used when the aneurysm extends to or into the iliac arteries (which is usually the case). (Courtesy of J. Golzarian, MD, Department of Radiology, Erasme Hospital, Brussels, Belgium.)

from abscesses. Postoperative hematomas and seromas should recede within weeks of surgery; therefore, regression of the size of a fluid collection is an important finding. Perigraft abscesses, however, persist and may increase in size. Graft stenosis is indicated by focal high velocity and flow disturbance. The technical details for diagnosing arterial stenosis are covered in Chapter 18. Occlusion is diagnosed by the absence of flow and the presence of echogenic material in the graft lumen. Aneurysms tend to occur at the anastomotic sites as late complications of arterial grafting. The graft/native vessel anastomosis may simply dilate, or the anastomosis may break down with subsequent formation of a pseudoaneurysm.

Complications of endoluminal prostheses include the following: (1) movement of the prosthesis; (2) continued or recurrent circulation of blood within the aneurysm but outside of the stent; (3) pseudoaneurysm formation; (4) thrombus formation within the stent, leading to stenosis or occlusion; and (5) arterial dissection. Reduced aneurysm size appears to be the norm after endoluminal stent placement and is a sign of successful treatment. Maintenance of pretreatment size or increase of aneurysm size after stenting suggests extrastent circulation. Careful postprocedure measurement of the aneurysm is important, therefore. Blood circulation around the stent (Fig. 27–19 [see p 403]) can come from several sources, including a defect in either the stent or the stent/arterial junction, and backflow through the inferior mesenteric artery, a lumbar artery, or an iliac artery. Rapid extrastent circulation of blood is easily recognized with color-Doppler ultrasonography, but low-velocity extrastent flow may be more difficult to detect. It appears that the source of extrastent circulation is better determined with CT than with ultrasound. Stent migration may be cephalad or caudad and may cause occlusion of branch vessels and extrastent circulation. Postoperative, baseline documentation of the stent position relative to the major aortic branches and the iliac artery bifurcation is of value, therefore, and follow-up examination should confirm the patency of major epigastric aortic branches and internal iliac arteries. Changes in the configuration of the stent are also important. Bulging of the stent, kinking, or fracture of the stent wires may predispose to stent migration or leakage. Thrombus formation within the stent is a potential problem. Thrombus may be visualized directly with ultrasound or indirectly through the detection of velocity elevation caused by narrowing of the stent lumen. Ultrasound examination of endoluminal prostheses should always include color-Doppler confirmation of stent patency and assessment for stenosis.

INFERIOR VENA CAVA

The IVC is evaluated with ultrasound mainly to determine whether this vessel is patent, and if it is not patent, to determine the cause of obstruction. The pathologic condition that most often affects the IVC is thrombosis. Thrombus usually propagates into the IVC from a tributary vessel, but thrombosis can also occur secondary to obstructive processes that reduce IVC flow. In current medical practice, IVC filter placement is a relatively common cause of IVC thrombosis. Neoplasia is probably the second most common pathologic condition affecting the IVC. Primary tumors of the IVC are rare, but extrinsic tumors that compress or invade the IVC are more common. These include renal cell carcinoma, hepatocellular carcinoma, and a host of other neoplasms that metastasize to paracaval lymph nodes. Congenital anomalies of the IVC are rare, but sonographers should be aware of several of the more common anomalies, as described later.

Ultrasound evaluation of the IVC[26, 34] is carried out in both longitudinal and transverse planes, but in my experience, longitudinal images (Fig. 27–20 [see p 403]) are most convenient and informative. Color-flow or Doppler evaluation is usually best accomplished with longitudinal images. Blood flow may be difficult to demonstrate on transverse scans because flow is perpendicular to the ultrasound beam. If the IVC is the focus of interest, the vessel should be examined in its entirety, including the suprahepatic, intrahepatic, and infrahepatic portions. If obstruction is found, an attempt should be made to determine its cause. If the IVC is thrombosed, the extent of thrombosis and involvement of tributary vessels should be ascertained, and a cause should be sought (e.g., compressive adenopathy).

The mean diameter of the IVC in normal individuals[27, 35] is 17.2 mm, as measured just below the renal veins during quiet respiration. The IVC ranges in diameter from 5 to 29 mm during quiet respiration, and the diameter increases about 10% during deep inspiration. The proximal portion of the IVC has a pulsatile flow pattern contributed by right atrial pressure changes occurring during each cardiac cycle and during respiration.[26, 34] Farther distal, near the confluence of the iliac veins, only respiratory variation may be observed. Partial obstruction of the IVC may eliminate normal flow variation. In such cases, Doppler flow signals are described as continuous, because a uniform flow velocity is present, without respiratory or cardiac variation.

Inferior Vena Cava Thrombosis

The ultrasound findings in acute IVC thrombosis[26–28, 34–36] are distention, absence of flow, and presence of echogenic material within the vein lumen. The echogenicity of thrombus varies with its age, as discussed in Chapter 23. In a typical case, the IVC is substantially or completely occluded by thrombus, but thrombus may occasionally propagate from a tributary vessel and float freely within the IVC without blocking flow.[29, 37] The pitfalls for sonographic diagnosis are the following: (1) acute IVC thrombosis may be so hypoechoic that it is overlooked in the absence of color-flow or Doppler examination, and (2) false-positive diagnosis of thrombosis may occur in very low flow states.

Inferior Vena Cava Filters

Ultrasonography is commonly used to evaluate devices, called *filters,* that prevent pulmonary embolization of thrombus originating in lower extremity or pelvic veins. Filters are placed in the IVC percutaneously, via the peripheral veins (usually femoral or jugular). Filter insertion may be complicated by thrombosis at the insertion site, inadequate position of the filter, IVC thrombosis, and pericaval hematoma resulting from perforation of the cava.[30–32, 38–40] IVC filters should be positioned below the renal veins (Fig. 27–21), and the IVC should be patent distal to the filter. Although the filters trap thrombus, ultrasound visualization of thrombus below the filter is considered abnormal.[32, 40]

As might be gleaned from the previous description, the most important functions of ultrasound after IVC filter insertion are to confirm that the IVC and introducer veins are patent and thrombus free, and to confirm the location of the filter relative to the renal veins.[26, 30–32, 34, 38–40] IVC perforation is uncommon, and although the resulting hematoma might be visible with ultrasound, CT is likely to be more useful for diagnosis of this complication.

Neoplastic Obstruction

Ultrasound diagnosis of neoplastic IVC obstruction is through the visualization of intraluminal tumor, or the visualization of an extrinsic tumor mass that obviously obstructs the IVC.[26, 28, 33, 34, 36, 41, 42] In the case of intraluminal tumor invasion (Fig. 27–22) the source of the tumor is usually readily apparent, as the tumor also obstructs either a renal vein or a hepatic vein. Neoplastic obstruction may cause secondary IVC thrombosis, but if thrombosis does not occur, flow may be reversed in the IVC inferior to the tumor, as a

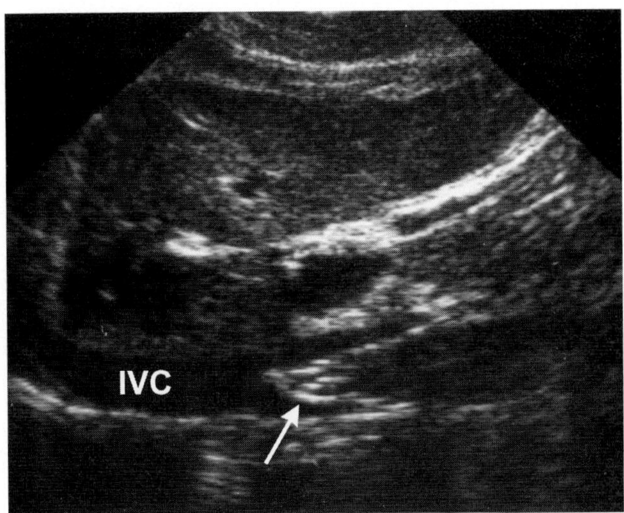

FIGURE 27–21 Inferior vena cava (IVC) filter. A longitudinal view of the IVC shows the proximal end of a filter device (*arrow*).

result of collateralization (Fig. 27–23). Alternatively, flow may be antegrade but at a very slow rate. In either case, the distal portion of the IVC is apt to be dilated. Primary IVC neoplasms are rare; of these, leiomyosarcoma is the most common.

Anomalies

Several anomalies of the IVC are noteworthy: duplication, left-sided IVC, absence of the intrahepatic portion, and membranous obstruction of the intrahepatic portion. Because these conditions are rare, they are considered only briefly.

Duplication occurs in the infrarenal portion of the IVC.[35,43] Two IVCs are seen, one on each side of the aorta. Each vessel continues cephalad as a direct extension of the ipsilateral iliac vein. In most cases, duplication ends at the level of the renal veins. The left IVC drains into the left renal vein and subsequently into the common IVC, which describes a normal course through the upper abdomen. A variant of this anomaly is a left-sided IVC (Fig. 27–24 [see p 404]) in which the left-sided IVC precursor persists rather than the right. The left-sided IVC may extend cephalad into the azygous system or may terminate at the left renal vein.

The intrahepatic portion of the IVC may be absent on a congenital basis.[36, 37, 44, 45] In such cases, flow from the renal veins and the lower extremities may be carried back to the heart by a number of conduits, but the most common are the azygos or hemiazygos veins. With the latter conduits, blood is subse-

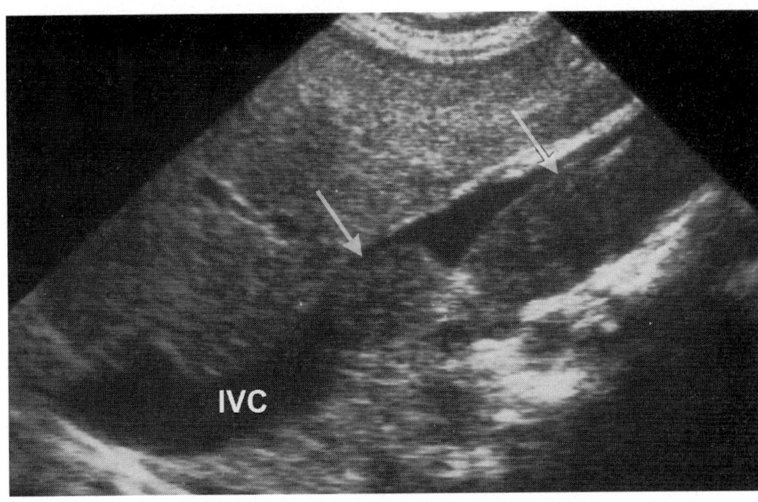

FIGURE 27–22 Extension of renal cell carcinoma (*arrows*) into the inferior vena cava (IVC).

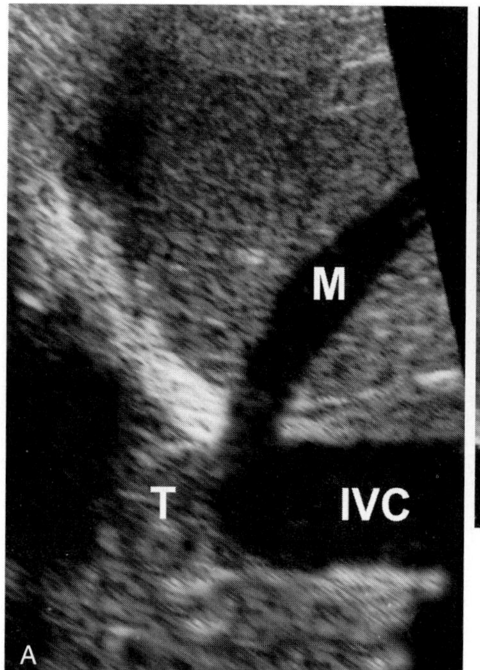

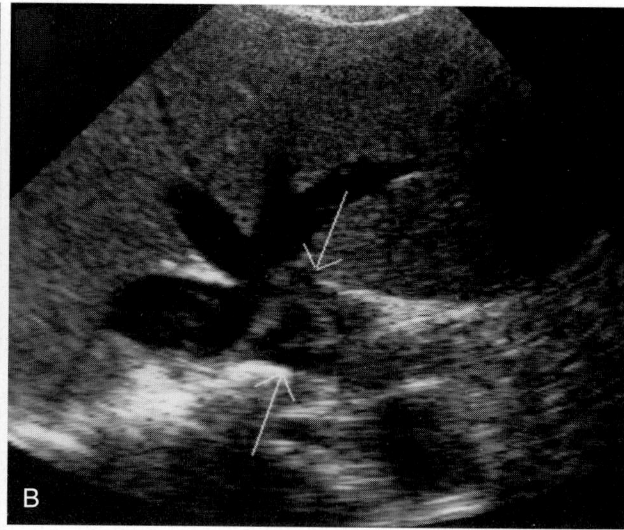

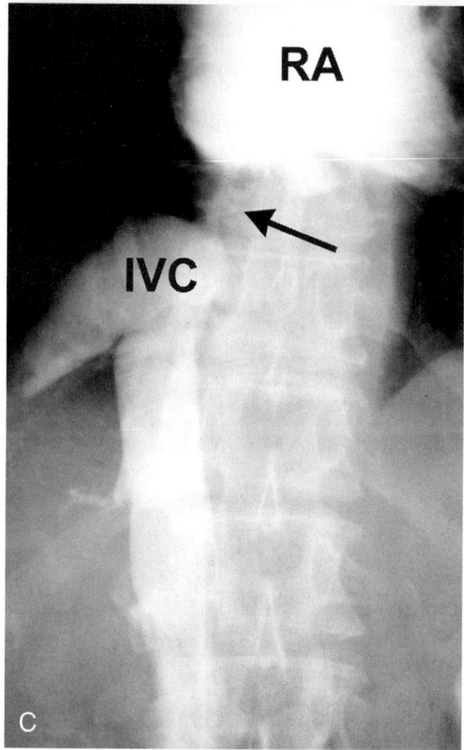

FIGURE 27–23 Inferior vena cava (IVC) occlusion. *A,* Localized growth of a hepatocellular carcinoma (T) obstructs the IVC at the diaphragm. Both the IVC and the middle hepatic vein (M) are markedly dilated. With real-time observation (not shown), blood flow from the hepatic veins was seen to move retrograde within the IVC. *B,* A transverse view shows the tumor mass (*arrows*) and marked distention of the hepatic veins. *C,* A venogram shows the obstructed segment of the IVC (*arrow*) located just below the right atrium (RA).

quently discharged into the superior vena cava, from whence it enters the right atrium. Ultrasound diagnosis is based on absence of the intrahepatic portion of the IVC and direct drainage of the hepatic veins into the right atrium, with or without a common trunk. The anomalous collateral route of the IVC may not be visible with ultrasound, but the diagnosis can be made with certainty based on the findings just described. This anomaly may be isolated and of no consequence, but it may also be a component of more serious conditions including congenital heart disease, cardiac situs anomalies, and visceral situs disorder.

Membranous obstruction of the IVC is rare in the United States, but this peculiar condition is the most common cause of hepatic outflow obstruction worldwide.[38, 39, 46, 47] The IVC is present in this condition but is interrupted by an oblique or transverse fibrous septum that is typically located just cephalad to the insertion of the right hepatic vein. The middle and left hepatic veins may insert above or below the membrane and therefore may or may not be obstructed. The right hepatic vein is almost always obstructed. Although membranous IVC obstruction is thought to be a congenital anomaly, it typically does not present until early or middle adulthood and may be an asymptomatic incidental finding. Typical presenting signs and symptoms are bilateral lower extremity swelling and signs of hepatic vein obstruction, as described in Chapter 29. Ultrasound findings are diagnostic. The obstructing membrane is visible at the diaphragm. Blood flow is reversed in the IVC, which is markedly dilated. The obstructed hepatic veins are dilated and demonstrate sluggish, continuous flow. Intrahepatic venous collateralization may be apparent, and findings of portal venous stasis may also be seen.

REFERENCES

1. Bluth EI: Ultrasound of the abdominal aorta. Arch Intern Med 144:377–380, 1984.
2. Steiner E, Rubens D, Weiss SL, et al: Sonographic examination of the abdominal aorta through the left flank: A prospective study. J Ultrasound Med 5:499–502, 1986.
3. Scott RAP, Ashton HA, Kay DN: Abdominal aortic aneurysm in 4237 screened patients: Prevalence, development and management over 6 years. Br J Surg 78:1122–1124, 1991.
4. Ricci MA, Kleeman M, Case T, Pilcher DB: Normal aortic diameter by ultrasound. J Vasc Technol 19:17–19, 1995.
5. Lederle FA, Johnson GR, Wilson SE, et al: Relationship of age, gender, race and body size to infrarenal aortic diameter. J Vasc Surg 25:595–601, 1997.
6. Hallett JW: Abdominal aortic aneurysm: Natural history and treatment. Heart Dis Stroke 1:303–308, 1992.
7. Blau SA, Kerstein MD, Deterling RA: Abdominal aortic aneurysm. *In* Kerstein MD, Moulder MD, Webb WR (eds): Aneurysms. Baltimore, Williams & Wilkins, 1983, pp 127–196.
8. DeSanctis RW, Doroghazi RM, Austen G, et al: Aortic dissection. N Engl J Med 317:1060–1067, 1987.
9. Garrett HE, Ilabaca PA: The ruptured abdominal aortic aneurysm. *In* Bergan JJ, Yao JST (eds): Aneurysms, Diagnosis and Treatment. New York, Grune & Stratton, 1982, pp 302–326.
10. Cronenwett JL, Murphy TF, Zelenock GB, et al: Actuarial analysis of variables associated with rupture of small abdominal aortic aneurysms. Surgery 98:462–483, 1985.
11. Scott RAP, Tisi PV, Ashton HA, Allen DR: Abdominal aortic aneurysm rupture rates: A 7-year follow-up study of the entire abdominal aortic aneurysm population detected by screening. J Vasc Surg 28:124–128, 1998.
12. Nevitt MP, Ballard DJ, Hallett JW: Prognosis of abdominal aortic aneurysms. N Engl J Med 321:1009–1014, 1989.
13. Bernstein EF, Chan EL: Abdominal aortic aneurysm in high-risk patients: Outcome of selective management based on size and expansion rate. Ann Surg 200:255–263, 1984.
14. Sterpetti AV, Shultz RD, Feldhaus RJ, et al: Abdominal aortic aneurysms in elderly patients: Selective management based on clinical status and aneurysmal expansion rate. Am J Surg 150:772–776, 1985.
15. LaRoy LL, Cormier PJ, Matalon TAS, et al: Imaging of abdominal aortic aneurysms. AJR Am J Roentgenol 152:785–792, 1989.
16. Hirose Y, Hamada S, Takamiya M, et al: Aortic aneurysms: Growth rates measured with CT. Radiology 185:249–252, 1992.
17. Paivansao M, Lahde S, Myllyla V, et al: Ultrasonography in the diagnosis of abdominal aortic aneurysms. Fortschr Röntgenstr 140:683–685, 1984.
18. Mower WR, Quiñones WJ, Gambhir SS: Effect of intraluminal thrombus on abdominal aortic aneurysm wall stress. J Vasc Surg 26:602–608, 1997.
19. Harter LP, Gross BH, Callen PW, et al: Ultrasonic evaluation of abdominal aortic thrombus. J Ultrasound Med 1:315, 1982.
20. King PS, Cooperberg PL, Madigan SM: The anechoic crescent in abdominal aortic aneurysms: Not a sign of dissection. AJR AM J Roentgenol 146:345–348, 1986.
21. Yucel EK, Fillmore DJ, Knox TA, Waltman AC: Sonographic measurement of abdominal aortic diameter: Interobserver variability. J Ultrasound Med 10:681–683, 1991.
22. Bundy AL, Ritchie WGM: Inflammatory aneurysm of the abdominal aorta. J Clin Ultrasound 12:102–104, 1984.
23. Cullenward MJ, Scanlan KA, Pozniak MA, et al: Inflammatory aortic aneurysm (periaortic fibrosis): Radiologic imaging. Radiology 159:75–82, 1986.
24. Clayton MJ, Walsh JW, Brewer WH: Contained rupture of abdominal aortic aneurysms: Sonographic and CT diagnosis. AJR Am J Roentgenol 138:154–156, 1982.
25. Rosen A, Korobkin M, Silverman PM, et al: CT diagnosis of ruptured abdominal aortic aneurysm. AJR Am J Roentgenol 143:265–268, 1984.
26. Falkoff GE, Taylor KJW, Morse S: Hepatic artery pseudoaneurysm: Diagnosis with real-time and pulsed Doppler US. Radiology 158:55–56, 1986.
27. Huey H, Cooperberg PL, Bogoch A: Diagnosis of giant varix of the coronary vein by pulsed-Doppler sonography. AJR Am J Roentgenol 143:77–78, 1984.
28. Mark A, Moss A, Lusby R, et al: CT evaluation of complications of abdominal aortic surgery. Radiology 145:409–414, 1982.
29. Hilton S, Megibow AJ, Naidich DP, et al: Computed tomography of the postoperative abdominal aorta. Radiology 145:403–407, 1982.

30. Fox AD, Whiteley MS, Murphy P, et al: Comparison of magnetic resonance imaging measurements of abdominal aortic aneurysms with measurements obtained by other imaging techniques and intraoperative measurements: possible implications for endovascular grafting. J Vasc Surg 24:632–638, 1996.
31. Blum U, Voshage G, Lammer J, et al: Endoluminal stent-grafts for infrarenal abdominal aortic aneurysms. N Engl J Med 336:12–20, 1997.
32. Golzarian J: Imaging of abdominal aortic aneurysms after endoluminal repair. Semin Ultrasound CT MRI 20:16–24, 1999.
33. Johnson BL, Harris EJ, Fogarty TJ, et al: Color duplex evaluation of endoluminal aortic stent grafts. J Vasc Technol 22:97–104, 1998.
34. Sandager GP, Flinn WR: Technical considerations for evaluation of the inferior vena cava. J Vasc Technol 19:263–268, 1995.
35. Sykes AM, McLoughlin RF, So CBB, et al: Sonographic assessment of infrarenal inferior vena caval dimensions. J Ultrasound Med 14:665–668, 1995.
36. Park JH, Lee JB, Han MC, et al: Sonographic evaluation of inferior vena caval obstruction: Correlative study with vena cavography. AJR Am J Roentgenol 145:757–762, 1985.
37. Sonnenfeld M, Finberg HJ: Ultrasonographic diagnosis of incomplete inferior vena caval thrombosis secondary to periphlebitis: The importance of a complete survey examination. Radiology 137:743–744, 1980.
38. Aswad MA, Sandager GP, Pais SO, et al: Early duplex scan evaluation of four vena caval interruption devices. J Vasc Surg 24:809–818, 1996.
39. Mohan CR, Hoballah JJ, Sharp WJ, et al: Comparative efficacy and complications of vena caval filters. J Vasc Surg 21:235–246, 1995.
40. Pasto ME, Kurtz AB, Jarrell BE, et al: The Kimray-Greenfield filter: Evaluation by duplex real-time pulsed Doppler ultrasound. Radiology 148:223–226, 1983.
41. Slovis TL, Philippart AI, Cushing B, et al: Evaluation of the inferior vena cava by sonography and venography in children with renal and hepatic tumors. Radiology 140:767–772, 1982.
42. Pussell SJ, Cosgrove DO: Ultrasound features of tumour thrombus in the IVC in retroperitoneal tumours. Br J Radiol 54:866–869, 1981.
43. Goss CM (ed): Gray's Anatomy, 29th American ed. Philadelphia, Lea & Febiger, 1973, p 705.
44. Garris JB, Hooshang K, Sample F: Ultrasonic diagnosis of infrahepatic interruption of the inferior vena cava with azygos (hemiazygos) continuation. Radiology 134:179–183, 1980.
45. Ritter SB, Bierman FZ: Noninvasive diagnosis of interrupted inferior vena cava: Gated pulsed Doppler application. Am J Cardiol 51:1796–1798, 1983.
46. Simson IW: Membranous obstruction of the inferior vena cava and hepatocellular carcinoma in South Africa. Gastroenterology 82:171–178, 1982.
47. Kimura C, Matsuda S, Koie H, Hirooka M: Membranous obstruction of the hepatic portion of the inferior vena cava: Clinical study of nine cases. Surgery 72:551–559, 1972.

Chapter 28

ULTRASOUND ASSESSMENT OF THE SPLANCHNIC ARTERIES

■ *William J. Zwiebel, MD*

SPLANCHNIC ARTERIES

The term *splanchnic arteries* refers to the vessels that supply the bowel with blood, principally the celiac artery, the superior mesenteric artery (SMA), and the inferior mesenteric artery (IMA). Stenosis or occlusion of the splanchnic arteries can cause acute or chronic bowel ischemia, but this is often prevented by collateralization. Although a variety of collateral routes may occur,[1] there are three principal collateral circuits: (1) the pancreaticoduodenal arcade, (2) the arc of Riolan, and (3) the marginal artery of Drummond. The pancreaticoduodenal arcade links the celiac artery and SMA circulations via arterial branches that encircle the duodenum and pancreas. The arc of Riolan and the marginal artery of Drummond link the SMA and the IMA circulations via mesenteric arterial branches.

Because of the potential for collateralization, splanchnic arterial occlusion is often asymptomatic. When mesenteric ischemic symptoms do occur, two of the three major splanchnic arteries are generally occluded or are highly stenotic. Indeed, autopsy studies have shown a 6 to 10% incidence of hemodynamically significant (50% or greater diameter), but asymptomatic, obstruction of the SMA or celiac artery.[1] The *two artery rule* of splanchnic obstruction does not hold up consistently, however, and some patients may exhibit mesenteric ischemia when only one major vessel is obstructed. Such patient-to-patient differences probably relate to variable potential for collateral development.

The presence of collateral circulation also makes it surprisingly easy to miss splanchnic artery occlusion during casual duplex ultrasound examination. For instance, if the celiac artery is not scrutinized, occlusion at the origin of this vessel may be overlooked when collateral flow is sufficient to produce normal Doppler signals within the hepatic and splenic arteries. In such cases, flow is reversed in the gastroduodenal and common hepatic arteries, but this may not be noticed by the sonographer.

A final important point about splanchnic arterial insufficiency concerns the arcuate ligament of the diaphragm, which crosses the anterior aspect of the aorta just *cephalad* to the celiac axis. In some patients, this ligament compresses and partially obstructs the celiac artery during expiration. A poorly defined complex of abdominal complaints, called the *median arcuate ligament syndrome,* has been attributed to obstruction of the celiac artery by this ligament, and surgical lysis of the ligament has been advocated in some cases.[1] Surgical treatment has met with variable success, however, ostensibly because celiac artery compression is not actually the cause of symptoms in many patients who are diagnosed with median arcuate ligament syndrome. Patients with this diagnosis have a high incidence of psychosocial disorders that are often the true cause of symptoms.[1] Furthermore, arcuate ligament compression of the celiac artery is evident angiographically in many *asymptomatic* patients.

Sonographers must be aware of median arcuate ligament compression of the celiac axis so as not to mistake this condition for significant, fixed stenosis of the celiac artery. A characteristic of the median arcuate ligament syndrome is marked reduction or disappearance of celiac obstruction with deep inspiration and return of the stenotic appearance with expiration. Sonographers should always test for median arcuate ligament compression by having the patient inhale deeply during color-flow imaging of the celiac artery origin.

Splanchnic Flow Characteristics

The anatomy and Doppler characteristics of the splanchnic arteries were discussed fully in Chapter 26, and readers should review this material if they are not already familiar with it. A high-resistance flow pattern is present in both the SMA and IMA in normal *fasting* patients.[1, 2] After the ingestion of a meal, intestinal blood flow increases markedly, and the high-resistance flow pattern gives way to a low-resistance flow pattern. The magnitude of this response varies with both the size and the composition of the meal. The timing of the response also varies, with peak mesenteric hyperemia occurring from 30 to 90 minutes after food is ingested.[1, 3]

In contrast to the situation in the SMA, a low-resistance flow pattern is present continually in the celiac artery, regardless of whether food has been ingested recently or not. The celiac artery has a low-resistance flow pattern because most of the blood in this vessel is directed to the liver and spleen, which have low-resistance capillary beds. No noticeable change in celiac flow resistance occurs after eating, because capillary resistance is not substantially affected by food ingestion.

Normal *fasting* values for SMA peak systolic velocity do not exceed 156 cm/sec (range of 96 to 156 cm/sec; mean values for peak systole 105 to 134 cm/sec). SMA end diastolic velocity ranges from 11 to 16 cm/sec.[3–8] With food ingestion, SMA peak systolic velocity increases about 40%. This is a relatively small change, because peak systole is already high in the high-resistance fasting flow state. *Mean* flow velocity increases much more (about 164%) after eating because of a massive increase in diastolic flow.[3]

Celiac artery peak systolic velocity in normal fasting subjects does not exceed 122 cm/sec in published reports, and end diastolic velocity ranges from 32 to 35 cm/sec.[3, 7] (The published range is 86 to 122 cm/sec for celiac peak systolic velocity. Mean values for peak systolic velocity range from 101 to 104 cm/sec.) Normal flow values have not been determined for the IMA.

MESENTERIC ISCHEMIA

Acute

Acute mesenteric ischemia is characterized by sudden onset of abdominal symptoms and inexorable progression to a life-threatening condition. Typically, acute ischemia is heralded by abdominal pain, followed by bowel evacuation, then by abdominal distention, fever, dehydration, acidosis, and death.[9] Acute mesenteric ischemia is a surgical emergency that is not generally of concern to vascular ultrasound practitioners because noninvasive tests have little or no role in its diagnosis or management. Certain findings on computed tomography are quite specific for acute mesenteric ischemia, but sensitivity is relatively low (64%).[10, 11] Nonetheless, computed tomography is currently the preferred method for diagnosis of acute mesenteric ischemia.

Chronic

Chronic mesenteric ischemia, as opposed to acute ischemia, is of considerable concern to vascular ultrasound practitioners because duplex ultrasonography has potential diagnostic value in this condition. Chronic mesenteric ischemia is characterized by postprandial abdominal pain that typically leads to conscious or unconscious dietary changes, including alteration of the size and contents of meals. These dietary changes reduce the severity of postprandial symptoms, but they typically cause substantial weight loss as well.[1] The astute physician may recognize more advanced symptoms of chronic mesenteric ischemia, but diagnosis at an earlier, less well-defined stage is unlikely. Therefore, an extensive diagnostic work-up is often pursued in patients with chronic mesenteric ischemia before the correct diagnosis is confirmed.

Catheter angiography is the definitive diagnostic method for chronic mesenteric ischemia, but less invasive diagnostic methods have become increasingly popular, including magnetic resonance angiography, computed tomographic angiography, and duplex ultrasonography. As of this writing, there are insufficient data in the medical literature to indicate which of these modalities is the best diagnostic approach, and it is likely that each will have a niche in the assessment of this condition. In this text, of course, I will concentrate on duplex ultrasonography, which has the advantages of being noninvasive, relatively inexpensive, and easy to perform.

Diagnostic Criteria

There are two aspects to duplex ultrasound diagnosis of mesenteric ischemia. The first is the assessment of the flow resistance pattern in the SMA (or IMA when it can be identified). The presence of a *low-resistance* flow pattern in the SMA or IMA in a *fasting* patient is proof-positive of mesenteric ischemia.[1] Recall that a high-resistance flow pattern is the norm in the SMA or IMA of a fasting patient. If the gut is ischemic, however, capillary beds are wide open, and a low-resistance pattern is present, even when the patient is fasting. This pattern would normally be seen only after food ingestion.

The second aspect of mesenteric ischemia diagnosis is direct duplex detection of stenosis or occlusion of the celiac artery, SMA, or IMA. Mesenteric ischemia is suggested when high-grade stenosis or occlusion of these vessels is detected in a patient with a typical symptom complex of mesenteric ischemia. Only stenoses causing 70% or greater diameter reduction (or occlusion) are thought to be clinically significant. Furthermore, the likelihood that mesenteric ischemia is the cause of symptoms increases if two (or rarely all three) major splanchnic arteries are obstructed.

Color-Doppler diagnosis of splanchnic artery stenosis is based on visualization of increased flow velocity and poststenotic flow disturbances (turbulence) (Figs. 28–1 through 28–4). Stenosis severity is quantified using Doppler spectrum analysis. Unfortunately, velocity criteria for specific levels of stenosis vary in published reports.[12–14] This inconsistency may be related to variations among ultrasound instruments as well as other factors, such as interobserver variability.[8] I can provide only general guidelines, therefore, concerning velocity criteria for splanchnic artery stenosis, and it will be necessary for the readers to verify these parameters within their own departments by correlating ultrasound findings with angiography or other diagnostic studies. As a rule of thumb, 70% or greater (diameter) *SMA* stenosis generates at least 275 cm/sec at peak systole and at least 45 cm/sec at end diastole in fasting patients. Seventy percent or greater (diameter) *celiac* artery stenosis generates peak systolic velocity of at least 200 cm/sec and end diastolic velocity of 55 cm/sec or greater. Velocity parameters for IMA stenosis have not been established.

Occlusion of a splanchnic artery is diagnosed with ultrasonography when blood flow is absent in a portion of the vessel on color-flow or spectral Doppler examination. A highly diagnostic finding in celiac artery occlusion is the detection of flow reversal in the gastroduodenal or common hepatic arteries. This finding appears to be 100% predictive for celiac artery occlusion (accompanied by collateral flow).[14] Collateralization may cause flow reversal in the SMA as well.

Diagnostic Accuracy

Published reports indicate that the celiac artery and SMA can be adequately examined with ultrasonography in greater than 90% of patients, making ultrasound a highly effective tool for assessing patients who may have mesenteric ischemia.[12–14] Denys and colleagues[2] reported that the IMA can be visualized with color-Doppler examination in 92% of normal, middle-aged subjects, but little information exists in the literature regarding ultrasound diagnosis of IMA obstruction.

For the SMA and celiac arteries, color-Doppler examination offers a high level of diagnostic accuracy. In published reports, Doppler sensitivity ranges from 89 to 100%, and Doppler specificity ranges from 91 to 96% for stenoses ranging from 50 or greater and 70 or greater diameter reduction (or occlusion). For the celiac artery, the reported sensitivity ranges from 87 to 93%, and specificity ranges from 80 to 100% for the same levels of obstruction.

EXAMINATION PROTOCOL

A standardized protocol should be established within each vascular laboratory for splanchnic arterial evaluation. A sample protocol is presented in Table 28–1. Please note that this protocol includes confirmation that the superior mesenteric, splenic, and portal veins are patent. Occlusion of the mesenteric veins may also produce mesenteric ischemic symptoms.

Text continued on page 428

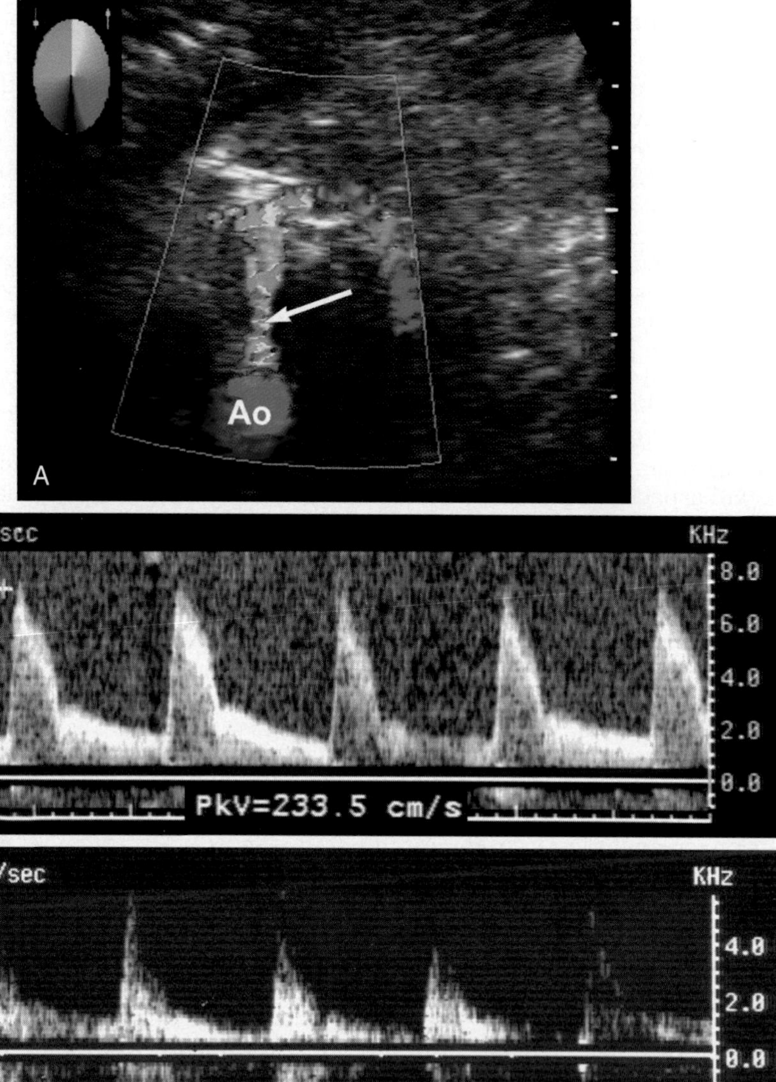

FIGURE 28–1 Celiac artery stenosis *A,* Considerable flow disturbance is evident in the celiac artery (*arrow*) and its branches. Ao = aorta. *B,* Doppler interrogation shows a peak systolic velocity of 233.5 cm/sec, exceeding the criteria for 70% diameter narrowing. End diastolic velocity was not measured but clearly exceeds 50 cm/sec. *C,* Flow is severely disturbed in the poststenotic region.

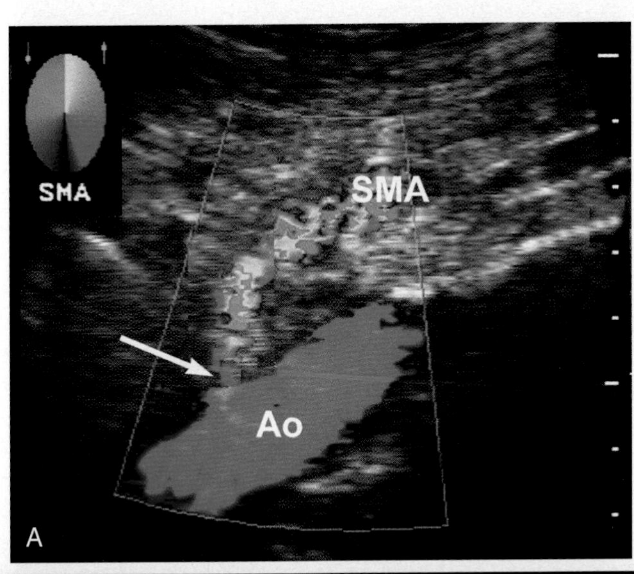

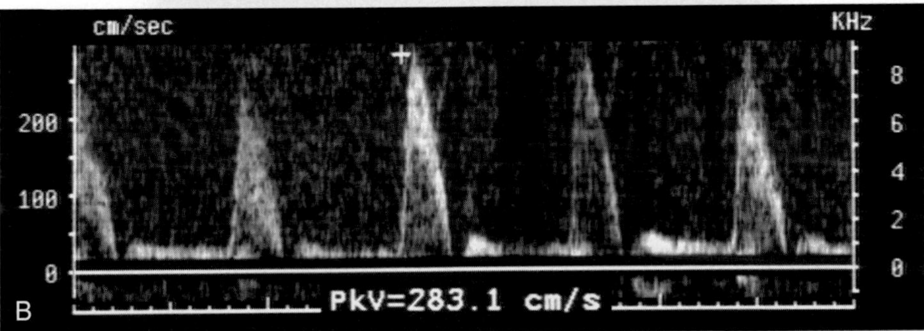

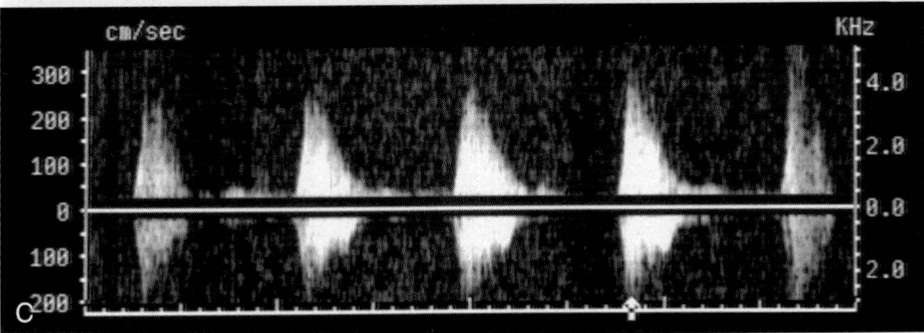

FIGURE 28–2 Superior mesenteric artery (SMA) stenosis *A,* The SMA appears narrowed (*arrow*) and blood flow is markedly disturbed. Ao = aorta. *B,* Peak systole is 283 cm/sec, slightly exceeding the criteria for significant SMA narrowing. *C,* Blood flow is quite disturbed in the poststenotic region. Diastolic flow is masked by the scale setting and the wall filter.

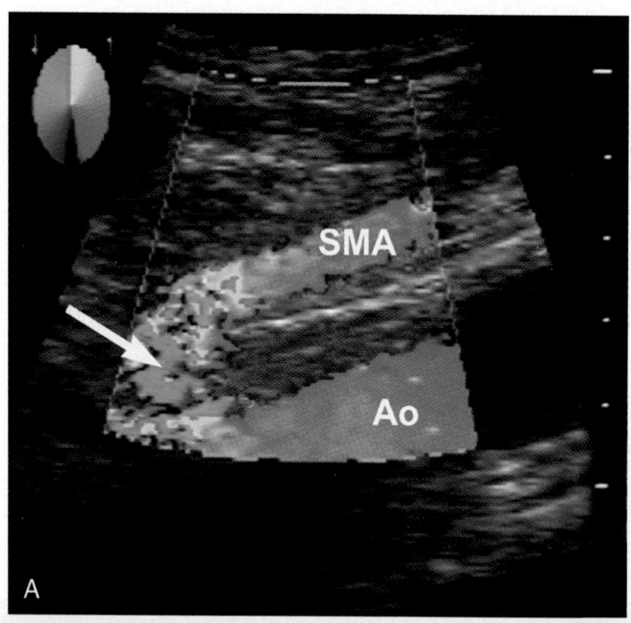

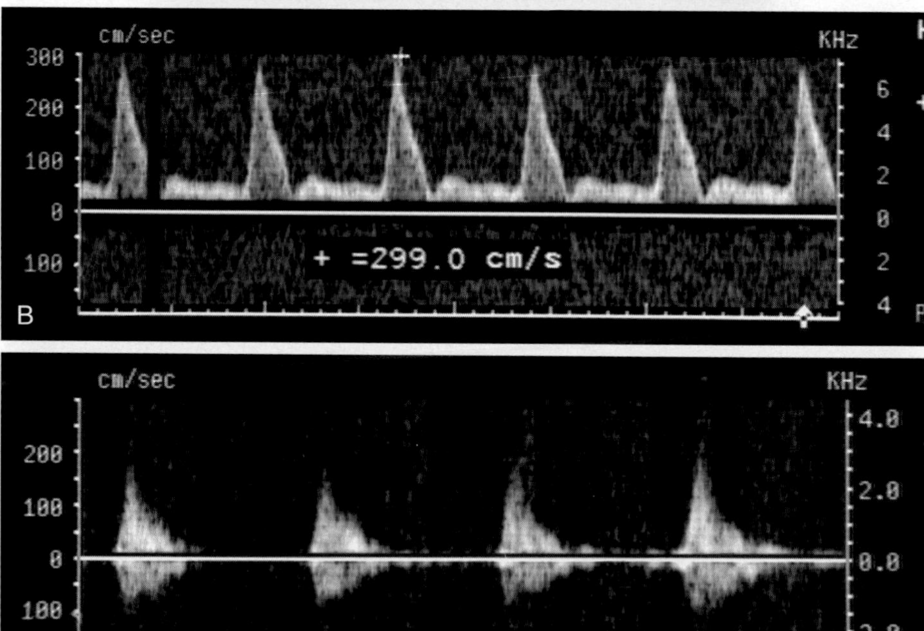

FIGURE 28–3 Superior mesenteric artery (SMA) stenosis *A,* The SMA is not appreciably narrowed on color-Doppler investigation, but considerable flow disturbance is evident. Ao = aorta *B,* Peak systolic velocity is measured at 299 cm/sec. End diastolic velocity was not measured but exceeds 50 cm/sec. *C,* flow is disturbed in the immediate poststenotic region. Low resistance is not evident for technical reasons.

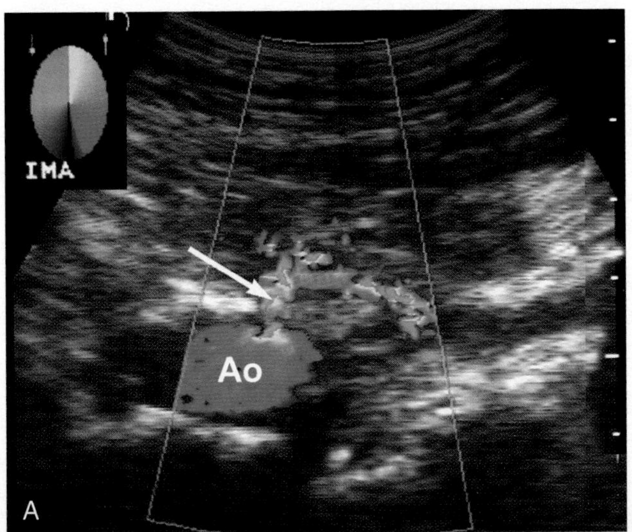

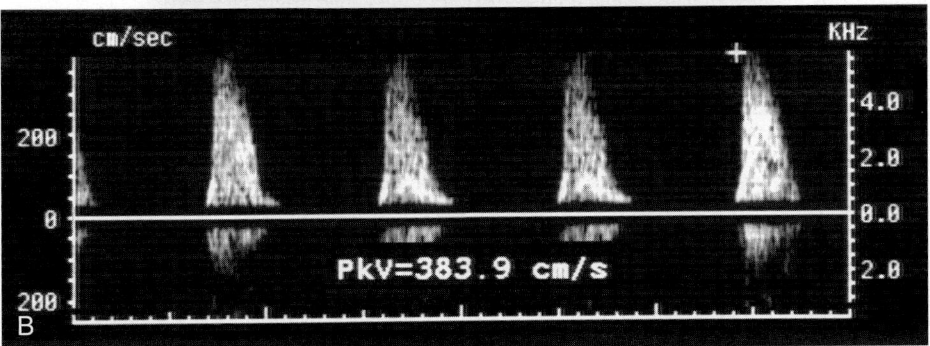

FIGURE 28–4 Inferior mesenteric artery (IMA) stenosis. *A,* An oblique view of the aorta (Ao) shows the origin of the IMA (*arrow*). Blood flow in the vessel appears disturbed. *B,* Peak systolic velocity was measured at 383.9 cm/sec. End diastolic velocity does not appear elevated for technical reasons.

TABLE 28-1 PROTOCOL FOR COLOR-FLOW EXAMINATION OF SPLANCHNIC VESSELS

Patient Preparation

Patient is examined fasting, in a supine position, and in quiet respiration.

Longitudinal Aorta and Great Vessel Origins

Document patency of the celiac and superior mesenteric arteries.

Look at the general condition of aorta and great vessels (atherosclerosis, aneurysm, and obstruction).

Celiac Artery

Document patency.

Look for high velocity or disturbed flow related to stenosis in the celiac artery, the splenic artery, or the common hepatic artery.

Note common hepatic artery flow direction.

Measure peak systolic velocity in stenotic areas, and assess flow disturbances.

If no stenosis, obtain representative celiac artery velocity and spectrum waveform.

Superior Mesenteric Artery

Document patency.

Look for high velocity or disturbed flow related to stenosis along as much of the artery as can be visualized.

Measure peak systolic velocity in stenotic areas, and assess poststenotic flow disturbance.

If no stenosis, document the presence of the normal (fasting) high-resistance flow pattern.

Inferior Mesenteric Artery

Locate the IMA if possible (look for a vessel heading obliquely to the left, just above the aortic bifurcation).

Repeat other steps as listed for the superior mesenteric artery.

Splanchnic Veins

Document the patency of the superior mesenteric vein, the splenic vein, and the portal vein.

Other Structures

Mesenteric ischemia symptoms are nonspecific, so it is advisable to examine the liver, gallbladder, pancreas, spleen, and kidneys, in addition to the great vessels. It is also advisable to check for para-aortocaval adenopathy.

Caveats

Watch out for reverse flow in the common hapatic artery and the gastroduodenal artery.

Do not be fooled by median arcuate ligament compression of the celiac artery (see text).

In most cases, we allow the patient to breath quietly during the examination. We position the Doppler sample volume such that it is over the vessel of interest during expiration. A few Doppler waveforms are recorded during each expiratory pause, and these are generally sufficient for diagnosis, even if they do not make pretty pictures.

REFERENCES

1. Moneta GL: Diagnosis of chronic intestinal ischemia. Semin Vasc Surg 3:176–185, 1990.
2. Denys AL, Lafortune M, Aubin B, et al: Doppler sonography of the inferior mesenteric artery: A preliminary study. J Ultrasound Med 14:435–439, 1995.
3. Moneta GL, Taylor DC, Helton WS, et al: Duplex ultrasound measurement of postprandial intestinal blood flow: effect of meal composition. Gastroenterology 95:1294–1301, 1988.
4. Jäger K, Bollinger A, Valli C, Ammann R: Measurement of mesenteric blood flow by duplex scanning. J Vasc Surg 3:426–429, 1986.
5. Bowersox JC, Zwolak RM, Walsh DB, et al: Duplex ultrasonography in the diagnosis of celiac and mesenteric artery occlusive disease. J Vasc Surg 14:780–788, 1991.
6. Aliotta A, Pompili M, Rapaccini GL, et al: Doppler ultrasonographic evaluation of blood flow in the superior mesenteric artery in celiac patients and in healthy controls in fasting conditions and after saccharose ingestion. J Ultrasound Med 16:85–91, 1997.
7. Mallek R, Mostbeck GH, Reinhard MW, et al: Duplex Doppler sonography of celiac trunk and superior mesenteric artery: Comparison with intra-arterial angiography. J Ultrasound Med 12:337–342, 1993.
8. Zoli M, Merkel C, Sabbà C, et al: Interobserver and inter-equipment variability of echo-Doppler sonographic evaluation of the superior mesenteric artery. J Ultrasound Med 15:99–106, 1996.
9. Bergan JJ: Diagnosis of acute intestinal ischemia. Semin Vasc Surg 3:143–148, 1990.
10. Taourel PG, Deneuville M, Pradel JA, et al: Acute mesenteric ischemia: Diagnosis with contrast-enhanced CT. Radiology 199:632–636, 1996.
11. Burkart DJ, Johnson CD, Reading CC, Ehman RL: MR measurements of mesenteric venous flow: Prospective evaluation in healthy volunteers and patients with suspected chronic mesenteric ischemia. Radiology 194:801–806, 1995.

12. Moneta GL, Yeager RA, Dalman R, et al: Duplex ultrasound criteria for diagnosis of splanchnic artery stenosis or occlusion. J Vasc Surg 14:511–520, 1991.
13. Moneta GL, Lee RW, Yeager RA, et al: Mesenteric duplex scanning: A blinded prospective study. J Vasc Surg 17:79–86, 1993.
14. Zwolak RM, Fillinger MF, Walsh DB, et al: Mesenteric and celiac duplex scanning: A validation study. J Vasc Surg 27:1078–1088, 1998.

Chapter 29

VASCULAR DISORDERS OF THE LIVER

■ *William J. Zwiebel, MD*

Vascular disorders of the liver are of considerable interest to ultrasound practitioners because the liver vessels are effectively imaged with ultrasonography in a high percentage of patients. As a result, ultrasonography is widely used for clinical assessment of hepatic vascular disorders.

This chapter considers the sonographic diagnosis of portal hypertension, portosystemic venous collaterals, therapeutic portosystemic shunts, portal vein occlusion, and hepatic vein occlusion.

PORTAL HYPERTENSION

The term *portal hypertension* refers to elevated pressure in the portal venous system, which results from impedance of blood flow through the liver. Increased splanchnic blood flow contributes to portal hypertension in some cases.[1–56] Cirrhosis is the usual cause of portal hypertension in Western nations. Other causes include hepatic vein occlusion, portal vein occlusion, and schistosomiasis.

Advances in ultrasound instrumentation have made direct, noninvasive interrogation of portal vein flow possible, and certain ultrasound parameters have been found valuable for diagnosis of portal hypertension, which include the following: (1) portal vein diameter; (2) response of the portal, splenic, or superior mesenteric veins to respiration; (3) portal flow direction; (4) portal flow velocity and waveforms; (5) spleen size; and (6) presence of portosystemic collaterals. Each of these parameters is discussed in this chapter.

Portal Vein Diameter

In normal individuals (Fig. 29–1), the portal vein diameter does not exceed 13 mm in quiet respiration and 16 mm in deep inspiration, as measured where the portal vein crosses anterior to the inferior vena cava (IVC).[6, 12–21] Respiration and patient position greatly affect the size of the portal vein and its tributaries; therefore, diagnostic measurements must be standardized by positioning the patient supine and using a state of quiet respiration. Under these circumstances, a portal vein diameter exceeding 13 mm (Fig. 29–2*A*) indicates portal hypertension with a high degree of specificity (100% reported) but with low sensitivity (45 to 50%).[20, 21] Sensitivity is increased by evaluating the response of the splenic or superior mesenteric veins to respiratory maneuvers. In normal individuals, the diameter of these veins increases by 20 to 100% from quiet respiration to deep inspiration (see Fig. 29–1*C, D*). An increase of less than 20% (see Fig. 29–2*B, C*) indicates portal hypertension with 81% sensitivity and 100% specificity.[21]

To understand the absence of respiratory response in portal hypertension, consider that elevated portal pressure has maximized portal vein distention. As a result, little or no further distention occurs when the hepatic vein outflow is restricted by sustained inspiration.

Portal Flow Direction and Velocity

In normal individuals, portal flow is hepatopedal (toward the liver) throughout the entire cardiac cycle. Mean flow velocity is about 15 to 18 cm/sec,[15, 16, 22–24] but the normal range is wide. Portal flow velocity varies with cardiac activity and respiration, giving the portal waveform an undulating appearance (see Fig. 29–1*B*).

With the development of portal hypertension, portal flow velocity may decrease and

Text continued on page 439

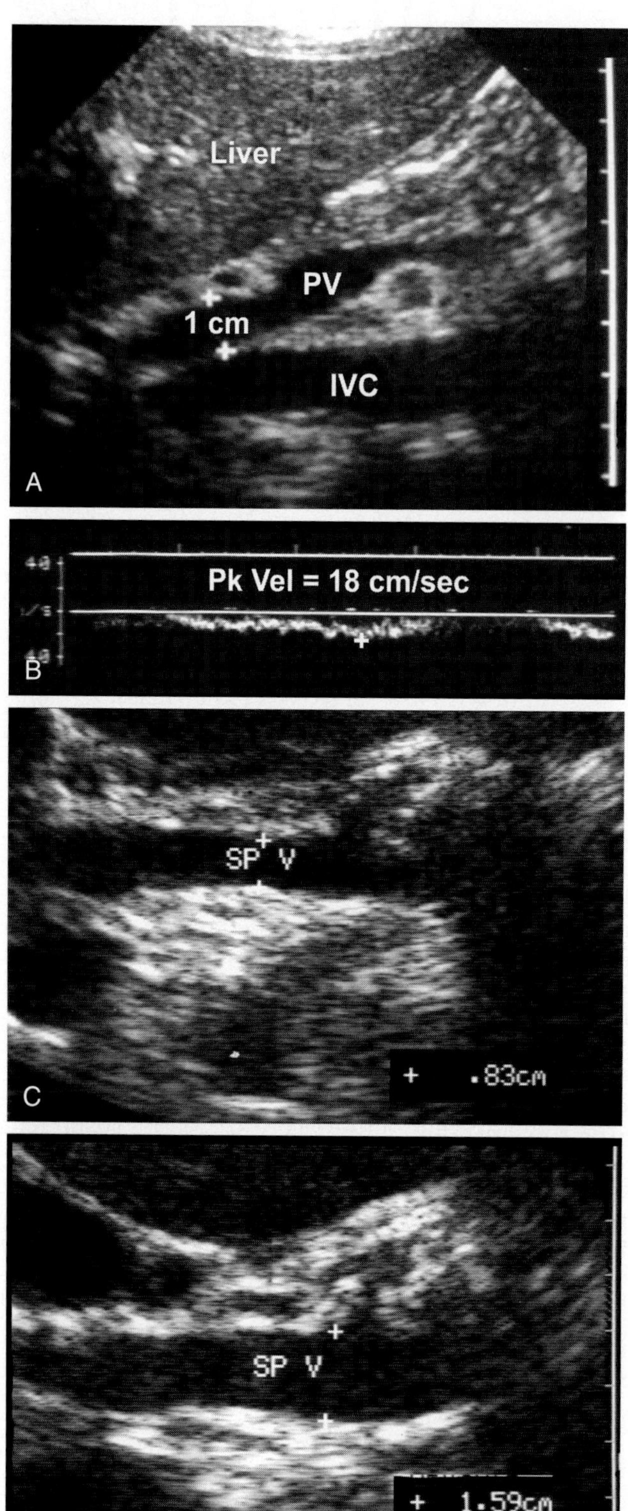

FIGURE 29–1 Normal portal vein features. *A,* The portal vein (PV) is measured where it crosses anterior to the inferior vena cava (IVC). With the patient supine and breathing quietly, the portal vein diameter (*cursors*) does not normally exceed 13 mm. *B,* Portal flow velocity undulates slightly in response to cardiac pulsation and respiration. Peak velocity (Pk Vel) is 18 cm/sec in this normal individual. In the same subject, the diameter of the splenic vein (SP V) increases more than 26% from quiet respiration (*C*) to deep inspiration (*D*).

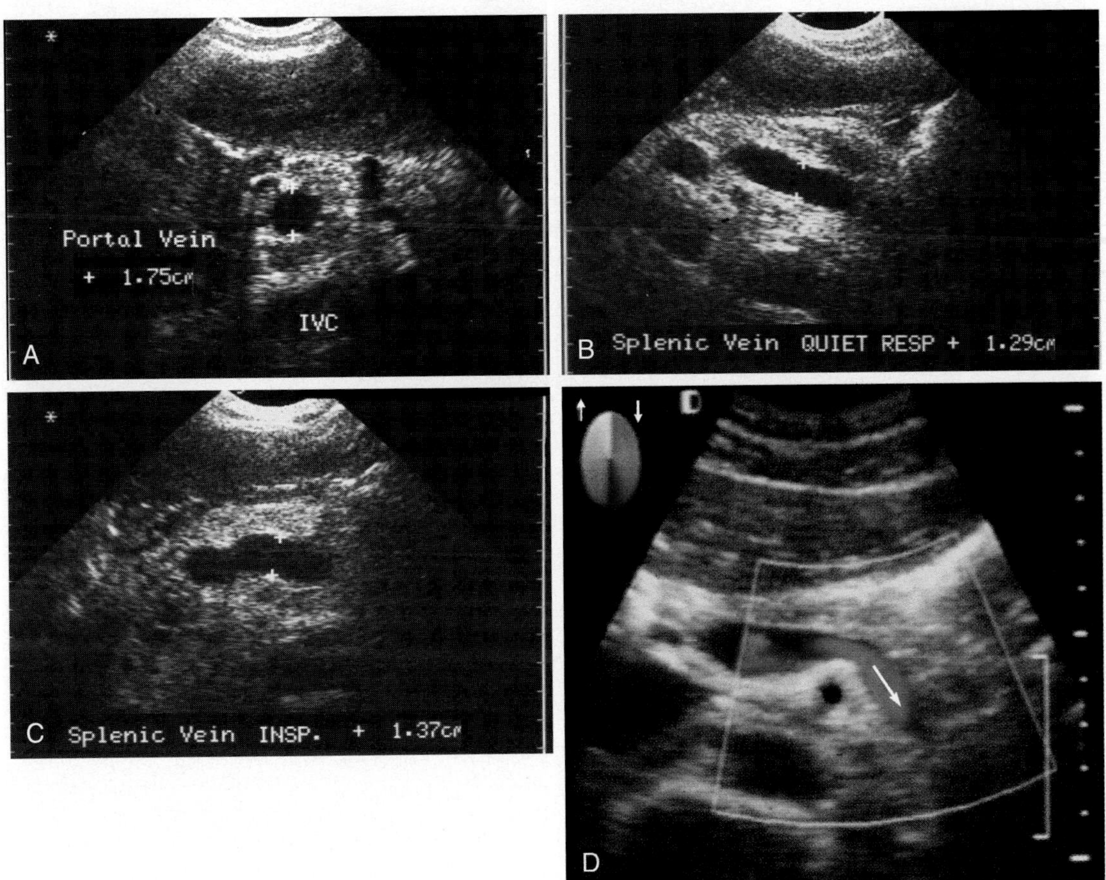

FIGURE 29–2 Features of portal hypertension. *A,* In this 48-year-old patient with alcohol-induced liver disease, the portal vein diameter (*cursors*) is 18 mm with the patient supine and breathing quietly. The diameter of the splenic vein increases only 6% from quiet respiration (*B*) to deep inspiration (*C*). *D,* In another patient with portal hypertension, splenic vein flow (*arrow*) is reversed (toward the spleen). (The spleen is not visible in this view.)

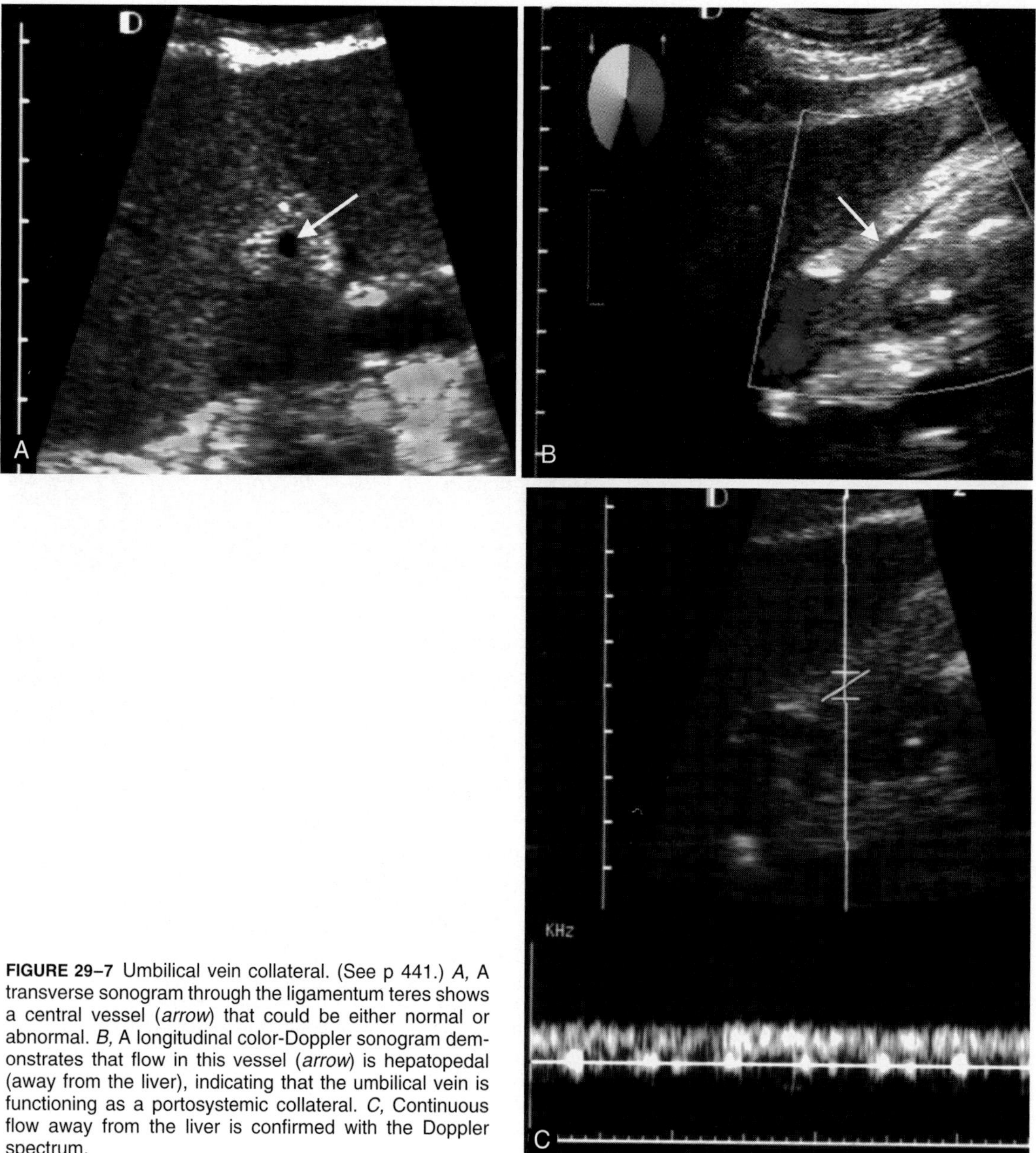

FIGURE 29–7 Umbilical vein collateral. (See p 441.) *A,* A transverse sonogram through the ligamentum teres shows a central vessel (*arrow*) that could be either normal or abnormal. *B,* A longitudinal color-Doppler sonogram demonstrates that flow in this vessel (*arrow*) is hepatopedal (away from the liver), indicating that the umbilical vein is functioning as a portosystemic collateral. *C,* Continuous flow away from the liver is confirmed with the Doppler spectrum.

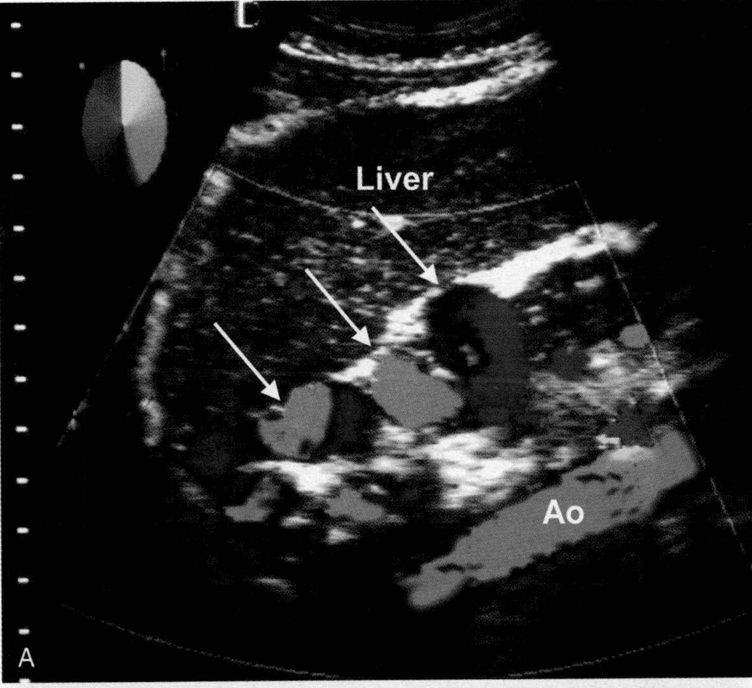

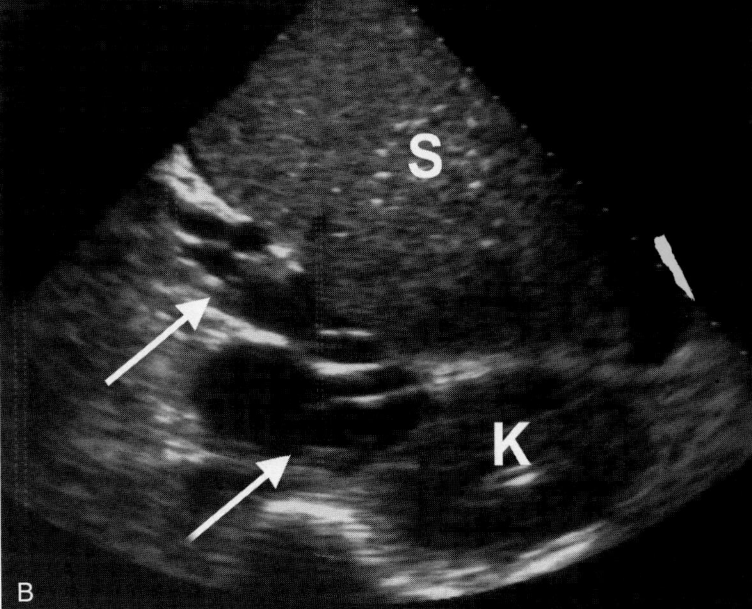

FIGURE 29–9 Splenic collaterals. (See p 441.) *A,* Large, tortuous collateral veins (*arrows*) are seen in the vicinity of the gastroesophageal junction on this longitudinal scan through the left lobe of the liver. These collaterals arise from the splenic hilum (not seen on this image). Ao = aorta. *B,* In this patient with congenital hepatic fibrosis, large splenorenal collateral veins (*arrows*) are seen to extend from the inferior end of the spleen (S) toward the left kidney (K).

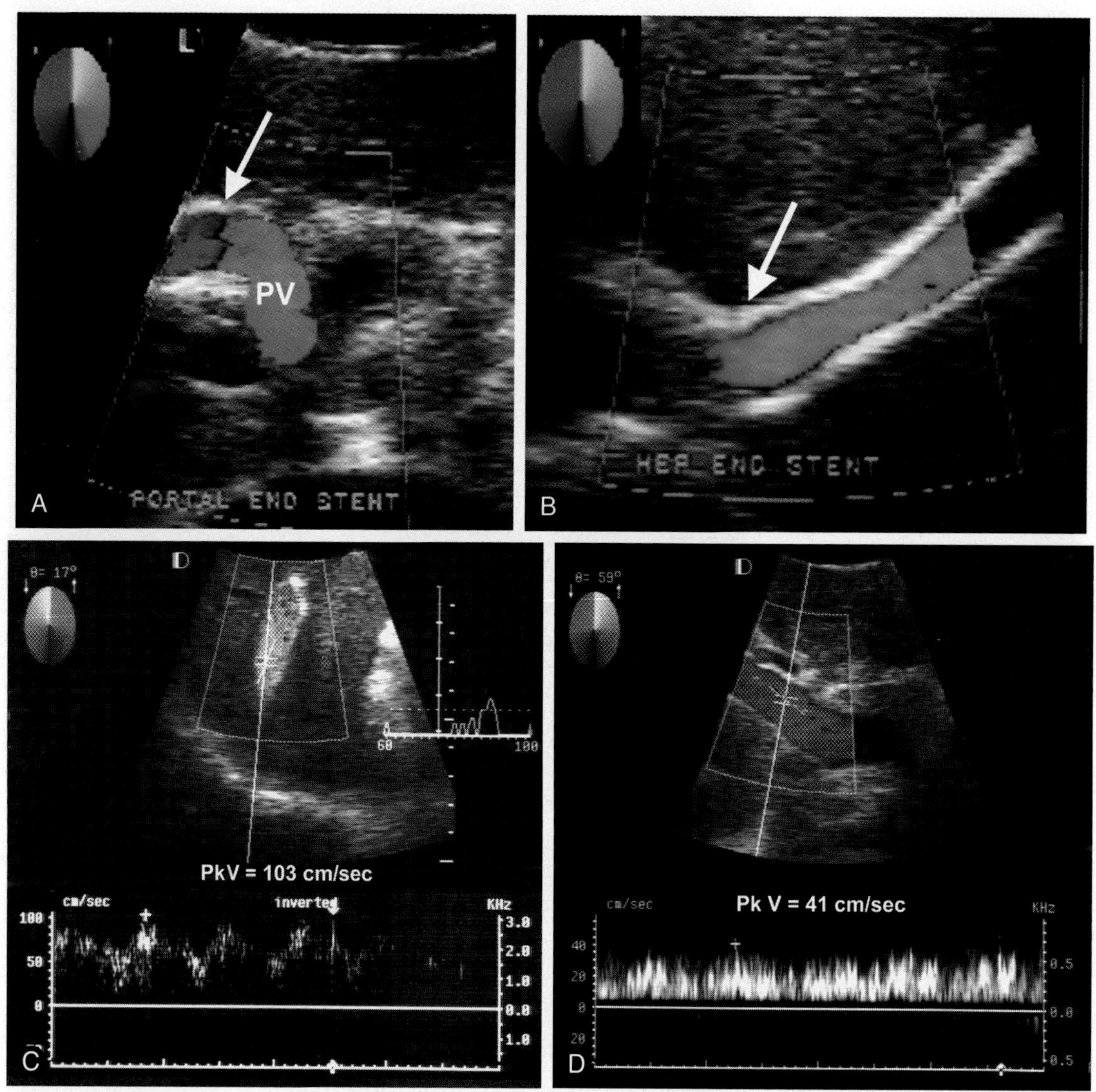

FIGURE 29–10 Normally functioning TIPS. (See p 443.) *A,* Color-Doppler image of the portal end of the shunt (*arrow*). PV = portal vein. *B,* Color-Doppler view of the hepatic vein end of the shunt (*arrow*), near the right atrium. *C,* Typical midshunt Doppler signal. Peak velocity (Pk V) is 103 cm/sec. *D,* A large volume of portal blood flow is indicated by a portal vein velocity (Pk V) of 41 cm/sec.

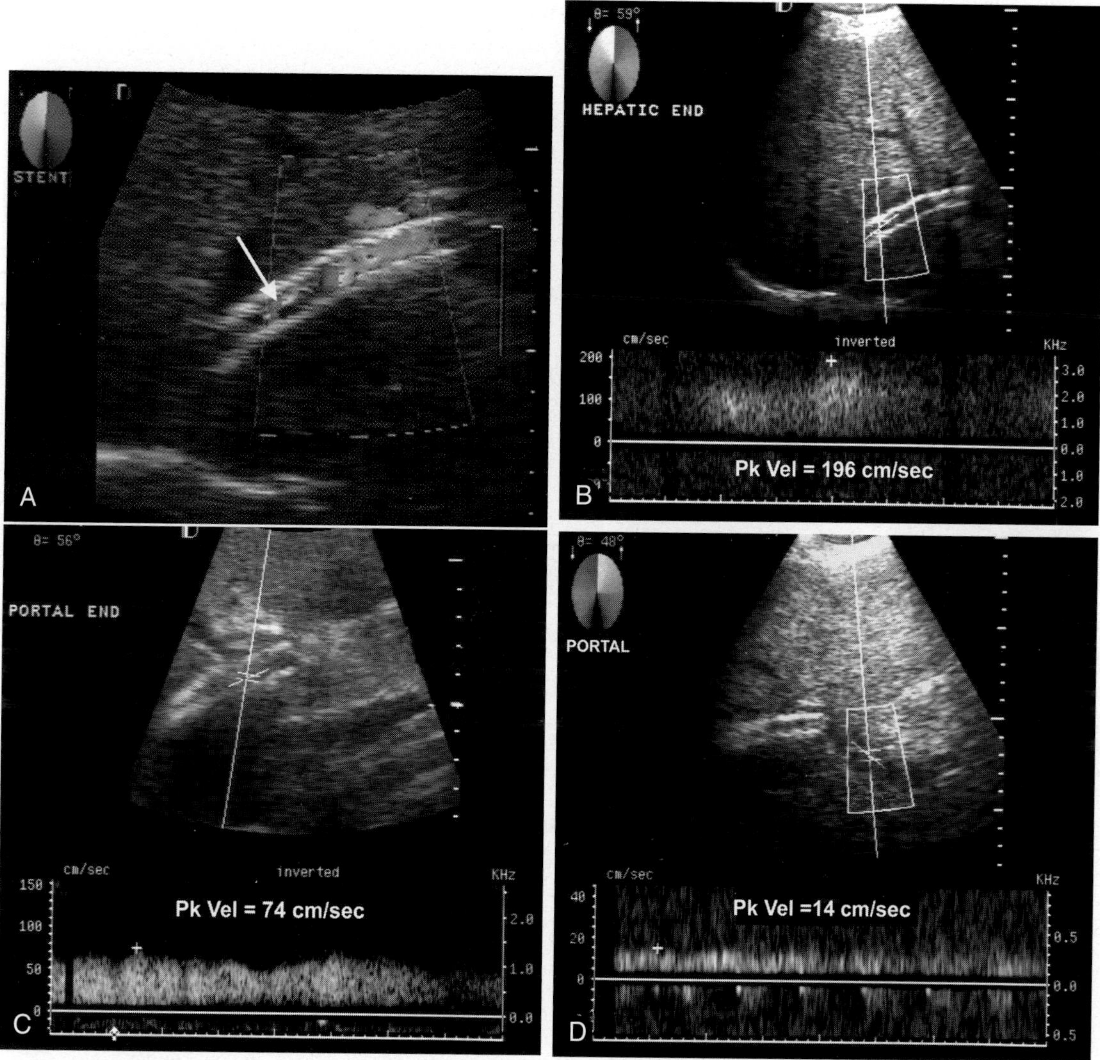

FIGURE 29–11 TIPS stenosis. (See p 444.) *A,* Near the hepatic vein end, the lumen of the shunt appears narrowed (*arrow*), and flow appears turbulent. *B,* The peak velocity (Pk Vel) in the narrowed segment is 196 cm/sec. This is more than 100 cm/sec greater than the velocity in the portal end (*C*), which is 74 cm/sec. *D,* Portal vein velocity is low (Pk Vel only 14 cm/sec).

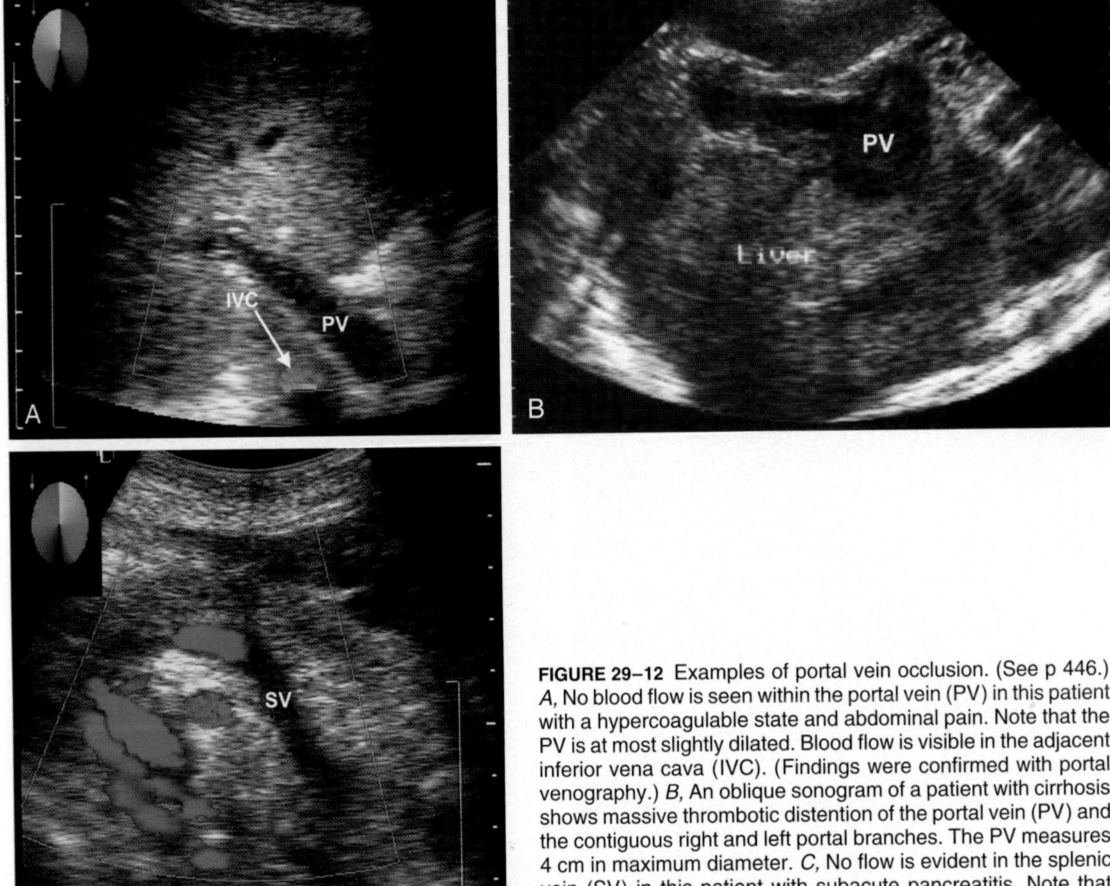

FIGURE 29–12 Examples of portal vein occlusion. (See p 446.) *A,* No blood flow is seen within the portal vein (PV) in this patient with a hypercoagulable state and abdominal pain. Note that the PV is at most slightly dilated. Blood flow is visible in the adjacent inferior vena cava (IVC). (Findings were confirmed with portal venography.) *B,* An oblique sonogram of a patient with cirrhosis shows massive thrombotic distention of the portal vein (PV) and the contiguous right and left portal branches. The PV measures 4 cm in maximum diameter. *C,* No flow is evident in the splenic vein (SV) in this patient with subacute pancreatitis. Note that flow is visible in other vessels at an equal depth.

velocity fluctuations may disappear (i.e., flow becomes continuous). Ultimately, as portal pressure increases, portal vein flow may become to-and-fro (biphasic), or the flow direction may reverse (hepatofugal flow) (see Fig. 29–2*D*). Concomitant flow reversal may occur in the splenic vein.

Flow reversal in the portal or splenic veins is a variable finding in portal hypertension, because flow direction in these vessels is influenced by collateral development. For instance, if splenorenal collaterals are the primary mode of portal decompression, flow may reverse in the portal vein. If, however, a large umbilical vein collateral is the primary mode of decompression, splenic and portal vein flow may well be normal (hepatopedal) because the diverting collateral (the umbilical vein) originates in the left portal system (discussed later). For the same reason, it is possible for flow to be simultaneously reversed in the right portal vein and normally directed in the left portal vein.

Congestive Index

Portal hypertension may also be recognized with the *congestive index,* which is the ratio of the portal vein area (cm^2) divided by the mean portal flow velocity (cm/sec).[22, 23] This ratio, which does not exceed 0.7 in normal individuals, is attractive because it takes into account two intersecting physiologic changes that occur in portal hypertension: portal vein dilatation and diminished flow velocity.

Cirrhotic Liver Morphology

Cirrhosis[57] is the nonspecific, end stage manifestation of hepatocyte injury, which leads, ultimately, to tissue necrosis, fibrosis, and attempted regeneration of liver tissue. There are numerous causes of cirrhosis. In Western nations, alcoholism is the principal etiology, but in Asia, Africa, and most developing countries, viral hepatitis is the usual cause. Although cirrhosis is an advanced form of hepatic fibrosis, *these disorders are not synonymous* and have markedly different clinical implications. Cirrhosis should be diagnosed with ultrasonography only when specific findings are identified, as discussed in the following. Cirrhosis is classified as *micronodular* or *macronodular,* depending on the size of regenerative nodules present. Macronodular cirrhosis is simply an advanced stage that has gone beyond the micronodular form.

The ultrasound findings that characterize cirrhosis[57–64] are illustrated in Figure 29–3. The following manifestations of cirrhosis are particularly noteworthy:

1. The attenuation of the cirrhotic liver is *similar* to that of the normal hepatic parenchyma. The cirrhotic liver may be slightly more echogenic than a normal liver, but the cirrhotic liver is not strongly echogenic and is easily penetrated by the ultrasound beam. (An exception to this rule occurs if fatty infiltration is superimposed on cirrhotic changes.)
2. In patients with advanced cirrhosis, the texture of the liver is more coarse than normal, and the surface is irregular because of the presence of regenerative nodules. Surface nodularity is most easily detected when ascites surrounds the liver and highlights its surface (see Fig. 29–3*A*). Even fine surface nodularity is abnormal and strongly suggests the diagnosis of cirrhosis.[58] Furthermore, nodularity is associated with sinusoidal obstruction and resultant portal hypertension. By identifying parenchymal nodules, one may distinguish between cirrhosis and other forms of liver disease, such as uncomplicated hepatic fibrosis and fatty liver.
3. Large regenerative nodules may occasionally be visualized as discrete, rounded structures within the liver parenchyma.[61–64] These nodules are either isoechoic or slightly hypoechoic relative to the surrounding hepatic tissue. Regenerative nodules are extremely numerous in cirrhotic livers, yet their visualization with ultrasonography is *rare*. Therefore, a regenerative nodule should not be the first thought when a discrete lesion is seen in a cirrhotic liver. Instead, the sonologist should think of neoplasia and particularly of hepatocellular carcinoma.
4. The number of visible portal or hepatic veins is reduced in cirrhotic livers, in proportion to the severity of disease. The loss of visible vessels appears to be a compressive phenomenon related to hepatic fibrosis, but the exact etiology is unknown.
5. Portal hypertension is an important concomitant finding in patients with diffuse

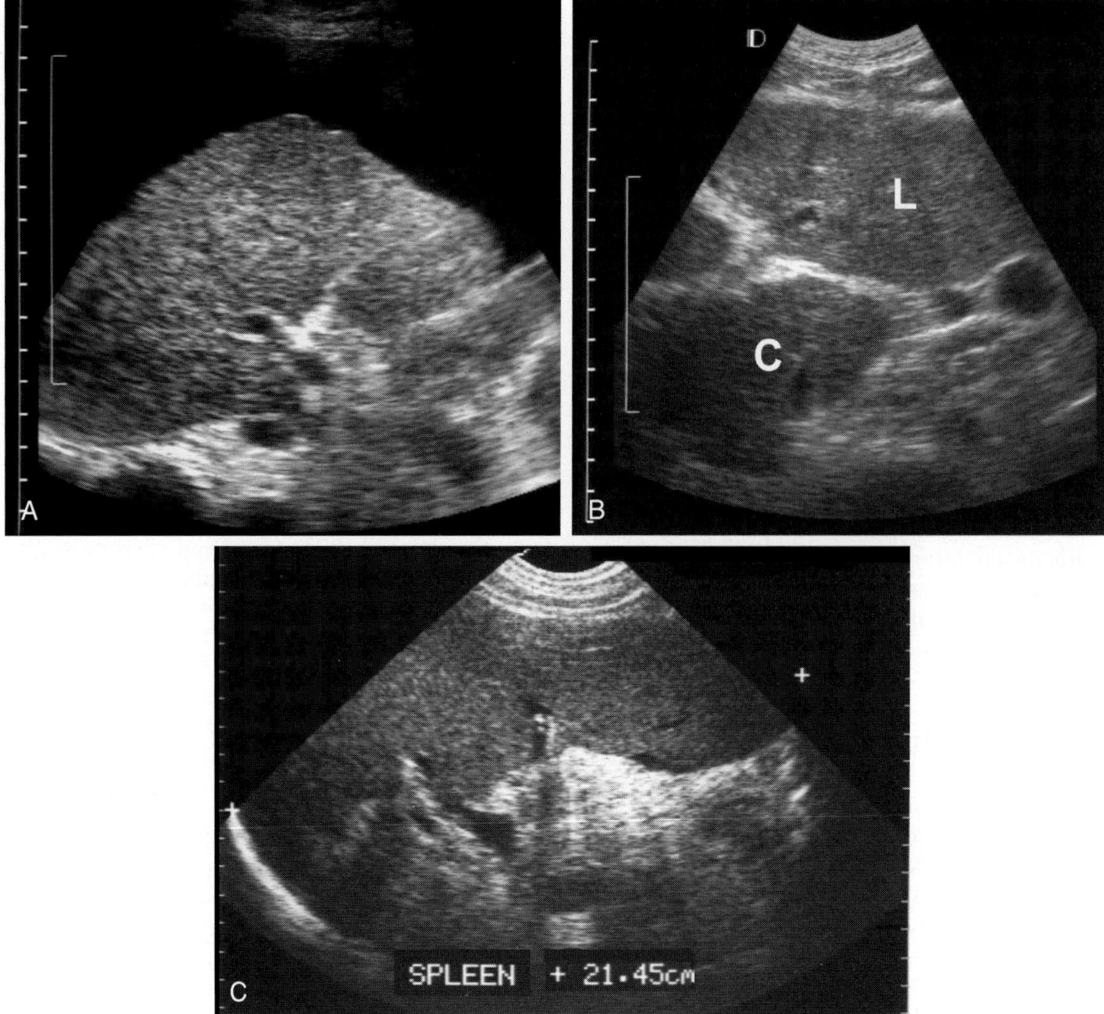

FIGURE 29–3 Morphologic findings associated with cirrhosis. *A,* The liver surface is nodular, and a large amount of ascites (black area) surrounds the liver. *B,* The left (L) and caudate (C) lobes of the liver are enlarged. *C,* The spleen is enlarged.

liver disease. The presence of portal hypertension confirms the diagnosis of cirrhosis and vice versa.

6. Cirrhosis may be accompanied by nonspecific, generalized shrinkage of the liver. In many cases, the right lobe shrinks more than the other lobes, and the caudate and left lobes enlarge as the right lobe shrinks[58–60] (see Fig. 29–3*B*). The cause of these morphologic changes is unknown. Cirrhosis may be diagnosed in some patients simply by comparing the maximum transverse dimension of the caudate and right lobes of the liver, as seen on transverse scans just below the portal bifurcation. If the caudate-to-right lobe ratio exceeds 0.65, cirrhosis may be diagnosed with 90 to 100% certainty.[57, 60] Unfortunately, this ratio is only 43% sensitive for cirrhosis.[60]

Spleen Size

An important manifestation of portal hypertension is splenomegaly (see Fig. 29–3*C*). The size of the spleen does not correlate well with the level of portal pressure; nonetheless, splenomegaly is a common feature of portal hypertension.[1, 2] The spleen is best measured in a coronal plane. A maximum cephalocaudal measurement exceeding 13 cm indicates enlargement with a high degree of reliability.[65]

Pitfalls of Portal Flow Assessment

Duplex ultrasound examination of the portal venous system (portal vein, splenic vein, and superior mesenteric vein) is successful in 93 to 95% of patients with suspected portal hypertension and portal vein occlusion,[8, 66] but portions of the portal venous system may be obscured by bowel gas in up to 10% of successful studies.[8] Even in successful studies, errors may be made, and the following pitfalls are particularly noteworthy:*

1. The direction of flow in the portal vein may be ambiguous or may spuriously appear to be reversed for technical reasons. Abnormal flow direction, therefore, should be confirmed with several interrogations of the portal vein, preferably from different transducer positions.
2. The portal vein may appear occluded on color-Doppler or spectral Doppler examination, even though it is patent, as discussed later.
3. Splenic vein occlusion or splenic flow reversal may be overlooked if only hilar branches are visualized and the splenic vein per se is not examined. This error occurs because blood flow, of necessity, must exit the spleen. Hence, flow in the hilar branches is always normally directed to the point where these branches communicate with collaterals.
4. Portal vein dilatation may be caused by severe congestive heart failure (CHF), because of transmission of back pressure from the right atrium through the hepatic circulation to the portal circulation.[25, 26] Such dilatation may be attributed mistakenly to cirrhosis. Two findings help to differentiate between CHF and true portal hypertension: in CHF, portal flow is often markedly pulsatile, and the IVC is dilated. Neither of these findings is a feature of portal hypertension related to liver disease.

PORTOSYSTEMIC VENOUS COLLATERALS

Portosystemic venous collaterals[2, 3, 6, 27–49] are important findings. In most cases, their presence is a clear indication of portal hypertension. The exception to this rule is collateralization related to venous occlusive disease, such as isolated splenic vein thrombosis. Portosystemic collaterals develop out of necessity in patients with portal hypertension, for blood from the gut must have an alternative means of reaching the heart when flow through the liver is restricted. The major portosystemic collateral routes are illustrated in Figure 29–4.

A systematic search is required for detecting portosystemic collaterals, as outlined in Table 29–1. Ultrasonography is reported to visualize 65 to 90% of portosystemic collaterals,[35, 36, 40, 41, 53] and virtually every collateral that may occur has been seen with ultrasonography.[6, 27–49] Only a few portosystemic collaterals are identified regularly, however, and these are described in Table 29–2 and Figures 29–4 through 29–9 (see also pp 434 and 435). Please review this material before proceeding as it is not repeated in the text.

Several caveats are noteworthy with respect to portosystemic collaterals:

1. The effectiveness of large collaterals in decompressing the portal system is subject to debate.[27, 33, 38, 41, 46, 67] Large collaterals do not clearly protect a patient from gastroesophageal hemorrhage.[68]
2. The *coronary vein* (also called the left gastric vein) may be seen in some normal individuals; therefore, the mere presence of a coronary vein does not indicate portal hypertension. The diameter of normal coronary veins does not exceed 4 mm, whereas a diameter exceeding 7 mm is evidence of an abnormal portal/systemic pressure gradient (exceeding 10 mm Hg). Hepatofugal coronary vein flow also indicates an abnormal portosystemic pressure gradient.[36, 42, 69]
3. *Umbilical vein* collateral flow* is an important feature of portal hypertension, for it carries a diagnostic specificity of 100%.[47, 48] An artery or vein of up to 2 mm in diameter may be present normally in the ligamentum teres; therefore, *the mere presence of a vessel in the ligamentum teres does not imply umbilical vein collateralization.*[43–48] The diagnosis of collateral flow requires documentation of venous flow *away from* the liver (see Fig. 29–5).

---

* References 2, 4–6, 8, 10, 24, 25, 32, 34–36, 50–79.

* Whether this is a recanalized portion of the umbilical vein or a paraumbilical vein is subject to debate.[46–48, 65]

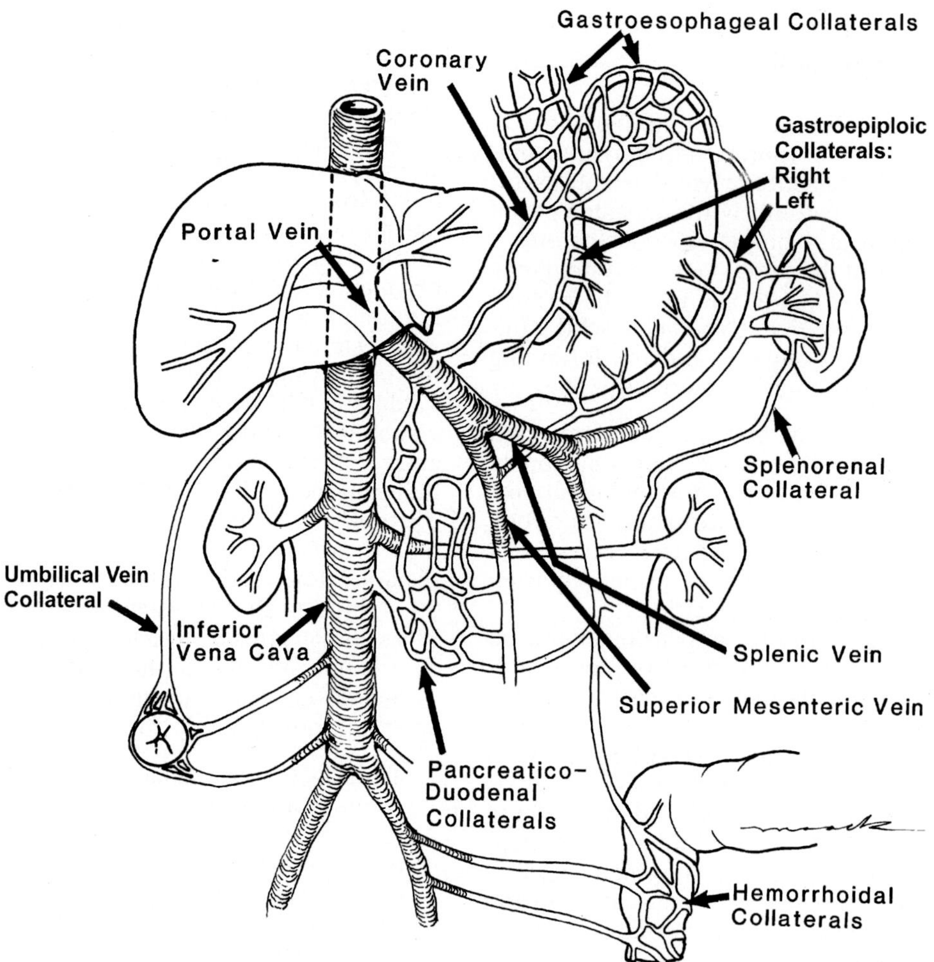

FIGURE 29–4 Major portosystemic collaterals.

It should be noted, however, that flow sometimes is hepatofugal in a normal ligamentum teres vein, but in such cases the velocity does not exceed 5 cm/sec.[44–46, 75]

4. Portosystemic collaterals may develop in response to venous occlusive disease unrelated to portal hypertension. The most common example is splenic vein occlusion, which is the most likely diagnosis when large splenosystemic collaterals are detected[49] (see Fig. 29–9). Differentiation between splenic vein thrombosis and portal hypertension is generally not a problem, because the presence or absence of a patent splenic vein can usually be documented with color-Doppler examination.
5. Large portosystemic collaterals at the esophagogastric junction may be mistaken for neoplastic masses, if color-Doppler examination is not performed.[32]

THERAPEUTIC PORTOSYSTEMIC SHUNTS

Portosystemic shunts may be created by transvascular or surgical means to decompress the portal venous system and thereby protect patients with portal hypertension from gastroesophageal bleeding. Duplex ultrasonography is an effective method for postprocedure assessment of shunt patency and function.[2, 6, 50–56] However, these shunts are frequently obscured by bowel echogenicity, and it is my personal preference to evaluate surgical portosystemic shunts with com-

TABLE 29–1 HOW TO SEARCH FOR PORTOSYSTEMIC COLLATERALS

Step 1	Begin with the splenic vein and note the direction of flow in this vessel. If flow is reversed (toward the spleen), splenogastric or splenorenal collaterals are likely to exist.
Step 2	Evaluate blood flow direction in the main portal vein and the right and left portal branches. A to-and-fro flow pattern or flow reversal indicates collateralization.
Step 3	Return to the left portal vein and follow it to the vicinity of the falciform ligament where an umbilical vein collateral may be visible (see Fig. 29–7).
Step 4	Look for a dilated coronary vein by locating the superior mesenteric vein-portal junction on longitudinal images. Move the scan plane slightly to the right and left until a *cephalad-directed* vessel is identified, as seen in Figure 29–5.
Step 5	Look for varices in the gallbladder wall and bed (see Fig. 29–6).
Step 6	With longitudinal scans, sweep along the left lobe of the liver, looking for gastric or gastroepiploic collaterals adjacent to the posterior surface of the liver (see Fig. 29–8).
Step 7	With longitudinal scans, look for collaterals in the vicinity of the gastroesophageal junction (see Fig. 29–9*A*).
Step 8	With the patient in the right lateral decubitus position and using coronal or transverse scans, look for splenorenal and splenogastric collaterals in the vicinity of the upper and lower poles of the spleen (respectively) (see Fig. 29–9*B*).

puted tomographic angiography or magnetic resonance angiography.

Percutaneous Transhepatic Shunts

Intrahepatic portacaval stents, installed percutaneously via the jugular vein, have become an important alternative to surgical portacaval shunts as a means of decompressing the portal venous system. As mentioned previously, the acronym TIPS is used for these shunts. The shunt is created with a metallic vascular stent that is readily seen and evaluated with duplex ultrasound, which is the preferred method of follow-up of TIPS patients[57, 66] (Fig. 29–10 [see p 436]). The goal of duplex examination is to confirm that the shunt is patent and to search for stenosis.

TIPS procedures are highly effective for reducing ascites, preventing hemorrhage from gastroesophageal varices, and improving the quality of life of patients with severe cirrhosis,[73–77] but the TIPS shunts are subject to a high rate of stenosis or occlusion. Either condition can result in recurrent gastrointestinal hemorrhage and ascites accumulation.

Primary patency of TIPS (without intervention to preserve or restore patency) ranges from 23 to 66% at 1 year.[78–81] With intervention for thrombosis or occlusion (balloon angioplasty and thrombolysis), the 1-year patency rate is increased to about 85%.[62] The importance of ultrasound shunt surveillance to detect stenosis is obvious from these statistics.

Occlusion or stenosis occurring within the first or second week after the TIPS procedure

TABLE 29–2 THE SONOGRAPHIC APPEARANCE OF PORTOSYSTEMIC COLLATERALS

Collateral	Appearance
Coronary vein	Prominent, *cephalad-directed* vessel that arises from the portal vein approximately opposite to the superior mesenteric vein. Visible on longitudinal images.
Gastroepiploic	Cephalad-directed vessels seen along the inferior border of the left lobe of the liver on longitudinal images.
Left gastroepiploic and gastroesophageal	Tortuous vessels near the upper pole of the spleen and the gastroesophageal junction. Seen primarily on coronal images.
Splenorenal	Tortuous, inferiorly directed vessels located between the spleen and the upper pole of the left kidney, possibly accompanied by left renal vein enlargement. Primarily seen on coronal images.
Umbilical vein	Solitary vessel that may be large, which originates from the ascending portion of the left portal vein. It courses inferiorly through the falciform ligament and along the anterior abdominal wall to the umbilicus. Seen on longitudinal or transverse images.

Adapted from Pollard, Nebesar RA: Altered hemodynamics in the Budd-Chiari syndrome demonstrated by selective hepatic and selective splenic angiography. Radiology 89:236–243, 1967; Menu Y, Alison D, Lorphelin J-M, et al: Budd-Chiari syndrome: US evaluation. Radiology 157:761–764, 1985.

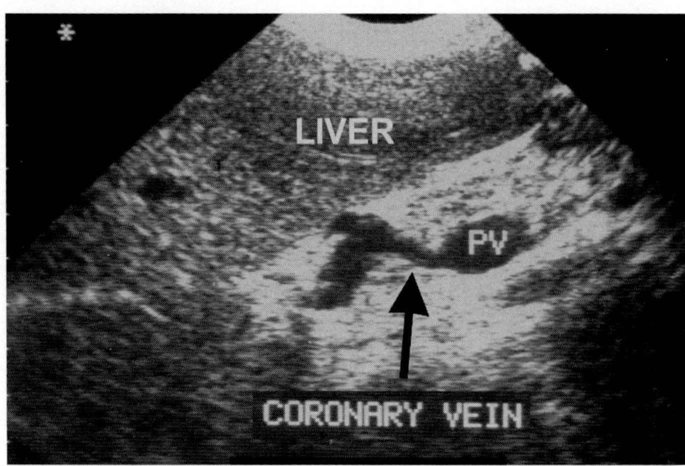

FIGURE 29–5 Coronary vein collateral. A longitudinal (parasagittal) sonogram shows a dilated coronary vein at its attachment to the portal vein (PV), near the portosplenic junction.

is the result of thrombosis and may occur from technical problems with the TIPS procedure. Occlusion or stenosis occurring later results from pseudointimal (neointimal) hyperplasia, in essence the proliferation of fibrous tissue in the stent wall.

The following examination protocol has been recommended for TIPS assessment.[65] In preparation for the TIPS procedure, a scan is performed to document patency and flow direction in the portal, splenic, and superior mesenteric veins and to confirm that the hepatic veins are patent. After the procedure, the shunt is scanned within the first 24 hours to document patency and to establish baseline flow velocities in the shunt and the portal vein. Follow-up examinations are then conducted at the discretion of the interventional radiologist. Regular follow-up is advisable, for reasons mentioned previously. Normal shunt findings include the following:

1. Slight protrusion of the proximal and distal ends of the shunt into the portal and hepatic veins (respectively).
2. Flow "filling" the stent from wall to wall.
3. Monophasic, slightly pulsatile flow with continuous flow throughout diastole.
4. Moderate-to-marked spectral broadening (turbulence).
5. Peak systolic velocity in the shunt of at least 50 to 60 cm/sec[72, 82–84] and normally ranging from 90 to 120 cm/sec.[82, 85, 86]
6. Similar velocity at proximal and distal ends of shunt.
7. Hepatopedal flow in the portal vein.
8. An increase in portal flow velocity as compared with preprocedure findings.
9. A portal vein velocity of at least 30 cm/sec, with a normal range of 37 to 47 cm/sec.[82, 85–88]

The most common location for shunt stenosis (Fig. 29–11 [see p 437]) is in the hepatic

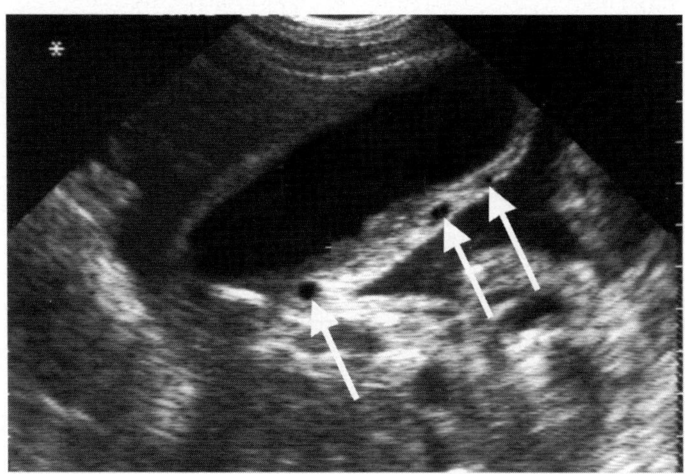

FIGURE 29–6 Gallbladder wall collateral. A longitudinal sonogram in a patient with cirrhosis shows large varices (*arrows*) within the gallbladder wall. Flow in these vessels was visualized on a computed tomogram (not shown). Ascites surrounds the gallbladder.

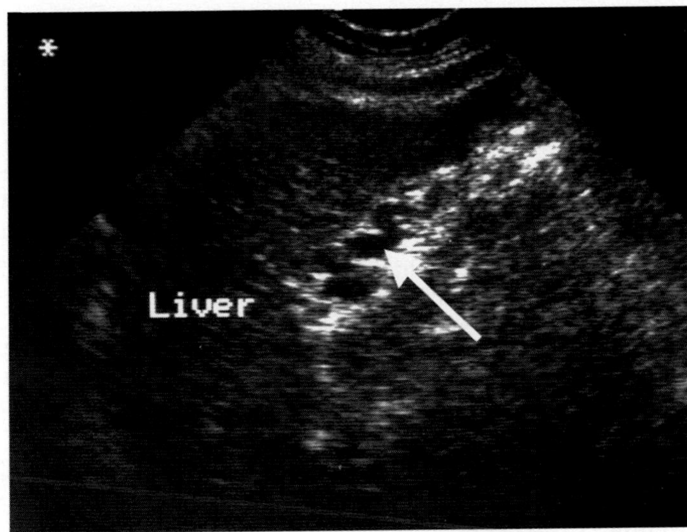

FIGURE 29–8 Left gastric collaterals. Collateral veins (*arrow*) are seen dorsal to the left lobe of the liver.

vein branch immediately adjacent to the stent, but stenosis can also occur at other locations in the shunt or diffusely throughout it. Shunt stenosis may occasionally be diagnosed directly with Doppler ultrasonography through detection of *localized* high-velocity flow and severe turbulence. Stenosis-related velocities as high as 400 cm/sec have been reported.[72] Shunt stenosis is also indicated by generalized reduced flow velocity *throughout* the stent, as compared with baseline values. A shunt velocity of less than 50 or 60 cm/sec (at any location) is highly specific for shunt malfunction and warrants close investigation of the shunt.[83–85, 88] A further indicator of shunt stenosis is an increase in velocity exceeding 100 cm/sec from a normal part of the shunt to a narrowed area.

A drop in portal vein flow velocity from the postprocedure baseline is highly suggestive of shunt malfunction.[85, 87, 88] This stands to reason, as portal vein flow should be at a high level if the shunt is patent. As noted previously, a portal vein flow velocity less than 30 cm/sec is of great concern.

Shunt occlusion is indicated by absence of flow in the shunt and return of portal flow velocity and direction to preprocedure status. Caution is advised in assessing the apparently occluded shunt, as *low-flow velocity in a highly stenosed stent may be difficult to detect with ultrasonography.* If flow is not detected with color-Doppler imaging, try spectral Doppler (which generally is more sensitive) before concluding that the shunt is occluded. Shunt occlusion should be confirmed angiographically, as a "trickle" of flow may be present that cannot be detected with ultrasonography. A highly stenosed or recently occluded shunt may be returned to patency, whereas a more chronically occluded stent cannot be repaired by any means.

Normal and abnormal values for TIPS are listed in Table 29–3.

TABLE 29–3 NORMAL AND ABNORMAL DOPPLER PARAMETERS FOR TIPS SHUNTS

Normal

1. Pulsatile flow in shunt
2. Peak systolic shunt velocity:
   At least 50–60 cm/sec
   Range 90–120 cm/sec
3. Velocity similar at portal and hepatic ends of shunt
4. Portal and splenic vein flow hepatopedal
5. Portal vein velocity:
   Substantially greater than preshunt value
   At least 30 cm/sec
   Range 37 to 47 cm/sec

Abnormal

1. Localized high velocity (stenosis) and flow disturbance (poststenosis)
2. Increase in velocity from one point to another in the shunt of more than 100 cm/sec
3. Visible diffuse narrowing with or without high velocity
4. Generalized low velocity throughout shunt (less than 50 cm/sec)
5. Continuous (nonpulsatile) flow in shunt
6. Decrease in portal vein velocity from postprocedure baseline
7. Portal vein velocity less than 30 cm/sec
8. Hepatofugal or to-and-fro portal or splenic vein flow
9. Absence of flow in shunt

PORTAL VEIN OCCLUSION

Pathology

Portal vein occlusion[2, 4–6, 10, 67–115] is principally caused by thrombosis or tumor invasion. Thrombosis may be precipitated by stagnant portal flow in patients with cirrhosis. Other causes include hypercoagulable states, surgery, and intraperitoneal inflammatory processes, such as pancreatitis and appendicitis. In appendicitis, the inflammatory process causes portal phlebitis, which in turn causes thrombus to form. Tumor invasion of the portal vein occurs most frequently with hepatocellular carcinoma and pancreatic carcinoma.[89–93, 100, 102–106]

Portal vein occlusion is usually permanent, but recanalization may occur in some cases of thrombosis. Portal flow may also be re-established via cavernous transformation (discussed later), and the use of TIPS shunting has been described for restoration of portal vein flow, if cavernous transformation has not occurred.[107] If portal flow is not adequately re-established, decompression of the portal system occurs via spontaneous portosystemic collaterals (see Fig. 29–4).

Acute Findings

The sonographic manifestations of acute portal vein occlusion[2, 6, 70–72, 74–82] are illustrated in Figure 29–12 (see p 438). These include failure to visualize the portal vein, detection of echogenic intraluminal material, absence of flow on color-Doppler examination, and other color-Doppler abnormalities discussed later.

The main portal vein is seen on 97% of upper abdominal sonograms;[95, 96] therefore, when a normal-appearing portal vein is not *readily* seen, portal vein occlusion should come to mind. The most important findings that corroborate the diagnosis of portal vein occlusion are absence of portal flow accompanied by echogenic material within the portal vein lumen. Occluding material, whether thrombus or tumor, is generally low or moderate in echogenicity. Recently formed thrombosis may be almost anechoic and may be overlooked in the absence of Doppler interrogation of flow. On color-Doppler examination, flow may be absent in an occluded portal vein, or a trickle of flow may be seen around the obstruction. Color-Doppler examination may be used to distinguish between tumor and thrombotic occlusion. Pulsatile or to-and-fro flow signals can be detected in vessels within the occluding tumor, whereas no flow signals or occasional continuous (nonpulsatile) flow is evident in thrombotic occlusion. If the portal vein is only partially blocked (see Fig. 29–12*A*), increased flow velocity and disturbed flow may be apparent at the site of obstruction. The occluding material frequently dilates the portal vein and its branches noticeably (see Fig. 29–12*B*). Massive dilatation, with a portal vein diameter exceeding 23 mm, suggests tumor, but this is not specific.[106] Thrombus may extend into the splenic or superior mesenteric veins (see Fig. 29–12*C*), and these tributaries should be evaluated to confirm the extent of occlusion.

Patent segments of the portal system distal* to an occluded portal vein are often dilated. Low-velocity, continuous flow may be present in these segments, rather than the normal phasic flow pattern. Intrahepatic collateral vessels may develop, connecting one portal segment with another.[110] Flow may be reversed in the splenic or superior mesenteric veins.

Chronic Findings

If portal vein thrombosis persists without substantial lysis, the portal vein undergoes fibrosis and may vanish from a sonographic perspective. Cavernous transformation of the portal vein is the principal manifestation of chronic portal vein thrombosis. Cavernous transformation produces a distinctive tangle of tortuous vessels in the porta hepatis, which appears within 6 to 20 days after acute occlusion[110] (Fig. 29–13). The uninitiated ultrasonographer may mistake these vessels for other pathology, including biliary dilatation. Duplex ultrasound examination should prevent such errors, however, by demonstrating venous flow in the collateral vessels. A secondary sign of chronic portal vein occlusion is the development of portosystemic collaterals. These are identical in location and appearance to those described previously (see Table 29–2 and Fig. 29–4). Intrahepatic collaterals may develop in spite of the presence

* The terms *distal* and *proximal* are used with respect to the heart. Proximal means closer to the heart, and distal means farther from the heart.

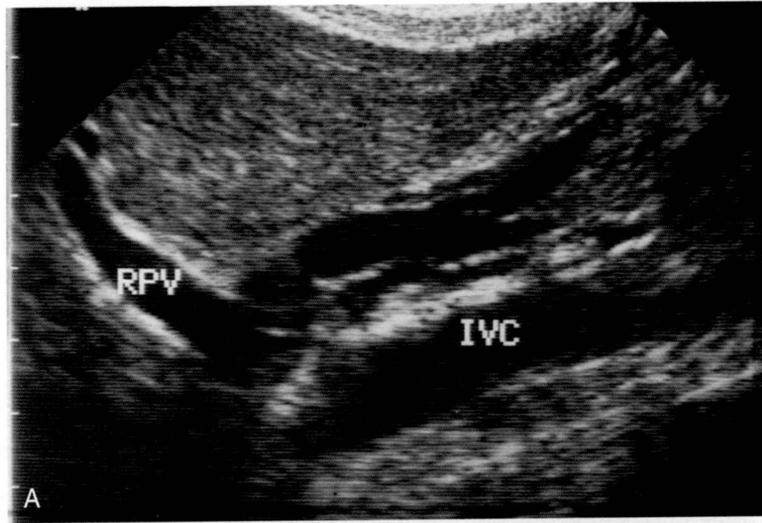

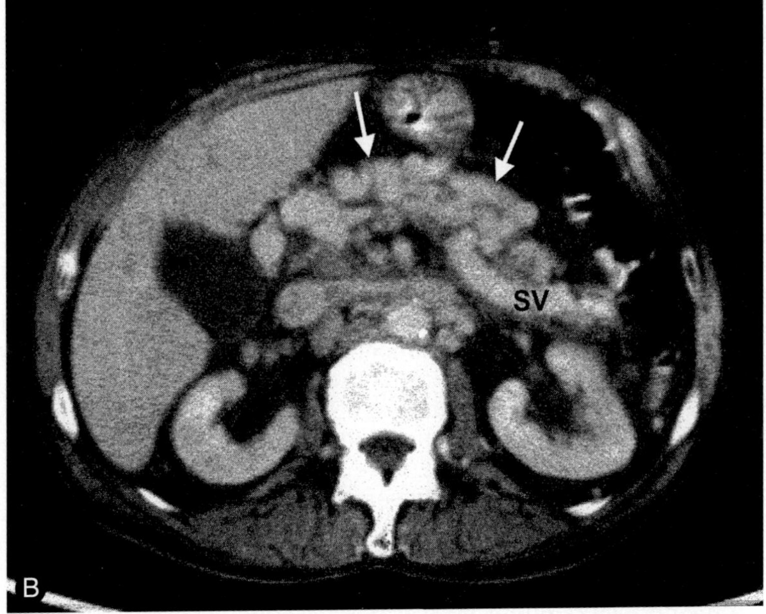

FIGURE 29–13 Cavernous transformation of the portal veins. *A,* An irregular tangle of vessels is seen at the porta hepatis in this patient with a remote history of portal vein thrombosis caused by abdominal sepsis. RPV = right portal vein; IVC = inferior vena cava. *B,* Contrast-enhanced computed tomography in the same patient shows a large tangle of collateral veins (*arrows*) in the vicinity of the pancreas that eventually coalesce as the splenic vein (SV).

of cavernous transformation.[110] Lobar atrophy may occur if only a portion of the intrahepatic portal system is occluded, but this usually occurs when concomitant biliary obstruction is present.[11]

Diagnostic Accuracy

The ultrasonographic diagnosis of portal vein occlusion is highly accurate (sensitivity 89 to 100% and specificity 96 to 100%).[98–105, 108, 115] Although diagnostic errors are uncommon, three pitfalls are particularly noteworthy. First, recently formed thrombus that is virtually anechoic may remain undetected, as noted previously. Second, patients with portal hypertension may have low-velocity or to-and-fro portal flow that is difficult to detect with Doppler ultrasonography, causing a false-positive impression of occlusion. Third, an inadequate Doppler angle may preclude detection of portal flow leading to a false-positive diagnosis.

HEPATIC VEIN OCCLUSION

A second venous occlusive disorder of the liver that may be detected sonographically is hepatic vein occlusion, which results in a clinical complex called the *Budd-Chiari syndrome.*[2, 5, 113–131]

Pathology

The term Budd-Chiari syndrome refers to clinical and histologic abnormalities occurring in response to acute obstruction of hepatic vein flow.[84–87] The clinical abnormalities are hepatomegaly (a result of congestion), abdominal pain (a result of hepatomegaly), abrupt development of ascites, and hepatocellular dysfunction (evidenced by biochemical tests). The histologic findings specific for Budd-Chiari syndrome are centrizonal sinusoidal distention and pooling of blood in the sinusoids.

The causes of the Budd-Chiari syndrome are numerous and vary in relation to the primary site of obstruction, which may be sinusoids, at the hepatic vein level, or in the IVC. The following imaging ramifications of these locations are noteworthy:

1. With sinusoidal occlusion,* the major hepatic veins may remain patent or may become occluded *secondarily,* as a result of sluggish blood flow. Ultrasonography can diagnose the sinusoidal form of the Budd-Chiari syndrome only when the hepatic veins undergo secondary thrombosis. Fortunately, the potential for false-negative studies is low, because sinosoidal occlusion is rare.
2. *Primary* hepatic vein occlusion is readily detected with ultrasonography. Such occlusion results either from thrombosis or from tumor invasion of the hepatic veins. Thrombosis is often related to cirrhosis (20% of cases)[83] or hypercoagulable disorders. Neoplastic invasion is most often seen with hepatoma.
3. IVC occlusion or stenosis *cephalad to* the hepatic veins causes the Budd-Chiari syndrome by inducing hepatic vein congestion (back pressure) or secondary hepatic vein thrombosis. This form of obstruction is readily detected with ultrasonography. IVC obstruction may have a variety of causes, including congenital stenosis or occlusion,* thrombosis from hypercoagulable states, and neoplastic invasion.
4. Finally, a Budd-Chiari–like syndrome may occur with excessive right atrial pressure, as seen with severe CHF or pericardial tamponade.

* Centrilobular venous occlusion is sometimes referred to by the confusing term *veno-occlusive disease of the liver.*

* This rare condition is attributed to congenital causes; nevertheless, the Budd-Chiari syndrome frequently does not occur until the fifth decade of life (40+).

Therapy

Certain cases of IVC occlusion are amenable to surgery, but in the past no treatment was available for primary hepatic vein occlusion. However, TIPS shunting has proved effective for cases of thrombotic occlusion, both in the acute and in the more chronic states.[131] It is likely that TIPS shunting will be used more commonly to treat hepatic veno-occlusive disease in the future.

Ultrasound Findings

The ultrasound findings associated with hepatic vein obstruction fall into three categories: (1) direct manifestations of hepatic vein or IVC occlusion, (2) secondary morphologic changes in the liver, and (3) secondary extrahepatic findings.

Direct Ultrasound Findings

The principal direct ultrasound manifestation of hepatic vein obstruction[2, 5, 6, 112, 117–130] (Fig. 29–14) is the presence of echogenic intraluminal material (thrombus or tumor) accompanied by absence of hepatic vein flow. If the hepatic vein is narrowed but not completely blocked, focal elevated velocity and poststenotic turbulence may be seen.

Frequently, distal portions of the hepatic veins (deep within the liver) remain patent, whereas proximal regions (near the IVC) are occluded. Continuous flow (see Fig. 29–14*D*), to-and-fro flow, or reversed flow patterns (rather than the normal, hepatofugal, pulsatile flow pattern) may be seen in the portions of the hepatic veins that remain patent deep within the liver. A characteristic finding in these cases is *bicolor* flow, in which one branch of a hepatic vein is blue, and the other

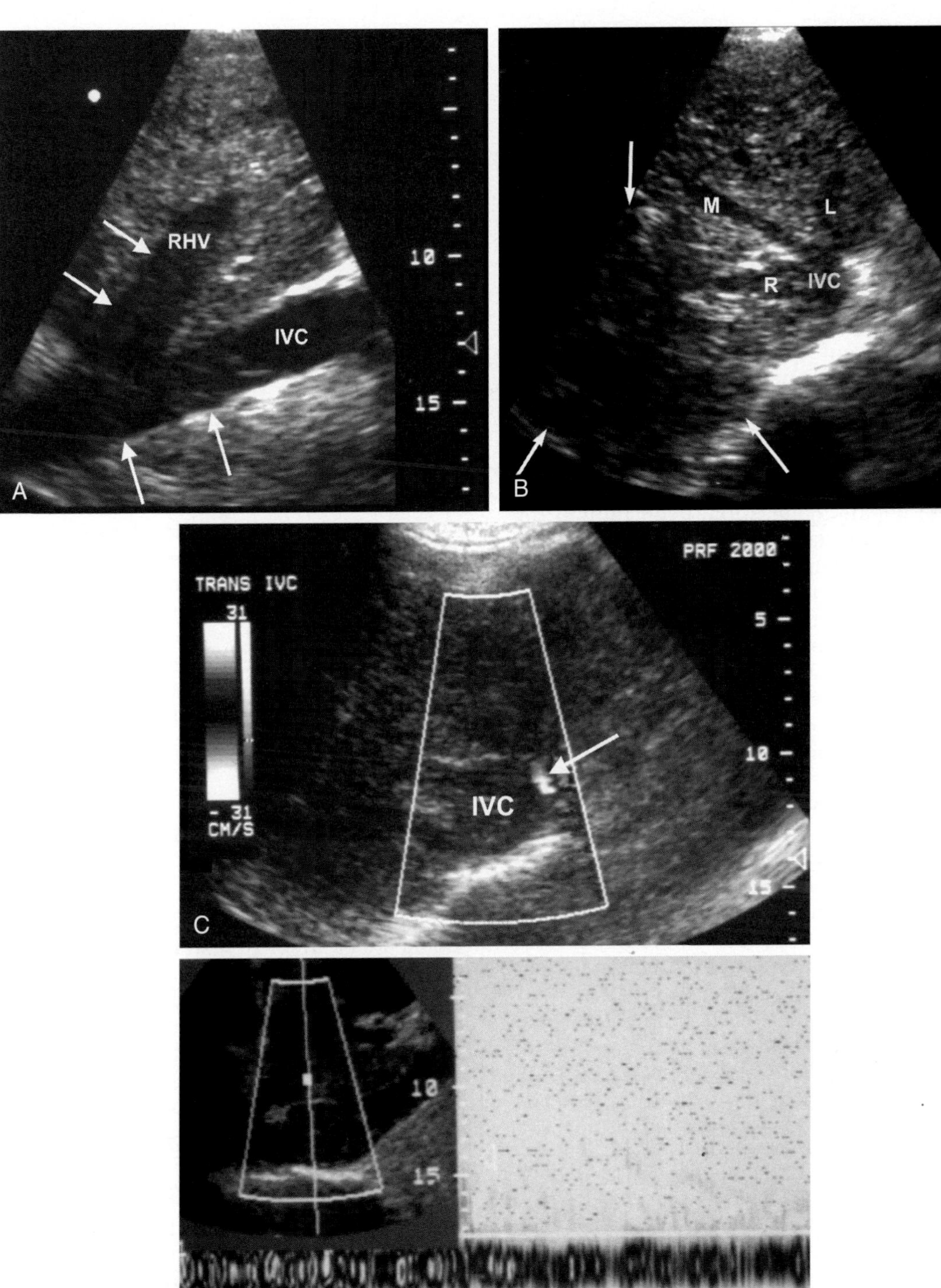

FIGURE 29–14 Hepatic vein occlusion. This elderly male alcoholic patient presented with classic features of the Budd-Chiari syndrome. *A,* A coronal image of the right lobe of the liver shows a faintly echogenic tumor (*arrows*) within the dilated right hepatic vein (RHV) and the inferior vena cava (IVC). *B,* A transverse scan shows the tumor-filled right hepatic vein (R) and IVC. A poorly defined hypoechoic area (*arrows*), representing hepatic edema, is seen in the posterior portion of the right hepatic lobe. The middle (M) and left (L) hepatic veins are patent, but this is inapparent on this gray-scale image. *C,* Blood flow from the middle and left hepatic veins passes through a narrow residual lumen (*arrow*) between the tumor mass and the wall of the IVC. (Black and white representation of a transverse color-Doppler image.) *D,* Doppler flow signals in the middle and left hepatic veins are continuous, consistent with significant obstruction.

is red. Flow is normally directed in one branch and reversed in the other (collateral) branch.

An important finding in hepatic vein occlusion is the visualization of intrahepatic collateral veins* (less than 1 cm and not following the usual course of hepatic vessels) that connect hepatic vein branches or connect the hepatic veins with portal or systemic veins. These collaterals may be seen as a tangle of small vessels or as larger vessels within the liver that do not follow the normal anatomic course of the hepatic veins. They may also be seen in a subcapsular location. It has been stated that intrahepatic collateralization is specific for hepatic vein occlusion. This is incorrect, as intrahepatic collateralization can also be seen (albeit uncommonly) with severe hepatic congestion, even though the hepatic veins are patent.[130] As noted previously, intrahepatic portal vein collateralization also occurs.

Portal flow abnormalities may also be present in cases of hepatic vein occlusion, including biphasic or reversed portal flow, decreased flow velocity, or secondary portal occlusion.

When IVC occlusion causes the Budd-Chiari syndrome,† direct ultrasound findings include the visualization of thrombus or tumor within the IVC lumen (see Figs. 29–14 and 27–23) possibly accompanied by absence of flow in one or more hepatic veins. If the IVC is stenosed but not occluded, high flow velocity may be seen in the stenotic lumen. Reversed flow may be evident in patient portion of the IVC and the iliac veins.

The occluding material in the IVC generates low-level echogenicity regardless of whether it is tumor or thrombus. Color-Doppler examination of the occluding material may help differentiate between tumor and thrombus, as discussed previously with respect to portal vein occlusion. Flow may be either absent or disturbed (in cases of stenosis) in the obstructed IVC segment. Caudal portions of the IVC and the iliac veins typically remain patent. These vessels are dilated, and they demonstrate flow abnormalities that may include a continuous flow pattern, flow reversal, and absence of the normal Valsalva response.

* These intrahepatic collaterals may communicate with nonoccluded hepatic veins, the portal vein, or even systemic veins.

† References 2, 5, 6, 113–117, 120–123, 125, 126.

The hepatic veins usually become occluded secondarily in patients with IVC obstruction, either from stasis-related thrombosis or from tumor extension (see Fig. 29–14). In some patients, however, the hepatic veins remain patent, and low-velocity antegrade flow is present in the hepatic veins, accompanied by *retrograde* flow in the patent portions of the IVC.

Secondary Morphologic Changes

Striking morphologic changes may occur in the liver in association with hepatic vein obstruction. Acutely, the portions of the liver subtended by obstructed veins are enlarged (swollen) and hypoechoic (see Fig. 29–14*B*). In the subacute and chronic phases, the affected areas become fibrosed and shrink in size, and these areas may be relatively echogenic, as compared with normal hepatic parenchyma. The caudate or left lobes of the liver may undergo striking compensatory enlargement, because these portions of the liver are relatively spared from the effects of venous back pressure.

Secondary Extrahepatic Manifestations

Ascites, pleural effusion, and gallbladder edema are commonly seen in the acute stage of the Budd-Chiari syndrome. Splenomegaly and portosystemic collaterals may be evident in chronic cases, in relation to persistent portal hypertension.

Problem of Nonvisualization

Nonvisualization of the hepatic veins is of little diagnostic value when Budd-Chiari syndrome is suspected, because the hepatic veins may sometimes be patent but invisible ultrasonographically. *In the author's opinion, Budd Chiari syndrome can be excluded only when the patency of the major hepatic vein branches can be confirmed unequivocally.* If large segments of the hepatic veins cannot be seen clearly (from the IVC to deep within the liver), no comment can be made with respect to Budd-Chiari syndrome, unless secondary findings, such as intrahepatic shunts, are seen. It is easy to locate and follow the hepatic veins in a young, healthy individual, but this task may be difficult or impossible in a patient with a shrunken, cirrhotic liver.

REFERENCES

1. Sherlock S, Dooley J: Diseases of the Liver and Biliary System, 9th ed. London, Blackwell Scientific Publications, 1993, pp 132–178.
2. Koslin DB, Mulligan SA, Berland LL: Duplex assessment of the splanchnic vasculature. Semin Ultrasound CT MRI 13:34–39, 1992.
3. Zwiebel WJ, Fruechte D: Basics of abdominal and pelvic duplex: instrumentation, anatomy, and vascular Doppler signatures. Semin Ultrasound CT MRI 13:3–21, 1992.
4. Ralls PW: Color Doppler sonography of the hepatic artery and portal venous system. AJR Am J Roentgenol 155:517–525, 1990.
5. Becker CD, Cooperberg PL: Sonography of the hepatic vascular system. AJR Am J Roentgenol 150: 999–1005, 1988.
6. Bolondi L, Mazziotti A, Arienti V, et al: Ultrasonographic study of portal venous system in portal hypertension and after portosystemic shunt operations. Surgery 95:261–269, 1984.
7. Taylor KJW, Burns PN: Duplex Doppler scanning in the pelvis and abdomen. Ultrasound Med Biol 11:643–658, 1985.
8. Patriquin H, Lafortune M, Burns PN, Dauzat M: Duplex Doppler examination in portal hypertension: Technique and anatomy. AJR Am J Roentgenol 149:71–76, 1987.
9. Zierler BK, Horn JR, Bauer LA, et al: Hepatic blood flow measurements by duplex ultrasound: How to minimize variability. J Vasc Technol 15:16–22, 1991.
10. Parvey HR, Eisenberg RL, Giyanani V, Krebs CA: Duplex sonography of the portal venous system: Pitfalls and limitations. AJR Am J Roentgenol 152: 765–770, 1989.
11. Bolondi L: The value of Doppler US in the study of hepatic hemodynamics (Consensus conference report, Bologna, Italy, 12 Sept 1989). J Hepatol 10: 353–355, 1990.
12. Strohm VWD, Wehr B: Korrelation zwischen Lebervenverchylubfrick und sonographich bestimmtem Durchmesser von Pfortader und Milz bei Leberkranken. Z Gastroenterol 17:695–703, 1979.
13. Rahim N, Adam EJ: Ultrasound demonstration of variations in normal portal vein diameter with posture. Br J Radiol 58:313–314, 1985.
14. Weinreb J, Kumari S, Phillips G, Pochaczevski R: Portal vein measurements by real-time sonography. AJR Am J Roentgenol 139:497–499, 1982.
15. Rabinovici N, Narot N: The relationship between respiration, pressure and flow distribution in the vena cava and portal and hepatic veins. Surg Gynecol Obstet 151:753–763, 1980.
16. Moriyasu F, Ban N, Nishida O, et al: Clinical application of an ultrasonic duplex system in the quantitative measurement of portal blood flow. J Clin Ultrasound 14:579–588, 1986.
17. Zoli M, Dondi C, Marchesini G, et al: Splanchnic vein measurements in patients with liver cirrhosis: A case-control study. J Ultrasound Med 4:641–646, 1985.
18. Goyal AK, Pokharna DS, Sharma SK: Ultrasonic measurements of portal vasculature in diagnosis of portal hypertension. A controversial subject reviewed. J Ultrasound Med 9:45–48, 1990.
19. Cottone M, D'Amico G, Maringhini A, et al: Predictive value of ultrasonography in the screening of non-ascitic cirrhotic patients with large varices. J Ultrasound Med 5:189–192, 1965.
20. Bolondi L, Gamrolfi L, Arienti V, et al: Ultrasonography in the diagnosis of portal hypertension: diminished response of portal vessels to respiration. Radiology 142:167–172, 1982.
21. Bolondi L, Mazziotti A, Arienti V, et al: Ultrasonographic study of portal venous system in portal hypertension and after portosystemic shunt operations. Surgery 95:261–269, 1984.
22. Moriyasu F, Ban N, Nishida O, et al: Portal hemodynamics in patients with hepatocellular carcinoma. Radiology 161:707–711, 1986.
23. Moriyasu F, Nishida O, Ban N, et al: "Congestion index" of the portal vein. AJR Am J Roentgenol 146:735–739, 1986.
24. Gaiani S, Bolondi L, Li Bassi S, et al: Effect of meal on portal hemodynamics in healthy humans and in patients with chronic liver disease. Hepatology 9:815–819, 1989.
25. Hosoki T, Arisawa J, Marukawa T, et al: Portal blood flow in congestive heart failure: Pulsed duplex sonographic findings. Radiology 174:733–736, 1990.
26. Duerinckx A, Grant EG, Perrella RR, et al: The pulsatile portal vein in cases of congestive heart failure: Correlation of duplex Doppler findings with right atrial pressures. Radiology 176:655–658, 1990.
27. DeCandio G, Campstelli A, Mosca F, et al: Ultrasound detection of unusual spontaneous portosystemic shunts associated with uncomplicated portal hypertension. J Ultrasound Med 4:297–305, 1985.
28. Patriquin H, Tessier G, Grignon A, Boisvert J: Lesser omental thickness in normal children: Baseline for detection of portal hypertension. AJR Am J Roentgenol 145:693–696, 1985.
29. Neumaier CE, Cicco GR, Derchi LE, Biggi E: The patent ductus venosus: An additional ultrasonic finding in portal hypertension. J Clin Ultrasound 11:231–233, 1983.
30. West MS, Garra BS, Horii SC, et al: Gallbladder varices: Imaging findings in patients with portal hypertension. Radiology 179:179–182, 1991.
31. Marchal GF, Van Holsbeeck M, Tschibwabwa-Ntumba E, et al: Dilatation of the cystic veins in portal hypertension: Sonographic demonstration. Radiology 154:187–189, 1985.
32. Brady TM, Gross BH, Glazer GM, Williams DM: Adrenal pseudomasses due to varices: Angiographic-CT-MRI-pathologic correlations. AJR Am J Roentgenol 145:301–304, 1985.
33. Di Candio G, Campatelli A, Mosca F, et al: Ultrasound detection of unusual spontaneous portosystemic shunts associated with uncomplicated portal hypertension. J Ultrasound Med 4:297–305, 1985.
34. Jüttner H-U, Jenney JM, Ralls PW, et al: Ultrasound demonstration of portosystemic collaterals in cirrhosis and portal hypertension. Radiology 142: 459–463, 1982.

35. Dökmeci AK, Kimura K, Matsutani S, et al: Collateral veins in portal hypertension: Demonstration by sonography. AJR Am J Roentgenol 137:1173–1177, 1981.
36. Dach JL, Hill MC, Palaez JC, et al: Sonography of hypertensive portal venous system: Correlation with arterial portography. AJR Am J Roentgenol 137:511–517, 1981.
37. Mori H, Hayashi K, Fukuda T, et al: Intrahepatic portosystemic venous shunt: Occurrence in patients with and without liver cirrhosis. AJR Am J Roentgenol 149:711–714, 1987.
38. Sie A, Johnson MB, Lee KP, Ralls PW: Color Doppler sonography in spontaneous splenorenal portosystemic shunts. J Ultrasound Med 10:167–169, 1991.
39. Subramanyam BR, Balthazar EJ, Raghavenadra BN, Lefleur RS: Sonographic evaluation of patients with portal hypertension. Am J Gastroenterol 78:369–373, 1983.
40. Subramanyam BR, Balthazar EJ, Madamba MR, et al: Sonography of porto-systemic collaterals in portal hypertension. Radiology 146:161–166, 1983.
41. Takayasu K, Moriyama N, Shima Y, et al: Sonographic detection of large spontaneous splenorenal shunts and its clinical significance. Br J Radiol 57:565–570, 1984.
42. Lafortune M, Marleau D, Breton G, et al: Portal venous system measurements in portal hypertension. Radiology 151:27–30, 1984.
43. Schabel S, Rittenberg GM, Javid LH, et al: The "Bull's-Eye" falciform ligament: A sonographic finding of portal hypertension. Radiology 136:157–159, 1980.
44. Saddekni S, Hutchinson DE, Cooperberg PL: The sonographically patent umbilical vein in portal hypertension. Radiology 145:411–443, 1982.
45. Aagaard J, Jensen LI, Sørensen TIA, et al: Recanalized umbilical vein in portal hypertension. AJR Am J Roentgenol 139:1107–1109, 1982.
46. Lafortune M, Constantin A, Breton G, et al: The recanalized umbilical vein in portal hypertension: A myth. AJR Am J Roentgenol 144:549–553, 1985.
47. Gibson RN, Gibson PR, Donlan JD, Clunie DA: Identification of a patent paraumbilical vein by using Doppler sonography: Importance in the diagnosis of portal hypertension. AJR Am J Roentgenol 153:513–516, 1989.
48. Mostbeck GH, Wittich GR, Herold C, et al: Hemodynamic significance of the paraumbilical vein in portal hypertension: Assessment with duplex US. Radiology 170:339–342, 1989.
49. Marn CS, Glazer GM, Williams DM, Francis IR: CT-angiographic correlation of collateral venous pathways in isolated splenic vein occlusion: New observations. Radiology 175:375–380, 1990.
50. Rice S, Lee KP, Johnson MB, et al: Portal venous system after portosystemic shunts or endoscopic sclerotherapy: Evaluation with Doppler sonography. AJR Am J Roentgenol 156:85–89, 1991.
51. O'Connor SE, LaBombard E, Musson AM, Zwolak RM: Duplex imaging of distal splenorenal shunts. J Vasc Technol 15:28–31, 1991.
52. Chezmar JL, Bernardino ME: Mesoatrial shunt for the treatment of Budd-Chiari syndrome: Radiologic evaluation in eight patients. AJR Am J Roentgenol 149:707–710, 1987.
53. Lafortune M, Patriquin H, Pomier G, et al: Hemodynamic changes in portal circulation after portosystemic shunts: Use of duplex sonography in 43 patients. AJR Am J Roentgenol 149:701–706, 1987.
54. Patriquin H, Lafortune M, Weber A, et al: Surgical portosystemic shunts in children: Assessment with duplex Doppler US. Radiology 165:25–28, 1987.
55. Grant EG, Tessler FN, Gomes AS, et al: Color Doppler imaging of portosystemic shunts. AJR Am J Roentgenol 154:393–397, 1990.
56. Bolondi L, Gaiani S, Mazziotti A, et al: Morphological and hemodynamic changes in the portal venous system after distal splenorenal shunt: An ultrasound and pulsed Doppler study. Hepatology 8:652–657, 1988.
57. Harbin WP, Robert NJ, Ferrucci JT: Diagnosis of cirrhosis based on regional changes in hepatic morphology. Radiology 135:273–283, 1980.
58. Di Lelio A, Cestari C, Lomazzi A, Beretta L: Cirrhosis: Diagnosis with sonographic study of the liver surface. Radiology 172:389–392, 1989.
59. Gore RM, Ghahremani GG, Joseph AE, et al: Acquired malposition of the colon and gallbladder in patients with cirrhosis: CT findings and clinical implications. Radiology 171:739–742, 1989.
60. Giorgii A, Amoroso P, Lettieri G, et al: Cirrhosis: Value of caudate to right lobe ratio in diagnosis with US. Radiology 161:443–445, 1986.
61. Freeman MP, Vick CW, Taylor KJW, et al: Regenerating nodules in cirrhosis: Sonographic appearance with anatomic correlation. AJR Am J Roentgenol 146:533–536, 1986.
62. Day DL, Letourneau JG, Allan BT, et al: Hepatic regenerating nodules in hereditary tyrosinemia. AJR Am J Roentgenol 149:391–393, 1987.
63. Murakami T, Kuroda C, Murakawa T, et al: Regenerating nodules in hepatic cirrhosis: MR findings with pathologic correlation. AJR Am J Roentgenol 155:1227–1231, 1990.
64. Giorgio A, Francica G, de Stefano G, et al: Sonographic recognition of intraparenchymal regenerating nodules using high-frequency transducers in patients with cirrhosis. J Ultrasound Med 10:355–359, 1991.
65. Senecal B: Sonographic anatomy of the normal spleen, normal anatomic variants, and pitfalls. *In* Bruneton JN (ed): Ultrasonography of the Spleen. Berlin, Springer-Verlag, 1988, pp 1–13.
66. Yeh H-C, Stancato-Pasik A, Ramos R, Rabinowitz JG: Paraumbilical venous collateral circulations: Color Doppler ultrasound features. J Clin Ultrasound 24:359–366, 1996.
67. Bach AM, Hann LE, Brown KT, et al: Portal vein evaluation with US: Comparison to angiography combined with CT arterial portography. Radiology 201:149–154, 1996.
68. Schmassmann A, Zuber M, Livers M, et al: Recurrent bleeding after variceal hemorrhage: Predictive value of portal venous duplex sonography. AJR Am J Roentgenol 160:41–47, 1993.
69. Morin C, Lafortune M, Pomier G, et al: Patent paraumbilical vein: Anatomic and hemodynamic variants and their clinical importance. Radiology 185: 253–256, 1992.
70. Wachsberg RH, Simmons MZ: Coronary vein diameter and flow direction in patients with portal hypertension: Evaluation with duplex sonography and correlation with variceal bleeding. AJR Am J Roentgenol 162:637–641, 1994.
71. Khedkar N, Traverso L, Walat S, et al: Transjugular intrahepatic portosystemic shunt (TIPS) duplex imaging. J Vasc Technology 17:192, 1993.

72. Chong WK, Malisch TW, Mazer MJ, et al: Transjugular intrahepatic portosystemic shunts: US assessment with maximum flow velocity. Radiology 189:789–793, 1993.
73. Nazarian GK, Ferral H, Bjarnason H, et al: Effect of transjugular intrahepatic portosystemic shunt on quality of life. AJR Am J Roentgenol 167:963–969, 1996.
74. Ochs A, Rossle M, Haag K, et al: The transjugular intrahepatic portosystemic stent-shunt procedure for refractory ascites. N Engl J Med 332:1192–1197, 1995.
75. Casarella WJ: Transjugular intrahepatic portosystemic shunt: A defining achievement in vascular and interventional radiology. Radiology 196:305, 1995.
76. Polak JF: Transjugular intrahepatic portosystemic shunt: Building on experience. Radiology 196:306–307, 1995.
77. Coldwell DM, Ring EJ, Rees CR, et al. Multicenter investigation of the role of transjugular intrahepatic portosystemic shunt in management of portal hypertension. Radiology 196:335–340, 1995.
78. Kerlan RK Jr, LaBerge JM, Gordon RL, Ring EJ: Transjugular intrahepatic portosystemic shunts: Current status. AJR Am J Roentgenol 164:1059–1066, 1995.
79. Ducoin H, El-Khoury J, Rosseau H, et al: Histopathologic analysis of transjugular intrahepatic portosystemic shunts. Hepatology 25:1064–1069, 1997.
80. Sterling KM, Darcy MD: Stenosis of transjugular intrahepatic portosystemic shunts: Presentation and management. AJR Am J Roentgenol 168:239–244, 1997.
81. Nazarian GK, Ferral H, Castañeda-Zúñiga WR, et al: Development of stenoses in transjugular intrahepatic portosystemic shunts. Radiology 192:231–234, 1994.
82. Foshager MC, Ferral H, Nazarian GK, et al: Duplex sonography after transjugular intrahepatic portosystemic shunts (TIPS): Normal hemodynamic findings and efficacy in predicting shunt patency and stenosis. AJR Am J Roentgenol 165:1–7, 1995.
83. Feldstein VA, Patel MD, LaBerge JM: Transjugular intrahepatic portosystemic shunts: Accuracy of Doppler US in determination of patency and detection of stenoses. Radiology 201:141–147, 1996.
84. Dodd GD III, Zajko AB, Orons PD, et al: Detection of transjugular intrahepatic portosystemic shunt dysfunction: Value of duplex Doppler sonography. AJR Am J Roentgenol 164:1119–1124, 1995.
85. Kanterman RY, Darcy MD, Middleton WD, et al: Doppler sonography findings associated with transjugular intrahepatic portosystemic shunt malfunction. AJR Am J Roentgenol 168:467–472, 1997.
86. Surratt RS, Middleton WD, Darcy MD, et al: Morphologic and hemodynamic findings at sonography before and after creation of a transjugular intrahepatic portosystemic shunt. AJR Am J Roentgenol 160:627–630, 1993.
87. Haskal ZJ, Carroll JW, Jacobs JE, et al: Sonography of transjugular intrahepatic portosystemic shunts: Detection of elevated portosystemic gradients and loss of shunt function. J Vasc Interv Radiol 8:549–556, 1997.
88. Murphy TP, Beechman RP, Kim HM, et al: Long-term follow-up after TIPS: Use of Doppler velocity criteria for detecting elevation of the portosystemic gradient. J Vasc Interv Radiol 9:275–281, 1998.
89. Grendell JH, Ockner RK: Mesenteric venous thrombosis. *In* Sleisinger MH, Fordtran JS (eds) Gastrointestinal Disease. Philadelphia, WB Saunders, 1983, pp 1557–1558.
90. Johnson CC, Baggenstoss AH: Mesenteric vascular occlusion: Study of 99 cases of occlusion of veins. Mayo Clin Proc 24:628–636, 1949.
91. North JP, Wollenman OJ: Venous mesenteric occlusion in course of migratory thrombophlebitis. Surg Gynecol Obstet 95:665–671, 1952.
92. Babcock DS: Ultrasound diagnosis of portal vein thrombosis as a complication of appendicitis. AJR Am J Roentgenol 133:317–319, 1979.
93. Verbanck JJ, Rutgeerts LJ, Haerens MH, et al: Partial splenoportal and superior mesenteric venous thrombosis. Gastroenterol 86:949–952, 1984.
94. Papanicolaou N, Harmatz P, Simeone JF, et al: Sonographic demonstration of reversible portal vein thrombosis following splenectomy in an adolescent. J Clin Ultrasound 12:575–577, 1984.
95. Merritt CBR: Ultrasonographic demonstration of portal vein thrombosis. Radiology 133:425–427, 1979.
96. Marx M, Scheible W: Cavernous transformation of the portal vein. J Ultrasound Med 1:167–169, 1982.
97. Subramanyam BR, Balthazar EJ, Lefleur RS, et al: Portal venous thrombosis: Correlative analysis of sonography, CT, and angiography. Am J Gastroenterol 79:773–776, 1984.
98. Kauzlaric D, Petrovic M, Barmeir J: Sonography of cavernous transformation of the portal vein. AJR Am J Roentgenol 142:383–384, 1984.
99. Weltin G, Taylor KJW, Carter AR, Taylor CR: Duplex Doppler: Identification of cavernous transformation of the portal vein. AJR Am J Roentgenol 144:999–1001, 1985.
100. Gansbeke FV, Avni EF, Delcour C, et al: Sonographic features of portal vein thrombosis. AJR Am J Roentgenol 144:749–752, 1985.
101. Tessler FN, Gehring BJ, Gomes AS, et al: Diagnosis of portal vein thrombosis: Value of color Doppler imaging. AJR Am J Roentgenol 157:293–296, 1991.
102. Wang L-Y, Lin Z-Y, Chang W-Y, et al: Duplex pulsed Doppler sonography of portal vein thrombosis in hepatocellular carcinoma. J Ultrasound Med 10:265–269, 1991.
103. Subramanyam BR, Balthazer EJ, Hilton S, et al: Hepatocellular carcinoma with venous invasion. Radiology 150:793–796, 1984.
104. Atri M, de Stempel J, Bret PM, Illescas FF: Incidence of portal vein thrombosis complicating liver metastasis as detected by duplex ultrasound. J Ultrasound Med 9:285–289, 1990.
105. Tanaka K, Numata K, Okazaki H, et al: Diagnosis of portal vein thrombosis in patients with hepatocellular carcinoma: Efficacy of color Doppler sonography compared with angiography. AJR Am J Roentgenol 160:1279–1283, 1993.
106. Tublin ME, Dodd GD, Baron RL: Benign and malignant portal vein thrombosis: Differentiation by CT characteristics. AJR Am J Roentgenol 168:719–723, 1997.
107. Blum U, Haag K, Rössle M, et al: Noncavernomatous portal vein thrombosis in hepatic cirrhosis: Treatment with transjugular intrahepatic portosystemic shunt and local thrombolysis. Radiology 195:153–157, 1995.
108. Chawla Y, Dilawari JB, Katariya S: Gallbladder varices in portal vein thrombosis. AJR Am J Roentgenol 162:643–645, 1994.

109. Furuse J, Matsutani S, Yoshikawa M, et al: Diagnosis of portal vein tumor thrombus by pulsed Doppler ultrasonography. J Clin Ultrasound 20:439–448, 1992.
110. De Gaetano AM, Lafortune M, Patriquin H, et al: Cavernous transformation of the portal vein: Patterns of intrahepatic and splanchnic collateral circulation detected with Doppler sonography. AJR Am J Roentgenol 165:1151–1155, 1995.
111. Hann LE, Getrajdman GI, Brown KT, et al: Hepatic lobar atrophy: Association with ipsilateral portal vein obstruction. AJR Am J Roentgenol 167:1017–1021, 1996.
112. Pollard JJ, Nebesar RA: Altered hemodynamics in the Budd-Chiari syndrome demonstrated by selective hepatic and selective splenic angiography. Radiology 89:236–243, 1967.
113. Chopra S: Budd-Chiari syndrome and veno-occlusive disease. *In* Disorders of the Liver. Philadelphia, Lea & Febiger, 1988.
114. Stanley P: Budd-Chiari syndrome. Radiology 170: 625–627, 1989.
115. Hommeyer SC, Teefey SA, Jacobson AF, et al: Venocclusive disease of the liver: Prospective study of US evaluation. Radiology 184:683–686, 1992.
116. Cho KY, Geisinger KR, Shields JJ, Forrest ME: Collateral channels and histopathology in hepatic vein occlusion. AJR Am J Roentgenol 139:703–709, 1982.
117. Murphy FB, Steinberg HV, Shires GT, et al: The Budd-Chiari syndrome: A review. AJR Am J Roentgenol 147:9–15, 1986.
118. Mathieu D, Vasile N, Menu Y, et al: Budd-Chiari syndrome: Dynamic CT. Radiology 165:409–413, 1987.
119. Harter LP, Gross BH, St Hilaire J, et al: CT and sonographic appearance of hepatic vein obstruction. AJR Am J Roentgenol 139:176–178, 1982.
120. Baert AL, Fevery J, Marchal G, et al: Early diagnosis of Budd-Chiari syndrome by computed tomography and ultrasonography: Report of five cases. Gastroenterology 84:587–595, 1983.
121. Makuuchi M, Hasegawa H, Yamazaki S, et al: Primary Budd-Chiari syndrome: Ultrasonic demonstration. Radiology 152:775–779, 1984.
122. Menu Y, Alison D, Lorphelin J-M, et al: Budd-Chiari syndrome: US evaluation. Radiology 157: 761–764, 1985.
123. Grant EG, Perrella R, Tessler FN, et al: Budd-Chiari syndrome: The results of duplex and colour Doppler imaging. AJR Am J Roentgenol 152:377–381, 1989.
124. Brown BP, Abu-Yousef M, Farner R, et al: Doppler sonography: A noninvasive method for evaluation of hepatic veno-occlusive disease. AJR Am J Roentgenol 154:721–724, 1990.
125. Hosoki T, Kuroda C, Tokunaga K, et al: Hepatic venous outflow obstruction: Evaluation with pulsed duplex sonography. Radiology 170:733–737, 1989.
126. Takayasu K, Moriyama N, Muramatsu Y, et al: Intrahepatic venous collaterals forming via the inferior right hepatic vein in 3 patients with obstruction of the inferior vena cava. Radiology 154:323–328, 1985.
127. Cho O-K, Koo J-H, Kim Y-S, et al: Collateral pathways in Budd-Chiari syndrome: CT and venographic correlation. AJR Am J Roentgenol 167: 1163–1167, 1996.
128. Kane R, Eustace S: Diagnosis of Budd-Chiari Syndrome: Comparison between sonography and MR angiography. Radiology 195:117–121, 1995.
129. Millener O, Grant EG, Rose S, et al: Color Doppler imaging findings in patients with Budd-Chiari Syndrome: Correlation with venographic findings. AJR Am J Roentgenol 161:307–312, 1993.
130. Middleton MA, Middleton WD: Intrahepatic venous collaterals in a patient with congestive heart failure. J Ultrasound Med 13:479–481, 1994.
131. Blum U, Rössle M, Haag K: Budd-Chiari syndrome: Technical, hemodynamic, and clinical results of treatment with transjugular intrahepatic portosystemic shunt. Radiology 197:805–811, 1995.

Chapter 30

DUPLEX EVALUATION OF NATIVE RENAL VESSELS AND RENAL ALLOGRAFTS

■ *William J. Zwiebel, MD*

This chapter focuses on duplex ultrasound assessment of the renal arteries and veins. Conditions affecting the native renal vessels are considered first, including renal artery stenosis and occlusion, renal vein thrombosis, and tumor invasion of the renal veins. Renal allografts are then considered, including vascular complications after transplantation and allograft rejection.

ANATOMY AND NORMAL VASCULAR SIGNATURES

The anatomy of the renal arteries and veins is presented in detail in Chapter 26; however, a few salient features bear emphasis.

1. The right renal artery arises from the aorta at an anterolateral location, not posterolateral as might be expected. The left renal artery generally arises at a lateral or posterolateral location.
2. The right renal artery is unique in that it passes posterior to the inferior vena cava (IVC). It is the only major vessel posterior to the IVC.
3. The origin of both renal arteries is slightly caudad to the superior mesenteric artery (SMA), which serves as a handy reference point for locating the renal arteries.
4. Duplicate main renal arteries and polar accessory renal arteries (Fig. 30–1) occur in about 12 to 22% of normal individuals.[1–8] Accessory renal arteries can arise from the aorta or the iliac arteries. Polar accessory renal arteries virtually always go unrecognized with ultrasonography, and even duplicated main renal arteries may be overlooked.[1–5, 9, 10, 12–16]
5. The left renal vein lies *between* the SMA and the aorta, in distinction to the splenic vein, which lies *anterior* to the SMA. The left renal vein may normally be quite large in a supine individual.
6. Blood flow in the renal artery and its branches normally has a low-resistance pattern; systolic waveforms are broad, and forward flow is present throughout diastole.
7. Renal vein flow is phasic, which means that the flow velocity varies with respiration and cardiac activity.

PRINCIPLES OF EXAMINATION

Duplex ultrasound examination of native renal vessels is technically demanding. Most sonographers are initially frustrated by difficulties with locating and following the renal arteries, and with obtaining Doppler signals from these vessels. With a little patience, however, a sonographer can become adept at this examination. Literature reports indicate that about 75 to 95% of main renal arteries can be adequately examined in adult patients.[9–12, 14]

My philosophy on renal artery duplex ultrasound examination is quite pragmatic. First, I do not believe there is any point in "beating a dead horse." If I cannot examine the renal arteries in a reasonable amount of

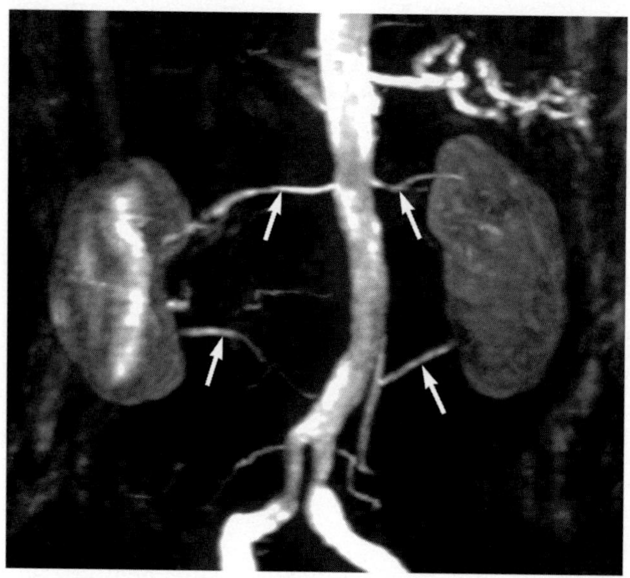

FIGURE 30–1 Multiple renal arteries. Each kidney in this hypertensive patient is supplied by two nonhilar accessory arteries (*arrows*). It is not likely that these would be visualized with ultrasound. (Gadolinium-enhanced magnetic resonance angiogram.)

time (about 20 minutes per artery), I give up. Second, I recognize that only the proximal 3 or 4 cm of each main renal artery can be visualized clearly in many adults, and I focus on these segments. I personally recommend duplex ultrasonography only for elderly patients who are apt to have atherosclerotic obstructive lesions, which are typically located proximally within the renal arteries (usually at the arterial origin).[10, 15] I have doubts about the value of renal artery duplex ultrasonography for younger adults who are more likely to have fibromuscular hyperplasia, because this condition may affect the distal renal artery or the segmental branches.[14, 17]

The technical difficulties associated with renal artery examination may be eased substantially by the use of ultrasound contrast (echo-enhancing) agents, which greatly increases the visibility of blood vessels. In addition to reducing examination time, the use of these agents may enhance ultrasound visualization of multiple renal arteries and hilar branches. Ultrasound contrast agents are being released for general clinical use concurrent with the publication of this textbook. Please see Chapter 5 for further details.

TECHNIQUE

Color-flow imaging is the mainstay of renal artery ultrasound examination. Color-flow imaging is used to locate the renal arteries and to detect flow disturbances that indicate stenosis. But color-flow imaging, when used alone, may give a false impression of renal artery stenosis because atherosclerotic plaques can cause flow disturbances in vessels that are not significantly stenotic. Doppler spectral analysis is used in conjunction with color-flow imaging, because Doppler analysis alone can quantify stenosis severity.

I recommend that you begin the renal artery examination by carefully examining each kidney. Left and right decubitus patient positions are preferred for this portion of the kidney examination (left decubitus for the right kidney and vice versa). Note the echogenicity and thickness of the renal parenchyma, and measure the kidney length (Fig. 30–2). Look for scarring, hydronephrosis, and renal masses. Next, evaluate the Doppler spectral waveforms in the segmental arteries in each kidney. For this part of the examination, use a low velocity range (such as that typically used for extremity veins) and a low wall filter setting. Adjust the spectral display so that the waveforms are large and easily measured.[18] Measure the acceleration time or index, the peak systolic velocity, and the pulsatility index,* and inspect the waveforms for side-to-side differences in pulsatility. Also examine the distal portions of the renal arteries as they enter the kidneys (if they are visible).

Begin the examination of the *proximal* renal arteries with a longitudinal view of the

* This parameter is not used for diagnosis of renal artery stenosis, but pulsatility may be elevated in parenchymal renal disease and urinary tract obstruction.

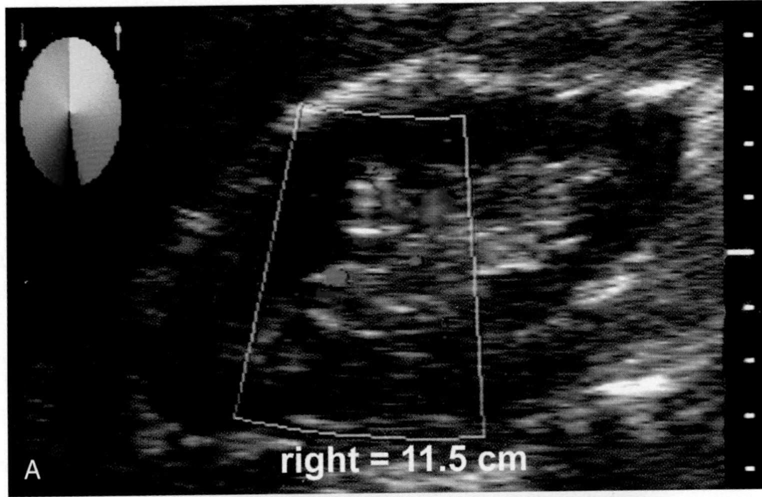

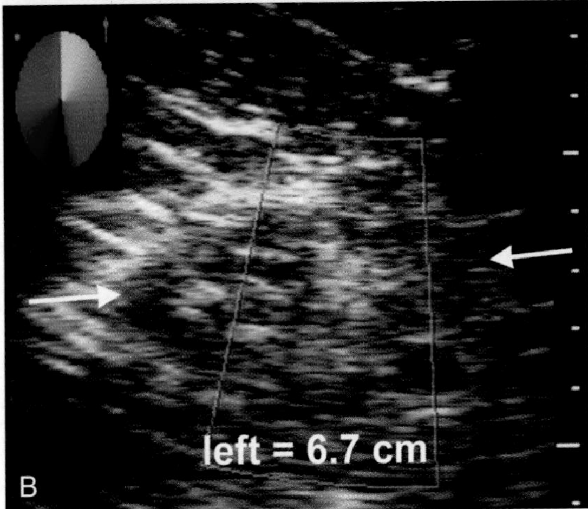

FIGURE 30–2 Occluded renal artery. *A,* The right kidney measures 11.5 cm in length and blood flow is readily visualized in the renal hilum with color-Doppler imaging. *B,* The left kidney is only 6.7 cm long, and no blood flow could be detected with color-Doppler imaging. Renal artery occlusion was confirmed angiographically.

abdominal aorta, which is obtained with the patient supine. Adjust gray-scale, color-flow, and Doppler settings. Adjustments preset by the instrument manufacturer usually suffice, but further refinement may be needed. When the instrument is properly adjusted, the aorta should be examined, with attention in elderly patients to atherosclerotic obstruction of the SMA, the celiac artery, and the aorta itself. Check also for aortic aneurysm, and then obtain an angle-corrected Doppler spectrum from the aorta at the approximate level of the renal arteries and the SMA. Measure the peak systolic velocity from this spectrum, which is used to determine the renal artery–to–aorta velocity ratio, as discussed later.

Next, locate the origin of the renal arteries on transverse images of the aorta.[19] Begin at the celiac axis or the SMA, because these are easily located, and move slightly caudad along the aorta until the origin of each renal artery is seen, as shown in Chapter 26. The right renal artery is often easier to identify than the left renal artery and is relatively easy to follow to the renal hilum. The left renal artery is harder to follow all the way to the kidney from an anterior approach. The distal portion of the left renal artery may be seen by positioning the patient in a *right* lateral decubitus position and scanning from a *left* posterolateral transducer approach,[20] using the left kidney as an acoustic window. An analogous approach can be used to visualize the distal right renal artery and its branches, with the patient in a *left* lateral decubitus position. In small children, both renal arteries can sometimes be viewed simultaneously from a coronal approach through the left kidney, as illustrated in Chapter 26.

Each renal artery should be examined with color-flow imaging from its origin to the hilum of the kidney (if possible). Look for areas of high-velocity flow or flow disturbances that might be related to stenosis, and interrogate these areas with spectral Doppler analysis. If there are no areas of abnormal flow, simply obtain representative systolic velocity measurements in the proximal and distal portions of the main renal artery.

VASCULAR DISORDERS

Renal Artery Stenosis

Stenosis or occlusion of a main renal artery or an accessory renal artery may cause renal ischemia, which in turn triggers the renin-angiotensin mechanism and causes hypertension. Renal artery stenosis can also cause or contribute to renal insufficiency by inducing renal parenchymal damage. The threshold level of renal artery stenosis that produces hypertension or ischemic damage is uncertain and probably varies from one patient to another. From a hemodynamic perspective, renal artery obstruction is considered hemodynamically significant (or flow reducing) when the lumen diameter is narrowed by 50 to 60%.

It is estimated that 10% of the United States population have hypertension, and 3 to 5% of this group have renal arterial disease.[1, 21] Although the latter percentages are small, renal artery disease represents the most common *correctable* cause of hypertension.[21] More recently, clinical interest has focused on the potential role of renal ischemia in the etiology of chronic renal insufficiency.[22, 23] Once again, the potential correctability of renal artery stenosis has been stressed. Few kidney diseases can be cured, and it is understandable that clinicians should be keenly interested in a potentially curable disorder such as renal artery stenosis. Does this mean, however, that we should seek to diagnose renal artery disease in every patient with hypertension or renal insufficiency? To do so could be expensive and not cost-effective;[24] furthermore, intervention for renal artery disease is risky and not always successful. Considering these points, I believe that renal artery stenosis should be sought only in the following selected groups of patients: (1) young patients with severe hypertension; (2) patients with rapidly accelerating hypertension or malignant hypertension; (3) patients with hypertension that is difficult to control in spite of a suitable three-drug treatment program; (4) patients with concomitant hypertension and deteriorating renal function; and (5) patients with renal insufficiency and discrepant kidney size (inferring renal artery stenosis).[1, 21–24]

Doppler Renal Artery Evaluation

Catheter angiography has traditionally been regarded as the definitive test for renal artery stenosis. Because this procedure is uncomfortable and carries some risk, a simple and effective noninvasive method has been sought for detecting renal arterial obstruction. Duplex sonography, magnetic resonance angiography, scintigraphy, and computed tomographic angiography have been investigated for this purpose,[1–51] but only duplex sonography is considered in detail in this chapter. The following general comments about duplex diagnosis of renal artery stenosis are noteworthy:

1. The principal ultrasound criterion for renal artery stenosis is Doppler-detected flow velocity elevation in the stenotic portion of the vessel[1, 11, 14, 15, 17, 29, 30] (Figs. 30–3 and 30–4). Flow velocity is increased in proportion to the severity of luminal narrowing; therefore, spectral Doppler measurements can be used to approximate stenosis severity. Narrowed areas detected with color-flow imaging must be carefully searched with the Doppler sample volume to ensure that the maximum flow velocity is identified.
2. Accurate assignment of the Doppler angle is essential for reliable measurement of stenosis-related velocity elevation, and a Doppler-to-vessel angle of 60 degrees or less is mandatory to ensure that velocity information is accurate.
3. Major stenoses are accompanied by poststenotic flow disturbance (turbulence). Although disturbed flow is a useful beacon for the presence of stenosis, it is neither quantitative nor specific. Only a rough correlation exists between the severity of disturbed flow and the severity of stenosis; furthermore, disturbed flow may occur without significant stenosis.
4. Arterial waveforms within the kidney (segmental or interlobar arteries) may be scrutinized for evidence of damping,

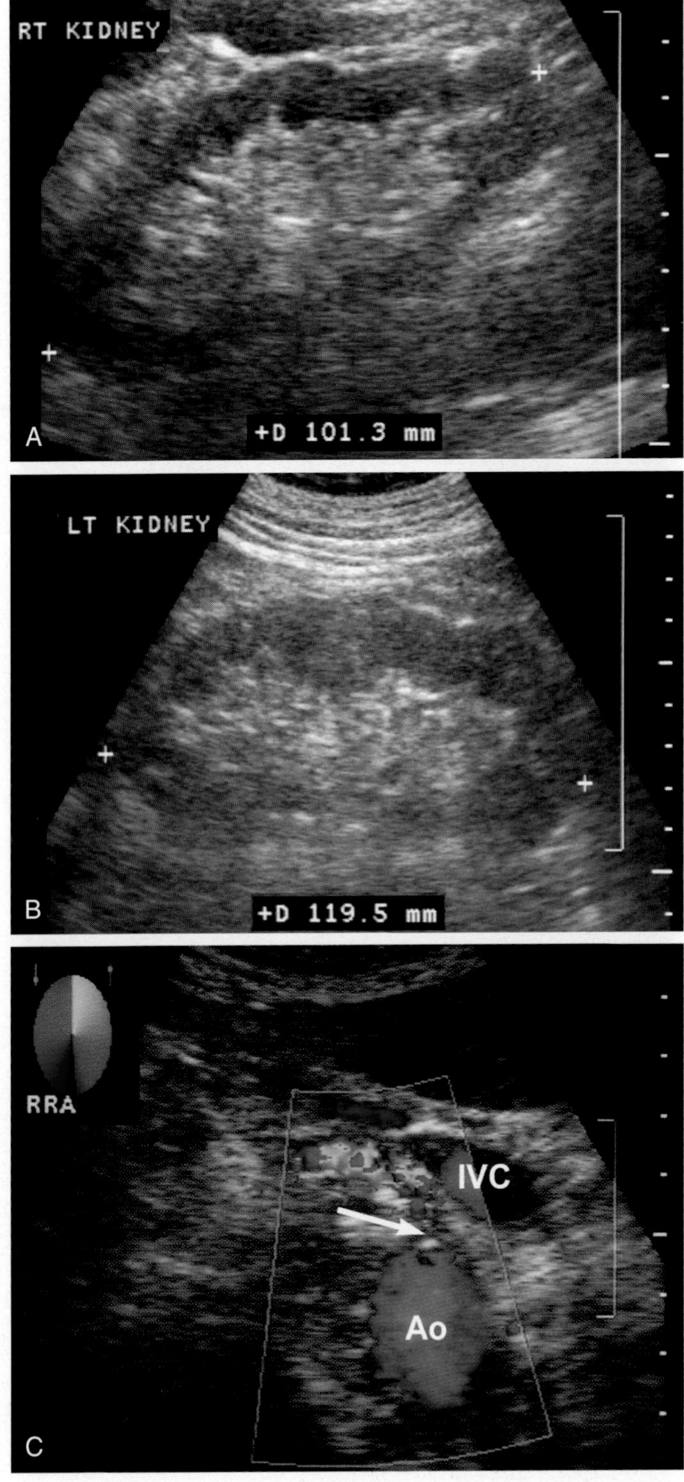

FIGURE 30–3 Renal artery stenosis. *A,* The right kidney measures 101.3 mm in length and the parenchyma appears a little thin. *B,* The left kidney measures 119.5 mm in length and the parenchyma appears thicker than on the right. *C,* A transverse view of the right renal artery origin (patient in left decubitus position) shows a stenosis (*arrow*) at the renal artery origin that produces considerable poststenotic flow disturbance. Ao = aorta; IVC = inferior vena cava.

Illustration continued on following page

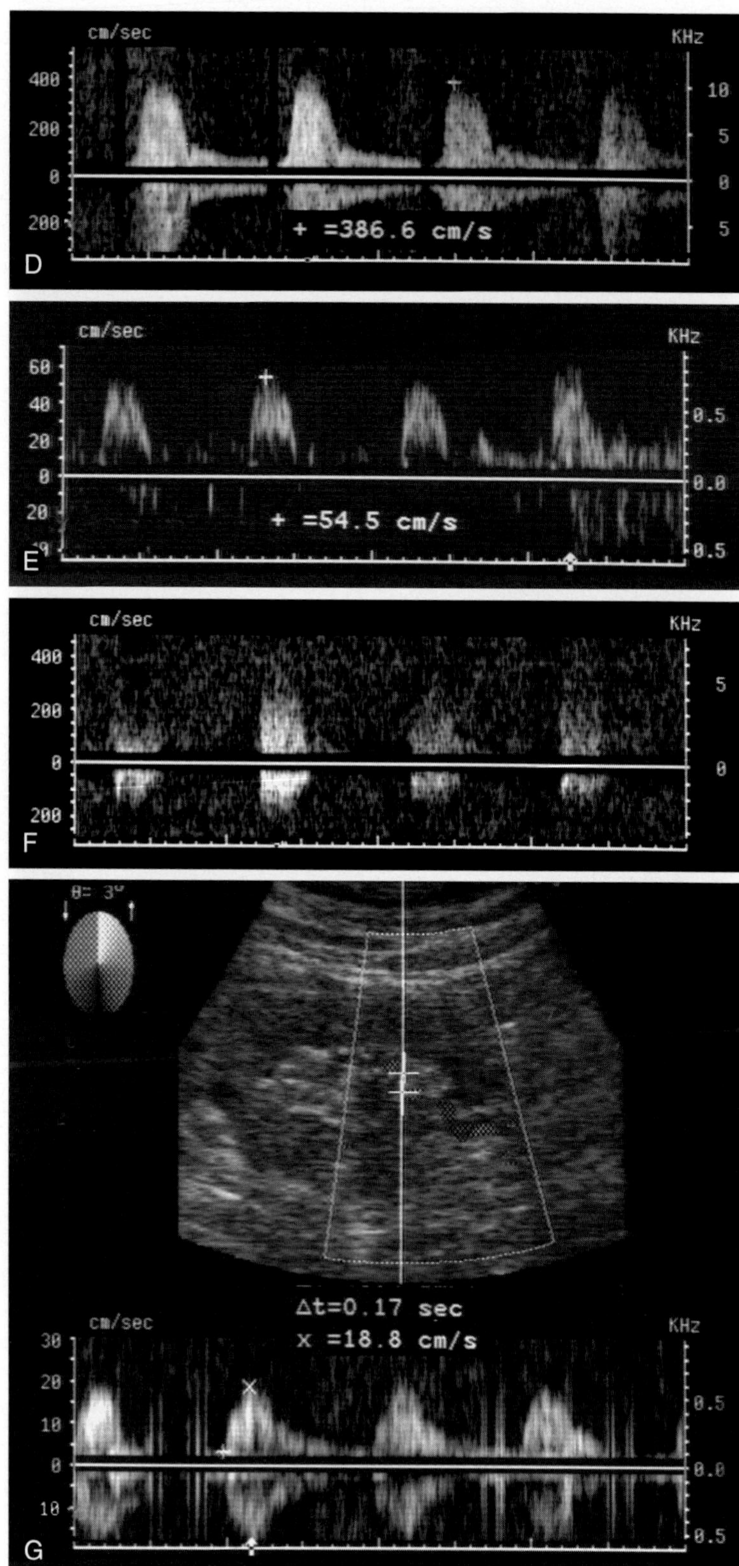

FIGURE 30–3 *Continued. D,* Peak systolic velocity at the right renal artery origin is 386.6 cm/sec, well above the 200 cm/sec cutoff for a hemodynamically significant stenosis. *E,* Peak systolic velocity in the aorta at the renal artery level is 54.5 cm/sec, making the renal artery/aortic ratio 7.0, which is well above the 3.5 cut-off for hemodynamic significance. *F,* Severe flow disturbance is evident just beyond the stenosis in the right renal artery. *G,* Systolic acceleration (0.17 second) is markedly prolonged in the right renal hilum.

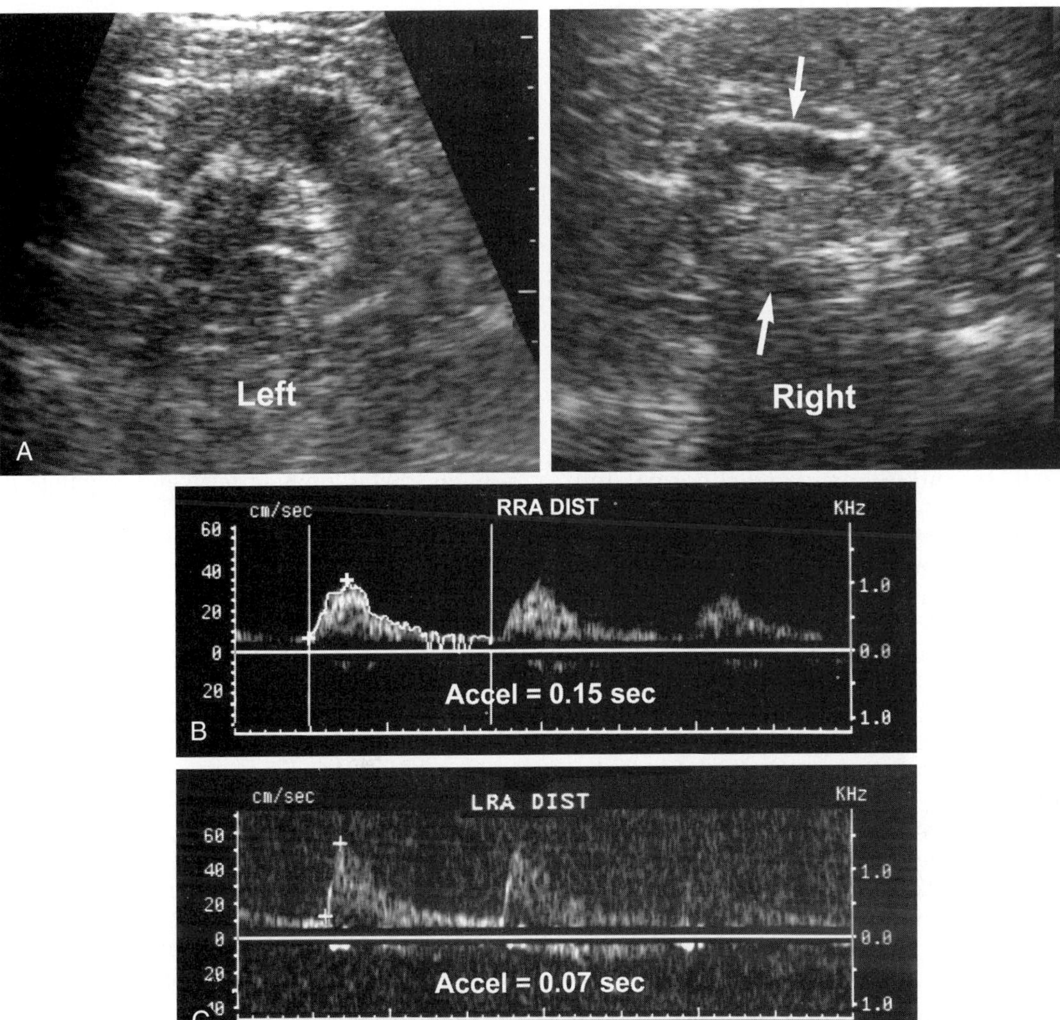

FIGURE 30–4 Abnormal intrarenal acceleration due to renal artery stenosis. *A,* At the same degree of magnification, the parenchyma of the right kidney (*arrows*) is visibly thinner than the parenchyma of the left kidney. *B,* Intrarenal systolic acceleration is visibly prolonged in the right kidney, and the acceleration time (0.15 second) is distinctly abnormal. Severe right renal artery stenosis was confirmed angiographically. *C,* Systolic acceleration is normal in the left kidney, which had a normal renal artery at angiography.

which is a downstream manifestation of renal artery stenosis. The most important downstream findings are the absence of an early systolic peak, a prolonged systolic acceleration time (see Fig. 30–4), or a reduced acceleration index.[6, 18, 29, 31–35]

Diagnostic Criteria

The peak systolic velocity in normal renal arteries ranges from 74 to 127 cm/sec in both adults and children.[17, 19, 36, 37] Numerous Doppler velocity criteria have been used in attempts to diagnose hemodynamically significant renal artery stenosis (defined generally as 50 to 60% (or greater) diameter reduction).* The most universally accepted Doppler criteria are (1) peak systolic velocity in the stenosis of 180 to 200 cm/sec or greater and (2) a renal/aortic ratio exceeding 3.3 or 3.5.[1–3, 10–13, 17] The latter is the ratio of peak systole in the stenotic portion of the renal artery divided by peak systole in the aorta at the renal artery level (see Fig. 30–3). In theory, the renal/aortic ratio compensates for he-

* References 1–5, 13, 15, 17, 19, 21, 32, 34, 35, 38–43.

modynamic variability, yet some authors have found peak systolic velocity measurements, used alone, to be more accurate than the renal/aortic ratio.[3]

Damping of *intrarenal* arterial signals is also an important criterion for diagnosis of renal artery stenosis. Damping is defined numerically with the acceleration index or the acceleration time (see Figs. 30–3 and 30–4). These measures are discussed further in Chapter 3. Both of these measures reflect the rate of systolic acceleration, which is slower than normal in patients with hemodynamically significant ipsilateral renal artery stenosis. An acceleration index less than 300 cm/sec or an acceleration time exceeding 0.07 second is considered abnormal and suggests a 60% or greater renal artery stenosis.[1, 2, 6, 15, 18, 31, 34, 43] Some authors use an acceleration time of 0.10 or 0.12 second as the cutoff for significant stenosis, which increases specificity.[1, 2, 43]

It has been suggested that the downstream effects of renal artery stenosis can be diagnosed merely by visual inspection of the shape of the segmental or interlobar Doppler waveforms.[18, 29, 43] Either the initial systolic peak is absent, or the systolic peak is grossly rounded in patients with severe ipsilateral stenosis, as illustrated in Figure 30–4*B*. However, the diagnostic accuracy of this method has been questioned, as discussed later.

Reported Results

A wide ranges of sensitivity (0 to 98%) and specificity (37 to 99%) have been reported for *direct* duplex detection of renal artery stenosis, based on either an elevated systolic velocity in the renal artery or an abnormal renal/aortic ratio.* The disparate results of these studies are a reflection of selection bias, examiner experience, and statistical methods. For instance, several of the more successful studies were potentially biased (exclusively or principally) because most or all of their patients were elderly individuals who, for the most part, have atherosclerotic stenoses at the renal artery origins. Because the origins of the renal arteries are the portions most easily visualized with ultrasonography, greater accuracy may be expected in this population than in younger individuals who may have more distal renal artery disease.[10–13] In addition, some studies included only successful Doppler examinations in statistical tabulation, whereas other studies included all examinations, regardless of the level of success.

In spite of the spread of reported results, it appears that *direct* duplex examination of the renal arteries is reasonably effective for diagnosis of clinically significant renal artery stenosis. With experience and good technique, the examiner is likely to attain sensitivity and specificity levels for adult patients in the vicinity of 90% for 60% (diameter) or greater stenosis in the proximal 4 cm (or so) of the main renal arteries. Diagnostic accuracy for distal renal artery and segmental branch lesions is not as good as that for more proximal stenoses, as discussed later.

Branch and Duplicate Artery Problems

In hypertensive patients, the documentation or exclusion of a renovascular etiology requires the assessment of the main renal artery, accessory renal arteries, or segmental renal arteries. Duplicated main (hilar) renal artery stenosis can clearly cause hypertension or ischemia. Polar accessory artery stenoses are thought to rarely cause hypertension and are probably not a significant cause of renal insufficiency.[1, 4, 6–8, 19]

As noted previously, atherosclerotic obstruction tends to occur at or near the origin of the renal arteries and is detected quite readily in main renal arteries with duplex sonography. Fibromuscular hyperplasia, however, can occur at any location from the origin of the vessel to the hilar branches and may involve multiple branches. Statistical details are limited, but my experience and that of others indicate that duplex results are poorer for distal renal artery and branch stenoses than they are for the more proximal portions of the main renal artery.[5, 14, 17] For instance, Hélénon and colleagues[14] reported a sensitivity level of only 60% for hilar branch stenoses, and Kliewer and associates[5] reported missing three branch vessel stenoses with duplex examination. Stenoses in hilar branch vessels can be repaired surgically or with angioplasty,[47] so their detection in hypertensive patients is important. For this reason, I advise the use of caution concerning

* References 1, 11, 12, 14, 19, 30, 32, 38–41, 44–46.

duplex ultrasound assessment of younger hypertensive patients who might have fibromuscular hyperplasia.[2–8, 14]

Angiographic studies show that 12 to 22% of kidneys are supplied by more than one renal artery. Kliewer and associates[5] found that 15% of kidneys had double main renal arteries and 13% had accessory arteries (usually at the poles of the kidney). Accessory arteries usually arise from the aorta but may also arise from the iliac arteries.

Unfortunately, the detection rate for multiple renal arteries with duplex ultrasonography (including color-flow imaging) is dismal. Hélénon and colleagues[14] reported detecting 30% of duplicate renal arteries with ultrasonography (but did not say whether these are double main renal arteries or polar arteries). Hélénon and colleagues[14] failed to detect 25% of main renal arteries, including duplicate arteries. Melany and coworkers[16] visualized several duplicate renal arteries with ultrasound contrast enhancement but failed to see three polar accessory arteries. In all other reports of which I am aware, no duplicate renal arteries were detected with ultrasound, and this includes main renal and polar artery duplication.[2–5, 9, 12–14] Failure to detect duplicate renal arteries adversely affects duplex accuracy, as evident in the study by Hansen and associates[12] in which duplex sensitivity for 60% (diameter) stenosis was 98% for single main renal arteries, but it was only 67% for all renal arteries, including duplicate vessels. Polar accessory renal arteries rarely cause hypertension or significant ischemia; hence, one could argue that their visualization is unimportant. Duplicated main renal arteries, however, can be repaired, and their detection *is* important. This limitation of sonography should be kept in mind, and other imaging studies should be considered in selected hypertensive patients even if duplex ultrasound examination is normal.

Intrarenal Waveform Assessment

An ideal survey method for renal artery stenosis would be accurate, quick, and easy. This is the appeal of Doppler assessment of intrarenal vessels for stenosis-related flow changes. For an experienced sonographer, the detection of intrarenal flow signals is relatively easy, and the examination is successful in most individuals.

It has long been recognized that renal artery stenosis can cause pulsus tardus and parvus changes in intrarenal flow signals,[48, 49] as illustrated in Figures 30–3 and 30–4 and defined in Chapter 3. It would be nice if one could simply look for such flow changes in the kidneys and thereby diagnose renal artery stenosis. Unfortunately, the accuracy of this diagnostic method is questionable. Several reports (based on acceleration time, acceleration index, and waveform shape changes) indicate Doppler sensitivity ranging from 89 to 95% and specificity ranging from 83 to 97% for renal artery stenoses exceeding 60 or 70% diameter reduction.[2, 18, 31, 34] In contrast, other literature reports, based on the same Doppler parameters, indicate poor results ranging from moderate accuracy to complete absence of correlation between Doppler and angiographic findings.[5, 6, 14, 29, 33, 44, 50]

In general, it appears that intrarenal waveform changes are more accurate for high-grade renal artery stenosis, which exceeds 70% diameter reduction, and such changes are not useful for detection of stenosis in the 50 to 60% range.[2, 5, 33] Even at high levels of stenosis, however, some patients do not have appreciable waveform changes. To make matters worse, damped intrarenal waveforms can occasionally be seen in the absence of significant renal artery stenosis. Such inconsistencies appear because intrarenal Doppler waveforms are influenced both by hemodynamic conditions in the renal parenchyma and by conditions within the main renal artery (i.e., renal artery stenosis).[51] The effects of renal artery stenosis can be overridden by flow conditions in the renal parenchyma, and vice versa, as discussed in the next section.

Because intrarenal Doppler waveform analysis has not been consistently accurate, I am uncomfortable with the exclusive use of These findings for the diagnosis of renal artery stenosis. However, I do evaluate acceleration and waveform shape in intrarenal arteries in conjunction with direct renal artery interrogation.

Doppler Waveform Abnormalities in Nonvascular Renal Disease

Flow resistance within the renal parenchyma may be increased by a variety of pathologic processes in addition to renal artery stenosis, including urinary tract obstruction and a host of acute and chronic parenchymal disorders.[70, 71] All of these conditions are associated with increased flow resistance in the parenchyma, which cause the Doppler waveforms to exhibit *increased pulsatility*. This may be evident on visual inspection of waveforms or through pulsatility measures such as the pulsatility index or resistivity index (defined in Chapter 3). Normally, a large amount of diastolic blood flow is evident on visual inspection of the intrarenal Doppler signals, and the pulsatility index in segmental or intralobar arteries does not exceed 0.7.

An increase in vascular resistance (and pulsatility) in renal pathology is an interesting finding, but it is of somewhat limited diagnostic value because it is multifactorial in origin. Increased pulsatility is of greatest diagnostic value when it is seen unilaterally, for in such cases, it implies acute urinary tract obstruction on the side with high pulsatility. High pulsatility may be apparent before significant urinary tract dilatation occurs.[70, 71]

Renal Artery Occlusion

Renal artery occlusion is diagnosed on the basis of the following findings: (1) absence of a visible main renal artery; (2) markedly reduced kidney size (smaller than 9 cm in length); and (3) either absence of detectable intrarenal blood flow or very low amplitude, damped intrarenal flow signals.[1, 3, 10, 11]

Diagnostic accuracy for renal artery occlusion is predicated on reasonable color-Doppler or spectral Doppler sensitivity at the level of the renal artery or kidney. That is, flow should be readily detected in other vessels at a similar depth or in the contralateral kidney before it is concluded that a renal artery is occluded (see Fig. 30–2). Although relatively few data exist in the medical literature, it appears that duplex diagnosis of renal artery occlusion is reasonably accurate. Thirty-eight of 41 occluded arteries were correctly diagnosed in three published series, for an overall accuracy rate of 93%.[3, 10, 11]

False-positive diagnosis of renal artery occlusion can occur when visualization of the main renal artery is poor or the kidney is small for reasons other than ischemia. False-negative results are caused by collateralization, which may occur via capsular or adrenal branches, and duplicate renal arteries. In the collateralized kidney, flow signals may well be present in the kidney parenchyma or in the renal hilum in spite of renal artery occlusion, and Doppler waveforms may even be normal in the kidney in some cases.

Renal Vein Thrombosis

Renal vein thrombosis appears to be an underdiagnosed vascular disease because of the nonspecificity of clinical and radiographic findings.[52–54] Acute renal vein thrombosis usually presents with pain and hematuria, and it may occasionally cause thromboembolic complications, such as pulmonary embolism. Chronic renal vein thrombosis may be asymptomatic or may present with nephrotic syndrome or hematuria.

The renal vein may be blocked by intraluminal thrombus formation or from extrinsic compression that may cause secondary venous thrombosis. Associated or predisposing conditions include pre-existing renal disease, hypercoagulable state, vena caval or ovarian vein thrombus (with extension to the renal veins), abdominal surgery, trauma, and dehydration. Primary renal disease is the most common predisposing factor, particularly the nephrotic syndrome and membranous glomerulonephritis.[54] Extrinsic retroperitoneal causes of renal vein thrombosis include acute pancreatitis, lymph node enlargement from a host of tumors, and retroperitoneal fibrosis. These conditions generally cause extrinsic compression of the vascular pedicle, predisposing to thrombosis.[52]

Renal vein thrombosis typically induces ischemic parenchymal damage in the kidney and acute renal failure.[52–54] The long-term effects of renal vein thrombosis are varied. The potential exists for recanalization of the renal vein or the development of venous collaterals, and, in some cases, the kidney returns to a normal sonograhic appearance. If the kidney is severely damaged, however, chronic changes become evident, including diminished kidney size and increased echogenicity (because of fibrosis).

The most easily detected ultrasound findings in *acute* renal vein occlusion[55–62] are kidney enlargement and altered parenchymal echogenicity, both of which are caused by parenchymal edema and in some cases by hemorrhage. Echogenicity changes may include the following: (1) hypoechoic cortex with decreased corticomedullary differentiation, (2) hyperechoic cortex with preservation of corticomedullary differentiation, and (3) mottled heterogeneity accompanied by the loss of normal intrarenal architecture. In some cases, echogenic linear streaks of unknown origin course through the renal parenchyma. These streaks are thought to be pathognomonic for renal vein thrombosis.[57, 58]

Kidney enlargement and altered parenchymal echogenicity are nonspecific findings, and the conclusive diagnosis of renal vein thrombosis depends on the direct identification of thrombus in the renal vein. With acute thrombosis, the renal vein is invariably enlarged, and Doppler signals are absent. A small trickle of flow may be present around the clot, and this may produce low-velocity, continuous (lacking phasic variation) Doppler signals, but normal phasic flow is absent. Recently formed thrombus is hypoechoic and in some cases is virtually anechoic. As a result, the thrombus may be invisible with gray-scale sonography and detectable only with color-flow or Doppler sonography. Two additional pitfalls are noteworthy. First, venous flow may be present within the kidney itself, even though the renal vein is occluded, because large collaterals may develop quickly. Second, very sluggish renal vein flow (as a result of more proximal obstruction or congestion) may mimic thrombosis because the Doppler signal may be difficult to detect at very slow flow rates.

Renal Vein Tumor Extension

Tumor extension into the renal vein is most commonly associated with renal cell carcinoma, although renal lymphoma, transitional cell carcinoma, and Wilms' tumor can also propagate along the renal veins. Venous invasion is common in renal cell carcinoma, with gross involvement of the main renal vein occurring in 21 to 35% of patients and caval tumor extension in 5 to 10% of patients.[61, 62] Vena caval invasion is approximately 3 times more common in right-sided tumors than those on the left, most likely because of the shorter length of the right renal vein.[61, 62] Preoperative diagnosis of venous tumor extension significantly influences surgical therapy. If no tumor is present, routine ligation of the renal vein may be performed through a flank incision, but if the renal vein is occluded by tumor and if the tumor extends into the IVC, a midline incision often is used, which may be extended cephalad to create a sternotomy if necessary.[62]

In most centers, contrast-enhanced computed tomography is the preferred method of investigation for intravenous tumor extension, supplemented when necessary with magnetic resonance imaging or sonography. The latter modality has cost and convenience advantages over magnetic resonance imaging and can often answer directed questions, such as the superior extent of the tumor within the IVC. Duplex sonography is not as accurate as computed tomography or magnetic resonance imaging for de novo detection of tumor extension into the renal vein, particularly on the left side where the vein is frequently obscured by bowel gas.[63–69] If the renal vein and IVC are well visualized, sonographic accuracy is good (96% sensitivity, 100% specificity), but renal vein visualization is inadequate in 34 to 54% of patients, and the IVC is inadequately seen in 4 to 21% of cases.[64, 67] Thus, the overall sensitivity of ultrasound for venous tumor extension may be as low as 18% for the renal veins and 33% for the IVC.[55]

As seen with ultrasound, an intravenous tumor[65–71] (Fig. 30–5) is typically homogeneous and is low or intermediate in echogenicity. The tumor-containing renal vein is almost always distended to a distinctly abnormal size, and even the IVC may be distended when a tumor is present. Doppler signals are absent within the tumor itself, but flow may be present around the tumor. Differentiation between intravenous tumor and thrombus may be difficult. Color-Doppler detection of small blood vessels within the tumor is definitive in some cases, however.

RENAL ALLOGRAFTS

The term *allograft* refers to any tissue transplanted from one human to another. The proper term for the transplanted kidney, therefore, is *renal allograft*. The allograft may be harvested (removed) from a living, related donor, or from a brain-dead donor. The term *cadaveric renal allograft* is used in the latter circumstance, even though the donor's heart

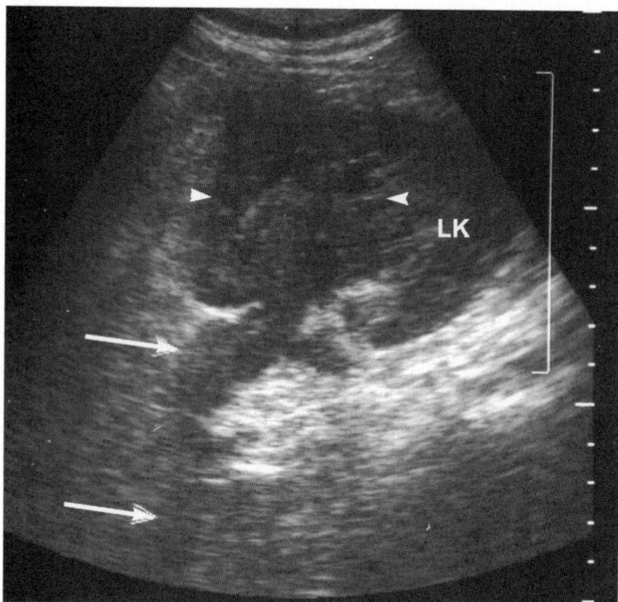

FIGURE 30–5 Renal vein tumor invasion from renal cell carcinoma. An ill-defined tumor mass (*arrowheads*) projects from the left kidney (LK). Tumor fills the left renal vein (*arrows*), which is visibly distended and slightly irregular. No blood flow could be detected in the vein with color-Doppler imaging (not shown).

continues to function at the time the kidney is removed.

The renal allograft is almost always placed in the right or left iliac fossa of the recipient. Usually the allograft is extraperitoneal (between the peritoneum and the iliacus muscle). In a child, the allograft may be placed intraperitoneally if it is too large for extraperitoneal transplantation. The allograft ureter is passed through an oblique tunnel in the muscular layer of the bladder, forming a nonrefluxing ureterovesical junction. The allograft artery is attached in one of three ways[72] (Fig. 30–6): (1) the end of the allograft artery to the side of the external iliac artery (end to side), (2) the end of the allograft artery to the end of an internal iliac branch (end to end), and (3) for multiple renal arteries or for a small renal artery from a child, a patch of the donor aorta containing the arterial orifice (Carrell's patch) is attached to an opening made in the external iliac artery. The renal vein anastomosis, in almost all cases, is end to side, with the cut end of the allograft vein attached to the side of the external iliac vein.

The native kidneys of the allograft recipient are usually left in place, but they are occasionally removed for a variety of reasons, including chronic or recurrent infection. Native kidneys are subject to the development of cysts and neoplasms in long-term dialysis patients, but these lesions do not result from renal transplantation per se.

Renal allografts are subject to a variety of complications including acute tubular necrosis (in the postoperative period), acute rejection, chronic rejection, infection, ureteral obstruction, ureteral reflex, vascular obstruction, and extrarenal fluid collections.[72–128]

Technical Considerations

Renal allografts are usually quite superficial in location, which necessitates the use of linear array or curved array transducers. These transducers provide a broad field of view and good near-field image quality.

From an ultrasound perspective, a transplanted kidney looks like a native kidney with several minor exceptions.[48, 49] First, anatomic detail is often clearer than in native kidneys because of the superficial location of the allograft. Second, the cortex may appear more echogenic than that of a normotopic kidney because of the lack of ultrasound attenuation by overlying structures (Fig. 30–7). Third, the allograft usually enlarges over a period of several months following transplantation, and such enlargement should not be mistakenly attributed to rejection. In adults, the volume of the allograft typically increases up to 30%,[49, 80] but this increase may be as great as 200% if a kidney from a young (and relatively small) donor is transplanted into a much larger recipient (e.g., an adult).[84]

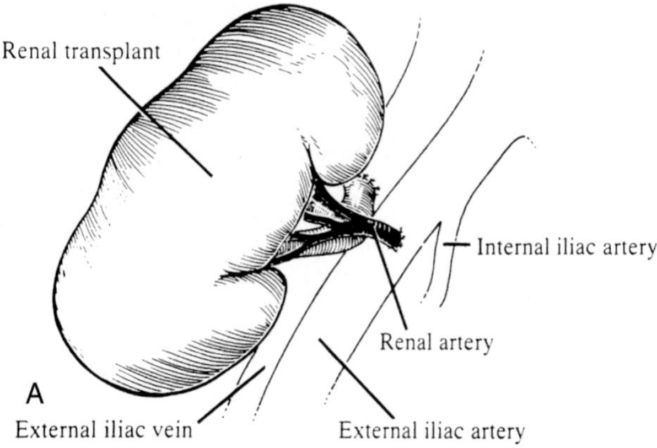

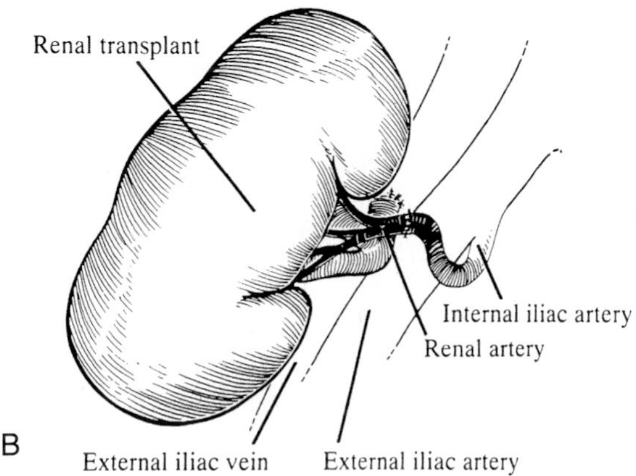

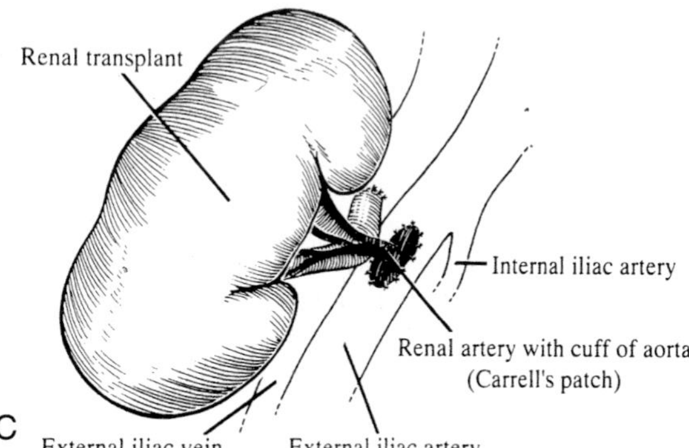

FIGURE 30–6 Allograft renal artery anastomoses. *A,* end-to-side anastomosis, allograft artery to external iliac artery. *B,* End-to-end anastomosis, allograft artery to internal iliac artery. *C,* Carrell's patch from the donor aorta.

Finally, slight dilatation of the allograft collecting system (hydronephrosis) is a common finding, particularly in the postoperative period. In most instances, such dilatation is not of urodynamic importance.

The sonographic diagnosis of allograft pathology is aided by a baseline scan conducted within the first 2 days after surgery. This scan represents an important standard against which later changes may be compared. Typically, a second scan is obtained at 1 to 2 weeks after transplantation, and a third scan is obtained at about 3 months.

Allograft Rejection and Acute Tubular Necrosis

Renal allograft rejection may produce a host of sonographic abnormalities, as listed

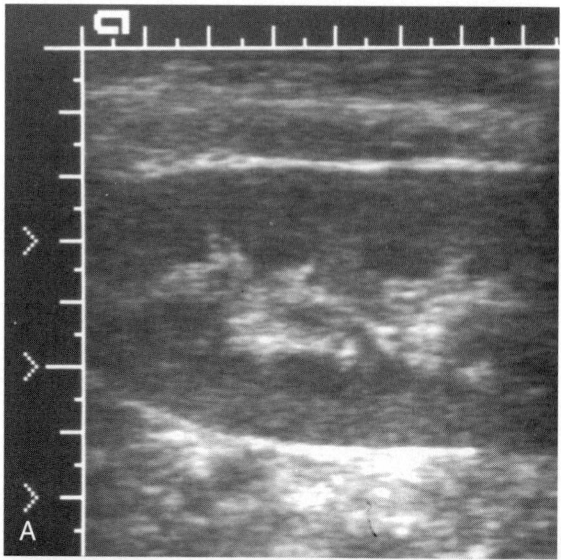

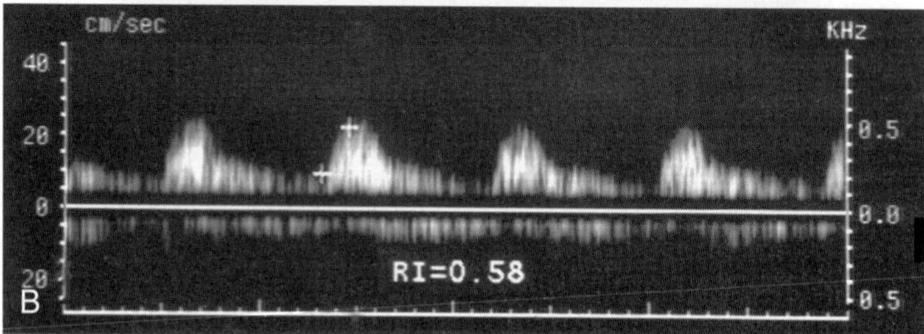

FIGURE 30–7 Normal renal allograft. *A,* A normally functioning renal allograft (1 month after surgery) demonstrates moderate cortical echogenicity and conspicuous pyramids typical of transplanted kidneys. *B,* a normal low-resistance flow pattern is seen intrarenally in the allgoraft.

in Table 30–1.[72, 74–90] The most common and important manifestations of allograft rejection (Fig. 30–8) are the following: (1) increased size of the graft (best appreciated through volume measurements), (2) increased cortical echogenicity, and (3) increased size or conspicuity of the renal pyramids.[78, 83, 87, 90] Additional important features of acute rejection are peripheral hypoechoic zones and diminished sinus echogenicity (see Fig. 30–8), but these are seen only in cases of severe rejection.[74, 76, 78, 81, 83, 90]

Doppler waveform abnormalities that indicate high peripheral arterial resistance (see Fig. 30–8*B*) also occur in renal transplant rejection. These flow abnormalities are evident in the segmental or interlobar arteries of the allograft, in both acute and chronic rejection.[91–111] As summarized in Table 30–2, the waveform changes associated with rejection include (1) absence of flow throughout diastole, (2) flow reversal in diastole, (3) a resistivity index* that equals or exceeds 0.7, and (4) a pulsatility index† that equals or exceeds 1.8.[91–93, 95–98, 101–108] Specificity for rejection is increased by using a resistivity index of 0.9 or greater as a sign of rejection.

In contrast to allograft rejection, postsurgical acute tubular necrosis (ATN), resulting from ischemia, does not generally alter the B-mode appearance of the renal allografts or the Doppler flow characteristics. Uncommonly, however, increased cortical echoge-

TABLE 30–1 SONOGRAPHIC MANIFESTATIONS OF RENAL ALLOGRAFT REJECTION

Increased allograft size (volume)
Increased cortical echogenicity (cellular infiltration)
Increased prominence of the renal pyramids*
Focal cortical hypoechoic regions (edema, necrosis)
Decreased echogenicity of the renal sinus (edema)
Increased flow resistance in parenchymal arteries

*Due to increased pyramid size and increased contrast between the hypoechoic pyramids and the echogenic cortex.

* The resistivity index is the peak systolic frequency minus the end diastolic frequency, divided by the peak systolic frequency.

† The pulsatility index is the peak systolic frequency minus the lowest diastole frequency (including reversed flow), divided by the mean frequency.

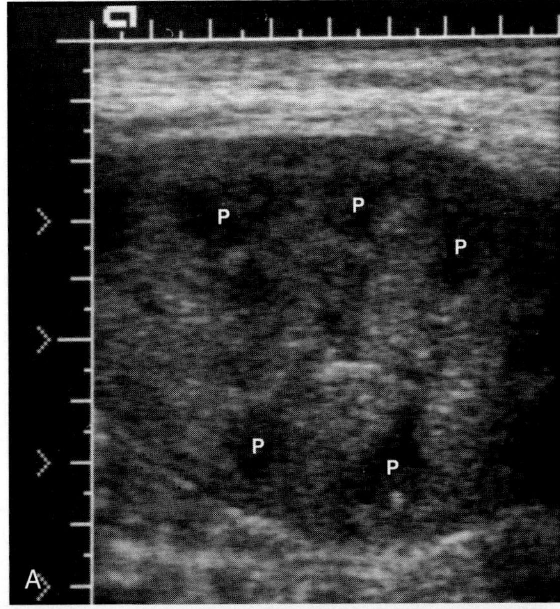

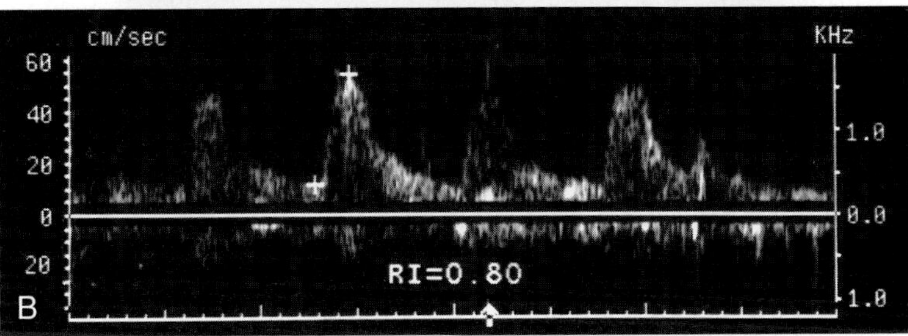

FIGURE 30–8 Renal transplant rejection. *A,* Prominent, enlarged medullary pyramids (P) stand out against echogenic renal cortex. The renal sinus is undefined because of edema within the sinus fat. The kidney has a globular shape caused by swelling. Renal volume, in this case, had increased 40% from the preceding study. *B,* Intrarenal Doppler waveforms are visibly pulsatile and the pulsatility index is high (0.80).

nicity and increased arterial pulsatility result from post-transplant ATN.

Accuracy for Rejection and Acute Tubular Necrosis

Initially it was hoped that sonography could be used to diagnose renal allograft rejection noninvasively and to differentiate between rejection and ATN in the postoperative period.* These hopes have faded with time, for experience has shown that ultrasonography is neither sensitive nor specific for allograft rejection.† To optimize specificity (to avoid false-positive diagnosis), *rejection should not be diagnosed sonographically unless several rejection-related abnormalities are present.*[80, 82, 83, 87, 90] Unfortunately, this requirement reduces the sensitivity for rejection to 70% or less. To make matters worse, sonographic changes seen with cyclosporine toxicity mimic those seen with rejection.[86, 96, 100, 111] (Cyclosporine is a commonly used immunosuppressant drug.)

In my opinion, ultrasound findings are most useful in cases of *severe* acute rejection. In such instances, the kidney is grossly enlarged, the pyramids are prominent, the renal sinus fat is hypoechoic, arterial flow resistance is elevated, and hypoechoic areas may be present in the renal cortex. I believe that

TABLE 30–2 DOPPLER FEATURES OF ALLOGRAFT REJECTION

High-resistance waveform appearance
Sharp, narrow systolic peaks
Second systolic peak higher than first
Minimal or absent diastolic flow
Flow reversal early in diastole
Pulsatility index ≥1.8
Resistivity index ≥0.7

* References 75–77, 79, 80, 92, 95, 96.

† References 74, 83, 86–91, 93, 96–106, 110, 128.

ultrasound findings are not very helpful when rejection is mild or moderate in severity. Furthermore, I think that the primary role of renal transplant sonography is not the detection of rejection, but the detection of other complications—particularly hydronephrosis and fluid collections.

Allograft Hydronephrosis

As noted previously, mild allograft hydronephrosis may occur normally during the first or second week after renal transplantation and probably results from postoperative edema at the insertion site of the ureter into the bladder. In some cases, mild hydronephrosis persists indefinitely, for no apparent reason. This finding is insignificant as long as urine output is good, renal function is satisfactory, and the degree of dilatation remains constant or regresses. The urodynamic significance of hydronephrosis may be evaluated with the Whitaker test,[100] scintigraphy, or pyelography in patients with abnormal renal function.

Moderate or severe hydronephrosis is a more disturbing finding, particularly if the degree of hydronephrosis increases over time. Functionally significant hydronephrosis in the immediate postoperative period usually results from surgical complications. Hydronephrosis appearing later is generally due to one of the following problems: (1) scarring at the ureterovesical junction, (2) obstructing debris (blood clots or fungal mycelia) within the ureter, (3) ureteral compression by extrinsic fluid collections, (4) bladder-emptying disorders, and (5) vesicoureteral reflux. Sonographic findings cannot differentiate among many of these causes.

Perigraft Fluid

Fluid collections are quite common after renal transplantation.[113–116] In the immediate postoperative period, a small volume of serous fluid (seroma) commonly accumulates adjacent to the allograft or in the operative wound, and this fluid should not be viewed with alarm as long as it does not increase in volume over time. Moderate to large collections are generally pathologic, regardless of when they appear, and these usually require further investigation with percutaneous aspiration or other means. The differential possibilities for perigraft fluid collections include serous fluid (seroma), blood (hematoma), pus (abscess), urine (urinoma), and lymph (lymphocele). Ultrasonography does not accurately differentiate among these collections in all cases, but an educated guess can be made by considering four factors: time of appearance (e.g., after surgery), symptoms, location, and sonographic appearance. These aspects of allograft-related fluid collections are outlined in Table 30–3.

Vascular Complications

The role of sonography in renal transplantation that is most germane to this text concerns the diagnosis of vascular problems.[114, 117–128] I believe that color-Doppler examination should be a routine component of renal allograft sonography, because such examination is relatively easy and yields valuable information. It is possible, in many cases, to trace the allograft vessels in their entirety, from the iliac anastomoses to the kidney,[127] and this should be the goal of the vascular examination, in addition to the assessment of arterial pulsatility, as discussed previously.

Vascular complications of renal allografts fall into four broad categories: arterial stenosis, vascular occlusion, arteriovenous fistula, and pseudoaneurysm.

Arterial Stenosis

The most common vascular complication of renal transplantation (about 10% of transplant patients) is arterial stenosis.[118] Typically, stenosis occurs within 3 years of transplantation and is heralded by hypertension.* Short segment stenosis at the allograft artery origin occurs early after transplantation and is almost always a surgical complication. On occasion, however, such a stenosis results from allograft artery rejection. Long segment, distal stenosis of the allograft artery is a later complication that usually results from intimal hyperplasia or scarring but may also result from rejection. In some cases, multiple

* In about 80% of cases, post-transplantation hypertension is caused by conditions other than renal artery stenosis.[59]

TABLE 30–3 DIAGNOSTIC FEATURES OF PERIGRAFT FLUID COLLECTIONS

Collection	Clinical Features	Sonographic Features
Seroma and hematoma	Asymptomatic; immediate postoperative period.	Anechoic or mixed echogenicity; adjacent to kidney or in wound; irregular shape; regresses in days or weeks.
Abscess	Fever, leukocytosis, pain; may be relatively asymptomatic because of immunosuppression; often postoperative, but may be later (weeks to months).	May be perinephric, in the parenchyma, or in the wound; usually well defined; contents anechoic to echogenic.
Urinoma	Pain, decreased renal output, fever; virtually always in immediate postoperative period.	Anechoic, often large, sometimes loculated; location variable; resembles lymphocele, but too early; scintigraphy is diagnostic.
Lymphocele	Asymptomatic or pain; may obstruct ureter by extrinsic compression; typically 1–2 mo or later after surgery, rarely earlier; attributed to interrupted allograft lymphatics.	Classically multilocular with thin septae and anechoic fluid; may be unilocular; classically located medially, between the allograft lower pole and the bladder.

distal stenoses are present. Stenosis of the recipient iliac artery is uncommon and almost invariably results from surgical injury.

The Doppler hallmark of renal artery stenosis is increased flow velocity in the stenotic segment, coupled with poststenotic disturbed flow. Arterial waveforms may be damped distal to very severe stenoses, but distal waveforms alone cannot be relied on to diagnose or exclude renal artery stenosis.[127] The quantification of allograft stenosis has not been worked out in any detail, but a few diagnostic parameters are available, as listed in Table 30–4.[117–122, 127]

Vascular Occlusion

Occlusion (thrombosis) of the allograft renal artery is an unusual complication (less than 1% of renal transplants)[118] that typically occurs acutely in the postoperative period, and is related to either rejection or technical factors. Arterial occlusion is readily detected with duplex sonography, because arterial and venous flow is absent in the allograft.[118, 119]

Occlusion (thrombosis) of the allograft vein is also a rare complication (less than 1% of cases) that occurs primarily in the immediate post-transplant period.[106] The kidney is enlarged, because of congestion, and the renal parenchyma typically has a nonhomogeneous appearance. Flow is absent in the renal vein, which may be visibly distended with thrombus. A characteristic feature of renal vein thrombosis is a peculiar *renal artery* waveform pattern consisting of sustained flow *reversal* in diastole.[118, 123] This finding has not been reported in other conditions.

TABLE 30–4 DIAGNOSTIC CRITERIA OF ALLOGRAFT RENAL ARTERIES

Normal flow parameters
1. Velocity: 80–118 cm/sec
2. Volume flow: 346–422 cc/min

Parameters for stenosis exceeding 50 or 60% decrease in diameter
1. Systolic velocity >190 cm/sec (+ poststenotic disturbed flow)
2. Systolic velocity ≥250 sm/sec, highly specific
3. Systolic velocity ratio* >3 (+ poststenotic disturbed flow)

* Ratio of stenotic zone peak systolic velocity to external iliac artery peak systolic velocity.

Data compiled from references 119–122 and 127.

Arteriovenous Fistula

Fistula formation between an artery and a vein may occur within the renal allograft as a result of biopsy trauma.[118, 124, 125] Many such parenchymal fistulae are asymptomatic, but others are associated with sustained hypertension. Color-Doppler sonography readily detects arteriovenous fistulae, because markedly disturbed flow within the fistula stands out like a beacon within the renal parenchyma. Additional findings are high-velocity flow in the artery that feeds the fistula, and a montage of color, called a *visible bruit,* in the parenchyma adjacent to the fistula.

Pseudoaneurysm

Most pseudoaneurysms in renal allografts occur within the renal parenchyma and result from arterial laceration during renal biopsy.[118, 125] These false aneurysms are represented on gray-scale images as well-defined, focal anechoic areas that are indistinguishable from renal cysts. Color-Doppler sonography shows blood flow in the pseudoaneurysm, confirming the diagnosis. In some cases, a characteristic high-velocity jet is visible in the aneurysm neck. Pseudoaneurysms may also occur at the renal artery–iliac artery anastomosis, but these are uncommon.[118]

REFERENCES

1. Dawson DL: Noninvasive assessment of renal artery stenosis. Semin Vasc Surg 9:172–181, 1996.
2. Baxter GM, Aitchison F, Sheppard D, et al: Colour Doppler ultrasound in renal artery stenosis: Intrarenal waveform analysis. Br J Radiol 69:810–815, 1996.
3. Miralles M, Cairols M, Cotillas J, et al: Value of Doppler parameters in the diagnosis of renal artery stenosis. J Vasc Surg 23:428–435, 1996.
4. Berland LL, Koslin DB, Routh WD, Keller FS: Renal artery stenosis: Prospective evaluation of diagnosis with color duplex US compared with angiography: Work in progress. Radiology 174:421–423, 1990.
5. Kliewer MA, Tupler RH, Hertzberg BS, et al: Doppler evaluation of renal artery stenosis: Interobserver agreement in the interpretation of waveform morphology. AJR Am J Roentgenol 162:1371–1376, 1994.
6. Kliewer MA, Hertzberg BS, Keogan MT, et al: Early systole in the healthy kidney: Variability of Doppler US waveform parameters. Radiology 205:109–113, 1997.
7. Bakker J, Beek FJA, Beutler JJ, et al: Renal artery stenosis and accessory renal arteries: Accuracy of detection and visualization with Gadolinium-enhanced breath-hold MR angiography. Radiology 207:487–504, 1998.
8. De Cobelli F, Vanzulli A, Sironi S, et al: Renal artery stenosis: Evaluation with breath-hold, three-dimensional, dynamic, Gadolinium-enhanced versus three-dimensional, phase-contrast MR angiography. Radiology 205:689–695, 1997.
9. Strotzer M, Felloner CM, Geissler A, et al: Noninvasive assessment of renal artery stenosis a comparison of MR angiography, color Doppler sonography, and intraarterial angiography. Acta Radiol 36:243–247, 1995.
10. Hoffmann U, Edwards JM, Carter S, et al: Role of duplex scanning for the detection of atherosclerotic renal artery disease. Kidney Int 39:1232–1239, 1991.
11. Olin JW, Piedmonte MR, Young JR, et al: The utility of duplex ultrasound scanning of the renal arteries for diagnosing significant renal artery stenosis. Ann Intern Med 122:833–838, 1995.
12. Hansen KJ, Tribble RW, Reavis S, et al: Renal duplex sonography: Evaluation of clinical utility. J Vasc Surg 12:227–236, 1990.
13. Kohler TR, Zierler RE, Martin RL, et al: Noninvasive diagnosis of renal artery stenosis by ultrasonic duplex scanning. J Vasc Surg 4:450–456, 1986.
14. Hélénon O, Rody FE, Correas JM, et al: Color Doppler US of renovascular disease in native kidneys. Radiographics 15:833–854, 1995.
15. Middleton WD: Doppler US evaluation of renal artery stenosis: Past, present, and future. Radiology 184:307–308, 1992.
16. Melany ML, Grant EG, Duerinckx AJ, et al: Ability of a phase shift US contrast agent to improve imaging of the main renal arteries. Radiology 205: 147–152, 1997.
17. Brun P, Kchouk H, Mouchet B, et al: Value of Doppler ultrasound for the diagnosis of renal artery stenosis in children. Pediatr Nephrol 11:27–30, 1997.
18. Stavros AT, Parker SH, Yakes WF, et al: Segmental stenosis of the renal artery: Pattern recognition of tardus and parvus abnormalities with duplex sonography. Radiology 184:487–492, 1992.
19. Strandness DE Jr: Duplex scanning in diagnosis of renovascular hypertension. Surg Clin North Am 70:109–117, 1990.
20. Isikoff MB, Hill MC: Sonography of the renal arteries: Left lateral decubitus position. AJR Am J Roentgenol 134:1177–1179, 1980.
21. Aristizabal D, Frohlich ED: Hypertension due to renal arterial disease. Heart Dis Stroke 1:227–234, 1992.
22. Wilcox CS: Ischemic nephropathy: Noninvasive testing. Semin Nephrol 16:43–52, 1996.
23. Meyrier A: Renal vascular lesions in the elderly: Nephrosclerosis or atheromatous renal disease? Nephrol Dial Transplant 11(suppl 9):45–52, 1996.
24. Blaufox MD, Middleton ML, Bongiovanni J, et al: Cost efficacy of the diagnosis and therapy of renovascular hypertension. J Nucl Med 37:171–177, 1996.
25. Silverman JM, Friedman ML, Van Allan RJ: Detection of main renal artery stenosis using phase-contrast cine MR angiography. AJR Am J Roentgenol 166:1131–1137, 1996.
26. Rubin GD, Walker PJ, Dake MD, et al: Three-dimensional spiral computed tomographic angiography: An alternative imaging modality for the abdominal aorta and its branches. J Vasc Surg 18:656–665, 1993.
27. Loubeyre P, Revel D, Garcia P, et al: Screening patients for renal artery stenosis: Value of three-dimensional time-of-flight MR angiography. AJR Am J Roentgenol 162:847–852, 1994.
28. Nally JV, Black HR: State-of-the-art review: Captopril renography—pathophysiological considerations and clinical observations. Semin Nucl Med 22:85–97, 1992.
29. Postma CT, Bijlstra PJ, Rosenbusch G, Thien T: Pattern recognition of loss of early systolic peak by Doppler ultrasound has a low sensitivity for the detection of renal artery stenosis. J Hum Hypertens 10:181–184, 1996.
30. Pederson EB, Egeblad M, Jorgensen J, et al: Diagnosing renal artery stenosis: A comparison between conventional renography, captopril renography and ultrasound Doppler in a large consecutive series of patients with arterial hypertension. Blood Press 5:342–348, 1996.
31. Nazzal MM, Hoballah JJ, Miller EV, et al: Renal hilar Doppler analysis is of value in the management of patients with renovascular disease. Am J Surg 174:164–168, 1997.

32. Handa N, Fukanaga R, Ogawa S, et al: A new accurate and non-invasive screening method for renovascular hypertension: The renal artery Doppler technique. J Hypertens Suppl 6:458–460, 1988.
33. Kliewer MA, Tupler RH, Carroll BA, et al: Renal artery stenosis: Analysis of Doppler waveform parameters and tardus-parvus pattern. Radiology 189:779–787, 1993.
34. Patriquin HB, LaFortune M, Jéquier J-C, et al: Stenosis of the renal artery: Assessment of slowed systole in the downstream circulation with Doppler sonography. Radiology 184:470–485, 1992.
35. LaFortune M, Patriquin HB, Demeule E, et al: Renal arterial stenosis: Slowed systole in the downstream circulation–experimental study in dogs. Radiology 184:475–478, 1992.
36. Stanley JC: Renal vascular disease and renovascular hypertension in children. Urol Clin North Am 11:451–463, 1984.
37. Strandness DE Jr: Duplex Scanning in Vascular Disorders. New York, Lippincott-Raven, 1990, p 240.
38. Greene ER, Venters MD, Avasthi PS, et al: Noninvasive characterization of renal artery blood flow. Kidney Int 20:523–529, 1981.
39. Taylor DC, Kettler MD, Moneta GL, et al: Duplex ultrasound scanning in the diagnosis of renal artery stenosis: A prospective evaluation. J Vasc Surg 7:363–369, 1988.
40. Avasthi PS, Voyles WF, Greene ER: Noninvasive diagnosis of renal artery stenosis by echo-Doppler velocimetry. Kidney Int 25:824–829, 1984.
41. Dubbins PA: Renal artery stenosis: Duplex Doppler evaluation. Br J Radiol 59:225–229, 1986.
42. Reid JH, Mackay S, Lantz BMT: Noninvasive blood flow measurements by Doppler ultrasound with applications to renal artery flow determination. Invest Radiol 15:323–331, 1980.
43. Isaacson JA, Neumyer MM: Direct and indirect renal arterial duplex and Doppler color flow evaluations. J Vasc Technol 19:309–316, 1995.
44. Isaacson JA, Zierler RE, Spittell PC, Strandness DE: Noninvasive screening for renal artery stenosis: Comparison of renal artery and renal hilar duplex scanning. J Vasc Technol 19:105–110, 1995.
45. Norris CS, Pfeiffer JS, Rittgers SE, Barnes RW: Noninvasive evaluation of renal artery stenosis and renovascular resistance. J Vasc Surg 1:192–201, 1984.
46. Rittgers SE, Norris CS, Barnes RW: Detection of renal artery stenosis: Experimental and clinical analysis of velocity waveforms. Ultrasound Med Biol 11:523–531, 1985.
47. Fujitani RM, Murray SP: Surgical methods for renal revascularization. Semin Vasc Surg 9:198–217, 1996.
48. Handa N, Fukunaga R, Etani H, et al: Efficacy of echo-Doppler examination for the evaluation of renovascular disease. Ultrasound Med Biol 14:1–5, 1988.
49. Nichols BT, Rittgers SE, Norris CS, Barnes RW: Non-invasive detection of renal artery stenosis. Bruit 8:26–29, 1984.
50. van der Hulst VPM, van Baalen J, Kool LS, et al: Renal artery stenosis: Endovascular flow wire study for validation of Doppler US. Radiology 100:165–168, 1996.
51. Bude RO, Rubin JM, Platt JF, et al: Pulsus tardus: Its cause and potential limitations in detection of arterial stenosis. Radiology 190:779–784, 1994.
52. Keating MA, Althausen AF: The clinical spectrum of renal vein thrombosis. J Urol 133:938–945, 1985.
53. Clark RA, Wyatt GM, Colley D: Renal vein thrombosis: An underdiagnosed complication of multiple renal abnormalities. Radiology 132:43–50, 1979.
54. Llach F, Papper S, Massry SG: The clinical spectrum of renal vein thrombosis: Acute and chronic. Am J Med 69:819–827, 1980.
55. Rosenberg ER, Traught WS, Kirks DR, et al: Ultrasonic diagnosis of renal vein thrombosis in neonates. AJR Am J Roentgenol 134:35–38, 1980.
56. Paling MR, Wakefield JA, Watson LR: Sonography of experimental acute renal vein occlusion. J Clin Ultrasound 13:647–653, 1985.
57. Metreweli C, Pearson R: Echographic diagnosis of neonatal renal venous thrombosis. Pediatr Radiol 14:105–108, 1984.
58. Lalmand B, Avni EF, Nasr A, et al: Perinatal renal vein thrombosis. J Ultrasound Med 9:437–442, 1990.
59. Rosenfield AT, Zeman RK, Cronan JJ, Taylor KJW: Ultrasound in experimental and clinical renal vein thrombosis. Radiology 137:735–741, 1980.
60. Taylor KJW, Burns PN: Duplex Doppler scanning in the pelvis and abdomen. Ultrasound Med Biol 11:643–658, 1985.
61. Goncharenko V, Gerlock AJ Jr, Kadir S, Turner B: Incidence and distribution of venous extension in 70 hypernephromas. AJR Am J Roentgenol 133:263–265, 1979.
62. Levine E: Malignant renal parenchymal tumors in adults. *In* Pollack HM (ed): Clinical Urography: An Atlas and Textbook of Urological Imaging. Philadelphia, WB Saunders, 1990, pp 1216–1291.
63. Goldstein HM, Green B, Weaver RM Jr: Ultrasonic detection of renal tumor extension into the inferior vena cava. AJR Am J Roentgenol 130:1083–1085, 1978.
64. Schwerk WB, Schwerk WN, Rodeck G: Venous renal tumor extension: A prospective US evaluation. Radiology 156:491–495, 1985.
65. Didier D, Racle A, Etievent JP, Weill F: Tumor thrombus of the inferior vena cava secondary to malignant abdominal neoplasms: US and CT evaluation. Radiology 162:83–89, 1987.
66. Dubbins PA, Wells I: Renal carcinoma: Duplex Doppler evaluation. Br J Radiol 59:231–236, 1986.
67. London NJM, Messios N, Kinder RB, et al: A prospective study of the value of conventional CT, dynamic CT, ultrasonography and arteriography for staging renal carcinoma. Br J Urol 64:209–217, 1989.
68. Roubidoux MA, Dunnick NR, Sostman HD, Leder RA: Renal carcinoma: Detection of venous extension with gradient-echo MR imaging. Radiology 182:269–272, 1992.
69. Thomas JL, Bernardino ME: Neoplastic-induced renal vein enlargement: Sonographic detection. AJR Am J Roentgenol 136:75–79, 1981.
70. Platt JF, Rubin JM, Ellis JH, DiPietro MA: Duplex Doppler US of the kidney: Differentiation of obstructive from nonobstructive dilatation. Radiology 171:515–517, 1989.
71. Platt JF, Ellis JH, Rubin JM, et al: Intrarenal arterial Doppler sonography in patients with nonobstructive renal disease: Correlation of resistive index with biopsy findings. AJR Am J Roentgenol 154:1223–1227, 1990.

72. Pozniak MA, Kelcz F, Dodd GD: Renal transplant ultrasound: Imaging and Doppler. Semin Ultrasound CT MR 12:319–334, 1991.
73. Lachance SL, Adamson D, Barry JM: Ultrasonically determined kidney transplant hypertrophy. J Urol 139:497–498, 1988.
74. Hillman BJ, Birnholz JC, Busch GJ: Correlation of echographic and histologic findings in suspected renal allograft rejection. Radiology 132:673–676, 1979.
75. Maklad NF, Wright CH, Rosenthal SJ: Gray scale ultrasonic appearances of renal transplant rejection. Radiology 131:711–717, 1979.
76. Hricak H, Toledo-Pereyra LH, Eyler WR, et al: The role of ultrasound in the diagnosis of kidney allograft rejection. Radiology 132:667–672, 1979.
77. Bricak H, Toledo-Pereyra LH, Eyler WR, et al: Evaluation of acute post-transplant renal failure by ultrasound. Radiology 133:443–447, 1979.
78. Singh A, Cohen WN: Renal allograft rejection: Sonography and scintigraphy. AJR Am J Roentgenol 135:73–77, 1980.
79. Frick MP, Feinberg SB, Sibley R, Idstrom ME: Ultrasound in acute renal transplant rejection. Radiology 138:657–660, 1981.
80. Hricak H, Cruz C, Eyler WR, et al: Acute post-transplantation renal failure: Differential diagnosis by ultrasound. Radiology 139:441–449, 1981.
81. Hricak H, Romanski RN, Eyler WR: The renal sinus during allograft rejection: Sonographic and histopathologic findings. Radiology 142:693–699, 1982.
82. Fried AM, Woodring JH, Loh FK, et al: The medullary pyramid index: An objective assessment of prominence in renal transplant rejection. Radiology 149:787–791, 1983.
83. Slovis TL, Babcock DS, Hricak H, et al: Renal transplant rejection: Sonographic evaluation in children. Radiology 153:659–665, 1984.
84. Babcock DS, Slovis TL, Han BK, et al: Renal transplants in children: Long-term follow up using sonography. Radiology 156:165–167, 1985.
85. Rosenfield AT, Zeman RK, Cicchetti DV, Siegel NJ: Experimental acute tubular necrosis. US appearance. Radiology 157:771–774, 1985.
86. Linkowski GD, Warvariv V, Filly RA, Vincenti F: Sonography in the diagnosis of acute renal allograft rejection and cyclosporine nephrotoxicity. AJR Am J Roentgenol 148:291–295, 1987.
87. Swobodnik WL, Spohn BE, Wechsler JG, et al: Real-time ultrasound evaluation of renal transplant failure during the early postoperative period. Ultrasound Med Biol 12:97–105, 1986.
88. Hoddick W, Filly RA, Backman U, et al: Renal allograft rejection: US evaluation. Radiology 161:469–473, 1986.
89. Hricak H, Terrier F, Marotti M, et al: Post-transplant renal rejection: Comparison of quantitative scintigraphy, US, and MR imaging. Radiology 162:685–688, 1987.
90. Cochlin DL, Wake A, Salaman JR, Griffin PJA: Ultrasound changes in the transplant kidney. Clin Radiol 39:373–376, 1988.
91. Rifkin MD, Needleman L, Pasto ME, et al: Evaluation of renal transplant rejection by duplex Doppler examination: Value of the resistive index. AJR Am J Roentgenol 148:759–762, 1987.
92. Taylor KJW, Morse SS, Rigsby CM, et al: Vascular complications in renal allografts: Detection with duplex Doppler US. Radiology 162:31–38, 1987.
93. Rigsby CM, Burns PN, Welton GG, et al: Doppler signal quantification in renal allografts: Comparison in normal and rejecting transplants with pathologic correlation. Radiology 162:39–42, 1987.
94. Sternberg HV, Nelson RC, Murphy FB, et al: Renal allograft rejection: Evaluation by Doppler US and MR imaging. Radiology 162:337–342, 1987.
95. Taylor KJW, Marks WH: Use of Doppler imaging for evaluation of dysfunction in renal allografts. AJR Am J Roentgenol 155:536–537, 1990.
96. Grant EG, Perrella RR: Wishing won't make it so: Duplex sonography in the evaluation of renal transplant dysfunction. AJR Am J Roentgenol 155:538–539, 1990.
97. Rigsby CM, Burns PN, Weltin GG, et al: Doppler signal quantification in renal allografts: Comparison in normal and rejecting transplants, with pathologic correlation. Radiology 162:39–42, 1987.
98. Genkins SM, Sanfilippo FP, Carroll BA: Duplex Doppler sonography of renal transplants: Lack of sensitivity and specificity in establishing pathologic diagnosis. AJR Am J Roentgenol 152:535–539, 1989.
99. Waltzer WC, Shabtai M, Anaise D, Rapaport FT: Usefulness and limitations of Doppler ultrasonography in the evaluation of postoperative renal allograft dysfunction. Transplant Proc 21:1901–1902, 1989.
100. Ward RE, Bartlett ST, Koenig JO, et al: The use of duplex scanning in evaluation of the posttransplant kidney. Transplant Proc 21:1912–1916, 1989.
101. Allen KS, Jorkasky DK, Arger PH, et al: Renal allografts: Prospective analysis of Doppler sonography. Radiology 169:371–376, 1988.
102. Harris DCH, Allen AR, Gruenewald S, et al: Doppler assessment in renal transplantation. Transplant Proc 21:1895–1896, 1989.
103. Townsend RR, Tomlanovich SJ, Goldstein RB, Filly RA: Combined Doppler and morphologic sonographic evaluation of renal transplant rejection. J Ultrasound Med 9:199–206, 1990.
104. Drake DG, Day DL, Letourneau JG, et al: Doppler evaluation of renal transplants in children: A prospective analysis with histopathologic correlation. AJR Am J Roentgenol 154:785–787, 1990.
105. Perchik JE, Baumgartner BR, Bernardino ME: Renal transplant rejection: Limited value of duplex Doppler sonography. Invest Radiol 26:422–426, 1991.
106. Kelcz F, Pozniak MA, Pirsch JD, Oberly TD: Pyramidal appearance and resistive index: Insensitive and nonspecific sonographic indicators of renal transplant rejection. AJR Am J Roentgenol 155:531–535, 1990.
107. Schwaighofer B, Kainberger F, Fruehwald F, et al: Duplex sonography of normal renal allografts. Acta Radiol 30:53–56, 1989.
108. Don S, Kopechy KK, Filo RS, et al: Duplex Doppler US of renal allografts: Causes of elevated resistive index. Radiology 171:709–712, 1989.
109. Warshauer DM, Taylor KJW, Bia MJ, et al: Unusual causes of increased vascular impedance in renal transplants: Duplex Doppler evaluation. Radiology 169:367–370, 1988.
110. Pozniak MA, Kelcz F, Stratta RJ, Oberley TD: Extraneous factors affecting resistive index. Invest Radiol 23:899–904, 1988.
111. Pozniak MA, Kelcz F, D'Alessandro A, et al: Sonography of renal transplants in dogs: The effect of acute tubular necrosis, cyclosporine nephro-

toxicity, and acute rejection on resistive index and renal length. AJR Am J Roentgenol 158:791–797, 1992.

112. Jaffe RB, Middleton AW Jr: Whitaker test: Differentiation of obstructive from nonobstructive uropathy. AJR Am J Roentgenol 134:9–15, 1980.
113. Siler TM, Campbell D, Wicks JD, et al: Peritransplant fluid collections. Radiology 138:145–151, 1981.
114. Coyne SS, Walsh JW, Tisnado WH, et al: Surgically correctable renal transplant complications: An integrated clinical and radiologic approach. AJR Am J Roentgenol 136:1113–1119, 1981.
115. Hildell J, Aspelin P, Nyman U, et al: Ultrasonography in complications of renal transplantation. Acta Radiol Diag 25:299–304, 1984.
116. Surratt JT, Siegel MJ, Middleton WD: Sonography of complications in pediatric renal allografts. Radiographics 10:687–699, 1990.
117. McGee GS, Peterson-Kennedy L, Astleford P, Yao JST: Duplex assessment of the renal transplant. Surg Clin North Am 70:133–141, 1990.
118. Dodd GD, Tublin ME, Shah A, Zajko AB: Imaging of vascular complications associated with renal transplants. AJR Am J Roentgenol 157:449–459, 1991.
119. Grenier N, Douws C, Morel D, et al: Detection of vascular complications in renal allografts with color Doppler flow imaging. Radiology 178:217–223, 1991.
120. Guzzo JA, Kupinski AM, Stone MP, et al: Evaluation of renal allograft blood flow rates by duplex ultrasonography. J Vasc Technol 14:232–234, 1990.
121. Snider JF, Hunter DW, Moradian GP, et al: Transplant renal artery stenosis: Evaluation with duplex sonography. Radiology 172:1027–1030, 1989.
122. Stringer DA, O'Halpin D, Daneman A, et al: Duplex Doppler sonography for renal artery stenosis in the post-transplant pediatric patient. Pediatr Radiol 19:187–192, 1989.
123. Reuther G, Wanjura D, Bauer H: Acute renal vein thrombosis in renal allografts: Detection with duplex Doppler US. Radiology 170:557–558, 1989.
124. Middleton WD, Kellman GM, Melson GL, Madrazo BL: Postbiopsy renal transplant arteriovenous fistulas: Color Doppler US characteristics. Radiology 171:253–257, 1989.
125. Hübsch PJS, Mostbeck G, Barton PP, et al: Evaluation of arteriovenous fistulas and pseudoaneurysms in renal allografts following percutaneous needle biopsy: Color-coded Doppler sonography versus duplex Doppler sonography. J Ultrasound Med 9:95–100, 1990.
126. MacLennan AC, Baxter GM, Harden P, Rowe PA: Renal transplant vein occlusion: An early diagnostic sign? Clin Radiol 50:251–253, 1995.
127. Baxter GM, Ireland H, Moss JG, et al: Colour Doppler ultrasound in renal transplant artery stenosis: Which Doppler index? Clin Radiol 50:618–622, 1995.
128. Hilborn MD, Bude RO, Murphy KJ, et al: Renal transplant evaluation with power Doppler sonography. Br J Radiol 70:39–42, 1997.

Chapter 31

ULTRASOUND AND DOPPLER EVALUATION OF THE PENIS

■ *Carol B. Benson, MD* ■ *Peter M. Doubilet, MD, PhD*

ANATOMY

The normal penis comprises three columns of spongy tissue, each encased by a dense fibrous sheath. Two of the columns, the paired corpora cavernosa, lie in parallel on the dorsal side of the penis. The corpora cavernosa contain multiple sinusoidal spaces with smooth muscle in their walls, and it is this spongy tissue that expands and fills with blood during an erection. The tunica albuginea is the dense fibrous sheath that encapsulates the sinusoidal tissue, providing structure and support when the penis is erect.

Along the ventral side of the penis runs the corpus spongiosum. This column of spongiosal tissue surrounds the urethra, which remains in a collapsed state except during active urination. The corpus spongiosum is usually smaller than the corpora cavernosa except at its distal end, where it broadens to form the glans penis. The spongiosal tissue of the corpus spongiosum expands somewhat with erection, but not to the extent that the cavernosal tissues expand. The three columns of tissue are surrounded by a layer of subcutaneous tissue and skin.

Arterial blood supply to the penis is via bilateral penile arteries, each a branch of the internal pudendal artery. The penile artery has two main branches, the dorsal artery and the cavernosal artery. The dorsal artery travels along the dorsal side of the penis, lateral to the midline dorsal vein, and supplies blood to the glans penis and the corpus spongiosum. It has few or no branches before it reaches the glans penis. The cavernosal artery travels centrally within the corpus cavernosum and supplies blood to the cavernosal sinusoids via multiple branches called *helicine arteries* that extend radially from the cavernosal artery (Fig. 31–1). Most men have a single cavernosal artery on each side; however, anatomic variants of cavernosal blood supply are common. In some cases, the cavernosal artery arises from the dorsal artery. In other cases, more than one cavernosal artery is present. During the generation of an erection, flow in the cavernosal arteries and helicine branches is markedly increased.

The venous drainage from the corpora cavernosa is via small veins that perforate the tunica albuginea to drain into the deep dorsal vein. Toward the base of the penis are small crural veins that drain into the deep pelvic veins to the internal pudendal vein. When the penis is erect and the corpora cavernosa are expanded, the small draining veins are occluded by stretching of the tunica albuginea.

ERECTILE FUNCTION

The physiologic process of a normal erection begins with increased parasympathetic motor nervous activity to the penis, involving sacral nerves two, three, and four. The parasympathetic motor activity causes the smooth muscle in the walls of the cavernosal sinusoids to relax, allowing the sinusoids to expand and decreasing the resistance to incoming blood flow. At the same time, the cavernosal arteries dilate and carry increased blood flow into the penis. The sinusoids fill with blood and the corpora cavernosa expand and stretch to become rigid. With expansion of the corpora cavernosa, the draining veins are occluded, preventing blood from leaving the dilated sinusoids. Once the cavernosal sinusoids are filled, the cavernosal arterial

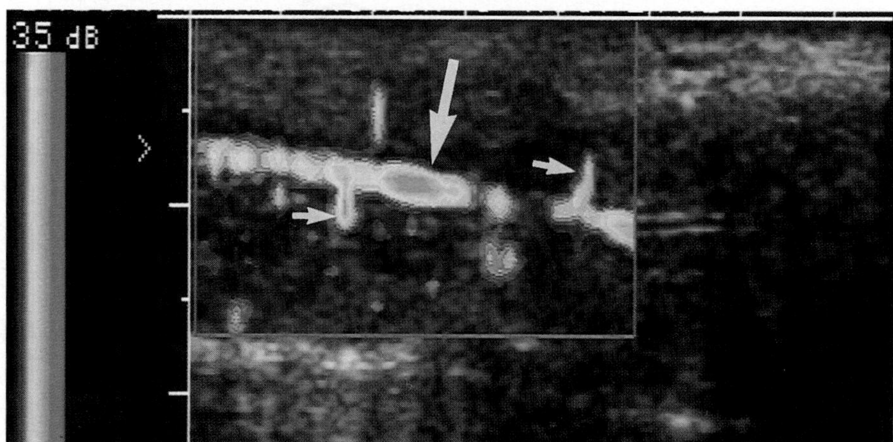

FIGURE 31–1 Cavernosal artery with helicine branches. Longitudinal power Doppler sonogram of the corpus cavernosum demonstrating flow in the cavernosal artery (*large arrow*) that runs through the middle of the corpus cavernosum. Small helicine branches (*small arrows*) extend radially from the cavernosal artery.

blood flow decreases, because of increased resistance within the corpora cavernosa. Continued parasympathetic nervous activity maintains the erection.[1]

Normal erectile function requires normal psychological health, normal endocrine balance, intact innervation to the penis, normal cavernosal sinusoids, adequate arterial blood supply, and normal venous occlusion with erection. Abnormalities of any of these systems may lead to erectile dysfunction. Impotence can be classified as organic, in which a physiologic abnormality is present, and psychogenic, in which impotence is due to psychological factors. Among men with previously normal erectile function who seek medical attention for impotence, an organic cause is found in 50 to 90%.[2–4]

The vast majority of patients with organic impotence have hemodynamic abnormalities: arterial insufficiency, venous incompetence, or both. Arteriogenic impotence occurs as a result of stenoses or occlusions that limit blood flow to the penis even in the presence of parasympathetic stimulation. If maximum flow is inadequate to fill the cavernosal sinusoids, tumescence and rigidity cannot occur. Without adequate filling of the corpora cavernosa, draining veins are not occluded but rather continue to carry blood away from the corpora cavernosa.[1, 5] Arteriogenic impotence occurs most commonly in men with risk factors for atherosclerosis, including diabetes mellitus, hypertension, hypercholesterolemia, and smoking.[6, 7]

Patients with mild to moderate arterial insufficiency in the absence of venous incompetence can often be successfully treated with self-injection therapy using prostaglandin E_1 or oral therapy with Viagra. Patients with severe arterial insufficiency usually require a penile implant to restore sexual function.[1]

Venous incompetence results from failure of occlusion of the draining veins, despite adequate filling of the cavernosal sinusoids. Patients may experience partial erections, but rigidity cannot be fully achieved or maintained.

Other penile abnormalities, including scarring within the corpora cavernosa or involving the tunica albuginea, may also cause impotence. Scarring or fibrosis of sinusoidal tissue prevents that area of the corpora from expanding when an erection is developing. The sinusoidal tissue around the scar fills with blood and pulls on the abnormal area, causing penile curvature. If the scarring is severe, expansion of the surrounding sinusoids may also cause pain, leading to detumescence.

When scarring affects the tunica albuginea that surrounds the corpora cavernosa, the tunica becomes thickened and may even calcify. Calcified plaques of the tunica are called *Peyronie's disease.* Plaques involving

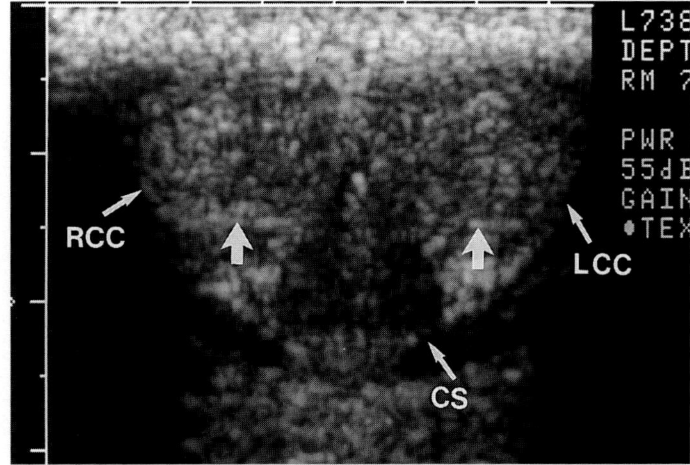

FIGURE 31–2 Normal nonerect penis. Transverse sonogram demonstrating two symmetric corpora cavernosa—right corpus cavernosum (RCC *arrow*) and left corpus cavernosum (LCC *arrow*)—dorsally and the corpus spongiosum (CS *arrow*) ventrally. The tunica albuginea is seen as a thin line (*thick arrows*) encapsulating the corpora cavernosa.

the tunica albuginea most often cause painless curvature with erection. Sometimes, as with cavernosal plaques, there may be enough pain from the plaque with an erection that detumescence results.

SONOGRAPHY

Sonographic evaluation of the penis is performed with high-frequency (7 to 10 MHz) linear transducers. The transducer is placed directly on the penis, and longitudinal and transverse images are obtained. The corpora of the normal penis have homogeneous echotexture. The two corpora cavernosa should be symmetric in size (Fig. 31–2). Within the corpora cavernosa the bright walls of the cavernosal arteries may be seen in some areas (Fig. 31–3). The tunica albuginea surrounding the cavernosal tissue appears as a thin echogenic line encasing the corpora (see Fig. 31–2). The corpus spongiosum is usually smaller than the corpora cavernosa but has similar echogenicity to the flaccid corpora. The urethra cannot be seen when it is collapsed.

When the penis is erect, the corpora cavernosa are larger, and the spongiosal tissue has a speckled appearance with small anechoic areas representing dilated sinusoids, separated by the brightly echogenic sinusoidal septa (Fig. 31–4). The cavernosal arteries are dilated and their walls are brightly echogenic (Fig. 31–5), because they are surrounded by blood-filled sinusoids.

Scarring of the corpora cavernosa or tunica albuginea can be diagnosed easily and accu-

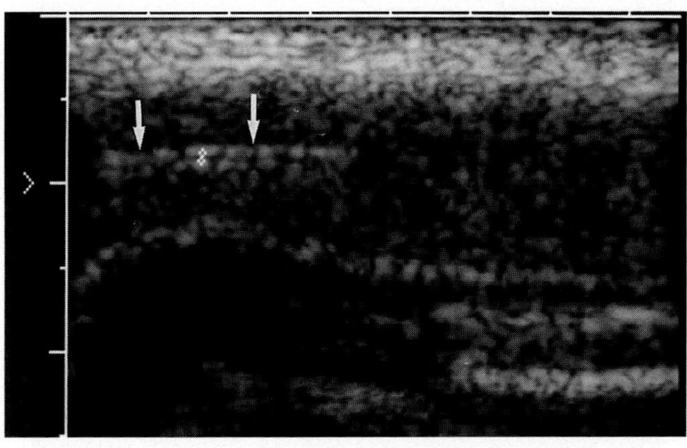

FIGURE 31–3 Cavernosal artery in nonerect penis. Longitudinal sonogram of the right corpus cavernosum demonstrating cavernosal artery (*calipers; arrows*) within sinusoidal tissue. The walls of the cavernosal artery are echogenic.

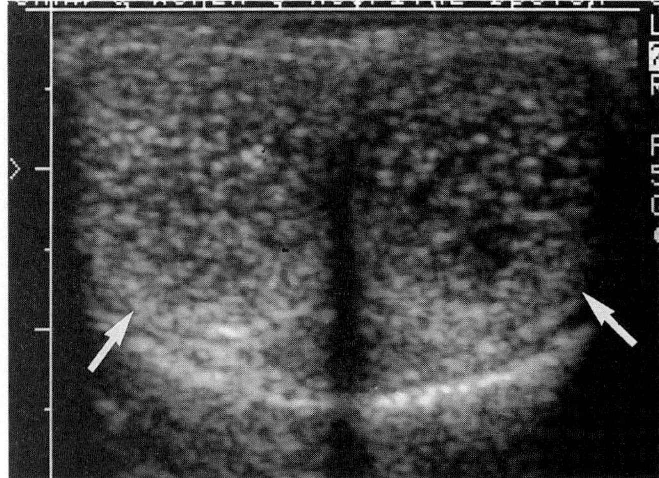

FIGURE 31–4 Erect penis. Transverse sonogram demonstrating the enlarged corpora cavernosa (*arrows*) with a speckled appearance because of blood-filled sinusoids.

rately by ultrasound. Scars of the corpora cavernosa appear as irregular echogenic areas within the corpora (Fig. 31–6). With an erection and dilatation of the surrounding sinusoids, the scars become more prominent and easier to delineate. Tunical plaques appear sonographically as focal areas of thickening of the tunica albuginea. Calcification in the plaque is brightly echogenic and casts an acoustic shadow (Fig. 31–7).

DOPPLER EVALUATION

Color-Doppler and pulsed Doppler assessments are used to evaluate the hemodynamic function of the penis. Doppler assessment is performed after intracavernosal injection of a vasoactive pharmacologic agent to induce and maintain an erection. Either papaverine or prostaglandin E_1, both of which induce an erection by causing sinusoidal smooth muscle relaxation and dilatation of the cavernosal arteries, can be used. The dose for papaverine is usually 30 to 60 mg, and that for prostaglandin E_1, 10 to 15 μg. The pharmacologic substance is injected directly into one corpus cavernosum using a small-gauge needle. A single injection acts on both corpora via multiple communications across the intercavernosal septum. Before injection, some examiners place a tourniquet at the base of the penis to prolong the local effect of the agent, leaving the tourniquet in place for 2 to 3 minutes until Doppler assessment is begun.

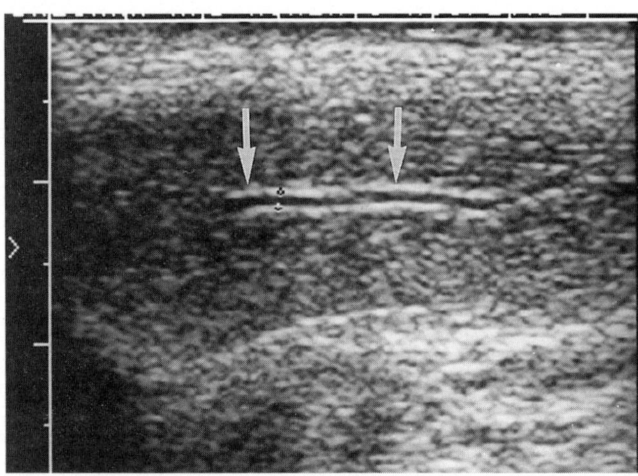

FIGURE 31–5 Cavernosal artery in erect penis. Longitudinal sonogram of the right corpus cavernosum demonstrating the cavernosal artery (*calipers; arrows*) with brightly echogenic walls running through blood-filled sinusoids.

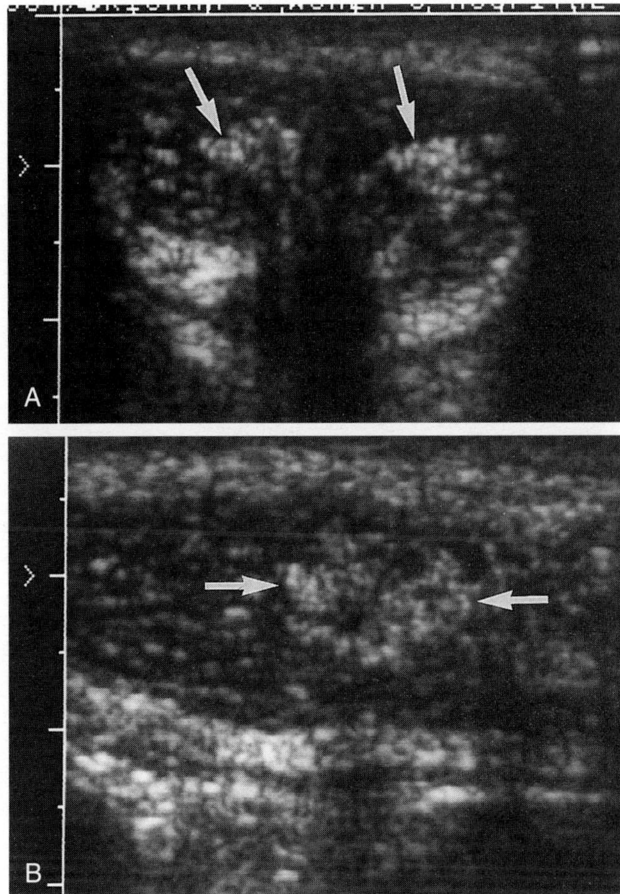

FIGURE 31–6 Sinusoidal scarring. *A*, Transverse sonogram demonstrating echogenic plaques (*arrows*) within both corpora cavernosa. *B*, Longitudinal sonogram demonstrating sinusoidal plaque (*arrows*).

Immediately after injection, some examiners use vibratory stimulation or ask the patient to manually stimulate the penis to promote the action of the drug.

Doppler assessment should begin 2 to 3 minutes after injection by obtaining Doppler waveforms from both cavernosal arteries and measuring the peak systolic velocity in each (Fig. 31–8). The waveforms are most easily obtained by scanning from the dorsal side of the penis, using color-Doppler assessment, if necessary, to help localize the cavernosal artery (Fig. 31–9). Arterial waveforms should be obtained at 2- to 3-minute intervals until the peak systolic velocity is above 35 cm/sec or has plateaued. Once the penis has reached maximal tumescence or the peak systolic velocity has plateaued, which usually occurs 8 to 10 minutes after injection but may be as long as 15 to 20 minutes in anxious patients,[8–11] the end diastolic velocity is measured from the cavernosal arterial waveform. At this time, flow is also assessed in the deep dorsal vein by scanning the vein from the ventral side of the penis using color-Doppler or pulsed Doppler assessments.[4, 8–10, 12–14]

The blood flow in men with normal hemodynamic function follows a predictable pattern during generation of an erection. Initially, in the flaccid state, Doppler waveforms of the cavernosal arteries demonstrate a high-resistance pattern, with low systolic peaks and absent or reverse diastolic flow (Fig. 31–10), and no flow is demonstratable in the deep dorsal vein. Two to 3 minutes after intracorporal injection of papaverine or prostaglandin E_1, the smooth muscles in the cavernosal sinusoids relax, leading to increased arterial inflow and a low-resistance arterial waveform, typified by high diastolic flow (Fig. 31–11). As the high flow continues in the cavernosal arteries and the sinusoids fill, the waveform changes to a higher resistance pattern with sharp systolic waveforms and diminished or absent diastolic flow

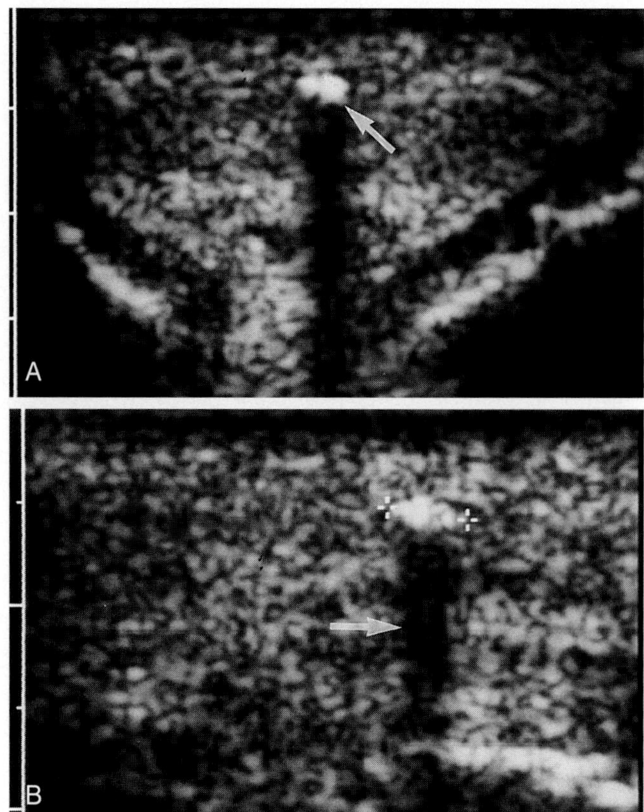

FIGURE 31–7 Peyronie's disease. *A,* Transverse sonogram demonstrating brightly echogenic calcified plaque (*arrow*) in midline, located dorsally between the corpora cavernosa. *B,* Longitudinal sonogram of calcified plaque (*calipers*) with acoustic shadowing behind calcification (*arrow*).

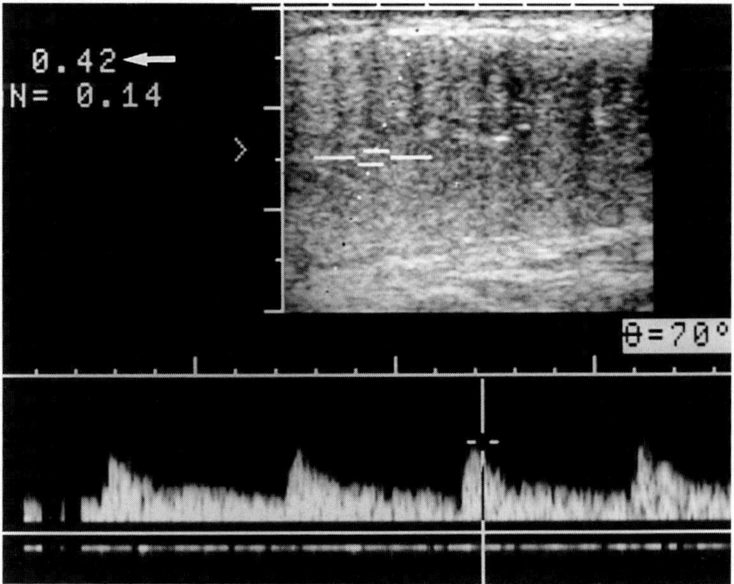

FIGURE 31–8 Normal cavernosal arterial waveform. Longitudinal sonogram with the Doppler waveform below, taken after injection of papaverine, demonstrating normal high velocities and low-resistance flow. Peak velocity is 42 cm/sec (0.42 m/sec, *arrow*).

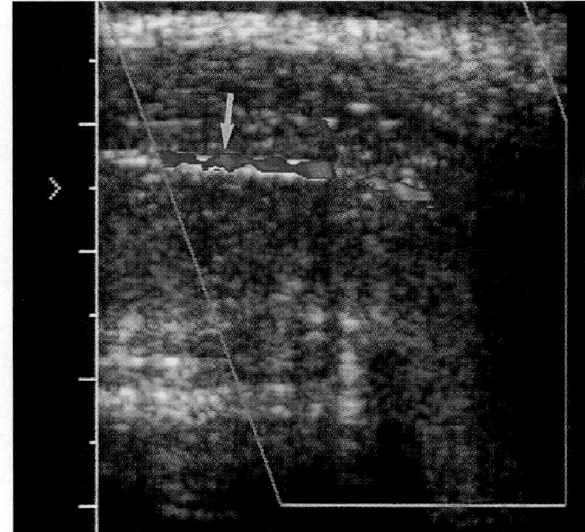

FIGURE 31–9 Color-Doppler assessment of cavernosal artery. Longitudinal sonogram with the color-Doppler image demonstrating flow in the cavernosal artery (*arrow*) located centrally within the corpus cavernosum.

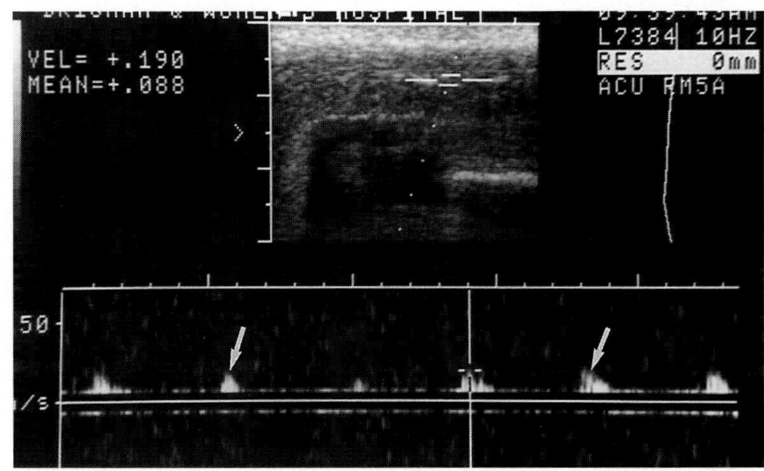

FIGURE 31–10 Cavernosal arterial waveform in the nonerect penis. Longitudinal sonogram with a Doppler waveform below demonstrating minimal arterial flow with short systolic peaks (*arrows*).

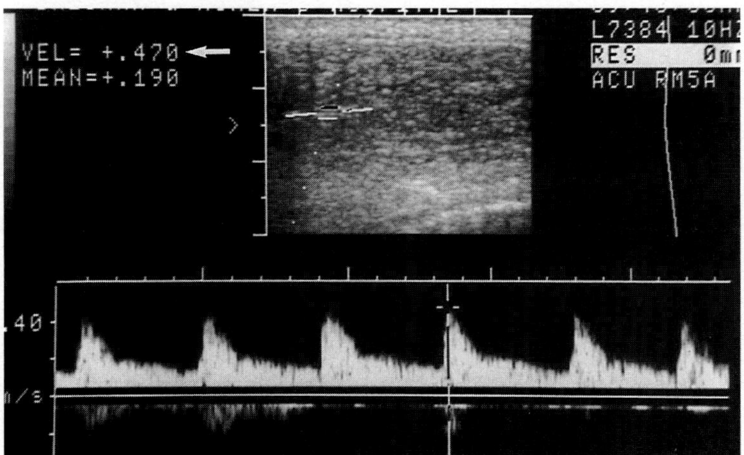

FIGURE 31–11 Cavernosal arterial waveform during the generation of erection. Longitudinal sonogram with a Doppler waveform below demonstrating low-resistance flow with normal systolic peak velocity of 47 cm/sec (0.47 m/sec, *arrow*).

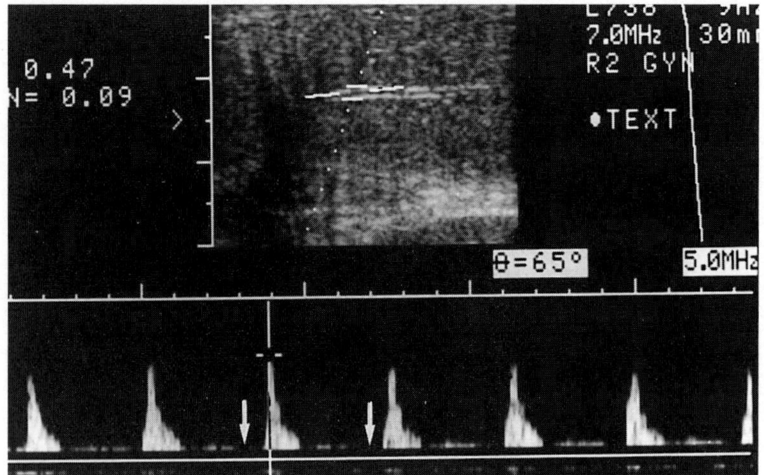

FIGURE 31–12 Cavernosal arterial waveform after full erection is achieved. Longitudinal sonogram with a Doppler waveform below demonstrating sharp systolic peaks with normal peak systolic velocity of 47 cm/sec and also absent end diastolic flow (*arrows*).

(Fig. 31–12). The peak systolic velocity increases over the first several minutes after injection, up to a maximum that exceeds 35 cm/sec in most normal men.[12, 15–17] Because some men who achieve normal erections have peak systolic velocities between 30 and 35 cm/sec, some researchers classify patients with peak flows of 30 cm/sec or greater as normal.[7, 9, 14] With full tumescence, peak systolic velocities decline and there is absent or even reverse end diastolic flow (Figs. 31–13 and 31–14). At this point, no flow should be seen in the deep dorsal vein with color-Doppler examination.

Deviation from this normal pattern may be diagnostic of arterial or venous disease. Arterial insufficiency is best diagnosed using the maximum cavernosal arterial systolic velocity, as good correlation has been demonstrated between this measurement and the arteriographic findings at angiography.[5, 18] The lower the peak systolic velocity, the greater the degree of severity of arterial disease. Patients with maximum systolic velocities somewhat below normal, in the range of 25 to 30 cm/sec, usually have mild to moderate arterial insufficiency. Patients with maximum velocities less than 25 cm/sec usually have severe arterial insufficiency (Figs. 31–15 and 31–16).[2, 7, 12, 14, 16, 19] A discrepancy in maximum velocities of greater than 10 cm/sec between right and left sides is also usually indicative of some degree of arterial insufficiency.

Although the maximum systolic velocity correlates fairly well with arterial function of

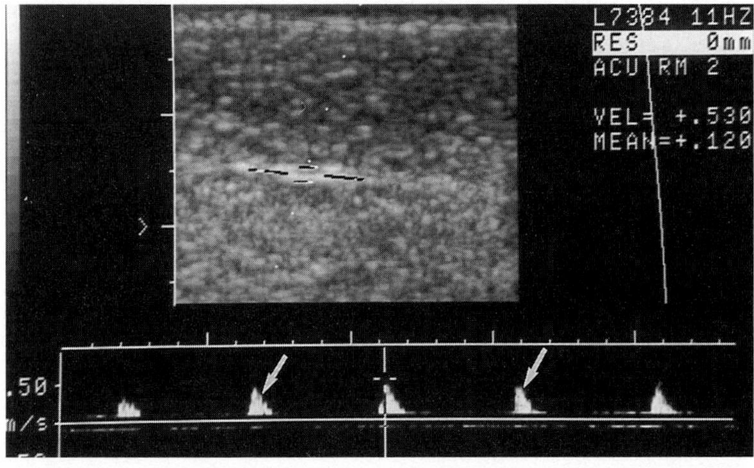

FIGURE 31–13 Cavernosal arterial waveform after full erection is achieved. Longitudinal sonogram with the Doppler waveform below demonstrating small systolic peaks (*arrows*) with normal peak systolic velocity of 53 cm/sec and also absent end diastolic flow.

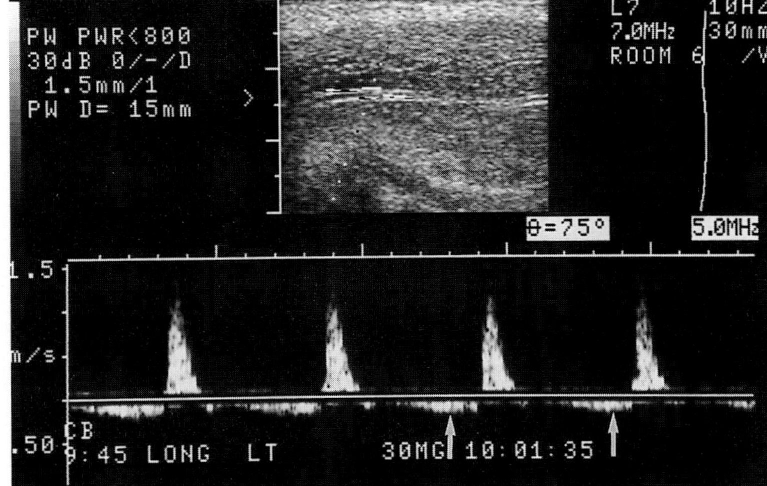

FIGURE 31–14 Cavernosal arterial waveform after full erection is achieved. Longitudinal sonogram with the Doppler waveform below demonstrating sharp systolic peaks and reverse end diastolic flow (*arrows*).

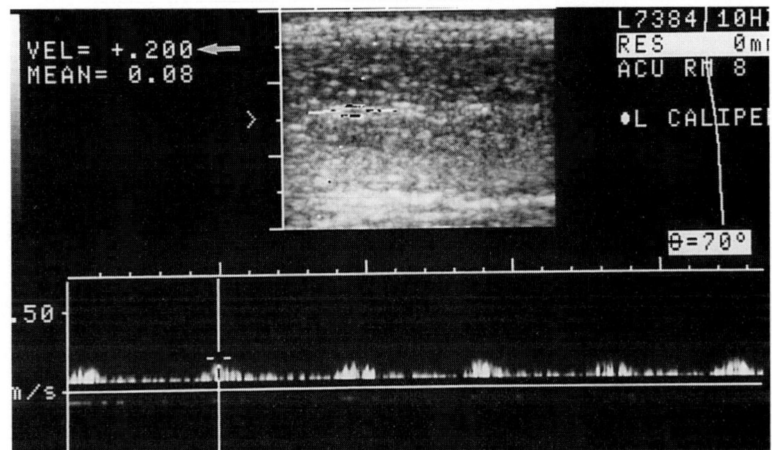

FIGURE 31–15 Cavernosal arterial waveform with arterial insufficiency. Longitudinal sonogram with the Doppler waveform below demonstrating an abnormally low peak systolic velocity of 20 cm/sec (0.20 m/sec, *arrow*).

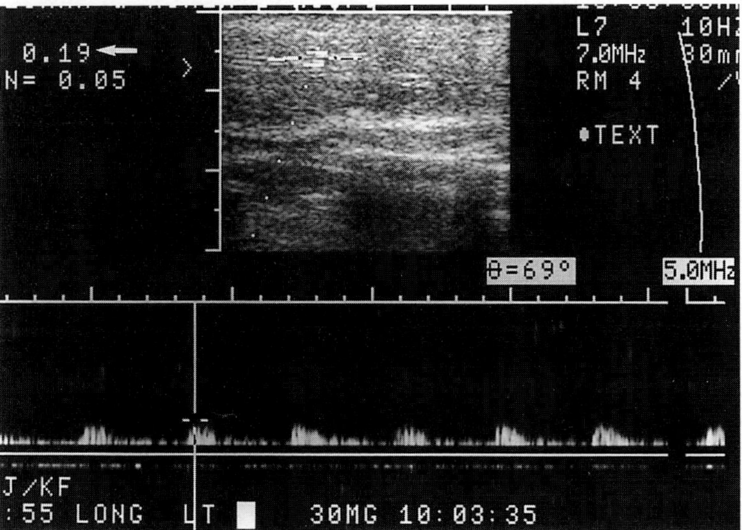

FIGURE 31–16 Cavernosal arterial waveform with arterial insufficiency. Longitudinal sonogram with the Doppler waveform below demonstrating an abnormally low peak systolic velocity of 19 cm/sec (0.19 m/sec, *arrow*).

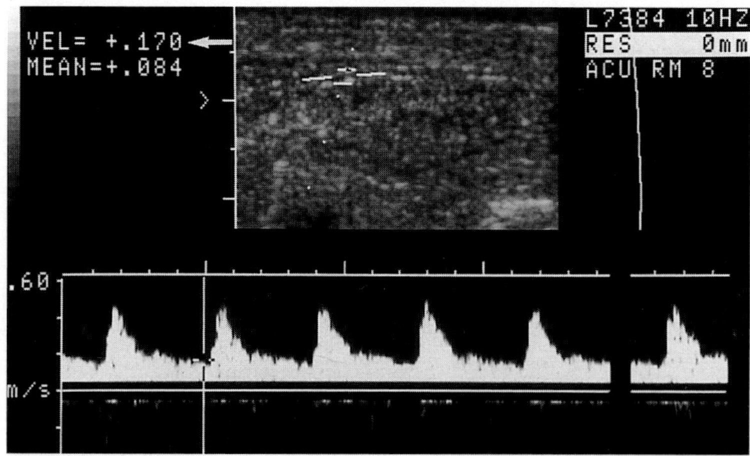

FIGURE 31–17 Venous incompetence. Longitudinal sonogram with the Doppler waveform below demonstrating persistent diastolic flow at 17 cm/sec (0.17 m/sec, *arrow*).

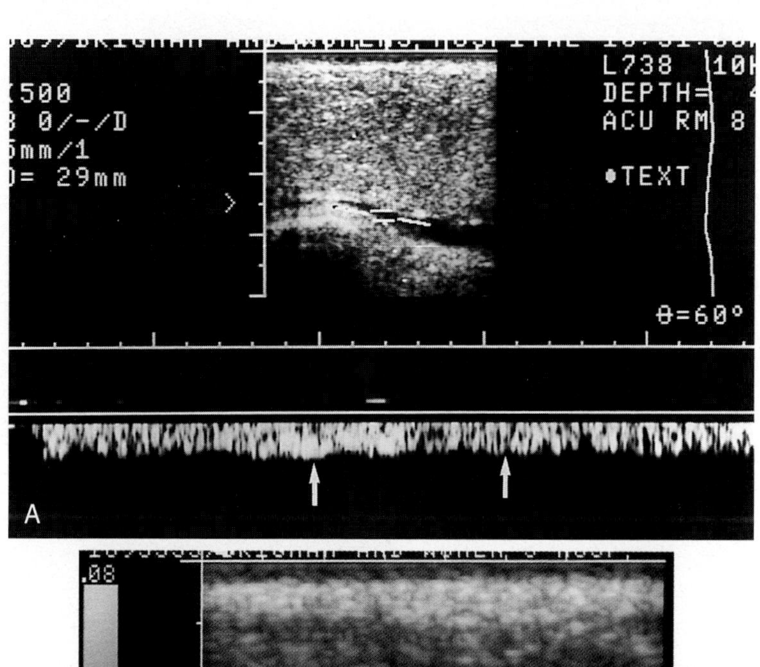

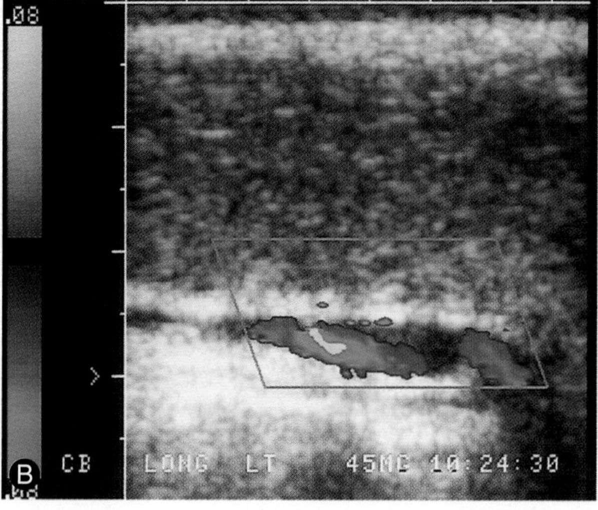

FIGURE 31–18 Venous incompetence. *A,* Longitudinal sonogram with the Doppler waveform below demonstrating flow in the dorsal vein (*arrows*). *B,* Longitudinal color-Doppler sonogram demonstrating flow in the dorsal vein.

the penis, there are limitations to this diagnostic method. Patient anxiety can diminish the arterial response to the vasoactive pharmacologic agents to the point that maximum velocities fall below the normal range despite normal arterial function. A similar decrease may be found in some patients with psychogenic impotence.[20] In general, the maximum systolic velocity is lower in patients with psychogenic impotence and normal arterial function than in normal patients.[17] Patients with variants of cavernosal arterial anatomy, such as duplicated cavernosal arteries on one side, may have peak systolic velocities less than 30 cm/sec despite normal arterial flow. For this reason, when more than one artery is seen, conclusions about arterial function cannot be drawn if the maximum systolic velocity is less than 30 cm/sec.[21]

Doppler sonography can also be helpful for diagnosing venous incompetence, as a number of findings suggest this diagnosis when arterial function is normal. This diagnosis should be suspected in any patient who fails to generate an adequate erection despite normal cavernosal arterial Doppler waveforms.[4, 12] The Doppler findings most suggestive of venous incompetence are flow in the dorsal vein or cavernosal arterial diastolic flow above 5 cm/sec (Fig. 31–17). Demonstration of dorsal vein flow, via either color-Doppler or pulsed Doppler assessment (Fig. 31–18), is consistent with dorsal venous incompetence.[12, 14, 22] Persistently high diastolic flow without evident dorsal venous flow suggests venous leakage through the crural veins, as flow in these veins cannot be detected by Doppler sonography.

Although Doppler sonography can suggest the diagnosis of venous insufficiency, it is not the modality of choice for evaluating this disorder. Cavernosometry and cavernosography are preferable. Cavernosometry, performed with vasoactive pharmacologic agents, is the most accurate method for making the diagnosis. When venous incompetence is found, cavernosography provides anatomic delineation of the abnormal venous pathways.[12, 22–25]

Venous competence can be assessed by Doppler only if arterial function is normal. Patients with arterial insufficiency may have too little arterial inflow to expand the sinusoids enough to occlude the draining veins, and hence these patients may have venous flow whether or not the veins are intrinsically competent. For this reason, the results of the Doppler assessment of the cavernosal arteries should be kept in mind when evaluating for venous leakage. If the maximum systolic velocities in the cavernosal arteries are within the normal range, then further assessment for venous competence can be performed. If a diagnosis of arterial insufficiency is made based on abnormally low peak systolic velocities, conclusions about venous competence cannot be drawn from the arterial waveform or Doppler assessment of the dorsal vein.[4]

REFERENCES

1. Krane RJ, Goldstein I, Tejada IS: Impotence. N Engl J Med 321:1648–1659, 1989.
2. Krysiewicz S, Mellinger BC: The role of imaging in the diagnostic evaluation of impotence. AJR Am J Roentgenol 153:1133–1139, 1989.
3. Paushter DM: Role of duplex sonography in the evaluation of sexual impotence. AJR Am J Roentgenol 153:1161–1163, 1989.
4. Benson CB, Vickers MA Jr, Aruny J: Evaluation of impotence. Semin Ultrasound CT MR 12:176–190, 1991.
5. Benson CB, Aruny JE, Vickers MA Jr: Correlation of duplex sonography with arteriography in patients with erectile dysfunction. AJR Am J Roentgenol 160:71–73, 1993.
6. Kaufman JM, Borges FD, Fitch WP, et al: Evaluation of erectile dysfunction by dynamic infusion cavernosometry and cavernosography (DICC). Urology 41:445–451, 1993.
7. Kadioglu A, Erdogru T, Tellaloglu S: Evaluation of penile arteries in papaverine-induced erection with color Doppler ultrasonography. Arch Esp Urol 48:654–658, 1995.
8. Govier FE, Asase D, Hefty TR, et al: Timing of penile color flow duplex ultrasonography using a triple drug mixture. J Urol 153:1472–1475, 1995.
9. Schwartz AN, Wang KY, Mack LA, et al: Evaluation of normal erectile function with color flow Doppler sonography. AJR Am J Roentgenol 153:1155–1160, 1989.
10. Meuleman EJH, Bemelmans BLH, Doesburg WH, et al: Penile pharmacological duplex ultrasonography: A dose-effect study comparing papaverine, papaverine/phentolamine and prostaglandin E_1. J Urol 148:63–66, 1992.
11. Shabsigh R, Fishman IJ, Quesada ET, et al: Evaluation of vasculogenic erectile impotence using penile duplex ultrasonography. J Urol 142:1469–1474, 1989.
12. Benson CB, Vickers MA: Sexual impotence caused by vascular disease: Diagnosis with duplex sonography. AJR Am J Roentgenol 153:1149–1153, 1989.
13. Broderick GA, Arger P: Duplex Doppler ultrasonography: Noninvasive assessment of penile anatomy and function. Semin Roentgenol 28:43–56, 1993.
14. Quam JP, King BF, James EM, et al: Duplex and color Doppler sonographic evaluation of vasculogenic impotence. AJR Am J Roentgenol 153:1141–1147, 1989.
15. Hampson SJ, Cowie AGA, Rickards D, Lees WR: Independent evaluation of impotence by colour Dop-

pler imaging and cavernosometry. Eur Urol 21:27–31, 1992.
16. Herbener TE, Seftel AD, Nehra A, Goldstein I: Penile ultrasound. Semin Urol 12:320–332, 1994.
17. Iacovo F, Barra S, Lotti T: Evaluation of penile deep arteries in psychogenic impotence by means of duplex ultrasonography. J Urol 149:1262–1264, 1993.
18. Mueller SC, Wallenberg-Pachaly H, Voges GE, Schild HH: Comparison of selective internal iliac pharmacoangiography, penile brachial index and duplex sonography with pulsed Doppler analysis for the evaluation of vasculogenic (arteriogenic) impotence. J Urol 143:928–932, 1990.
19. Mueller SC, Lue TF: Evaluation of vasculogenic impotence. Urol Clin North Am 15:65–76, 1988.
20. Allen RP, Engel RME, Smolev JK, Brendler CB: Comparison of duplex ultrasonography and nocturnal penile tumescence in evaluation of impotence. J Urol 151:1525–1529, 1994.
21. Mancini M, Bartolini M, Maggi M, et al: The presence of arterial anatomical variations can affect the results of duplex sonographic evaluation of penile vessels in impotent patients. J Urol 155:1919–1923, 1996.
22. Vickers MA, Benson CB, Richie JR: High resolution ultrasonography and pulsed-wave Doppler for detection of corporo-venous incompetence in erectile dysfunction. J Urol 43:1125–1127, 1990.
23. Gall H, Sparwasser DH, Stief CG, et al: Diagnosis of venous incompetence in erectile dysfunction. Urology 35:235–238, 1990.
24. Rudnick J, Bodecker R, Weidner W: Significance of intracavernosal pharmacological injection test, pharmacocavernosography, artificial erection and cavernosometry in the diagnosis of venous leakage. Urol Int 46:338–343, 1991.
25. Vickers MA, Benson CB, Dluhy R, Ball R: The current cavernosometric criteria for corporo-venous dysfunction are too strict. J Urol 147:614–617, 1991.

Index

Note: Page numbers in *italics* refer to illustrations; page numbers followed by t refer to tables.

E

T

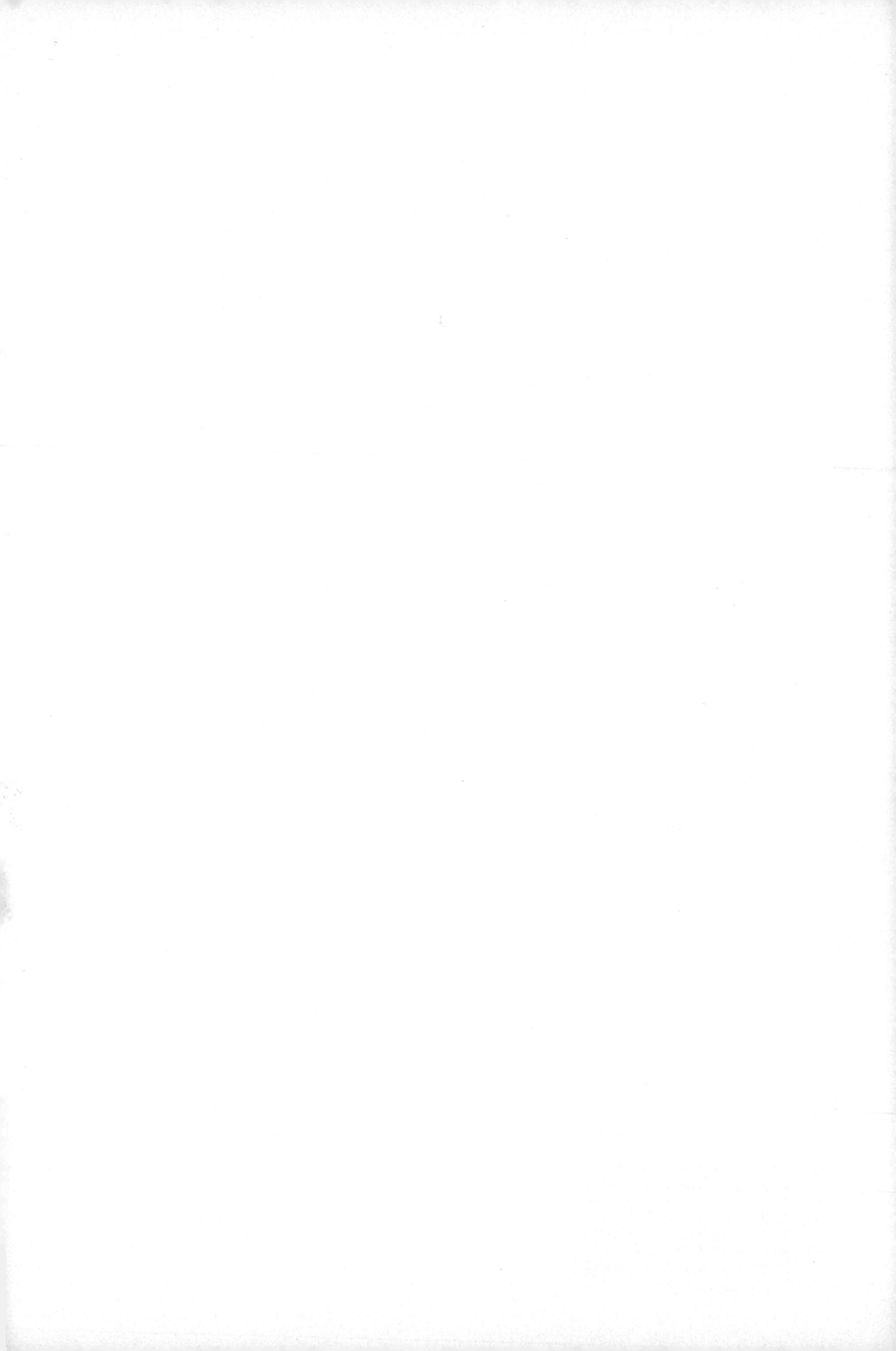

ISBN 0-7216-6949-2